UI

Γ

iative Medicine

This i
self

This book is dedicated to the memory
of my mother Katharine
1914–59

Palliative Medicine

Evidence-based symptomatic and supportive care for patients with advanced cancer

Roger Woodruff

FOURTH EDITION

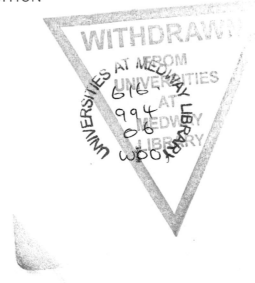
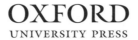

OXFORD

UNIVERSITY PRESS

OXFORD
UNIVERSITY PRESS

253 Normanby Road, South Melbourne, Victoria 3205, Australia

Oxford University Press is a department of the University of Oxford.
It furthers the University's objective of excellence in research, scholarship,
and education by publishing worldwide in

Oxford New York

Auckland Cape Town Dar es Salaam Hong Kong Karachi
Kuala Lumpur Madrid Melbourne Mexico City Nairobi
New Delhi Shanghai Taipei Toronto

With offices in

Argentina Austria Brazil Chile Czech Republic France Greece
Guatemala Hungary Italy Japan Poland Portugal Singapore
South Korea Switzerland Thailand Turkey Ukraine Vietnam

OXFORD is a trade mark of Oxford University Press
in the UK and in certain other countries

National Library of Australia
Cataloguing-in-Publication data:

Woodruff, Roger.
  Palliative medicine: evidence-basd symptomatic and supportive care
  for patients with advanced cancer.

  4th edition.
  Bibliography.
  Includes index.
  ISBN 0 19 551677 X

  1. Palliative treatment. 2. Cancer—Palliative treatment.
  3. Pain—Treatment. I. Title.

362.175

Typeset by OUPANZS
Printed through Bookpac Production Services, Singapore

Preface to the Fourth Edition

In the ten years since the publication of the first edition of *Palliative Medicine*, palliative care has continued to flourish, and in many parts of the world it has become an accepted part of mainstream medical care. The features that distinguish palliative care—attention to the whole person and to all aspects of their suffering, and a multidisciplinary approach to care—are better appreciated and are being applied in other branches of medicine. There is increasing recognition of the interaction between the various aspects of a patient's suffering—pain, other physical symptoms, psychological, social, cultural, and spiritual—none of which can be treated in isolation. All must be addressed, not as an elaborate or fashionable form of practice but as a clinical necessity, and a multidisciplinary approach is a prerequisite for successful palliative care.

As with the previous editions, this book is primarily concerned with the treatment of pain and other medical problems experienced by patients with advanced cancer. These patients deserve excellent medical care, which must be appropriate to the stage of the disease and their prognosis. It is hoped this book will allow a better understanding of the causes of common problems, and provide a rational approach to assessment and treatment. At the same time, the importance of psychosocial and non-physical aspects of suffering, and the need for a holistic and multidisciplinary approach to care, are stressed. In this edition the text has been completely revised and updated and there are new sections on assessing outcomes of palliative care, barriers to the provision of care, advance care planning, selective COX-2 inhibitors, transmucosal fentanyl, NMDA receptor antagonists, and the demoralization syndrome.

The knowledge base in palliative medicine has grown rapidly and the electronic revolution of the last decade has made it much more accessible. The principles of evidence-based medicine are required to make the best use of this knowledge and in this edition the results of more than 350 randomized controlled trials (RCTs), dozens of systematic reviews, and 45 Cochrane reviews are highlighted. None is perfect and the results must always be interpreted according to each individual patient's particular circumstances, but they constitute the best evidence base that there is for the teaching and practice of clinical palliative medicine. Where relevant, the instruments used to detect and rate symptoms or adverse effects of treatment are included, as there is great need for descriptions to be standardized as palliative medicine goes forward. Also new in this edition, the text is extensively referenced, inviting the reader to further explore the literature.

In caring for patients with cancer, the importance of providing comprehensive symptomatic and supportive care long before the terminal phase of the illness is more widely appreciated. The artificial demarcation between active treatment of the disease and care for the dying is slowly disappearing, and it is hoped that the information in this book will be just as useful in oncology wards as it is in palliative care units.

Optimal palliative care should be available to all patients with terminal illness. It should provide excellent medical care, be multidisciplinary in nature and holistic in focus, and there should be a partnership of care between the patient and family and the professional carers. It is hoped that this book, in some small way, may contribute to the delivery of better care to more patients with advanced cancer.

Roger Woodruff
Melbourne, August 2003

Acknowledgments

The contribution of many professional colleagues to the production of this book is gratefully acknowledged. I owe much to one of my early medical teachers, the late Dr Walter Moon, who practised palliative care long before it was given that name.

My most grateful thanks go to my wife Prudence, not only for all her help in completing the manuscript but also for unending encouragement, support and patience.

Contents

SECTION IV PSYCHOSOCIAL ASPECTS OF CARE

SECTION V COMPLEMENTARY AND ALTERNATIVE THERAPIES

Abbreviations

The following abbreviations are used in the text.

Routes of administration

CSCI	continuous subcutaneous infusion
EP	epidural
IM	intramuscular
II	intrathecal
IV	intravenous
PO	oral
PR	rectal
SC	subcutaneous
SL	sublingual
TM	transmucosal
TD	transdermal

Time

sec	second
min	minute
h	hour
d	day
w	week
m	month

Measures

μg	microgram
mg	milligram
g	gram
kg	kilogram
fl	fentilitre
μl	microlitre
ml	millilitre
dl	deciliter
l	litre
m^2	metre squared, a measure of body surface area

Measures of radiation

Gy	Gray (100 rad)
MBq	megabecquerel
mCi	millicurie

Preparation

cap	capsule
inj	injection
mixt	mixture
supp	suppository
tab	tablet
IR	immediate release
SR	sustained release

Frequency of administration

PRN (*pro re nata*)	as required
q (*quantum*)	frequency e.g. q4h is every 4 hours

Procedures

ECG	electrocardiography
EMG	electromyography
CT scan	computerised tomography
MRI scan	magnetic resonance imaging

Organizations

ASCO	American Society of Clinical Oncology
ECOG	Eastern Cooperative Oncology Group
EORTC	European Organisation for Research and Treatment of Cancer
NCI	National Cancer Institute (USA)
NCI CTC	NCI Common Toxicity Criteria
RTOG	Radiation Therapy Oncology Group

Clinical trials

RCT	randomized controlled trial
n	number
pS	statistically significant ($p \leq .05$)
pNS	not statistacally significant ($p > .05$)

Section I

An introduction to palliative care

To cure, occasionally
To relieve, often
To comfort, always

Anonymous
(16th Century)

Death should simply become
a discreet but dignified exit
of a peaceful person
from a helpful society...
without pain or suffering
and ultimately without fear.

Philippe Ariès, 1977
The Hour of Our Death

1

Palliative care

Palliative care has been described as a new medical specialty. It is not. It is probably the oldest, for in centuries gone by physicians and nurses frequently had only palliation to offer for diseases like cancer. The misunderstanding arises because many doctors and nurses practising today were educated in an era of technologically sophisticated medicine, when matters relating to the care of the terminally ill received little or no attention. What is new are the medical and scientific advances of the last few decades, which are of great benefit in the practice of palliative care. Better knowledge about disease processes and the causation of symptoms, together with advances in pharmacology, surgery and radiotherapy, have enhanced the medical care we are able to deliver. Add to this an improved understanding about the importance and optimal management of the psychosocial suffering associated with advanced disease, and it is possible to provide comprehensive care covering all aspects of patients' disease and suffering. This is modern palliative care.

History

Palliative care has been practised since antiquity and, until relatively recently, palliation was all that could be offered to most patients with cancer. Early palliative care was multidisciplinary in fashion, relying not only on the physician but also nurses, clergy, nuns, family members and other lay persons. Hospice facilities for the care of the dying were established in France, Ireland, England, Australia and the United States in the late nineteenth and early twentieth centuries, principally by various Catholic Orders. The emphasis in these institutions was on physical, psychological and spiritual comfort, and respect for the individual.

During the first half of the twentieth century the care of the terminally ill became increasingly neglected in mainstream medicine and nursing. The success of the early hospices may have been one factor in reducing the level of education in the care of the terminally ill given to doctors and nurses. Discussion of death and dying became medically and socially unacceptable

Table 1.1 Comments on mainstream medical care for the terminally ill

We emerge deserving of little credit; we who are capable of ignoring the conditions which make muted people suffer. The dissatisfied dead cannot noise abroad the negligence they have experienced.

J. Hinton[1]

... medical inpatients being treated with narcotic analgesics for pain showed that 32% of the patients were continuing to experience severe distress ... and another 41% were in moderate distress ... Physicians who exaggerated the dangers of addiction were more likely to prescribe lower doses of drugs, even for patients with terminal malignancy.

R. M. Marks and E. J. Sachar[2]

... I observed the desperate need of the hospital staff to deny the existence of terminally ill patients on their ward.

Elizabeth Kubler-Ross[3]

In modern hospitals, dying is often made unnecessarily wretched. Physical symptoms are inadequately treated. Depression and anxiety commonly go untreated. The dying person is isolated physically and emotionally, surrounded by biased and misleading systems of communication, in a social setting that gives very low priority to the individual's own personality and inner experiences, and in a seriously deficient physical environment.

M. A. Simpson[4]

and dying patients were seen as medical failures. The situation was aggravated in the 1960s and 1970s with the introduction of chemotherapy for the treatment of cancer and the expectation that many cancers could be cured. Sadly, this has not as yet been realized.

During the 1950s and 1960s there was increasing awareness of the need for better care for the terminally ill. The medical profession and the hospital system were criticized from within and without (Table 1.1). Criticisms included lack of care and attention, unrelieved pain, disease-orientated management to the exclusion of psychosocial and spiritual problems, and the lack of skilled personnel to provide care in the home environment.

In response to these needs, a movement developed, dedicated to improving the care and support provided for the terminally ill and their families, popularly known as the 'hospice movement'. The founders of the organizations in this movement were nurses, social workers, concerned lay people and a few committed medical practitioners. This hospice movement frequently operated quite separately from mainstream medicine and, as it had limited medical input, was not truly multidisciplinary. It was perceived by some as a challenge to orthodox medical care. From this movement came expressions such as 'caring versus curing', 'a good death', 'death with dignity' and 'the family as unit of care'. In retrospect, this movement should be acknowledged for making the medical and nursing professions more aware of the real needs of the terminally ill, particularly the psychosocial and spiritual aspects of care. They have in turn been criticized (Table 1.2) but the better aspects of their programmes have been incorporated in modern multidisciplinary palliative care.

The evolution of modern multidisciplinary palliative care can be seen in five stages, which are not necessarily sequential or exclusive (Table 1.3). The opening of St Christopher's Hospice in London in 1967 by Dr Cicely Saunders was probably the most important. This was a free-standing hospice providing for the first time comprehensive and multidisciplinary palliative care for patients with advanced cancer. The aim was to give appropriate attention to the psychological, social and spiritual aspects of care whilst simultaneously providing excellent medical treatment. There was also a major commitment to research and teaching.

Table 1.2 Comments on the early hospice movement

There is far too much talk in death and dying circles in this country about psychological and emotional problems, and far too little about making the patient comfortable. Any group concerned with service to the dying should be talking about smoothing sheets, rubbing bottoms, relieving constipation, and sitting up at night. Counselling a person who is lying in a wet bed is ineffective.

If people are cared for with common sense and basic professional skills, with detailed attention to self-evident problems and physical needs, then patients and families themselves cope with many of their emotional crises. Without pain, well nursed, with bowels controlled, mouth clean and a caring friend available, the psychological problems fall into manageable perspective.

Sylvia Lack[5]

During the past decade an unprecedented public and professional interest has developed around issues involving death and dying. Persons of differing backgrounds and with different objectives are rushing onto this scene in rapidly increasing numbers. Some of these persons have little understanding of the medical complexities of dying and no clinical experience with dying patients.

R. P. Hudson[6]

[Hospices] will have to be on their guard against ... psychobabble enthusiasts who will not roll up their sleeves to *nurse* the patient.

R. Lamerton[7]

The demonstrable benefits of this multidisciplinary approach to care quickly led to the same principles being applied to the palliative care delivered in the domiciliary setting. In contrast to earlier services, this involved specialist nurses educated and experienced in palliative care, working with the patient's own medical practitioner, and with the assistance and back-up of a multidisciplinary palliative care team.

The success of St Christopher's and other free-standing hospices paved the way for the establishment of hospices or hospice wards within general hospitals, making multidisciplinary palliative care available to many more terminally ill patients. This was a significant development as it was acknowledgement of the need for multidisciplinary palliative care within the hospital system. It also brought palliative care service personnel back to the general hospital campus, to work alongside their colleagues in mainstream medicine, to the benefit of both. This professional contact helped dispel misconceptions about palliative care and demonstrate that it was a genuine sub-specialty of medicine.

Table 1.3 The development of modern multidisciplinary palliative care

Establishment of inpatient hospice care
    providing comprehensive multidisciplinary care including excellent medical treatment

Development of multidisciplinary domiciliary palliative care
    involving nurses trained in palliative care and the patient's own doctor, with support from a multidisciplinary palliative care team

Establishment of hospital-associated hospices and hospice wards
    acceptance of multidisciplinary palliative care back into 'mainstream' hospital medicine

Development of consultative palliative care services in general hospitals
    allowing earlier involvement by multidisciplinary palliative care and education by example

Education of all health care professionals in the essentials of multidisciplinary palliative care

The development of consultative palliative care services in general hospitals has further increased the availability of palliative care. These multidisciplinary teams provide consultative advice and assistance regarding the palliative care aspects of patient management. Patients are more likely to be referred earlier, rather than only when all avenues of anticancer treatment are exhausted. Consultative services are also more likely to receive referrals from doctors who wish to remain involved in a patient's management. These services have been termed 'symptom control teams' or 'terminal care support teams' but these terms should be avoided because they imply a restriction of function—to just symptoms or to just dying patients—rather than the complete spectrum of multidisciplinary palliative care. The presence of palliative care service personnel on general wards, demonstrating that there is a more comprehensive way of managing the terminally ill and providing practical education by example, has further improved the status of palliative care.

The ultimate objective should be for all doctors, nurses and health care professionals to understand and appreciate the goals and benefits of multidisciplinary palliative care. A start has been made with the inclusion of palliative care in undergraduate medical and nursing curricula, but it will take time before the majority of health care professionals are educated about the needs of patients with advanced cancer and their families.

Definition

There is no one entirely satisfactory definition of palliative care. In North America, the term 'hospice' has been used to describe palliative care, but to many people hospice still means the building or institution where the patients are housed. The Oxford dictionary defines palliate as 'to alleviate symptoms' and 'to mitigate suffering', which makes it an entirely appropriate term. A simple and useful definition, modified from one developed by Derek Doyle and his colleagues, is

> Palliative care is the care of patients with progressive, far-advanced disease and a short life expectancy, for whom the focus of care is the relief and prevention of suffering and the quality of life.

This definition focuses on the quality of whatever life remains for the patient. It is person-oriented, not disease-oriented. It is not primarily concerned with either life prolongation (or with life shortening) or with producing long-term disease remission. It is holistic in approach and aims to address all the patient's problems, both physical and psychosocial. A multidisciplinary approach involving doctors, nurses and allied health personnel is employed to cover all aspects of care. The message of palliative care is that whatever the disease, however advanced it is, whatever treatments have already been given, there is always something that can be done to improve the quality of the life remaining to the patient.

A short life expectancy is variously defined but is usually understood to be less than a year, often less than six months. Difficulties related to accurate prognostication are discussed in Chapter 2. The definition does not mention the site of care, for the principles of palliative care are the same whether the patient is at home or in a hospital or hospice. The terms *dying* and *terminal* are not used because the principles and practices of palliative care should be employed long before the final days or weeks of life; *terminal care* and *care of the dying* are two stages in the continuum of palliative care. The World Health Organization definition of palliative care[8] is shown in Table 1.4.

Table 1.4 WHO definition of palliative care[8]

Palliative care is an approach that improves the quality of life of patients and their families facing the problems associated with life-threatening illness, through the prevention and relief of suffering by means of early identification and impeccable assessment and treatment of pain and other problems, physical, psychosocial and spiritual.

Palliative care

provides relief from pain and other distressing symptoms

affirms life and regards dying as a normal process

intends neither to hasten or postpone death

integrates the psychological and spiritual aspects of patient care

offers a support system to help patients live as actively as possible until death

offers a support system to help the family cope during the patient's illness and in their own bereavement

uses a team approach to address the needs of patients and their families, including bereavement counselling, if indicated

will enhance quality of life, and may also positively influence the course of illness

is applicable early in the course of illness, in conjunction with other therapies that are intended to prolong life, such as chemotherapy or radiation therapy, and includes those investigations needed to better understand and manage distressing clinical complications

Palliative care and suffering

Suffering may be defined as the distress associated with events that threaten the intactness or wholeness of the person. It involves some symptom or process that threatens the patient because of fear, the meaning of the symptom, and concerns about the future.[9, 10] The aim of palliative care is to provide integrated and comprehensive care to prevent and relieve all aspects of a patient's suffering. Suffering needs be distinguished from the pain or other symptoms with which it may be associated, for several reasons. First, suffering is experienced by persons, whole persons, and not just by a body or a mind. Second, suffering may result from interruption or interference with any aspect of the person—physical, psychological, social, cultural or spiritual—and not just pain or other symptoms. Third, there is great indi-

Figure 1.1 The causes of suffering

Pain
Physical symptoms
Psychological problems
Social difficulties
Cultural factors
Spiritual concerns

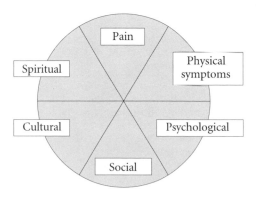

Figure 1.2 Total suffering

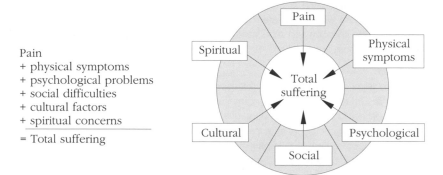

Pain
+ physical symptoms
+ psychological problems
+ social difficulties
+ cultural factors
+ spiritual concerns
_____
= Total suffering

vidual variation in the amount of suffering caused by a particular pain or threat. Last, it is acknowledged that there may be little if any suffering associated with the pain and physical distress of acute illnesses that are of limited duration and the significance of which is easily comprehended by the patient. However, this last distinction is usually not applicable in palliative care where problems are usually both chronic and progressive and of obvious significance to the patient, and some degree of suffering is almost universal.

The aetiology of suffering is a complex issue about which many philosophical, psychological and theological treatises have been written. In clinical practice it is helpful to have a simple classification so that the complex problems presented by patients may be disentangled, in order to provide comprehensive palliation and relief of suffering. The causes of suffering may be grouped by their physical, psychological, social, cultural or spiritual origin (Figure 1.1). For patients with advanced cancer, suffering may result from any or all of the various causes and the effects are additive. The term *Total suffering* is used to describe the sum total of a patient's suffering, which is what has to be addressed in palliative care (Figure 1.2).

Aspects of suffering and the components of palliative care

The components of palliative care, or the aspects of care and treatment that need to be addressed, follow logically from the causes of suffering (Figure 1.3). Each has to be addressed in the provision of comprehensive palliative care. Treatment of pain and physical symptoms are addressed first because it is not possible to deal with the psychosocial aspects of care if the patient has unrelieved pain or other distressing physical symptoms.

Figure 1.3 Aspects of suffering and the components of palliative care

Suffering	*Care*
pain + other physical symptoms + psychological problems + social difficulties + cultural issues + spiritual concerns	treatment of pain + other physical symptoms + psychological problems + social difficulties + cultural issues + spiritual concerns
= Total suffering	= Multidisciplinary palliative care (Total care)

The majority of patients with advanced cancer suffer pain to some degree. It is usually chronic, progressive, of obvious significance to the patient, and frequently associated with suffering. Other physical symptoms and psychosocial problems will also cause suffering. Cultural factors and religious difficulties may be the source of suffering. All patients with a terminal illness experience some spiritual (or existential) suffering, although in the presence of pain or physical symptoms it may go unsaid or unheard.

Interdependence of the various causes of suffering

The various aspects of suffering (Figure 1.2) are interdependent. Untreated or unresolved problems relating to one cause of suffering may cause or exacerbate other aspects of suffering. In practical terms, this means that the treatment of any one problem has to take account of the effects that each of the other aspects of suffering may have. To take pain as an example, unrelieved pain can cause or aggravate problems related to any or all of the other causes of suffering, including other physical symptoms, anxiety or depression, social, cultural and spiritual problems (Figure 1.4a). The importance of these interrelationships is that these other components of suffering will not be treated successfully until the pain is relieved. Conversely, pain may be aggravated by problems relating to other causes of suffering, including physical symptoms, anxiety or depression, social problems, cultural attitudes or spiritual concerns (Figure 1.4b). In this situation, no amount of well-prescribed analgesia will relieve the patient's pain until the other aspects of suffering that are aggravating the problem of pain are addressed. Thus, successful pain control requires attention to some or all of the other aspects of care and suffering and this makes a multidisciplinary approach to assessment and treatment mandatory; failure to do this often results in unrelieved pain. Each aspect of suffering and care is subject to the same interrelationships.

Figure 1.4 Interdependence of the various causes of suffering. (a) Unrelieved pain may cause or aggravate problems related to any of the other aspects of suffering. (b) Unresolved problems relating to other aspects of suffering may cause or aggravate pain.

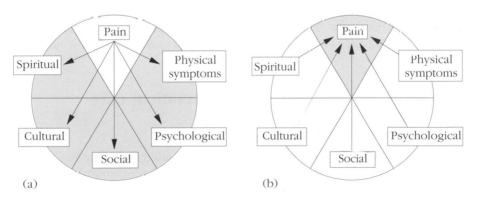

Multidisciplinary approach to palliative care

As already described, successful palliative care requires attention to all aspects of a patient's suffering. Optimal care requires input or assistance from a range of medical, nursing and allied health personnel—a multidisciplinary approach.

Table 1.5 The multidisciplinary team

Medical staff
Nursing staff
Social worker
Physiotherapist
Occupational therapist
Dietician
Psychologist (or liaison psychiatrist)
Chaplain (or pastoral care worker)
Volunteers
Other personnel, as required

Family members
Patient

Established palliative care services work as a multidisciplinary or interprofessional team. Multidisciplinary is the term that used to be applied to palliative care teams, but if the individuals work independently and there are no regular team meetings, patient care may become fragmented and conflicting information given to patients and families. The term interprofessional is now used for teams that meet on a regular basis to discuss patient care and develop a unified plan of management for each patient (Table 1.5). As all treatment must be with the patient's consent and in accordance with their wishes, they may be considered a 'member' of the team although they do not participate in team meetings. Similarly, members of the patient's family can be considered 'members', as they have an important role in the patient's overall care and their opinions should be included when formulating a plan of management. The availability of the experience and expertise of all members of the team ensures that all aspects of care are satisfactorily addressed. Volunteers play an important role in many palliative care services.[11]

In situations where there is no established palliative care service, the same principles should apply. It is the responsibility of the physician managing the patient to assess all areas of potential suffering and to seek appropriate advice and assistance with the non-medical aspects of care.

Integration of palliative care into clinical care

Palliative care is *active* therapy

Many health care workers believe that palliative care is the 'soft option' adopted when 'active' therapy stops. This is untrue. Palliative care, addressing all the patient's physical and psychosocial problems, is very active therapy; in some situations, it is tantamount to intensive care, though different from what is seen in an intensive care unit. Symptomatic and supportive palliative care should be practised before the terminal phase of the illness, in some instances at the same time as anticancer therapy. Even when 'active' anticancer treatment is no longer being given, palliative care remains medically *active* therapy. Active interventions such as medical treatment for hypercalcaemia, radiotherapy for pain or spinal cord compression, and surgery for fractures or visceral obstruction are common.

Seamless integration

Palliative care has in the past been regarded as the care employed when all avenues of anti-cancer treatment are exhausted and further active medical treatment considered inappropriate (Figure 1.5).

Figure 1.5 A traditional view of palliative care. Symptomatic and supportive palliative care is withheld until all avenues of anticancer treatment are exhausted and the treatment of other medical problems considered inappropriate.

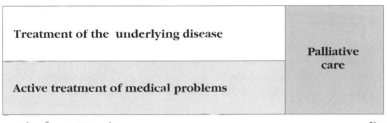

The principles and practices of multidisciplinary palliative care should be initiated at such time as a patient with cancer is symptomatic of active, progressive, incurable disease, and should *never* be withheld until such time as all modalities of anticancer treatment have been exhausted (Figure 1.6). Palliative care should be regarded as active therapy that is complementary to active treatment of the underlying disease. It should be implemented long before the terminal phases of the disease and integrated in a seamless manner with other aspects of care. It employs a holistic approach to care, encompassing all aspects of a patient's

Figure 1.6 A modern view of palliative care. Symptomatic and supportive palliative care is complementary to, and seamlessly integrated with, active treatment of the underlying disease.

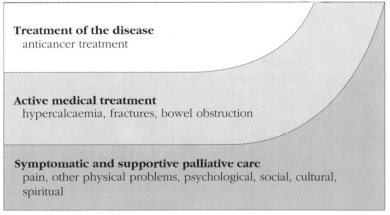

suffering, which is a prerequisite for successful palliative care but is often lacking in modern disease-orientated medicine.

Palliative care and active anticancer treatment

The early and complementary introduction of palliative care into patients' management, whilst some are continuing to receive chemotherapy or other 'active' anticancer treatment, constitutes good medical practice (Figure 1.7).[12, 13] The anticancer treatment in this situation, given to improve either the length or quality of life, is in fact palliative. Whether or not it is categorized as part of the patient's palliative care does not matter provided the symptomatic and supportive aspects of multidisciplinary palliative care are not delayed or omitted. For patients referred earlier in the course of their terminal illness, palliative care may contribute little to their medical management but will address the psychosocial aspects of care that might not otherwise receive the attention they deserve in a disease-orientated oncology clinic. Patients with a prognosis of six months or less may require the full resources of the palliative care team. As illustrated in Figures 1.6 and 1.7, the need for palliative care will increase as the disease progresses.

Figure 1.7 Integration of palliative care in the management of cancer.

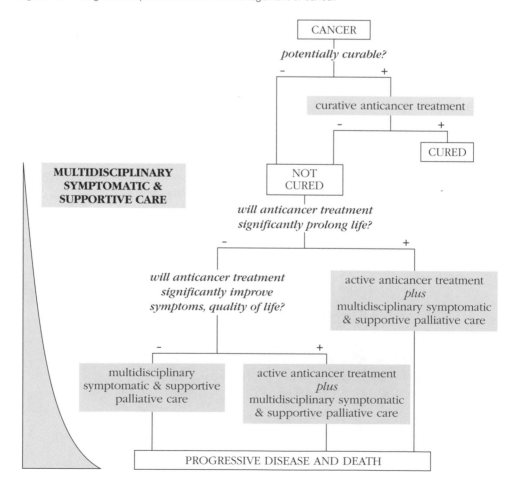

Palliative care is not just terminal care. There must be no return to the days when referral to palliative care was only made when all modalities of anticancer treatment were exhausted and the patient was dying.

Models of care

Palliative medicine is practised in hospitals, hospices and in the home.[14] The principles of care are discussed in Chapter 2 and are the same in each environment.

In hospitals, a palliative care service may either manage patients or provide a consultative advisory service.[15] Most of the diagnoses necessitating palliative care are made in hospitals and the presence of a palliative care service allows earlier involvement. The advantage of a consultative service is that, whilst endeavouring to ensure that a patient receives appropriate and comprehensive care, it fosters palliative care skills for other health care professionals.

Hospices provide an excellent and less institutionalized alternative to hospitals for patients who cannot be cared for at home. However, if they are free-standing, the patient has to be moved from one institution to another and this will cause some disruption of care and the patient has to adjust to a new treatment team. Palliative care units associated with hospitals are preferable to free-standing hospices because of the ready access to hospital facilities and expertise that are important for palliative treatment, such as orthopaedic surgery and radiotherapy.

Palliative care in the patient's home, sometimes more difficult for the family and the treatment team, has a number of advantages (Table 1.6).[16] A patient's condition, both physical and psychological, can improve after discharge home and a number of studies have documented that home is the site of care preferred by both patient and family.[17]

Table 1.6 Home care

Advantages of home	Disadvantages of hospital
comfort	rigid time-tables
privacy	impersonal care
familiarity	loss of control
security	unnecessary monitoring of vital signs
autonomy	investigations of questionable value
reduced focus on illness	financial cost
close to family, friends	travelling distance for family, friends
allows family involvement in care	

Palliative Day Care services aim to enhance the quality of life of patients at home by providing social interaction and support, creative and therapeutic activities, clinical surveillance and physical care, as well as some respite for home carers.[18–21]

Assessing outcomes

The assessment of palliative care is complex and subject to practical and methodological difficulties. Not least, a variety of different study end-points have been used including quality

Table 1.7 Benefits of palliative care services in hospitals [33]

Increased patient and family satisfaction
Improved pain and symptom management
Facilitating understanding of the diagnosis and prognosis; negotiating goals of care
Safe and effective discharge planning; lower readmission rates
Less burden and stress on other staff
Decreased length of stay
Reduced hospital costs

of life (QoL), pain and symptom control, patient and family satisfaction, the patient being cared for in the place of their choice, and health care costs. Systematic reviews of randomized controlled trials (RCTs)[22–25] highlighted these problems and found there was little high-quality evidence on which to base conclusions. In general, the reviews suggest that multidisciplinary palliative care provides similar or improved clinical outcomes compared to standard care. Reviews of the effectiveness of palliative care in hospital[26–28] and at home[29–31] are generally positive. Studies that examined health care costs showed a reduction in hospital inpatient days with equal or lower costs.[32]

A review of the benefits of a hospital-based palliative care service is summarized in Table 1.7.[33] Facilitating the understanding of the diagnosis and prognosis, and negotiating realistic goals of care, both of which can be very time consuming, are possibly the most important.

Quality of life (QoL)

Quality of life (QoL) is part of the definition of palliative care but is difficult to measure in clinical practice.[34–37] A number of QoL instruments have been developed (Table 1.8), primarily for use in clinical trials of cancer treatment. The need for more clinically interpretable measures is a matter of continuing discussion,[38, 39] and most instruments are too long to be completed by terminally ill patients. Their use in palliative care has also been questioned because they are focused more on the intensity of symptoms than the impact of the symptoms on the respondent, and may therefore not be measuring what is most important for the patient's QoL. Five important determinants of patient's QoL are the patient's own state (including physical and cognitive functioning, psychological state, and physical condition), the quality of palliative care, the physical environment, relationships, and outlook.[40] Modifications to standard QoL

Table 1.8 Quality of Life instruments

Functional Living Index—Cancer (FLIC)[43]
EORTC QLQ C-30[44]
Support Team Assessment Schedule (STAS)[45]
Functional Assessment of Cancer Therapy Scale (FACT)[46]
McGill Quality of Life Questionnaire[47]
Schedule for the Evaluation of Individual Quality of Life (SEIQoL)[41]
Quality of Life in Life-Threatening Illness—Patient Version (QOLLTI-P)[40]

instruments are being made to make them more useful in the palliative care setting.[34, 40] Another approach is used in the Schedule for the Evaluation of Individual Quality of Life (SEIQoL), which asks respondents to nominate the five life areas that are most important to their QoL.[41] A measure of the quality of dying and death has also been proposed.[42]

Place of care

Surveys of palliative care patients indicate that care at home is the most common preference,[17] and the numbers of patients dying at home has been used as a measure of the effectiveness of community-based palliative care services. However, the progressive decline in home-death rates that has been observed recently[48] should not be regarded as a failure of home care. Palliative care at home allows many patients to spend more quality time out of hospital, even if they are admitted to inpatient services during the final hours or days.

Patients' expectations

Whilst research continues into the meaningful measurement of QoL of palliative care patients, assessment of palliative care should take account of patients expectations and what they consider to be important.[49] For patients, good end-of-life care includes adequate pain and symptom management, avoiding inappropriate prolongation of dying, achieving a sense of control, relieving burden, strengthening personal relationships, and affirmation of the whole person.[50, 51] Perceptions of what constitutes 'good' and 'bad' deaths may differ between patients and staff.[52]

Evaluation of care

There is increasing pressure in all fields of medicine to assess the quality and effectiveness of care, and palliative care is no exception. Assessments, including quality assurance, audit and accreditation are necessary for both professional and political reasons. Formal objective evaluation permits self-assessment by individuals or whole services, to ensure agreed standards are achieved and maintained. The assessments encourage critical evaluation of the outcome of care, fostering continual improvement. In the political sphere, palliative care services need to be able to prove the value of the service they provide, given the finite resources that are available.

Quality assurance

The measurement of quality of health care is complex. It encompasses a number of features (Table 1.9), which may be viewed from a different perspective by patients and families, by professional carers, or by administrators and politicians. There is also need to consider those aspects of care that are peculiar to palliative care—the appropriateness of care and the empowerment of patients and families to be involved in decision making.

The measurement of quality is related to the achievement of specific aims, objectives, standards and targets. Quality assurance is the definition of standards, the measurement of

Table 1.9 Quality of health care

Effectiveness—achieving the intended benefits
Acceptability and humanity—to the consumer and to the provider
Equity and accessibility—the provision and availability of services to all
Efficiency—avoidance of waste

Table 1.10 Simplified example of a standard of care

Function
symptom control
Goal
all patients will have their symptoms controlled to a level that is acceptable to them
Structure criteria
patient is able to discuss symptoms with a member of the team
multidisciplinary team available for symptom control
Process criteria
patient's symptoms managed according to agreed quality guidelines
multidisciplinary team involved
Outcome criteria
patient confirms symptoms are controlled to an acceptable degree
documentation of involvement of the multidisciplinary team

their achievement, and the mechanisms to improve performance. Audit is one component of quality assurance.

Standards of practice for palliative care have been developed in a number of countries.[53–55] Slightly differing methodologies are used but the principles are similar. For each function there is a goal statement. The measures necessary to achieve and document each goal are described in terms of the structure, process, and outcome model. Structure includes the personnel, physical, and financial resources required. Process represents the essential steps that need to be taken. Outcome is the result of the changes made to the antecedent care. A simplified example of a standard of care for symptom control is shown in Table 1.10. Outcome focused standards of practice are now accepted as more important and meaningful. Many early standards of practice focused on structure and process but, unless the desired outcome is achieved, structure and process are of less importance.

The Liverpool Care Pathway for the Terminal/Dying Phase is an evidence-based standard of care for the optimal management of dying patients.[56, 57]

The development and adoption of uniform standards of care will provide a basis for self-assessment as well as facilitating external accreditation. Self-assessment will highlight areas worthy of audit, the results of which will identify problems related to structure (resource needs) and process (treatment protocol modification). This cycle of review and modification is termed continuous quality improvement or CQI.

Audit

Clinical audit is the systematic, critical analysis of the quality of clinical care including the procedures used for diagnosis and treatment, the use of resources, and the resulting outcome and quality of life for the patient. It is usually focused on a particular aspect of care that is problematic, but any service function affecting the outcome of patient care can be subject to audit. Examples include administrative functions (e.g. admission policies), communication within and without the service, or treatment of specific clinical problems. Audit and quality improvement are used to raise standards of care.[58–61] The process of audit involves the measurement, improvement and then re-measurement of a particular aspect of care, known as the audit cycle (Table 1.11).

Table 1.11 The audit cycle

Select topic for audit
Standards or targets are defined and agreed, based on best current practice from the literature
Survey of recent or current results
Implementation of protocol modifications
Reassessment to determine if standards or targets have been achieved

A considerable number of validated measurement tools exist that can be used in audit.[58, 62–64] Their use standardizes measurement and allows comparisons between different services. Some are focused on particular symptoms such as pain or anxiety, whilst others provide a more global or QoL assessment. These instruments can be used for baseline measurements and re-used to evaluate the effect of interventions.

Barriers to palliative care

Despite its demonstrated benefits, many patients with advanced cancer do not receive palliative care,[65] and some are referred too late in the course of their disease to benefit from treatment. The reasons for this may relate to the physician, the patient, or to social factors (Table 1.12). Doctors may be reluctant to refer patients to palliative care, or transfer them only when they are terminally ill, because of poor prognostication or because they lack the communication skills to discuss end-of-life issues.[66] Prognostication and communication are discussed in Chapter 2. Patients may be unwilling to accept palliative care if they believe their prognosis is better than what they are told, or if they have unrealistic expectations that their disease will respond to experimental therapies or alternative medicine.[67, 68] If there has been no advance care planning, disagreements between the patient and family about

Table 1.12 Barriers to palliative care

Physician
late referral
poor prognostication
lacks communication skills to address end-of-life issues
reluctant to refer
doesn't understand or believe in palliative care
loss of control, loss of income
lack of institutional standards for end-of-life care
Patient
believe prognosis better than what they are told
unrealistic expectation of disease response
patient–family disagreement about treatment options
lack of advance care planning
Social factors
ethnic minorities, language barriers
rural communities
poor or underprivileged

treatment options may prevent the introduction of palliative care.[69] However, the SUPPORT study demonstrated that facilitating advance care planning and doctor–patient communication was insufficient to change patients' attitudes or physicians' practices, and that other means are necessary to improve access to, and acceptance of, good palliative care.[70] There may be limited access to palliative care services for patients who live in rural communities, and for those who are poor or underprivileged. Cultural and language barriers may prevent patients from ethnic minorities receiving palliative care.[71] Continued education and research are required to overcome these barriers, so that the majority of patients with advanced cancer receive appropriate palliative care.

Future directions

Multidisciplinary palliative care has developed rapidly in the last thirty years. The features that distinguish palliative care—attention to the whole person and to all aspects of a patient's suffering, and a multidisciplinary approach to care—have improved the standards of care for patients with advanced and incurable cancer as evaluated by pain and symptom control, patient and family satisfaction, quality of life and other measures. With further improvement in medical treatments and continued development of our understanding of the psychosocial aspects of care, the standards will continue to improve in the future.

The need for palliative care is enormous and will continue to increase. The existence of an increasingly aged population and the fact that the proportion of cancers that are cured has remained relatively constant, have resulted in an increasing number of patients with incurable cancer. Even though the number of palliative care services has increased dramatically in recent years, only a relatively small proportion of patients with advanced cancer are being accommodated. The solution requires both the further development of services as well as the education of all health care professionals in the essentials of palliative care.

References

1   Hinton, J. (1967). *Dying*. Penguin Books.
2   Marks, R.M. and Sachar, E.J. (1973). Undertreatment of medical inpatients with narcotic analgesics. *Annals of Internal Medicine* 78, 173–81.
3   Kubler-Ross, E. (1973). *On Death and Dying*. Tavistock Publications.
4   Simpson, M.A. (1976). Planning for terminal care. *Lancet* 2, 192–3.
5   Lack, S.A. (1976). Philosophy and organisation of a hospice program. In *Psychosocial Care of the Dying Patient* (ed. C. Garfield). San Francisco, University of California Press.
6   Hudson, R.P. (1978). Death, dying, and the zealous phase. *Annals of Internal Medicine* 88, 696–702.
7   Lamerton, R. (1980). *Care of the Dying*. Penguin Books.
8   World Health Organization (2002). *National cancer control programmes: policies and managerial guidelines. 2nd edition.* Geneva, WHO.
9   Cassell, E.J. (1991). *The Nature of Suffering and the Goals of Medicine.* New York, Oxford University Press.
10 Cassell, E.J. (1999). Diagnosing suffering: a perspective. *Annals of Internal Medicine* 131, 531–4.
11 Doyle, D. (ed.) (2002). *Volunteeers in Hospice and Palliative Care.* Oxford, Oxford University Press.
12 Dudgeon, D.J., et al. (1995). When does palliative care begin? A needs assessment of cancer patients with recurrent disease. *Journal of Palliative Care* 11, 5–9.
13 American Society of Clinical Oncology (1998). Cancer care during the last phase of life. *Journal of Clinical Oncology* 16, 1986–96.

14 Bosanquet, N. and Salisbury, C. (ed.) (1999). *Providing a Palliative Care Service*. Oxford, Oxford University Press.

15 Dunlop, R.J. and Hockley, J.M. (ed.) (1998). *Hospital-based Palliative Care Teams: The Hospital/hospice Interface*. Oxford, Oxford University Press.

16 Doyle, D. and Jeffrey, D. (2000). *Palliative Care in the Home*. Oxford, Oxford University Press.

17 Higginson, I.J. and Sen-Gupta, G.J.A. (2000). Place of care in advanced cancer: A qualitative systematic literature review of patient preferences. *Journal of Palliative Medicine* 3, 287–300.

18 Higginson, I.J., et al. (2000). Palliative day care: what do services do? Palliative Day Care Project Group. *Palliative Medicine* 14, 277–86.

19 Hearn, J. and Myers, K. (ed.) (2001). *Palliative Day Care in Practice*. Oxford, Oxford University Press.

20 Goodwin, D.M., et al. (2002). What is palliative day care? A patient perspective of five UK services. *Supportive Care in Cancer* 10, 556–62.

21 Goodwin, D.M., et al. (2003). Effectiveness of palliative day care in improving pain, symptom control, and quality of life. *Journal of Pain and Symptom Management* 25, 202–12.

22 Rinck, G.C., et al. (1997). Methodologic issues in effectiveness research on palliative cancer care: a systematic review. *Journal of Clinical Oncology* 15, 1697–1707.

23 Hearn, J. and Higginson, I.J. (1998). Do specialist palliative care teams improve outcomes for cancer patients? A systematic literature review. *Palliative Medicine* 12, 317–32.

24 Goodwin, D.M., et al. (2002). An evaluation of systematic reviews of palliative care services. *Journal of Palliative Care* 18, 77–83.

25 Higginson, I.J., et al. (2003). Is there evidence that palliative care teams alter end-of-life experiences of patients and their caregivers? *Journal of Pain and Symptom Management* 25, 150–68.

26 Ellershaw, J.E., Peat, S.J. and Boys, L.C. (1995). Assessing the effectiveness of a hospital palliative care team. *Palliative Medicine* 9, 145–52.

27 Higginson, I.J., et al. (2002). Do hospital-based palliative teams improve care for patients or families at the end of life? *Journal of Pain and Symptom Management* 23, 96–106.

28 Homsi, J., et al. (2002). The impact of a palliative medicine consultation service in medical oncology. *Supportive Care in Cancer* 10, 337–42.

29 Smeenk, F.W., et al. (1998). Effectiveness of home care programmes for patients with incurable cancer on their quality of life and time spent in hospital: systematic review. *British Medical Journal* 316, 1939–44.

30 Grande, G.E., et al. (2000). A randomized controlled trial of a hospital at home service for the terminally ill. *Palliative Medicine* 14, 375–85.

31 Ringdal, G.I., Jordhoy, M.S. and Kaasa, S. (2002). Family satisfaction with end-of-life care for cancer patients in a cluster randomized trial. *Journal of Pain and Symptom Management* 24, 53–63.

32 Raftery, J.P., et al. (1996). A randomized controlled trial of the cost-effectiveness of a district coordinating service for terminally ill cancer patients. *Palliative Medicine* 10, 151–61.

33 Center to Advance Palliative Care (2000). The Case for Hospital-Based Palliative Care. <www.capc.org>

34 Cohen, S.R. (2001). Defining and measuring quality of life in palliative care. In *Topics in Palliative Care. Volume 5* (ed. E. Bruera and R. Portenoy). New York, Oxford University Press.

35 Salek, S., et al. (2002). The use of quality-of-life instruments in palliative care. *European Journal of Palliative Care* 9, 52–6.

36 Cohen, S.R. (2003). Assessing quality of life in palliative care. In *Issues in Palliative Care Research* (ed. R. Portenoy and E. Bruera). New York, Oxford University Press.

37 Kaasa, S. and Loge, J.H. (2003). Quality of life in palliative care: principles and practice. *Palliative Medicine* 17, 11–20.

38 Browman, G.P. (1999). Science, language, intuition, and the many meanings of quality of life. *Journal of Clinical Oncology* 17, 1651–3.

39 Kornblith, A.B. (2001). Does palliative care palliate? *Journal of Clinical Oncology* 19, 2111–13.

40 Cohen, S.R. and Leis, A. (2002). What determines the quality of life of terminally ill cancer patients from their own perspective? *Journal of Palliative Care* 18, 48–58.

41 Waldron, D., et al. (1999). Quality-of-life measurement in advanced cancer: assessing the individual. *Journal of Clinical Oncology* 17, 3603–11.

42 Curtis, J.R., et al. (2002). A measure of the quality of dying and death. Initial validation using after-death interviews with family members. *Journal of Pain and Symptom Management* 24, 17–31.

43 Schipper, H., et al. (1984). Measuring the quality of life of cancer patients: the Functional Living Index—Cancer: development and validation. *Journal of Clinical Oncology* 2, 472–83.

44 Aaronson, N.K., et al. (1993). The European Organization for Research and Treatment of Cancer QLQ–C30: a quality-of-life instrument for use in international clinical trials in oncology. *Journal of the National Cancer Institute* 85, 365–76.

45 Higginson, I.J. and McCarthy, M. (1993). Validity of the support team assessment schedule: do staffs' ratings reflect those made by patients or their families? *Palliative Medicine* 7, 219–28.

46 Cella, D.F., et al. (1993). The Functional Assessment of Cancer Therapy scale: development and validation of the general measure. *Journal of Clinical Oncology* 11, 570–9.

47 Cohen, S.R., et al. (1995). The McGill Quality of Life Questionnaire: a measure of quality of life appropriate for people with advanced disease. A preliminary study of validity and acceptability. *Palliative Medicine* 9, 207–19.

48 Higginson, I.J., Astin, P. and Dolan, S. (1998). Where do cancer patients die? Ten-year trends in the place of death of cancer patients in England. *Palliative Medicine* 12, 353–63.

49 Emanuel, L.L., et al. (2000). What terminally ill patients care about: toward a validated construct of patients' perspectives. *Journal of Palliative Medicine* 3, 419–31.

50 Singer, P.A., Martin, D.K. and Kelner, M. (1999). Quality end-of-life care: patients' perspectives. *Journal of the American Medical Association* 281, 163–8.

51 Steinhauser, K.E., et al. (2000). Factors considered important at the end of life by patients, family, physicians, and other care providers. *Journal of the American Medical Association* 284, 2476–82.

52 Payne, S.A., Langley-Evans, A. and Hillier, R. (1996). Perceptions of a 'good' death: a comparative study of the views of hospice staff and patients. *Palliative Medicine* 10, 307–12.

53 Palliative Care Australia (1999). Standards for Palliative Care Provision. 3rd edition. <www.pallcare.org.au/publications/index.html>

54 National Health Service (2000). Manual of Cancer Services Standards. <www.doh.gov.uk/cancer/mcss.htm>

55 Canadian Hospice Palliative Care Association (2001). A Model to Guide Hospice Palliative Care: Based on National Principles and Norms. <www.chpca.net/pub_and_press_releases/norms.htm>

56 Ellershaw, J. and Ward, C. (2003). Care of the dying patient: the last hours or days of life. *British Medical Journal* 326, 30–4.

57 Ellershaw, J. and Wilkinson, S. (ed.) (2003). *Care of the Dying. A Pathway to Excellence*. Oxford, Oxford University Press.

58 Higginson, I.J. and Hearn, J. (2000). Palliative care audit: tools, objectives, and models for training in assessment, monitoring and review. In *Topics in Palliative Care. Volume 4* (ed. R. Portenoy and E. Bruera). New York, Oxford University Press.

59 Lynn, J., Schuster, J.L. and Kabcenell, A. (2000). *Improving Care for the End of Life. A Sourcebook for Health Care managers and Clinicians.* New York, Oxford University Press.

60 Bookbinder, M. and Romer, A.L. (2002). Raising the standard of care for imminently dying patients using quality improvement. *Journal of Palliative Medicine* 5, 635–44.

61 Higginson, I.J. (2003). Clinical and organisational audit in palliative medicine. In *Oxford Textbook of Palliative Medicine, 3rd edition* (ed. D. Doyle, G. Hanks, N. Cherny and K. Calman). Oxford, Oxford University Press.

62 Hearn, J. and Higginson, I.J. (1997). Outcome measures in palliative care for advanced cancer patients: a review. *Journal of Public Health and Medicine* 19, 193–9.

63 Teno, J.M. (2002). Outcomes assessment in palliative care. In *Principles and Practice of Palliative Care and Supportive Oncology* (ed. A.M. Berger, R.K. Portenoy and D.E. Weissman). Philadelphia, Lippincott, Williams and Wilkins.

64 Teno, J.M. (2003). Toolkit of Instruments to Measure End-of-Life Care (TIME). <www.chcr. brown.edu/pcoc/toolkit.htm>

65 McCarthy, E.P., et al. (2003). Barriers to hospice care among older patients dying with lung and colorectal cancer. *Journal of Clinical Oncology* 21, 728–35.

66 von Gunten, C.F. (2002). Discussing hospice care. *Journal of Clinical Oncology* 20, 1419–24.

67 Weeks, J.C., et al. (1998). Relationship between cancer patients' predictions of prognosis and their treatment preferences. *Journal of the American Medical Association* 279, 1709–14.

68 Navari, R.M., Stocking, C.B. and Siegler, M. (2000). Preferences of patients with advanced cancer for hospice care. *Journal of the American Medical Association* 284, 2449.

69 Phipps, E., et al. (2003). Approaching the end of life: attitudes, preferences, and behaviors of African-American and white patients and their family caregivers. *Journal of Clinical Oncology* 21, 549–54.

70 The SUPPORT Principal Investigators (1995). A controlled trial to improve care for seriously ill hospitalized patients. The study to understand prognoses and preferences for outcomes and risks of treatments (SUPPORT). *Journal of the American Medical Association* 274, 1591–8.

71 Chan, A. and Woodruff, R.K. (1999). Comparison of palliative care needs of English- and non-English speaking patients. *Journal of Palliative Care* 15, 26–30.

2

Principles of palliative care

Attitude to care	Advance care planning
Communication	Managing stress
Palliative care	

The aim of palliative care is to relieve and prevent suffering for patients with incurable disease. The treatment required incorporates the whole spectrum of care—medical, nursing, psychological, social, cultural and spiritual. A holistic approach, incorporating these wider

Table 2.1 Principles of palliative care

Attitude to care
    caring attitude
    commitment
    consideration of individuality
    cultural considerations
    consent
    choice of site of care

Communication
    communication amongst health care professionals
    communication with patients and families

The care
    clinical context: appropriate treatment
    comprehensive and multidisciplinary
    care excellence
    consistent
    co-ordinated
    continuity
    crisis prevention
    caregiver support
    continued reassessment

Advance care planning

aspects of care, is good medical practice and in palliative care it is essential. The principles of palliative care (Table 2.1) might simply be regarded as those of good medical practice.

Attitude to care

Caring attitude

A caring attitude involves sensitivity, sympathy and compassion, and demonstrates concern for the individual. There is concern for all aspects of a patient's suffering and not just the medical problems. It also implies a non-judgmental approach in which personality, intellect, ethnic origin, religious belief or any other individual factors do not prejudice the delivery of optimal care.

A caring attitude is essential for successful palliative care. A correct physical diagnosis and the prescription of appropriate treatment may be quite ineffective unless other aspects of a patient's suffering are considered. A caring attitude is difficult to teach; it is fortunate that caring individuals are drawn to the practice of palliative care, and it is the responsibility of those experienced in the field to lead by example.

Commitment

Palliative care is a form of intensive care, though much different from what is seen in a hospital intensive care unit. It requires a definite commitment by the staff for treatment to be successful. Dealing constantly with patients with advanced cancer can be stressful and considerable dedication is required to support patients with the complex and difficult psychosocial problems, some of which are not resolvable.

Consideration of individuality

Each patient is a unique individual. The practice of categorizing patients by their type of cancer, based on the similarity of the medical problems encountered, fails to recognize the individual psychosocial features and problems that makes every patient different. These unique characteristics can greatly influence suffering and need to be taken into account when planning the palliative care for individual patients.

Cultural considerations

Ethnic, racial, religious and other cultural factors may have a profound effect on a patient's suffering. Cultural differences are to be respected and treatment planned in a culturally sensitive manner.

Consent

The consent of a patient, or those to whom the responsibility is delegated, is necessary before any treatment is given or withdrawn. The majority of patients want shared decision making and physicians tend to underestimate this.[1] Having assessed what treatment is appropriate or inappropriate, this is discussed with the patient. In most instances, adequately informed patients will accept the recommendations made. The key word is *informed*—whether the patient and family have been honestly apprised of the stage of the cancer. If informed patients want more or less treatment than was envisaged as appropriate, there is an obligation to consider their wishes. Informed consent is particularly relevant in palliative care because of the additional suffering that may result from continuing active treatment that is inappropriate to the stage of the patient's disease and prognosis.

Choice of site of care

The patient and family need to be included in any discussion about where a patient is to be managed. Patients with a terminal illness should be managed at home by their own doctor, with the support of a domiciliary palliative care service, whenever possible.

Communication

Good communication between all those involved in a patient's care is essential and is fundamental to many of the aspects of palliative care discussed in this chapter. Communication is less likely to be a problem if there is an established palliative care service conducting regular team meetings. Where no such service exists, it is the responsibility of the treating doctor to ensure adequate communication with all other personnel involved in a patient's care.

Good communication with the patient and family is vital. Communication between patients with advanced cancer and their doctors has become more open during the last thirty years and more patients are now wishing to be better informed about their disease and to participate more actively in their own care.[1] At the same time, discussion of terminal diagnoses and death remains unacceptable to some people. Moderate or severe communication problems between patients and their professional carers occur in 10–20% of cases.[2]

In palliative care, there is frequent need for discussions of very sensitive matters including breaking bad news, transferring from oncology to palliative care, communicating a prognosis, and discussing a do-not-resuscitate (DNR) order. To be effective, these interviews need to be structured,[3, 4] and the necessary communication skills are able to be learned.[5, 6]

Breaking bad news

There are some basic rules that must be followed when talking with patients for the purpose of breaking bad news (Table 2.2). First, the discussion is conducted in person and never on the telephone. Second, at least one family member or friend should accompany the patient. The patient will feel supported by the presence of family members or a friend, and there will be better retention of the medical information presented. It will also prevent any conspiracy of silence or breakdown of communication within the family caused by one person not knowing what another has been told. The nurse and the social worker are included in the interview if they are to be involved in the patient's subsequent care. Third, the interview allows sufficient time for as much discussion as the patient or family wish. They may need time to absorb the information given and a second interview may need to be arranged at which they can present questions. Fourth, the physician or counsellor should not stand over the patient's bed but should be seated, so that level eye contact with the patient can be made. Last, the interviews are conducted in private surroundings with as few interruptions as possible.

Communication should always be directly with the patient, who should be accompanied or supported by at least one family member or friend. The exceptions to this rule are patients who are semiconscious or demented and those who have made it clear that they wish to know no more about their disease and have delegated responsibility to a family member. Relatives who request that patients not be told of their diagnosis should be resisted. Many patients have suspicions or fears about their diagnosis and to withhold information will

Table 2.2 Communicating with patients

Basic rules
> conduct the interview in person (not by telephone)
> ensure privacy, prevent interruptions
> sitting down (not standing over the bed)
> allow enough time
> at least one family member or friend should accompany the patient

Provide information
> the medical situation
> what treatment can be offered
> the possible benefits and burdens of any treatments
> avoid precise prognostication
> as much or as little information as they want

Information should be conveyed
> in a caring and sympathetic way, not abruptly or bluntly
> in a way they can understand
> clearly (avoiding euphemisms)
> truthfully
> in a positive manner
> use independent interpreters rather than let the family translate

compound their anxiety. In addition, patients who are not informed about their situation cannot participate in any meaningful way in discussions about their treatment.

Information is delivered in a caring and sympathetic way and never abruptly. For patients for whom only symptomatic and supportive care is available, information is conveyed in a positive manner and hope never denied. The information given must be clear, unambiguous and presented in a way the patient can understand. Euphemisms such as 'growth' or 'spots' are avoided as they may be misinterpreted by the patient. Printed fact sheets are useful. Where language barriers exist, independent interpreters are used in preference to family members, as it is well known that the latter frequently alter what is said.

Patients should be informed of their situation in a truthful way. Lies inevitably cause distress or distrust at a later stage.[7, 8] The facts are delivered in a gentle and sensitive manner, tailored to the patient's intellectual and emotional state; being abrupt or blunt or totally negative is inexcusable. Patients and families will cope better, given time and support, knowing what they have to deal with, rather than the uncertainty of not knowing. Honesty will strengthen the doctor–patient relationship, improve patient co-operation and, at such time as there is disease progression, there will be less anguish and suffering. The patient is told not only the diagnosis, but also what treatment can be offered. If they are to receive palliative anticancer treatment, this is discussed; if they are to receive only symptomatic and supportive care, then this is discussed in a positive manner. *Never* is a patient told 'nothing more can be done', as it is never true and may be interpreted as abandonment of care. If further chemotherapy or radiotherapy will not be of benefit, the patient is informed of this and the positive aspects of continuing symptomatic and supportive care are stressed.

Patients vary greatly in how much they want to know. Lack of information causes anxiety, but so may too much. How much a patient is told is individually determined. It depends on a number of factors including intellect, emotional state, social and cultural background, family support, and their ability to cope. It is usually possible to allow the patient to determine how much information is discussed. If patients want to know more they will ask; in this situation all their questions are answered. Patients not wanting more information usually make this obvious by lack of questions and their general attitude; this can be confirmed by indirect questions and they are reassured that any questions they might have in the future will be answered.

Structuring the interview. After ensuring that the physical environment is appropriate, there should be a clear statement of the purpose of the meeting (Table 2.3). Then the patient should be asked to relate what they understand about their current situation and their expectations for the future. Factual information may need to be given if they do not fully appreciate their medical condition. Then realistic possibilities and goals can be discussed in the context of their view of the present and future. Talking with patients in this manner allows them to feel they are participating and not just being lectured to, and helps them to maintain hope of achieving realistic and personally meaningful goals.

Table 2.3 Structuring the interview

Appropriate setting (see Table 2.2)
Introduce the discussion   *e.g.* we need to talk about what is happening with your illness
Ask what the patient and family know   *e.g.* tell me what you know about your illness
Find out what they are expecting or hoping for   *e.g.* tell me what you see happening in the future
Provide information, if necessary (see Table 2.2)
Discuss realistic possibilities in the context of their view of the present and future
Respond sympathetically to emotional reactions
Agree upon a plan, with provision that it can be modified if circumstances change

Transferring to palliative care

If palliative care is introduced early in the course of advanced cancer, patients are less likely to be distressed when told that further anticancer therapy has no realistic chance of being of benefit. For others, being told there is no more chemotherapy and that they are to be transferred to palliative care can be most distressing. A survey of medical oncologists reported that discussing no further chemotherapy and moving to palliative care was the most difficult of 'bad news' conversations.[9] It often falls to the palliative care staff to discuss what palliative care means and this should be done in the context of the patient's understanding of their medical situation and their visions of the future (Table 2.4).[10] If the patient is accepting that further anticancer therapy is not of benefit, palliative care can be discussed in terms of helping them achieve their personal goals. If they are not willing to accept the discontinuation of anticancer therapy, discussions about palliative care are not likely to be useful. Patients moving to palliative care should be reassured that it is about maximizing quality of life and not 'giving up'.

Prognostication

Prognostication for individual patients with advanced cancer is notoriously inexact. Surveys show physicians' estimates to be accurate in only 20–40% of cases, although the accuracy

Table 2.4 Discussing palliative care

Appropriate setting
    privacy, sitting down, adequate time, prevent interruptions, patient accompanied

Introduction
    e.g. we need to talk about your current problems and our goals for your care

Find out what the patient understands
    e.g. tell me what you understand about your current medical problems

Find out what the patient expects, what their goals are
    e.g. what do you see happening in the future? Or what things are important for you?

Discuss palliative care in the context of how it can help them achieve their goals
    e.g. you have told me you would like to … Palliative care may be able to help you achieve what you want

Emphasize the positive aspects of palliative care
    e.g. living as well as possible, for as long as possible; not 'giving up'

Respond sympathetically to emotional reactions

Agree upon a plan, which might include:
    convening a family meeting
    organizing them to meet someone from palliative care

increases to about 70% if the life expectancy is less than 14 days.[11, 12] Survival estimates based on readily available laboratory and clinical data produce results similar to the physicians' estimates, and combining the two may give the most accurate results.[13, 14] Estimates given to patients are frequently optimistic or over-estimates.[11, 15] Physicians feel poorly prepared for prognosticating and find it stressful.[16]

There are some general guidelines for how to respond when patients or families ask for a prognosis (Table 2.5).[17] The uncertainty of predicting an individual's prognosis needs to be explained and a realistic time range given. Attempts at precise prognostication should be avoided as they are invariably wrong and, whether the original time given was too long or too short, it will compound the suffering of the patient and the family. It is better to give a 'best' and 'worst' estimate that, depending on the stage of the patient's disease, may encompass a considerable range of time. Patients with a short life expectancy should be encouraged to try and do the things that are important to them as well as getting their personal affairs in

Table 2.5 Communicating prognoses

Explain the uncertainty in estimating an individual patient's prognosis

Give a realistic time range

Provide realistic hope—helping them to achieve what is important for them

Recommend that family relationships and worldly affairs be attended to

Be prepared to answer questions about the process of dying

Provide on-going support and counselling

Reassure about continuity of care

order. Patients asking about their prognosis may also be asking how they are going to die. Patients who have reached the point of specifically asking about their life expectancy should be provided with access to on-going counselling, as they are likely to benefit from continuing open discussions.

Do-Not-Resuscitate (DNR) orders

For patients with advanced cancer, cardiopulmonary resuscitation (CPR) is rarely successful.[18] In one study, 2% of 406 patients survived to discharge from hospital;[19] in another, 6% of 83 patients survived 6 weeks.[20] However, some institutions require that it be discussed with the patient before a DNR order is given. This is clearly inappropriate for patients who are actively dying, for whom CPR would be completely futile; if the patient or family raises the issue, the importance of patient comfort and dignity, as well as the futility of CPR, should be stressed. For patients with a longer life expectancy (months), discussion about CPR should be in the context of their understanding of their clinical situation and their expectations (Table 2.6).[21] Most patients with advanced cancer know their disease is not curable and hope that their death will be peaceful and painless. In this situation, CPR performed immediately after they have died can be viewed as undignified and not in keeping with how they wish to be treated. Patients should be reassured that all their other medical therapy will be continued. Only if necessary should the futility and indignity of CPR, or the likely scenario should they survive CPR, be discussed.

Table 2.6 Discussing Do-Not-Resuscitate (DNR) orders

Appropriate setting
    privacy, sitting down, adequate time, prevent interruptions

Introduction
    e.g. we need to discuss something that we discuss with all patients admitted to the hospital

Find out what the patient understands
    e.g. what do you understand about your current medical problems?

Find out what the patient expects, what their goals are
    e.g. what do you see happening in the future?

Discuss a DNR order in the context of the patient's view of their future
    e.g. you have told me you would like ... so CPR would not seem appropriate if you die

If necessary, discuss
    futility of CPR (chances of surviving to discharge)
    indignity of CPR
    being on a respirator in ICU and unable to communicate

Respond sympathetically to emotional reactions

Reassure patient that all other medical care will continue

Patients' assessment of communication

The views of patients provide some guidance on how best to communicate with them. Satisfaction with interviews during which bad news was delivered related to the environment, to what the physician said, and to how it was said.[22, 23] Another study defined six domains that were important in communicating with patients with advanced disease: being honest and straightforward, being willing to talk about dying, giving bad news in a sensitive way, listening to patients, encouraging questions from patients, and being sensitive to when patients are ready to talk about death.[24]

The care

Clinical context: appropriate treatment

All palliative treatment should be appropriate to the stage of the patient's disease and the prognosis. Over-enthusiastic therapy and patient neglect are equally deplorable. Palliative care has been accused of the medicalization of death, and care must be taken balancing technical intervention with a humanistic orientation to dying patients.[25] The prescription of appropriate treatment is particularly important in palliative care because of the unnecessary additional suffering that may be caused by inappropriately active therapy or by lack of treatment. When palliative care includes active anticancer treatment, limits should be observed, appropriate to the patient's condition and prognosis. Where symptomatic and supportive palliative measures are employed, all efforts are directed at the relief of suffering and quality of life, and not necessarily at the prolongation of life. Prognostication or the assessment of what stage a patient has reached in the course of a terminal illness may be inexact, making the prescription of appropriate treatment difficult in some circumstances. There is no easy solution and decisions are based on good clinical judgment and experience.

Comprehensive multidisciplinary care

The goal of palliative care is to provide total or comprehensive care for all aspects of a patient's suffering, which necessitates a multidisciplinary approach. Comprehensive care is the cornerstone of palliative care and the treatment of the whole person and all aspects of suffering cannot be achieved in part or by fragments. To provide medical treatment without knowledge or attention to the psychosocial aspects of suffering is unlikely to be successful. Similarly, to provide psychosocial and spiritual support, without attention to the medical needs, will likewise be unsuccessful.

The non-medical or psychosocial aspects of care require particular attention and may be less easily discussed.[26] There are guidelines suggesting how to explore issues of suffering and dignity with patients.[27, 28]

Care excellence

Palliative care should deliver the best possible medical, nursing and allied health care that is available and appropriate. Wherever possible it should be evidence-based, although the evidence base for palliative medicine is still in its infancy. Optimal care should be available to all patients but is particularly important for those terminally ill. In hospitals, it is commonplace for terminally ill patients to be relegated to side rooms, out of sight. That they and their family deserve more privacy is commendable; that they receive less care and attention is inexcusable.

The delivery of excellent care depends on caring and commitment, which are important considerations in staff selection. It also depends on the skills and experience of the team members, their commitment to maintaining quality standards of care, and their involvement in the continual assessment of the results of therapy.

Consistent medical care

Consistent medical management requires that an overall plan of care be established for each patient. This is communicated by the doctor to the patient and the family and to all staff involved in the patient's care. The doctor should be able to predict if changes are likely in the pattern of care, avoiding sudden or unexpected alterations. Medical care is most likely to be inconsistent when the patient is transferred to another institution or discharged home.

Sudden or unexpected changes in medical management can be distressing for the patient and family. For example, the abrupt cessation of active anticancer treatment, sometimes accompanied by the statement 'nothing more can be done', can be devastating. Similarly, the patient admitted to hospital to die but suddenly commenced on intravenous therapy for asymptomatic hypercalcaemia, can be distressing for the family.

Co-ordinated care

Co-ordination of care involves the effective organisation of the work and efforts of the members of the palliative care team, to provide maximal support and care to the patient and family. The activities of the multidisciplinary team require good leadership and a good team spirit. Care planning meetings, to which all members of the team can contribute, and at which the views of the patient and the family are presented, are used to develop a plan of care for each individual patient. Having established this plan of care and goals for the management of each patient, there is less likely to be any conflict or duplication of effort amongst team members, and communication with people outside the team will be clear.

Continuity of care

The provision of continuous symptomatic and supportive care from the time the patient is first referred until death is basic to the aims of palliative care. Problems arise when patients are moved from one place of care to another and ensuring continuity of all aspects of care is most important. A synopsis of the patient's current condition and treatment, present and anticipated problems, and goals and prognosis should be available to the doctor and other staff assuming responsibility for the patient's care on the day the patient is transferred. Continuity of care depends primarily on effective co-ordination and good communication.

Crisis prevention

Good palliative care involves careful planning to prevent physical and emotional crises that occur with progressive cancer. Many of the clinical problems that occur with disease progression can be anticipated and some can be prevented by appropriate treatment. Patients and their families should be forewarned of likely problems, and contingency plans made to minimize physical and emotional distress. Prevention of crises is particularly important in the home care situation.

Caregiver support

The relatives of patients with advanced cancer are subject to considerable emotional and physical stress, especially if the patient is being managed at home.[29, 30] Particular attention must be paid to their needs as the success or failure of palliative care may depend on the caregivers' ability to cope. Emotional and social support, help with daily tasks, and the temporary hospitalization of the patient to allow the caregiver a period of respite, are some of the measures that can be considered.

Continued reassessment

All patients with advanced cancer have progressive disease and increasing and new clinical problems are to be expected. This applies as much to psychosocial issues as it does to pain and other physical symptoms. Continued reassessment is therefore a necessity, both to adjust treatments already instituted and to manage new problems.

Advance care planning

Advance care planning involves a number of processes—informing the patient, eliciting preferences, and identifying a surrogate decision maker to act if the patient is no longer able to make decisions about their own care. The principle is not new and it is common for patients aware of approaching death to discuss with their carers how they wish to be treated. However, these wishes have not always been respected, especially if the patient is urgently taken to hospital or if there is disagreement amongst family members about what is appropriate treatment.

Advance care planning is a means for patients to record their end-of-life values and preferences, including their wishes regarding future treatments (or avoidance of them).[31] It usually involves discussions with family members, or at least with the person who is to be the surrogate decision maker. The 'Respecting Choices' program in Wisconsin employs trained personnel to facilitate the discussions and record the outcomes, which are in writing and signed, and kept in the front of the patient's file.[32, 33] It is important for the surrogate decision maker to be involved in the discussions in order that they have explicit knowledge of the patient's wishes; otherwise they may feel burdened by the responsibility.[34] There is less conflict between patients and their families if advance care planning has been discussed.[35]

Routine advance care planning for all patients with recurrent cancer would greatly facilitate their management. The patient would be reassured that their wishes would be respected even if they were no longer able to make decisions. There would be less decision making in crisis and no family arguments about what treatment the patient should receive. As the process becomes more widely accepted, it is to be hoped that it will become unacceptable for oncologists not to go through advance care planning with their patients who develop recurrent cancer.[36]

Coping with stress

Working in palliative care *is* stressful, although possibly no more than in other specialties.[37–39] Some claim that hospice work may be associated with less stress, due to the various anti-stress defences built into the work. It has been reported that palliative care workers in hospices suffer less stress than their colleagues who work in hospitals.[40] The obvious source of stress would seem to be working with dying patients, with at least some of whom there will be emotional involvement, but surveys suggest more stress is attributable to organizational and social issues.

Sources of stress

Poor management in terms of general administration, fiscal policy or resource allocation may all lead to staff stress (Table 2.7). In palliative care, it is important that management acknowledge the achievements of the staff and provide an environment that encourages the development of new skills. Poor team leadership with unclear goals and role conflict between team members will cause stress.

Table 2.7 Sources of stress

Organizational	poor administration lack of goal definition financial constraints lack of resources, poor allocation failure to recognize clinical team's achievements no opportunity to develop new skills
Team	poor leadership poor definition of goals unreasonable clinical workloads poor communication role ambiguity: interdisciplinary conflict
Patients	difficult patients difficult families identifying with patients
Unrealistic goals	attempting to solve all problems dealing with chronic family problems
Personal	stresses at home: personal, marital those at home become disinterested

Many patients and families cared for by palliative care services are described as 'difficult', which is not surprising given the problems they face. This will lead to stress if there are too many difficult problems or too many deaths close together. All health care professionals tend to identify with some patients, whose subsequent death may be stressful. Working with the dying heightens workers' awareness of their own losses and their own mortality.

Palliative care workers are often expected to provide solutions to all problems, regardless of the fact that many of these are long standing and predate the diagnosis of cancer. Chronic problems related to marital discord, family dynamics, personality disorders, and alcohol or substance abuse are not problems with which the palliative care team should have to deal and attempts to do so will result in frustration and stress.

Stress at work may aggravate problems in the health care professional's personal life, and vice versa. Stress at work may cause or aggravate problems at home—personal, marital or to do with children. People with problems at home will perform and cope less well at work, a vicious circle being created. Another source of stress is if people at home, who have been regularly used to 'unload' work-related stress, become disinterested and discontinue their role.

Diagnosis of stress

The features of a stressful work place include hostility and rivalry between team members, lack of respect for the team leader, high staff turnover and sickness rates, associated with a general lethargy and lack of enthusiasm.

Some of the physical, psychological and behavioural features of stress are listed in Table 2.8. Stress can manifest as either over-involvement in work with a feeling of being indispensable, or as apathy and disinterest in the emotional needs of patients (distancing). If not detected and addressed, these features of stress may progress to psychiatric illness including depression and alcoholism.[41]

Table 2.8 Features of stress

Physical	Psychological	Behavioural
insomnia	apathy	over-involvement
tension headache	loss of enthusiasm	indispensability
exhaustion	depression	distancing
fatigue	irritability, frustration	
weight change	anger	
GI disturbances	conflicts with staff	
	poor self-esteem	
	guilt—failure to achieve or complete	
	feeling inadequate	
	cynicism	

Prevention of stress

The prevention of stress in palliative care workers is important for job satisfaction and team morale. More importantly, it is necessary for the delivery of optimal care to patients and their families. Whatever the prime cause of stress in palliative care workers, it is the responsibility of the organization and team to ensure that adequate support systems are available in the work environment. At the same time, the workers have to take some responsibility for their own psychological health.

Organizational. The strength and unity of the treatment team is most important in preventing stress. A good team will have more open communication and there will be fewer contentious issues. Team members will be able to share their fears and vulnerabilities with each other. Good management to avoid overburdening individuals with too much work on a daily basis is important. Formal supervision by a superior, to indicate areas worthy of development, can be beneficial; supervision performed in an insensitive manner can be a source of stress. Encouragement to take rostered days off and holidays on schedule are important and guard against over-involvement. Informal one-on-one debriefing needs to be available at any time a team member has been involved with an unusually stressful episode. If a treatment team is working successfully, individuals should enjoy feelings of satisfaction from their work. To be confident that they are good at their job should result in some pride and pleasure.

Individual. A wide range of activities is advocated to help the individual palliative care worker avoid becoming stressed. They include regular physical exercise, involvement in the creative arts, relaxation activities such as yoga or meditation, and regular involvement in something totally unrelated to palliative care.

References

1   Bruera, E., et al. (2001). Patient preferences versus physician perceptions of treatment decisions in cancer care. *Journal of Clinical Oncology* 19, 2883–5.
2   Higginson, I.J. and Costantini, M. (2002). Communication in end-of-life cancer care: a comparison of team assessments in three European countries. *Journal of Clinical Oncology* 20, 3674–82.

3   von Gunten, C.F., Ferris, F.D. and Emanuel, L.L. (2000). The patient–physician relationship. Ensuring competency in end-of-life care: communication and relational skills. *Journal of the American Medical Association* 284, 3051–7.

4   Von Roenn, J.H. and von Gunten, C.F. (2003). Setting goals to maintain hope. *Journal of Clinical Oncology* 21, 570–4.

5   Jenkins, V. and Fallowfield, L. (2002). Can communication skills training alter physicians' beliefs and behavior in clinics? *Journal of Clinical Oncology* 20, 765–9.

6   Maguire, P. and Pitceathly, C. (2002). Key communication skills and how to acquire them. *British Medical Journal* 325, 697–700.

7   Smith, T.J. (2000). The art of oncology: when the tumor is not the target. Tell it like it is. *Journal of Clinical Oncology* 18, 3441–5.

8   Fallowfield, L.J., Jenkins, V.A. and Beveridge, H.A. (2002). Truth may hurt but deceit hurts more: communication in palliative care. *Palliative Medicine* 16, 297–303.

9   Baile, W.F., et al. (2002). Oncologists' attitudes toward and practices in giving bad news: an exploratory study. *Journal of Clinical Oncology* 20, 2189–96.

10 von Gunten, C.F. (2002). Discussing hospice care. *Journal of Clinical Oncology* 20, 1419–24.

11 Christakis, N.A. and Lamont, E.B. (2000). Extent and determinants of error in doctors' prognoses in terminally ill patients: prospective cohort study. *British Medical Journal* 320, 469–72.

12 Higginson, I.J. and Costantini, M. (2002). Accuracy of prognosis estimates by four palliative care teams: a prospective cohort study. *BMC Palliative Care* 1, 1.

13 Knaus, W.A., et al. (1995). The SUPPORT prognostic model. Objective estimates of survival for seriously ill hospitalized adults. Study to understand prognoses and preferences for outcomes and risks of treatments. *Annals of Internal Medicine* 122, 191–203.

14 Vigano, A., et al. (2000). Clinical survival predictors in patients with advanced cancer. *Archives of Internal Medicine* 160, 861–8.

15 Lamont, E.B. and Christakis, N.A. (2001). Prognostic disclosure to patients with cancer near the end of life. *Annals of Internal Medicine* 134, 1096–1105.

16 Christakis, N.A. and Iwashyna, T.J. (1998). Attitude and self-reported practice regarding prognostication in a national sample of internists. *Archives of Internal Medicine* 158, 2389–95.

17 Loprinzi, C.L., Johnson, M.E. and Steer, G. (2000). Doc, how much time do I have? *Journal of Clinical Oncology* 18, 699–701.

18 Ebell, M.H., et al. (1998). Survival after in-hospital cardiopulmonary resuscitation. A meta-analysis. *Journal of General Internal Medicine* 13, 805–16.

19 Wallace, S.K., et al. (2002). Outcome and cost implications of cardiopulmonary resuscitation in the medical intensive care unit of a comprehensive cancer center. *Supportive Care in Cancer* 10, 425–9.

20 Varon, J., et al. (1998). Should a cancer patient be resuscitated following an in-hospital cardiac arrest? *Resuscitation* 36, 165–8.

21 von Gunten, C.F. (2001). Discussing do-not-resuscitate status. *Journal of Clinical Oncology* 19, 1576–81.

22 Parker, P.A., et al. (2001). Breaking bad news about cancer: patients' preferences for communication. *Journal of Clinical Oncology* 19, 2049–56.

23 Ptacek, J.T. and Ptacek, J.J. (2001). Patients' perceptions of receiving bad news about cancer. *Journal of Clinical Oncology* 19, 4160–4.

24 Wenrich, M.D., et al. (2001). Communicating with dying patients within the spectrum of medical care from terminal diagnosis to death. *Archives of Internal Medicine* 161, 868–74.

25 Clark, D. (2002). Between hope and acceptance: the medicalisation of dying. *British Medical Journal* 324, 905–7.

26 Detmar, S.B., et al. (2000). How are you feeling? Who wants to know? Patients' and oncologists' preferences for discussing health-related quality-of-life issues. *Journal of Clinical Oncology* 18, 3295–301.

27 Cassell, E.J. (1999). Diagnosing suffering: a perspective. *Annals of Internal Medicine* 131, 531–4.

28   Chochinov, H.M., et al. (2002). Dignity in the terminally ill: a cross-sectional, cohort study. *Lancet* 360, 2026–30.

29   Aranda, S.K. and Hayman-White, K. (2001). Home caregivers of the person with advanced cancer: an Australian perspective. *Cancer Nursing* 24, 300–7.

30   Borneman, T. and Ferrell, B. (2001). Care of the elderly with advanced diseases: caregiver issues. In *Topics in Palliative Care. Volume 5* (ed. E. Bruera and R. Portenoy). New York, Oxford University Press.

31   Fried, T.R., et al. (2002). Understanding the treatment preferences of seriously ill patients. *New England Journal of Medicine* 346, 1061–6.

32   Hammes, B.J. and Rooney, B.L. (1998). Death and end-of-life planning in one midwestern community. *Archives of Internal Medicine* 158, 383–90.

33   Hammes, B.J. (2001). What does it take to help adults successfully plan for future medical decisions? *Journal of Palliative Medicine* 4, 453–6.

34   Hines, S.C., et al. (2001). Improving advance care planning by accommodating family preferences. *Journal of Palliative Medicine* 4, 481–9.

35   Phipps, E., et al. (2003). Approaching the end of life: attitudes, preferences, and behaviors of African–American and white patients and their family caregivers. *Journal of Clinical Oncology* 21, 549–54.

36   Lynn, J. and Goldstein, N.E. (2003). Advance care planning for fatal chronic illness: avoiding commonplace errors and unwarranted suffering. *Annals of Internal Medicine* 138, 812–18.

37   Vachon, M.L. (1995). Staff stress in hospice/palliative care: a review. *Palliative Medicine* 9, 91–122.

38   Vachon, M.L. (1998). Staff burn-out: diagnosis, management and prevention. In *Topics in Palliative Care. Volume 2.* (ed. E. Bruera and R. Portenoy). New York, Oxford University Press.

39   Vachon, M.L. (2003). The stress of professional caregivers. In *Oxford Textbook of Palliative Medicine, 3rd edition* (ed. D. Doyle, G. Hanks, N. Cherny and K. Calman). Oxford, Oxford University Press.

40   Graham, J., et al. (1996). Job stress and satisfaction among palliative physicians. *Palliative Medicine* 10, 185–94.

41   Meier, D.E., Back, A.L. and Morrison, R.S. (2001). The inner life of physicians and care of the seriously ill. *Journal of the American Medical Association* 286, 3007–14.

3

Ethics in palliative care

Principles of medical ethics	Consent
Partnership of care	Appropriate therapy
Disclosure	Euthanasia and physician-assisted suicide

Health care professionals in all fields of medicine are increasingly involved in issues relating to the ethical aspects of the care they provide.[1] In palliative care issues relating to the appropriateness of therapy, disclosure and informed consent, 'living wills' and advance directives, as well as physician-assisted suicide and euthanasia, have all come to the fore.

Principles of medical ethics

There are four main principles of medical ethics that should guide doctors and other health care professionals in their work and decision making (Table 3.1).

Table 3.1 Principles of medical ethics

Beneficence
Non-maleficence
Respect for autonomy
Justice

Beneficence means to produce benefit, to do good, to always act in the best interests of the patient. Non-maleficence means to minimize or do no harm. The principle of autonomy acknowledges patients' rights of self-determination, for competent patients to decide what treatment they do or do not wish to have, without prejudice. Implicit in autonomy is that treatment is only given with patients' informed consent. Autonomy may be viewed as the obverse of paternalism, once an accepted part of health care, in which patients were expected to be submissive, unquestioning and compliant, and the doctor made all the decisions and shielded the patient from distress. The principle of justice involves the equitable allocation of health care resources according to need. It requires that health care professionals act fairly and without discrimination, for any reason.

In clinical situations where there is apparent conflict between different principles, it is necessary to assess which is the more important. In most cases these can be easily resolved by giving priority to what is in the best interests of the individual patient and assessing the benefits and potential burdens for each proposed therapy. Many potential dilemmas are avoided if there is a partnership of care, incorporating patient autonomy, between patients and their professional carers.

Partnership of care

In palliative care, the relationship between patients and their doctors, or between the patients and their families or carers and the whole health care team, should be a partnership of care.

The relationship between patients and their professional carers is always biased in favour of the professionals, although a partnership of care provides the opportunity to redress some of the imbalance. It is the professional carers who decide what information is discussed and what treatment options are offered, and they often act as the gatekeeper to resources. Patients, besides suffering the effects of their disease, lack medical knowledge and may have less social or intellectual skills. In other words, no matter how much we try to enhance patient autonomy and empowerment there will always be some inequality.

A partnership is the model of care that is most likely to result in the delivery of optimal care, with minimum conflict, whilst respecting patient autonomy. In a partnership of care, the doctor and health care team provide medical knowledge and experience of what options and supports are available to achieve this; and patients bring their personal values, priorities, goals and life plans. The parties work together towards the mutual goal in a constructive or creative manner; confrontation is avoided. Decisions regarding goals of care, treatment options, place of care and other issues are made jointly, and responsibility for the outcome of the decisions is shared. Patients need to feel they can trust the doctor and health care team who, in turn, must be honest and have genuine commitment to doing what is in patients' best interests. There needs to be mutual respect and open communication in both directions.

Disclosure

Good communication is a cornerstone of palliative care and includes the provision of information about the disease and prognosis (see Communication, Chapter 2). Without information, patients cannot participate in their own treatment planning, they cannot give informed consent to treatment, and cannot make suitable plans for themselves and their families. Problems related to disclosure should not arise if there is a continuing partnership of care in which management questions are discussed openly, with appropriate sensitivity. The patient's family or carers should also be involved in all discussions, further avoiding any conflict about disclosure.

It is the responsibility of the doctor to personally discuss the results of investigations and it must be done in a sensitive, understandable and unhurried manner. The information should always be given to the patient, with family members or carers present to listen and to provide support. Exceptions to this are patients who are not competent and those who have delegated the responsibility to a family member. Patients should be told as little or as much as they want to know and, if treatment decisions are involved, as much as is needed to make their consent informed.

When relatives request the patient not be told. Relatives sometimes request that the patient not be told of the diagnosis or prognosis. In general, such requests should be resisted. When made, requests need to be carefully and sensitively discussed to determine the motives or reasons behind them and to explain the possible adverse consequences. Requests based on lack of knowledge or misconceptions about the medical situation can usually be resolved by the provision of accurate information. Misguided requests, resulting from a relative's personal difficulty in dealing with the diagnosis, require appropriate counselling. It needs to be pointed out that most patients know or strongly suspect the nature of their illness, and that the fear and anxiety of not knowing may be a greater burden than dealing with the actual situation. Relatives requesting non-disclosure need to be told that patients will be answered honestly if they ask direct questions.

Consent

All treatment requires a patient's informed consent except for those who are not competent or have specifically delegated the responsibility to another person. For patients to be informed requires effective communication, as discussed in the previous section. A partnership of care between the patient and the health care professionals, with all management decisions made jointly, will largely circumvent problems related to patient autonomy and informed consent.

Advance directives or 'living wills'. Advance directives are written documentation of patients' views regarding the extent of medical care they might wish to have in given circumstances. They usually stipulate that extraordinary means should not be used to keep a patient alive if there is no hope of recovery. If patients have written advance directives, this should be known to all involved in their care, and the principle of their wishes upheld. However, no matter what care is put into the wording of advance directives, there is often confusion or doubt about the real meaning of them in particular clinical situations.[2,3] Terms such as 'active treatment', 'extraordinary means' and 'terminal illness' can be interpreted various ways. In the palliative care setting, if there is a partnership of care between patients and their professional carers, matters pertinent to advance directives should not arise.

Advance care planning. This is a more specific means for patients to record their end-of-life preferences, including their wishes regarding future treatments (or avoidance of them). It includes the appointment of a surrogate decision maker to act if the patient is no longer able to make decisions about their own care. It is discussed in Chapter 2.

Appropriate therapy

Questions regarding appropriate therapy frequently arise in palliative care. For patients who are not terminally ill, the question may be whether treatment to prolong life is warranted or should all therapy be directed solely at symptom control. For patients with more advanced disease, there may be difficulty deciding whether their life expectancy warrants recommending a course of palliative radiotherapy.

Benefits and burdens

Whether or not it is appropriate to offer (or withhold/withdraw) a particular treatment depends on the balance between the potential benefits and the possible burdens and risks of that treatment (the benefits to burdens/risks calculus) (Table 3.2). Assessment of the appropriateness of a particular treatment will depend on individual clinical circumstances and is

Table 3.2 Some considerations regarding appropriate therapy

Patient condition	general condition stage of the disease life expectancy
Treatment	aim of the treatment success rate of the treatment adverse effects
Potential benefits	prolongation of life improved symptom control improved quality of life less distressing terminal events, death
Potential burdens	poor/worse quality of life more distressing terminal events, death prolonging dying ('prescribing a lingering death') hastening death ('double effect')

often difficult and complex. In addition, a decision to offer (or withhold) a particular treatment may need to be reviewed regularly as a patient's condition changes.

Potential benefits include prolongation of life or improved control of symptoms. If prolongation of life is the goal, the benefits and quality of the life prolonged must be considered. However, it is not possible to assess the quality of another person's life, or the value of that life to them. The quality of life following a particular treatment may appear poor to some but be perfectly acceptable to a patient with particular values or goals. There is also a risk that a life-prolonging intervention will lead to more unpleasant terminal events and death. Treatment given to improve symptoms may inadvertently either hasten death or prolong the dying process.

Treatments that are futile need not be discussed with patients. However, with the exception of treatments that have no chance of success because they are physiologically impossible, the exact definition of futile is difficult because the potential benefits, including quality of life, are subjective. Treatments with no chance of benefit need not be discussed; to do so would be dishonest and engender false hope. Therapies offering a chance of significant benefit, whether associated with small or large burdens and risks, are discussed appropriately with the patient. Whether or not to discuss treatments offering a small chance of benefit, but associated with high burdens or risks, is a matter of judgment and depends on individual clinical circumstances.

The outcome of giving (or withholding/withdrawing) a particular treatment is always uncertain and both the patient and the treatment team must be prepared to review and, if necessary, modify or reverse any treatment decision. Another approach is to embark on a time-limited trial, in which treatment is given for a specified period of time, and then discontinued if it is not producing the desired benefit.

Stopping anticancer therapy

Most patients with advanced cancer reach a stage where anticancer treatment no longer controls the progression of their disease. Unfortunately, many patients are told 'there is nothing more that can be done', a statement that is never true and that may be interpreted as abandonment of care. Patients vary in their acceptance that anticancer treatment is of no further benefit; those insistent on continuing active therapy should be informed of the benefits and risks of treatments that are available or offered enrolment in an experimental clinical trial.

Treating the terminally ill

The guidelines in Table 3.2 will help with decisions about withholding or withdrawing treatment in patients who are terminally ill. Whether or not a terminally ill patient should receive antibiotics for chest infection can be problematic. It requires judgment about the patient's nearness to death, their wishes and those of their family, and the expected benefits from the patient's point of view. If antibiotics will merely prolong the dying process, they are probably best withheld; alternatively, if they will help relieve distressing symptoms not responsive to other measures, such as pyrexia, delirium or excessive sweating, they may be of benefit. Another example is the treatment of renal failure due to ureteric obstruction in patients with advanced pelvic disease. If the patient was terminally ill due to the effects of cancer before renal failure supervened, active therapy is probably best withheld; if the patient was previously relatively well and has a reasonable life expectancy except for the effects of renal failure, consideration for stenting or nephrostomy insertion is appropriate.

Artificial nutrition

Anorexia and weight loss occur in most patients with advanced cancer and are the cause of much anxiety. Requests for artificial feeding, usually from family members, are common.

As discussed in Chapter 28, continuing weight loss in the majority of patients with advanced cancer is primarily due to the metabolic abnormalities that characterize the anorexia-cachexia syndrome and not to starvation. There is no evidence that enteral or parenteral nutrition have any effect on these metabolic abnormalities and should be considered futile.[4] The use of enteral and parenteral nutrition for patients with cancer has been reviewed and there is no evidence of any significant benefit with respect to survival, tumour response, or the toxicity associated with radiation or chemotherapy.[5-7] Parenteral nutrition requires regular monitoring, a central venous catheter, and is associated with an increased incidence of infections; enteral feeding is associated with abdominal pain, distention, and diarrhoea.

Few patients with advanced cancer and cachexia complain of hunger and they are well satisfied with small amounts of food.[8] Treatment is with adequate explanation, a trial of a corticosteroid or progestogen, and dietary measures such as small frequent meals and being given what food they want, when they want it. Family members need to be counselled not to try and force patients to eat more than they want.

Whilst artificial feeding is not of benefit for patients with the anorexia-cachexia syndrome, it is certainly justified for patients who would otherwise be at risk of starvation.[9, 10] Patients with upper gastrointestinal obstruction, not terminally ill from their cancer, warrant feeding via a nasogastric tube or gastrostomy. Patients undergoing treatment that will prevent them eating for two weeks or more (e.g. extensive surgery, radiotherapy) should be considered for parenteral nutrition. Whether patients with persistent or recurrent small bowel obstruction warrant parenteral nutrition is a matter of judgment and depends on individual clinical circumstances. If there is uncertainty, a time-limited trial can be offered.

Artificial hydration

Artificial hydration should be considered for patients who are unable to take or retain adequate oral fluids and have symptoms or signs of dehydration, providing they are not imminently dying. Symptoms of dehydration include thirst and a dry mouth, cognitive impairment and delirium, lethargy, malaise and postural hypotension. In palliative care, subcutaneous hydration (hypodermoclysis) has been shown to be safe and effective and can be employed at home.[11] Infusions of 500ml over one hour can be given 2 or 3 times a day via a subcutaneous butterfly needle that can be left in place for an average of 5 days. An RCT has shown that routine use of hyaluronidase is not necessary for successful subcutaneous hydration (Table 3.3),[12] but it may be useful for a minority of patients who tolerate infusions poorly due to swelling or pain. If there is uncertainty whether hydration will be of clinical benefit, a time-limited trial can be offered.

The use of artificial hydration in patients who are in the last days of life is controversial,[9, 13–15] and decisions have to be individualized.[16] On the one hand, it is argued that decreasing oral intake in the last days is a normal physiological part of the dying process and may be of benefit to the terminally ill. Reduced urine output requires less movement needed to void and incontinence is less likely; less pulmonary secretions reduce dyspnoea and terminal congestion; less gastrointestinal secretions make nausea less likely; and oedema and effusions may be less troublesome. Artificial hydration might have the opposite effects and worsen the patient's situation. In addition, it may give an ambiguous message or false hope to a patient or family, and the equipment used may act as a physical barrier between patient and relatives at a time when physical contact is important.

Against this it is argued that artificial hydration will improve symptom control, cognitive function, and avoid opioid toxicity. Symptoms of thirst and a dry mouth occur frequently in this population, but may be due to a range of other causes besides dehydration including medications, stomatitis, xerostomia, and mouth breathing.[17] Observational studies have shown a lack of correlation between thirst and biochemical markers of dehydration,[18–20] and the incidence of thirst may remain high despite artificial hydration.[21] Other studies have shown that the symptoms of terminal dehydration can be well managed with good mouth care, sips of fluid, and keeping the lips moist.[8, 22] The state of consciousness was not improved by artificial hydration in one study;[23] the reported reduction in the incidence of agitated delirium associated with the more frequent use of subcutaneous hydration in another may be explained by simultaneous implementation of early opioid rotation.[24] A recently published RCT reported no improvement in thirst, cognitive function or delirium after 48 hours of subcutaneous hydration (Table 3.3).[25]

Table 3.3 Artificial hydration: RCTs

Author	n	Intervention	Outcome
Bruera[12]	21	500mL SC fluid over 1h ± 150units hyaluronidase	no difference in pain, swelling, rash, leakage, or patient preference
Cerchietti[25]	42	IL/d SC fluid x 2d vs no SC fluid	no improvement in thirst, cognition or delirium

Decisions regarding artificial hydration in the terminally ill must be individualized, but it should probably be avoided except in exceptional circumstances. Keeping the mouth and lips moist is important and can be done by the family. Gentle explanations that extra fluids will not be of benefit and may cause harm are given to the patient and family. Demands for artificial hydration from anxious relatives, who insist that something must be done, require explanation and negotiation; if unsuccessful, a small volume subcutaneous infusion may resolve the situation without causing the patient any significant distress.

'Do-Not-Resuscitate' (DNR) orders

This is discussed in Chapter 2. For patients with advanced cancer, cardiopulmonary resuscitation (CPR) is rarely successful.[26] In one study, 2% of 406 patients survived to discharge from hospital;[27] in another, 6% of 83 patients survived 6 weeks.[28] However, some institutions require that it be discussed with the patient before a DNR order is given. This is clearly inappropriate for patients who are actively dying, for whom CPR would be completely futile. In this situation, it is more appropriate to stress patient comfort and dignity and reassure the family that nothing will be done to prolong the dying process.[29] Some have recommended that instead of withholding CPR with a DNR order, the letters AND should be used, standing for 'allow natural death'. Others have claimed that DNR orders might deny patients hope; for patients with terminal cancer, this would be false hope. If there is a partnership of care between patients and their professional carers, and decisions concerning treatment and the goals of therapy are jointly made, differences about whether patients are 'for resuscitation' or 'not for resuscitation' rarely arise.

Euthanasia and physician-assisted suicide

Many who work in palliative care have become involved in the continuing debate over the legalization of euthanasia and physician-assisted suicide (PAS).[30–34] Euthanasia is regarded by some as the antithesis of good palliative care (Figure 3.1).

Figure 3.1   Diagrammatic comparison of euthanasia and successful palliative care

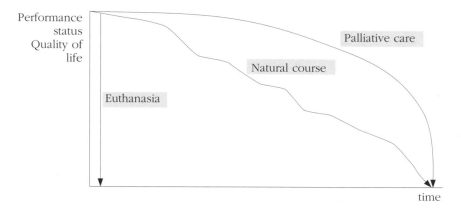

Euthanasia. Euthanasia is defined as a deliberate intervention undertaken with the express intention of ending a life so as to relieve intractable suffering. If performed at the dying person's request or with that person's consent, it is voluntary; otherwise it is non-voluntary. The terms 'active' and 'passive' are ambiguous and misleading.

Physician-assisted suicide (PAS). In PAS, the physician provides the knowledge and necessary means (equipment, drugs) but the patient performs the act. It is similarly a deliberate act with the express intention of ending life, and raises the same clinical and moral issues as euthanasia.

Withholding or withdrawing medical treatment. Decisions about appropriate therapy may be difficult and need to be based on individual clinical circumstances. Terminally ill patients should not be subjected to futile therapies, and decisions not to employ such treatment constitute good medical practice. There is no requirement or justification to sustain life at all costs and a doctor has no right to prescribe a prolonged or lingering death. Withholding or withdrawing futile treatment from the terminally ill does not shorten life or hasten death; it does not artificially prolong life. It does not constitute euthanasia, as the intention is to allow death to occur naturally, not to deliberately terminate life.

'**Double effects**'. The principle of 'double effect' was used to describe the situation where medications given for the relief of distressing pain or symptoms might hasten the moment of death. Providing that appropriate drugs are given for appropriate medical reasons and in appropriate doses, this cannot be considered euthanasia. In this situation, the hastening of death may or may not be foreseen, but it is never intended; in euthanasia, the sole aim of the treatment is to terminate the life of the patient. However, there is no evidence that good palliative medicine shortens life and effective symptom control is just as likely to extend it as shorten it. A systematic review of the literature reported no evidence that analgesics or sedatives used in terminal care hastened death.[35] Referring to 'double effects' may therefore be perpetuating a myth.[36, 37]

Arguments for and against

The reasons for requests for euthanasia and PAS, and the effect that appropriate palliative care might have, are summarized in Table 3.4.

Pain and physical symptoms can be well controlled for the great majority of patients with standard therapies;[38, 39] for patients with difficult or complex problems, the expertise of an experienced interdisciplinary team may be required for optimal management. Patients' attitudes to euthanasia change when a positive attitude and effective symptom control are introduced.[40, 41]

There is a high incidence of depression and depressive symptoms in patients with advanced cancer who request assisted death.[42–46] The diagnosis of depression in the terminally ill can be very difficult,[47] and a number of studies document that doctors not trained in psychiatry miss up to half of the cases of major depression in the medically ill.[48] Treatment of the depression is reported to lessen the desire for hastened death in patients with cancer[49] and geriatric patients.[50, 51]

Other patients may request euthanasia for a variety of reasons—loss of dignity, unworthy dying, dependency and being a burden, hopelessness, and tiredness of life—that are best

Table 3.4 Euthanasia and PAS: reasons and responses

Unrelieved pain and physical symptoms
should not occur given optimal interdisciplinary palliative care
Severe anxiety and depression
should be controlled given optimal interdisciplinary palliative care
Intolerable suffering, existential distress
should be controlled given appropriate interdisciplinary palliative care
Carer fatigue
is preventable
Autonomy and self-determination
the existence of a right to request and receive euthanasia is controversial
Iatrogenic – the 'nothing more can be done' syndrome
would not occur if patients were referred to a palliative care service

grouped as existential distress.[43, 45, 52–54] The 'demoralization syndrome' encompasses the hopelessness, loss of meaning, and existential distress manifest by these patients.[55, 56] Therapeutic approaches have been developed to address problems related to dignity, integrity and remorse, as well as issues of hopelessness and meaninglessness. Cognitive techniques can help patients modify the appraisal of their lives, diminish distress and enhance a positive attitude. Socialization and interest in art and music or other hobbies will reduce boredom and loneliness and enhance the quality of life. Insight-directed therapy can help patients acknowledge that there are meaningful tasks to be done, joys to be shared, things to be said or completed, relationships to be savoured and differences to be settled. Given appropriate therapy, refractory existential distress is rare.

Requests for euthanasia, direct or implied, may result from family fatigue and exhaustion. This may occur if there is continuing inadequate relief of the patient's suffering, if there are inadequate resources and support to carry out home care, or if the family carers have unrealistic expectations of themselves.[57, 58] These issues are all preventable or manageable given timely implementation of co-ordinated, multiprofessional care for the patient and family together.

The principles of individual autonomy and self-determination lead some to believe that there is a fundamental right to request and receive euthanasia; others argue that such a right does not exist.[30, 31, 33, 34] The ideal of total individual autonomy is at odds with a modern society, in which innumerable laws and regulations exist, accepted by society as a whole, that limit individual autonomy for the purpose of protecting the rights of others. The essential issue is whether exercise of one individual's autonomy will compromise the rights of others and the high incidence of non-voluntary euthanasia in the Netherlands would certainly suggest that it does. Opponents of legalized euthanasia have expressed concern that the vulnerable—the elderly, lonely, sick and those who feel a burden—would feel pressure, whether real or imagined, to request early death. Palliative care, focused on the needs and wishes of the patients and their families, can do more for individuals' autonomy and self-respect.

The rising tide of public opinion is based on fear and medical ignorance. There is a widespread public perception, fostered by groups such as the Voluntary Euthanasia Society, that the treatment of pain and suffering is frequently ineffective and that euthanasia is the only means of ensuring adequate relief of suffering. The results of public opinion polls are questionable unless very sophisticated and complete questions are asked. If healthy adults are given the choice of themselves or their loved ones dying with unrelieved pain and suffering or legalizing euthanasia, most caring people will vote for euthanasia. But what would they choose if offered elective death or comprehensive palliative care with good symptom control and relief of suffering?

The attitudes of the doctor and other professional carers can have a profound influence on the generation of hope or hopelessness in the patient and family. Doctors feeling isolated and exasperated in the face of severe suffering will project their helplessness onto the patient and family. Doctors who regard death as a medical or professional failure are likely to withdraw from the care of terminally ill, often saying that 'nothing more can be done'. These iatrogenic causes of requests for euthanasia require professional education. There should be professional pride in the effective palliation of symptoms and supporting patients and families through a terminal illness. Patients with uncontrolled suffering require the resources and expertise of an experienced interdisciplinary palliative care team. Uncontrolled suffering in the terminally ill should be considered a medical emergency and not an indication for euthanasia.

Dealing with requests for assisted dying

Requests for euthanasia or PAS indicate significant suffering or fear of future suffering and need be dealt with in a calm and sympathetic manner. On occasions, requests are the result of transient changes in mood and can be dealt with appropriately. If the request is persistent and durable, the underlying reasons motivating the request need to be identified.[59] The patient should be asked about their expectations and fears, their sense of meaning and quality of life, their goals and unfinished business, and about family concerns and whether they feel a burden. They should also be assessed for symptoms of depression or the demoralization syndrome.[55, 60] Pain and physical symptoms need to be under optimal control and the patient reassured about continuing control in the future. It may require time and a number of conversations to identify the reasons behind a patient's request, which can then be addressed in an appropriate manner.

Desire for euthanasia or PAS may fluctuate with time.[42, 44, 61] In the research context, two tools have been developed for measuring the desire for assisted death: the Desire for Death Rating Scale (DDRS)[42] and the Schedule of Attitudes toward Hastened Death (SAHD).[62]

Euthanasia and PAS in practice

Euthanasia or PAS have been introduced into clinical practice in the Netherlands, in Oregon in America, and in the Northern Territory in Australia.

The Netherlands. The practice of euthanasia and PAS has been permitted in the Netherlands for many years and has now been formally legalized. Strict guidelines were introduced in 1991 permitting euthanasia or PAS for patients with intolerable suffering and no prospect of improvement who made voluntary and durable requests. Second opinions had to be obtained and all cases had to be reported to the authorities.[63] Examination of the reports published by the Dutch themselves show that the tolerance of voluntary euthanasia has led to non-voluntary euthanasia for patients who never requested it.[33, 34, 64–66] The proportion of patients with a prognosis of six months or more rose from 8% in 1990 to 20% in 1995.[64, 65] Euthanasia is reported for patients with depression [67] and mental handicap.[68] Second opinions were not obtained in many cases [65] and the majority of cases were not reported to the authorities.[69]

The Northern Territory. Euthanasia and PAS were legalized in the Northern Territory for a nine-month period in 1996–97. A review of the seven patients with cancer who died under the provisions of the legislation showed a high incidence of social isolation, hopelessness, depression and demoralization.[70]

Oregon. PAS has been a legal option available to terminally ill patients in Oregon since 1997. Patients requesting PAS presented multiple concerns including being a burden, loss of autonomy, and inability to participate in enjoyable activities.[71] During the first four years of the program, only 70 patients with cancer (of more than 20,000 deaths from cancer during that time) died by PAS, and nearly half of those who received palliative care dropped their request for PAS.[72]

Effects of euthanasia

The effects of legalizing euthanasia and PAS are summarized in Table 3.5.

Euthanasia shortens the period of pre-mortem suffering and gives the patient a measure of control over the process of dying. But other patients will have their autonomy compromised. The Dutch reports show that voluntary euthanasia leads to non-voluntary euthanasia, and almost half

Table 3.5 Effects of legalizing euthanasia

Patients
  voluntary euthanasia leads to non-voluntary euthanasia
  euthanasia for the terminally ill leads to euthanasia for people not terminally ill
  euthanasia for terminal illness leads to euthanasia for treatable conditions like depression
  the vulnerable in society may feel pressure to request euthanasia
  patients likely to undergo euthanasia will not receive palliative care

Professional
  will not encourage good medical practice and palliative care
  distrust in the doctor–patient relationship

Society
  discourages a caring attitude towards the elderly, the sick and other vulnerable people
  devaluation of human life

of the patients treated by euthanasia made no explicit request for it. There is evidence from the Netherlands that the vulnerable—the aged, the sick and those who feel a burden—may experience pressure to request euthanasia.[73,74] Patients likely to proceed with euthanasia are unlikely to have their pain and suffering addressed in a comprehensive or caring way.

Euthanasia will encourage poor medical practice. Patients who are likely to receive euthanasia in days or weeks are not likely to receive comprehensive or multidisciplinary care. The principles of palliative care will be lost and there will be no professional pride in the skilful palliation of symptoms and supporting the patient and family through a terminal illness.

Patients may come to distrust their professional carers and may be fearful of the wishes of their relatives in a society where it is known non-voluntary euthanasia is practised.

Euthanasia will save society an enormous amount of money, presently spent on the care of patients with terminal diseases. But vulnerable people in society are more likely to feel that they are a burden, rather than people who matter.

Euthanasia will devalue human life. Regardless of any religion, it is justifiable to assert that life has value and meaning. The terminal stages of life may be a time of reconciliation and personal growth, particularly if pain and physical symptoms are controlled.

Legalized euthanasia or palliative care

Euthanasia and PAS are quicker, easier and cheaper. However, the laws that have been put in place to police the practice are quite inadequate,[34] and expert opinion from around the world suggests that euthanasia cannot be controlled by anything less than complete prohibition.

A preferable option would be to ensure that comprehensive multidisciplinary palliative care, which is of proven benefit in the relief of suffering of the terminally ill, be universally available and accessible to all patients who need it.

References

1   Randall, F. and Downie, R.S. (1999). *Palliative Care Ethics*. Oxford, Oxford University Press.
2   Ewer, M.S. and Taubert, J.K. (1995). Advance directives in the intensive care unit of a tertiary cancer center. *Cancer* 76, 1268–74.
3   Gilbert, J. (1996). The benefits and problems of living wills (advance statements about medical treatment) in cancer patients. *Progress in Palliative Care* 4, 4–6.

4   Rabeneck, L., McCullough, L.B. and Wray, N.P. (1997). Ethically justified, clinically comprehensive guidelines for percutaneous endoscopic gastrostomy tube placement. *Lancet* 349, 496–8.

5   Klein, S. and Koretz, R.L. (1994). Nutrition support in patients with cancer: what do the data really show? *Nutrition in Clinical Practice* 9, 91–100.

6   Flatow, F.A. and Long, S. (2001). Specialized care of the terminally ill. In *Cancer. Principles and Practice of Oncology. 6th edition* (ed. V.T. De Vita, S. Hellman and S.A. Rosenberg). Philadelphia, Lippincott Williams Wilkins.

7   Smith, J.S. and Souba, W.W. (2001). Nutritional support. In *Cancer. Principles and Practice of Oncology. 6th edition.* (ed. V.T. De Vita, S. Hellman and S.A. Rosenberg). Philadelphia, Lippincott Williams Wilkins.

8   McCann, R.M., Hall, W.J. and Groth-Juncker, A. (1994). Comfort care for terminally ill patients. The appropriate use of nutrition and hydration. *Journal of the American Medical Association* 272, 1263–6.

9   MacDonald, N. (1998). Ethical issues in hydration and nutrition. In *Topics in Palliative Care. Volume 2* (ed. E. Bruera and R. Portenoy). New York, Oxford University Press.

10   Keeley, P. (2002). Feeding tubes in palliative care. *European Journal of Palliative Care* 9, 229–31.

11   Fainsinger, R.L., et al. (1994). The use of hypodermoclysis for rehydration in terminally ill cancer patients. *Journal of Pain and Symptom Management* 9, 298–302.

12   Bruera, E., et al. (1999). A randomized controlled trial of local injections of hyaluronidase versus placebo in cancer patients receiving subcutaneous hydration. *Annals of Oncology* 10, 1255–8.

13   Dunphy, K., et al. (1995). Rehydration in palliative and terminal care: if not—why not? *Palliative Medicine* 9, 221–8.

14   Viola, R.A., Wells, G.A. and Peterson, J. (1997). The effects of fluid status and fluid therapy on the dying: a systematic review. *Journal of Palliative Care* 13, 41–52.

15   Bruera, E. and MacDonald, N. (2000). To hydrate or not to hydrate: how should it be? *Journal of Clinical Oncology* 18, 1156–8.

16   National Council for Hospice and Specialist Palliative Care Services and the Association for Palliative Medicine (1997). Artificial hydration (AH) for people who are terminally ill. *European Journal of Palliative Care* 4, 124.

17   Huang, Z. and Ahronheim, J.C. (2002). Issues in nutrition and hydration. In *Principles and Practice of Palliative Care and Supportive Oncology* (ed. A.M. Berger, R.K. Portenoy and D.E. Weissman). Philadelphia, Lippincott, Williams and Wilkins.

18   Burge, F.I. (1993). Dehydration symptoms of palliative care cancer patients. *Journal of Pain and Symptom Management* 8, 454–64.

19   Ellershaw, J.E., Sutcliffe, J.M. and Saunders, C.M. (1995). Dehydration and the dying patient. *Journal of Pain and Symptom Management* 10, 192–7.

20   Morita, T., et al. (2001). Determinants of the sensation of thirst in terminally ill cancer patients. *Supportive Care in Cancer* 9, 177–86.

21   Musgrave, C.F., Bartal, N. and Opstad, J. (1995). The sensation of thirst in dying patients receiving i.v. hydration. *Journal of Palliative Care* 11, 17–21.

22   Vullo-Navich, K., et al. (1998). Comfort and incidence of abnormal serum sodium, BUN, creatinine and osmolality in dehydration of terminal illness. *American Journal of Hospice and Palliative Care* 15, 77–84.

23   Waller, A., Hershkowitz, M. and Adunsky, A. (1994). The effect of intravenous fluid infusion on blood and urine parameters of hydration and on state of consciousness in terminal cancer patients. *American Journal of Hospice and Palliative Care* 11, 22–7.

24   Bruera, E., et al. (1995). Changing pattern of agitated impaired mental status in patients with advanced cancer: association with cognitive monitoring, hydration, and opioid rotation. *Journal of Pain and Symptom Management* 10, 287–91.

25   Cerchietti, L., et al. (2000). Hypodermoclysis for control of dehydration in terminal-stage cancer. *International Journal of Palliative Nursing* 6, 370–4.

26 Ebell, M.H., et al. (1998). Survival after in-hospital cardiopulmonary resuscitation. A meta-analysis. *Journal of General Internal Medicine* 13, 805–16.

27 Wallace, S.K., et al. (2002). Outcome and cost implications of cardiopulmonary resuscitation in the medical intensive care unit of a comprehensive cancer center. *Supportive Care in Cancer* 10, 425–9.

28 Varon, J., et al. (1998). Should a cancer patient be resuscitated following an in-hospital cardiac arrest? *Resuscitation* 36, 165–8.

29 National Council for Hospice and Specialist Palliative Care Services and the Association for Palliative Medicine (1997). CPR for people who are terminally ill. *European Journal of Palliative Care* 4, 125.

30 Angell, M. (1997). The Supreme Court and physician-assisted suicide—the ultimate right. *New England Journal of Medicine* 336, 50–3.

31 Doyal, L. (2001). Why active euthanasia and physician assisted suicide should be legalised. *British Medical Journal* 323, 1079–80.

32 Emanuel, E.J. (2001). Euthanasia: where the Netherlands leads will the world follow? No. Legalisation is a diversion from improving care for the dying. *British Medical Journal* 322, 1376–7.

33 Foley, K. and Hendin, H. (2002). *The Case Against Assisted Suicide. For the Right to End-of-Life Care*. Baltimore, Johns Hopkins University Press.

34 Keown, J. (2002). *Euthanasia, Ethics and Public Policy. An Argument Against Legalisation*. Cambridge, Cambridge University Press.

35 Sykes, N., et al. (2003). The use of opioids and sedatives at the end of life. *Lancet Oncology* 4, 312–18.

36 Anderson Fohr, S. (1998). The double effect of pain medication: separating myth from reality. *Journal of Palliative Medicine* 1, 315–28.

37 Thorns, A., et al. (2000). Opioid use in last week of life and implications for end-of-life decision-making. *Lancet* 356, 398–9.

38 Jacox, A., et al. (1994). *Management of Cancer Pain. Clinical Practice Guideline No. 9*. Rockville, MD: Agency for Health Care Policy and Research, U.S. Department of Health and Human Services.

39 Goudas, L., et al. (2001). *Management of cancer pain*. Rockville, MD: Agency for Healthcare Research and Quality. <http://www.ahrq.gov/clinic/tp/canpaintp.htm>

40 Zylicz, Z. (1995). 'Death on Request' and Dutch euthanasia policy. *Progress in Palliative Care* 3, 43–4.

41 Severson, K.T. (1997). Dying cancer patients: choices at the end of life. *Journal of Pain and Symptom Management* 14, 94–8.

42 Chochinov, H.M., et al. (1995). Desire for death in the terminally ill. *American Journal of Psychiatry* 152, 1185–91.

43 Wilson, K.G., et al. (2000). Attitudes of terminally ill patients toward euthanasia and physician-assisted suicide. *Archives of Internal Medicine* 160, 2454–60.

44 Emanuel, E.J., Fairclough, D.L. and Emanuel, L.L. (2000). Attitudes and desires related to euthanasia and physician-assisted suicide among terminally ill patients and their caregivers. *Journal of the American Medical Association* 284, 2460–8.

45 Breitbart, W., et al. (2000). Depression, hopelessness, and desire for hastened death in terminally ill patients with cancer. *Journal of the American Medical Association* 284, 2907–11.

46 Tiernan, E., et al. (2002). Relations between desire for early death, depressive symptoms and anti-depressant prescribing in terminally ill patients with cancer. *Journal of the Royal Society of Medicine* 95, 386–90.

47 Chochinov, H.M., et al. (1994). Prevalence of depression in the terminally ill: effects of diagnostic criteria and symptom threshold judgments. *American Journal of Psychiatry* 151, 537–40.

48 Ryan, C.J. (1996). Depression, decisions and the desire to die. *Medical Journal of Australia* 165, 411.

49 Kugaya, A., et al. (1999). Successful antidepressant treatment for five terminally ill cancer patients with major depression, suicidal ideation and a desire for death. *Supportive Care in Cancer* 7, 432–6.

50 Ganzini, L., et al. (1994). The effect of depression treatment on elderly patients' preferences for life-sustaining medical therapy. *American Journal of Psychiatry* 151, 1631–6.

51 Hooper, S.C., et al. (1996). Major depression and refusal of life-sustaining medical treatment in the elderly. *Medical Journal of Australia* 165, 416–19.

52 Kelly, B., et al. (2002). Terminally ill cancer patients' wish to hasten death. *Palliative Medicine* 16, 339–45.

53 Suarez-Almazor, M.E., et al. (2002). Attitudes of terminally ill cancer patients about euthanasia and assisted suicide: predominance of psychosocial determinants and beliefs over symptom distress and subsequent survival. *Journal of Clinical Oncology* 20, 2134–41.

54 Virik, K. and Glare, P. (2002). Requests for euthanasia made to a tertiary referral teaching hospital in Sydney, Australia in the year 2000. *Supportive Care in Cancer* 10, 309–13.

55 Kissane, D.W., Clarke, D.M. and Street, A.F. (2001). Demoralization syndrome—a relevant psychiatric diagnosis for palliative care. *Journal of Palliative Care* 17, 12–21.

56 Clarke, D.M. and Kissane, D.W. (2002). Demoralization: its phenomenology and importance. *Australian and New Zealand Journal of Psychiatry* 36, 733–42.

57 Covinsky, K.E., et al. (1994). The impact of serious illness on patients' families. SUPPORT Investigators. Study to Understand Prognoses and Preferences for Outcomes and Risks of Treatment. *Journal of the American Medical Association* 272, 1839–44.

58 Borneman, T. and Ferrell, B. (2001). Care of the elderly with advanced diseases: caregiver issues. In *Topics in Palliative Care. Volume 5* (ed. E. Bruera and R. Portenoy). New York, Oxford University Press.

59 Bascom, P.B. and Tolle, S.W. (2002). Responding to requests for physician-assisted suicide: 'These are uncharted waters for both of us...'. *Journal of the American Medical Association* 288, 91–8.

60 Chochinov, H.M., et al. (1999). Will to live in the terminally ill. *Lancet* 354, 816–19.

61 Wolfe, J., et al. (1999). Stability of attitudes regarding physician-assisted suicide and euthanasia among oncology patients, physicians, and the general public. *Journal of Clinical Oncology* 17, 1274.

62 Rosenfeld, B., et al. (2000). The schedule of attitudes toward hastened death: Measuring desire for death in terminally ill cancer patients. *Cancer* 88, 2868–75.

63 Walton (1995). Dilemmas of life and death: Parts 1 & 2. *Journal of the Royal Society of Medicine* 88, 311–15 and 372–6.

64 van der Maas, P.J., et al. (1991). Euthanasia and other medical decisions concerning the end of life. *Lancet* 338, 669–74.

65 van der Maas, P.J., et al. (1996). Euthanasia, physician-assisted suicide, and other medical practices involving the end of life in the Netherlands, 1990–1995. *New England Journal of Medicine* 335, 1699–705.

66 Onwuteaka-Philipsen, B.D., et al. (2003). Euthanasia and other end-of-life decisions in the Netherlands in 1990, 1995, and 2001. *Lancet* 2003; 362: 395–99.

67 Groenewoud, J.H., et al. (1997). Physician-assisted death in psychiatric practice in the Netherlands. *New England Journal of Medicine* 336, 1795–801.

68 van Thiel, G.J., et al. (1997). Retrospective study of doctors' 'end of life decisions' in caring for mentally handicapped people in institutions in The Netherlands. *British Medical Journal* 315, 88–91.

69 van der Wal, G., et al. (1996). Evaluation of the notification procedure for physician-assisted death in the Netherlands. *New England Journal of Medicine* 335, 1706–11.

70 Kissane, D.W., Street, A. and Nitschke, P. (1998). Seven deaths in Darwin: case studies under the Rights of the Terminally Ill Act, Northern Territory, Australia. *Lancet* 352, 1097–102.

71 Hedberg, K., Hopkins, D. and Southwick, K. (2002). Legalized physician-assisted suicide in Oregon, 2001. *New England Journal of Medicine* 346, 450–2.

72 Ganzini, L., et al. (2000). Physicians' experiences with the Oregon Death with Dignity Act. *New England Journal of Medicine* 342, 557–63.

73 Hendin, H. (1997). *Seduced by Death*. New York, W. W. Norton.

74 Hendin, H. (2002). The Dutch experience. In *The Case Against Assisted Suicide. For the Right to End-of-Life Care* (ed. K. Foley and H. Hendin). Baltimore, Johns Hopkins University Press.

Pain

Pain is perfect misery, the worst of evils

John Milton (1608–74)

For all the happiness mankind can gain
Is not in pleasure, but in rest from pain

John Dryden (1631–1700)

Pain is a more terrible lord of mankind than even death itself

Albert Schweitzer (1875–1965)

Pain lengthens time

Anita Hart Balter, 1990

4

Pain

Pain is one of the most common symptoms in patients with advanced cancer; it is certainly the most feared. Satisfactory pain control should be possible for about 90% of patients with advanced cancer using drugs and other treatments that are readily available, together with appropriate attention to the psychosocial aspects of care.[1-3] Unfortunately, cancer-related pain is often poorly treated and the results achieved in routine clinical practice are much less satisfactory.[4]

Unrelieved pain is a major cause of suffering and poor quality of life in patients with advanced cancer. It is associated with psychological distress and depression, impaired physical functioning and social interaction, as well as insomnia and fatigue. Improved treatment results in measurable and significant changes in pain relief, pain severity, psychological distress, and quality of life.[5]

The aim of palliative care is to allow patients with advanced cancer to be pain-free or for their pain to be sufficiently controlled that it does not interfere with their ability to function

Table 4.1 Prerequisites for good pain control for patients with advanced cancer

Accurate and detailed assessment of each pain

Knowledge of types of pains suffered by patients with cancer

Different therapeutic approach to chronic pain

Knowledge of which treatment modalities to use

Knowledge of the actions and adverse effects of analgesics and other treatment modalities

Assessment and treatment of other aspects of suffering that may aggravate pain
  physical, psychological, social, cultural, spiritual

Treatment of pain as part of a co-ordinated plan of total care

Continued reassessment

or detract from their quality of life. The prerequisites for good pain control (Table 4.1) are the subject of this and the following chapters.

Incidence

The incidence of pain increases as cancer progresses. Moderate or severe pain occurs in about one-third (30–40%) of patients at the time of diagnosis, between one- and two-thirds (40–70%) receiving active anticancer treatment, and in more than two-thirds (60–100%) with advanced or terminal cancer.[6–8]

Certain cancers are more likely to be associated with pain than others. The available data has been collated by Bonica (Table 4.2).[9] There is some variation with regard to pain severity and stage of disease between the various reports included, but the results are in keeping with the clinical observation that some types of cancer are more likely to be associated with pain.

Most cancer patients have more than one pain. About one-third of patients reported a single pain, one-third had two pains, and one-third had three pains or more.[10]

Certain groups of patients—females, minorities, and the elderly—have a higher incidence of cancer-related pain,[3, 11–13] suggesting they may be underserved or inadequately treated.

Table 4.2 Incidence of pain by primary site of cancer

% Patients with pain	Site
>80	bone, pancreas, oesophagus
71–80	lung, stomach, hepatobiliary, prostate, breast, cervix, ovary
61–70	oropharynx, colon, brain, kidney/bladder
51–60	lymphoma, leukaemia, soft tissue

Adapted from: J. J. Bonica, The Management of Pain, Lea and Febiger, Philadelphia, 1990

Definitions

The most widely accepted definition of pain is that given by the International Association for the Study of Pain (IASP):[14] 'Pain is an unpleasant sensory and emotional experience associated with actual or potential tissue damage, or described in terms of such damage. Pain is always subjective.' The rider that pain is always subjective is very important and emphasizes that matters of psychosocial or spiritual concern can modify the sensation of pain. Aristotle alluded to the concept that pain was a somatopsychic phenomenon when he described it as a 'passion of the soul'.

A more practical definition is 'Pain is what the patient says hurts'. It emphasizes that a patient's pain is what they describe and not what others think it ought to be.

The terminology used in the description of pain is complex and may be confusing. Some commonly used terms are listed in Table 4.3.

Pain and suffering

The terms *pain* and *suffering,* sometimes used interchangeably or synonymously, need to be clearly distinguished. Suffering has been defined as the condition or distress associated with events that threaten the intactness or wholeness of the person.[15] Suffering may be caused by

Table 4.3 Pain terminology

Reduced sensation	
anaesthesia	absence of sensation
analgesia	absence of pain in response to a stimulus that is normally painful
hypoaesthesia	diminished sensitivity to stimulation, excluding the special senses
hypoalgesia	diminished sensitivity to a stimulus that is normally painful
Increased sensation	
allodynia	pain due to a stimulus that does not normally cause pain
hyperaesthesia	increased sensitivity to stimulation, excluding the special senses
hyperalgesia	increased sensitivity to a stimulus that is normally painful
hyperpathia	increased reaction to a stimulus, particularly a repetitive one, in association with an increased pain threshold
Abnormal sensation	
anaesthesia dolorosa	pain in an area which is anaesthetic
central pain	pain associated with a lesion of the central nervous system
deafferentation pain	pain due to complete or partial nerve lesions
dysaesthesia	an unpleasant abnormal sensation, spontaneous or provoked
neuropathic pain	pain due to damage or dysfunction of a nerve
paraesthesia	an abnormal sensation, spontaneous or provoked
sympathetic type pain (causalgia)	a syndrome of sustained burning pain, allodynia and hyperpathia following a traumatic nerve lesion, often combined with vasomotor and sudomotor dysfunction and later trophic changes
Other terms	
breakthrough pain	pain occurring during the time of action of an administered analgesic
incident pain	pain occurring only in certain circumstances (e.g. movement, standing)
myofascial pain	a muscular disorder characterized by the presence of a localized tender point (trigger point), stimulation of which causes local pain that radiates in a non-dermatomal manner
neuralgia	pain in the distribution of a nerve or nerves
neuritis	inflammation of a nerve or nerves
neuropathy	disturbance of function (with or without pain) in a nerve or nerves
nociceptive pain	pain resulting from chemical or physical stimulation of peripheral nerve endings (nociceptors)
pain threshold	the least stimulus that produces pain
pain tolerance	the level of pain that a subject is prepared to tolerate
sensory threshold	the least stimulus that can be recognized

Adapted from: IASP Subcommittee on Taxonomy. Pain 1979; 6: 249–52.
J. J. Bonica, The Management of Pain, Lea and Febiger, Philadelphia, 1990

any of a number of factors, of which pain is one, or any combination of them and the sum of these effects is referred to as Total Suffering (Figure 4.1).

Pain frequently causes suffering although there may be little or no suffering associated with the pain of acute illness or experiences like childbirth, which are of limited duration and of obvious significance to the patient. In the palliative care setting, where pain is usually chronic and progressive and of obvious significance to the patient, some degree of suffering is common.

The relationship between pain and suffering is further complicated by the interdependence and interrelationships between the various causes of suffering. Unrelieved pain can exacerbate problems related to other causes of suffering (Figure 4.2a). More importantly,

Figure 4.1 Total suffering

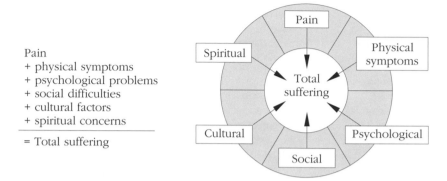

Pain
+ physical symptoms
+ psychological problems
+ social difficulties
+ cultural factors
+ spiritual concerns

= Total suffering

pain may be caused or aggravated by problems related to any of the other causes of suffering (Figure 4.2b). These interrelationships have important implications for clinical practice (Table 4.4). The most important is that when pain is caused or aggravated by problems related to other causes of suffering, no amount of well-prescribed analgesia will relieve the pain until the underlying problems are addressed. These interrelationships underline the need for a holistic and multiprofessional approach to care and explain why a patient's pain cannot be treated in isolation.

Figure 4.2 Interdependence of the various causes of suffering. (a) Unrelieved pain may cause or aggravate problems related to any of the other aspects of suffering. (b) Unresolved or untreated problems relating to other aspects of suffering may cause or aggravate pain.

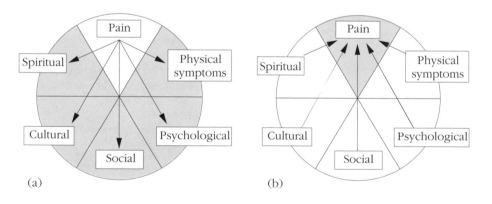

(a)   (b)

Table 4.4 Clinical implications of the relationship between pain and suffering

Pain is only one potential cause of suffering   treatment of pain alone will not relieve all a patient's suffering
Pain may cause or aggravate psychosocial problems causing suffering   pain must be controlled for psychosocial problems to be treated successfully
Pain may be caused or aggravated by psychosocial causes of suffering   psychosocial problems must be resolved for pain to be treated successfully
Pain cannot be treated in isolation and requires a holistic and multiprofessional approach

Neurophysiology

The neurophysiology of pain is complex and our understanding of it is continually improving.[16-19] Pain is caused by stimulation of free nerve endings (nociceptors), causing impulses to be carried along the peripheral nerve to the dorsal horn of the spinal cord. There they synapse with cells of the spinothalamic tract, which carry the impulses up the spinal cord, through the brain stem to the thalamus. From the thalamus, impulses are delivered to various areas of the cerebral cortex, which allow the perception of, and reaction to, pain (Figure 4.3).

Free nerve endings in the skin and connective tissues (somatic nociceptors) and viscera (visceral nociceptors) may be stimulated physically (pressure, heat, visceral distention) but are more commonly activated by chemical stimuli consequent upon tissue injury or inflammation. Tissue injury results in the production and accumulation of a variety of algesic substances that have been shown to affect nociceptors including prostaglandins, bradykinin, serotonin, histamine, and potassium and hydrogen ions.

Prostaglandins play a major role in the tissue injury-nociceptive pain cycle, which explains the usefulness of prostaglandin synthetase inhibitors in the treatment of pain. The algesic substances may also affect other nerve endings, such as those responsible for heat or pressure, reducing the stimulation threshold and facilitating activation.

Figure 4.3 A simplified diagram of pain pathways

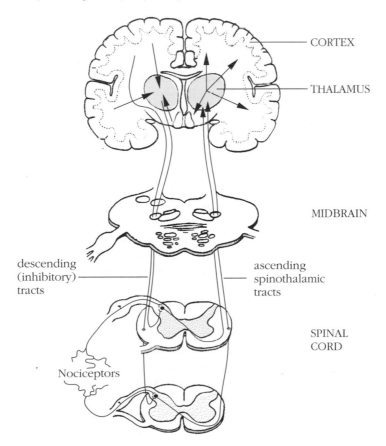

CORTEX

THALAMUS

MIDBRAIN

descending (inhibitory) tracts

ascending spinothalamic tracts

SPINAL CORD

Nociceptors

Nerve fibres from somatic nociceptors pass along peripheral nerves and enter the spinal cord by the dorsal root. In the case of fibres from visceral nociceptors, about 20% enter by the ventral route, which explains why surgical sectioning of the dorsal roots (dorsal rhizotomy) may fail to control visceral pain. Visceral and somatic afferent fibres converge on the same neurons in the spinal cord, the ascending spinal fibres being common for impulses from both viscera and skin. This is the anatomical basis for referred pain, in which visceral pain is accompanied by pain in particular dermatomes.

In the dorsal horn of the spinal cord the afferent sensory nerves synapse with fibres of the ascending spinothalamic tract, either directly or via a complex system of connecting fibres or interneurons, employing a variety of neurotransmitters including substance P and glutamate. The presynaptic terminal of the afferent sensory fibre contains opioid receptors that bind endogenous opioid substances (endorphins) or exogenous opioid medications. Such binding reduces or blocks the release of neurotransmitter by the afferent sensory fibre, reducing or relieving the sensation of pain. This is the prime site of action of exogenous opioid drugs. Similarly, activation of the inhibitory neurons in the dorsal horn, known to have endorphins as neurotransmitters, will reduce pain. The inhibitory neurons are stimulated by activity in the descending pathways from the brain or by activity in other sensory fibres in the same segment, explaining why massage, heat or electrical stimulation applied to a painful area may reduce pain. Other receptors in the dorsal horn may have an opposite effect. Activation of the N-methyl D-aspartate (NMDA) receptors sensitizes dorsal horn cells and will facilitate or perpetuate the sensation of pain (the 'wind-up' phenomenon) and may be responsible for the reduced opioid sensitivity of neuropathic pain. The NMDA receptor antagonist, ketamine, can be effective in relieving pain in this situation.

The ascending spinothalamic tract is the major connection for transmission of information regarding pain to the brain, but there are several other ascending pathways that are involved to a lesser extent. These additional pathways explain why surgical interruption of the spinothalamic tract does not produce complete pain relief.

Pain impulses transmitted to the thalamus are relayed to several areas of the cerebral cortex: the sensory areas of the parietal lobe, which allow localization and interpretation of the pain; the limbic system, which is involved in both the affective and autonomic response to the pain; the temporal lobe, which is involved in pain memory; and the frontal lobe, where cognitive function assesses the significance of the pain and the emotional response to it.

The major endogenous mechanism of pain inhibition is the suppression of pain impulses at the dorsal horn by pathways descending from the midbrain and brain stem. These centres receive input from the cortex, the thalamus and other midbrain centres and, by a variety of descending pathways, stimulate the inhibitory interneurons in the dorsal horn of the spinal cord, producing analgesia or reducing pain. The neurotransmitters involved with the descending inhibitory pathways are noradrenaline and serotonin. This is a possible explanation why drugs that block presynaptic re-uptake and augment the postsynaptic action of these substances, such as amitriptyline, may augment analgesia.

Neuropathic pain results from damage to nerves or neural tissue rather than the stimulation of nociceptors by tissue injury or inflammation. Pain results from spontaneous electrical activity of the damaged nerves or to increased sensitivity to exogenous stimuli; the neural pathways involved are the same as for nociception. Damage to sensory afferent fibres results in a significant reduction in the number of opioid receptors in the presynaptic terminals of the affected fibres in the dorsal horn, possibly explaining the reduced opioid sensitivity of neuropathic pain. Damage to sympathetic nerve fibres may lead to sympathetic type pain in which neuropathic pain is accompanied by signs of autonomic dysfunction, including vasomotor instability and sudomotor (sweating) changes.

Although all the anatomical, physiological and pharmacological relationships involved in pain remain incompletely documented, it is apparent that the major site of modulation of pain impulses is in the dorsal horn of the spinal cord, as was originally proposed in the 1960s by Melzack and Wall in their 'gate control' theory. The modulation of pain in the dorsal horn of the spinal cord provides a basis for explaining why painful stimuli can be modified by cortical, subcortical and other spinal activity, including psychological factors, pain at other sites and simultaneous stimulation of sensory fibres in the same peripheral nerve.

Chronic pain leads to other changes in the nervous system. Alterations in receptors and transmitters occur in the spinal cord and brain that may lead to perpetuation of pain or reduced opioid sensitivity.[16, 18, 19] The physiological changes remain incompletely defined at present but the clinical inference is obvious—chronic pain should be well controlled, as quickly as possible.

Classifications of pain

The various classifications of pain are listed in Table 4.5.

Table 4.5 Classifications of pain experienced by patients with cancer

Temporal	Pathophysiological	Aetiological
acute	nociceptive	due to cancer
chronic	somatic	due to therapy
incident	visceral	due to general illness but not cancer
	neuropathic	unrelated to cancer or therapy
	central	
	peripheral	
	sympathetic	
	psychogenic	

Acute and chronic pain

The distinction between acute and chronic pain is important in the management of patients with advanced cancer. They have different physical signs and psychological associations and require different approaches to treatment (Table 4.6).

Acute pain is usually due to a definable acute injury or illness.[20] It has a definite onset and its duration is limited and predictable (Figure 4.4). It is associated with clinical signs of sympathetic overactivity: tachycardia, tachypnoea, hypertension, sweating, pupillary dilatation and pallor. These signs, commonly seen in the hospital emergency department, are considered characteristic of a patient 'obviously in pain'. Acute pain is usually associated with anxiety rather than other psychological changes. However, if acute pain indicates progression of cancer (or is thought to by the patient), it may be associated with the signs of depression and withdrawal more commonly seen with chronic pain. Patients able to be told that their illness and pain are transitory usually exhibit an understanding, positive attitude. Treatment is directed at the acute illness or injury causing pain, with or without the short-term use of analgesics.

Chronic pain results from a chronic pathological process.[21] It has a gradual or ill-defined onset, continues unabated and may become progressively more severe. The patient appears depressed and withdrawn and, as there are usually no signs of sympathetic overactivity, they

Table 4.6 Acute and chronic pain

	Acute	**Chronic**
Onset	well-defined	ill-defined
Cause	acute injury or illness	chronic process
Duration	days/weeks predictable limited	months/years unpredictable unlimited
Physiological	sympathetic over-activity 'obviously in pain'	no sympathetic over-activity 'not obviously in pain'
Affective	anxiety	depression other psychological changes
Cognitive	positive response to transient illness meaningful	lacks positive meaning* meaningless
Behavioural	inactivity until recovery	changes in lifestyle changes in functional ability withdrawn
Treatment	treatment of injury, illness temporary use of analgesics	treatment of underlying cause regular analgesics to prevent pain psychosocial supportive care

* chronic pain may have definite negative meaning if it is a sign of progression of cancer

are frequently labelled as 'not looking like somebody in pain'. Patients with chronic pain have symptoms of depression with lethargy, apathy, anorexia and insomnia. Personality changes may occur due to progressive alterations in lifestyle and functional ability. For patients with chronic pain of non-malignant origin, the pain is said to lack positive meaning; for patients with chronic pain related to cancer, the pain usually has definite negative implications with regard to their prognosis and life expectancy. Chronic pain related to cancer requires treatment of the underlying disease where possible, regular use of analgesics to control pain and

Figure 4.4 Acute and chronic pain

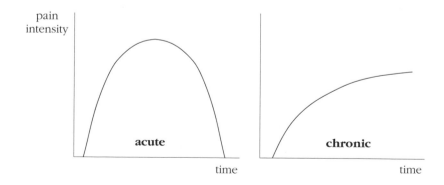

to prevent its recurrence, as well as psychological and social supportive care. Successful treatment is often associated with dramatic improvement in the patient's well being.

Patients with chronic pain due to cancer must be distinguished from patients with chronic pain of non-malignant origin, who often have definite psychiatric and social problems. Patients with non-malignant pain may exhibit 'pain behaviour' due to dependency on their painful situation and its rewards, and they fail to respond to the supportive care measures and analgesia that will benefit most patients with pain due to cancer. Operant conditioning and similar methods used for patients with chronic non-malignant pain have little or no place in the treatment of patients with advanced cancer and pain.

Establishing the dividing line between acute and chronic pain is difficult. Non-malignant pain is traditionally classified as chronic if it persists longer than the expected healing time for the causative injury or illness. However, there is evidence that all of the pathophysiological changes associated with chronic pain—central sensitization, hyperalgesia, novel gene expression, synaptic remodeling ('plasticity'), 'pain memory' formation, and behavioural adjustment—are initiated within days of acute, ongoing tissue injury.[20] This argues against the use of an arbitrary time interval to separate acute and chronic pain. For patients with documented malignancy, and in the absence of an acute injury or illness that will heal or respond to therapy, pain lasting more than two weeks should be considered as chronic and treated accordingly.

Incident pain occurs only in certain circumstances, such as pain that occurs after a particular movement or on standing. It should be regarded as chronic pain but, because of its intermittent nature, it should be managed with local measures where possible.

Nociceptive, neuropathic and psychogenic pain

Nociceptive or physiological pain is produced by stimulation of specific sensory receptors or nociceptors located in the tissues. The neural pathways involved are normal and intact. Somatic pain from the skin and superficial structures is usually well localized and described as aching, sharp, throbbing or pressure-like. Visceral pain from deep-seated structures is less well localized and felt over a larger area, and there is often referred pain to cutaneous sites. It may be described as a deep aching or throbbing pain, which may be sharp if organ capsules are involved. Obstruction of hollow viscera causes gnawing or colicky pain.

Neuropathic pain is caused by peripheral or central nervous system injury.[18, 22, 23] Neuropathic pain from a lesion involving the central nervous system is referred to as central pain and is non-dermatomal in distribution. The pain from peripheral nerve lesions, sometimes referred to as deafferentation pain, is dermatomal in distribution. Pain occurs because the injured nerves react abnormally to stimuli or discharge spontaneously. Neuropathic pain is most often described as a burning or stinging feeling or as a shooting, lancinating pain. Terms used to qualitatively describe neuropathic pain, such as dysaesthesia and allodynia, are listed in Table 4.3.

Damage to sympathetic nerves may lead to sympathetic-type pain. It is characterized by burning pain and allodynia, similar to deafferentation pain. There are signs of sympathetic dysfunction in the affected area including vasomotor instability (erythema, pallor, oedema), sudomotor (sweating) abnormalities, and trophic changes (thinning of the skin and atrophy of the subcutaneous tissue). Sympathetic pain is less sensitive to non-opioid and opioid analgesics but often responds to a regional sympathetic nerve block.

Psychogenic pain refers to pain for which there is no physical basis, in patients who have other evidence of psychopathology. Psychogenic pain does not occur as a consequence of cancer.

Causes

The various causes of pain in patients with cancer and the approximate frequency with which they occur are shown in Table 4.7.[10] These figures obviously depend on the stage of the patient's disease; for example, a terminally ill patient will not have pain caused by anti-cancer treatment but is likely to have more pain related to general illness and debility.

Table 4.7 Causes of pain

Tumour infiltration	70–80%
Associated with treatment	10–20%
Due to general illness but not cancer	10–20%
Unrelated to cancer or its treatment	10%

Pain caused by tumour infiltration

Tumour infiltration causes pain by variety of means. Bone metastases are the most frequent cause of pain directly attributable to cancer. Bone metastases cause pain by local bone destruction, pathological fractures, infiltration of surrounding tissues, secondary muscle spasm, or by compression of neurological structures including the spinal cord and peripheral nerves.

Compression and infiltration of a peripheral nerve causes a dull ache or a constant superficial burning pain in the area of sensory loss, sometimes associated with hyperaesthesia, dysaesthesia and lancinating pain. Infiltration of the brachial or lumbosacral plexus will produce pain and diminished sensation in the distribution of the relevant nerve roots as well as motor signs.

Soft tissue infiltration causes pain because of local tissue destruction and by infiltration of pain-sensitive tissues such as fascia or periosteum. It also causes pain by compression or infiltration of nerves and vessels. Infiltration of the skin and mucous membranes causes local pain sometimes aggravated by secondary infection.

Infiltration of viscera causes poorly localized, deep-seated aching pain, often accompanied by pain referred to cutaneous sites. Involvement of the tissue capsule produces more severe sharp pain, which is well localized and associated with local tenderness. Infiltration of hollow viscera will cause colic and pain that is poorly localized and frequently associated with referred pain.

Pain associated with treatment

Diagnostic and staging procedures, surgery, chemotherapy and radiotherapy may all cause pain (Table 4.8).

Pain related to debilitating disease

A small proportion of pains experienced by patients with advanced cancer relate to the effects of debilitating disease (Table 4.9).

Myofascial pain originates from a muscle and its surrounding fascia. It is characterized by a localized tender point (trigger point), stimulation of which produces local pain that radiates in a non-dermatomal manner. Myofascial pain is common in the general population but occurs more frequently in patients with advanced cancer, especially those who are debilitated or cachectic.

Table 4.8 Examples of pain caused by treatment

Diagnostic and staging procedures

Surgery
    neuropathy after thoracotomy, neck dissection, mastectomy
    postamputation stump pain, phantom limb pain

Chemotherapy
    mucositis
    phlebitis, tissue necrosis (extravasation)
    neuropathy (vinca alkaloids)
    myalgia, arthralgia (corticosteroid withdrawal)

Radiotherapy
    mucositis, neuropathy, myelopathy

Table 4.9 Examples of pain related to debilitating disease

Constipation	Musculoskeletal pain
Pressure sores	secondary to inactivity
Gastric distention	myofascial pain
Reflux oesophagitis	caused by unusual activity
Bladder spasms (with catheterization)	Infection
Thrombosis and embolism	Post-herpetic neuralgia
Mucositis	

Pain unrelated to cancer or treatment

A small proportion of pains reported by patients with advanced cancer are unrelated to the cancer or therapy. Most frequently encountered are the various forms of arthritis and pain due to ischaemic heart disease and peripheral vascular disease.

References

1   Jacox, A., et al. (1994). *Management of Cancer Pain. Clinical Practice Guideline No. 9.* Rockville, MD: Agency for Health Care Policy and Research, U.S. Department of Health and Human Services.

2   Jadad, A.R. and Browman, G.P. (1995). The WHO analgesic ladder for cancer pain management. Stepping up the quality of its evaluation. *Journal of the American Medical Association* 274, 1870–3.

3   Goudas, L., et al. (2001). *Management of cancer pain.* Rockville, MD: Agency for Healthcare Research and Quality. <www.ahrq.gov>

4   Cleeland, C.S., et al. (1994). Pain and its treatment in outpatients with metastatic cancer. *New England Journal of Medicine* 330, 592–6.

5   Chang, V.T., Hwang, S.S. and Kasimis, B. (2002). Longitudinal documentation of cancer pain management outcomes. A pilot study at a VA medical center. *Journal of Pain and Symptom Management* 24, 494–505.

6   Foley, K.M. (2001). Management of Cancer Pain. In *Cancer. Principles and Practice of Oncology. 6th edition* (ed. V.T. De Vita, S. Hellman and S.A. Rosenberg). Philadelphia, Lippincott Williams Wilkins.

7   Carr, D., et al. (2002). *Management of Cancer Symptoms: Pain, Depression, and Fatigue. Evidence Report/Technology Assessment No. 61.* Rockville, MD: Agency for Healthcare Research and Quality. <www.ahrq.gov>

8   Cherny, N. (2002). Cancer pain: principles of assessment and management. In *Principles and Practice of Palliative Care and Supportive Oncology* (ed. A.M. Berger, R.K. Portenoy and D.E. Weissman). Philadelphia, Lippincott, Williams and Wilkins.

9   Bonica, J.J. (ed.) (1990). *The Management of Pain. 2nd edition.* Philadelphia, Lea and Febiger.

10   Grond, S., et al. (1996). Assessment of cancer pain: a prospective evaluation in 2266 cancer patients referred to a pain service. *Pain* 64, 107–14.

11   Cleeland, C.S., et al. (1997). Pain and treatment of pain in minority patients with cancer. The Eastern Cooperative Oncology Group minority outpatient pain study. *Annals of Internal Medicine* 127, 813–16.

12   Bernabei, R., et al. (1998). Management of pain in elderly patients with cancer. SAGE Study Group. Systematic Assessment of Geriatric Drug Use via Epidemiology. *Journal of the American Medical Association* 279, 1877–82.

13   Anderson, K.O., et al. (2000). Minority cancer patients and their providers: pain management attitudes and practice. *Cancer* 88, 1929–38.

14   IASP Subcommittee on Taxonomy (1979). Pain terms: a list with definitions and notes on usage. Recommended by the IASP Subcommittee on Taxonomy. *Pain* 6, 249.

15   Chapman, C.R. and Gavrin, J. (1999). Suffering: the contributions of persistent pain. *Lancet* 353, 2233–7.

16   Besson, J.M. (1999). The neurobiology of pain. *Lancet* 353, 1610–15.

17   Cervero, F. and Laird, J.M. (1999). Visceral pain. *Lancet* 353, 2145–8.

18   Woolf, C.J. and Mannion, R.J. (1999). Neuropathic pain: aetiology, symptoms, mechanisms, and management. *Lancet* 353, 1959–64.

19   Regan, J.M. and Peng, P. (2000). Neurophysiology of cancer pain. *Cancer Control* 7, 111–19.

20   Carr, D.B. and Goudas, L.C. (1999). Acute pain. *Lancet* 353, 2051–8.

21   Ashburn, M.A. and Staats, P.S. (1999). Management of chronic pain. *Lancet* 353, 1865–9.

22   Moulin, D.E. (1998). Neuropathic cancer pain: syndromes and clinical controversies. In *Topics in Palliative Care. Volume 2* (ed. E. Bruera and R. Portenoy). New York, Oxford University Press.

23   Martin, L.A. and Hagen, N.A. (1997). Neuropathic pain in cancer patients: mechanisms, syndromes, and clinical controversies. *Journal of Pain and Symptom Management* 14, 99–117.

5

Factors that modify the perception of pain

The concept of Clinical Pain

Pain is always subjective and the perception of pain may be modified by problems or influences related to any or all of the potential causes of suffering—pain, other physical symptoms, psychological problems, social difficulties, cultural issues and spiritual concerns. Physical pain (the pain due to cancer, treatment or unrelated causes) can be modified by any of these factors, resulting in the final Clinical Pain (Figure 5.1). These modifying factors may

Figure 5.1   The concept of Clinical Pain

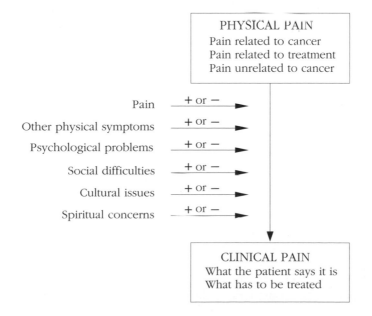

have a positive or negative effect on the perception of pain, making it either better or worse. In clinical practice the modifying factors usually aggravate pain, either by decreasing the pain threshold or increasing the sensitivity to pain. Sometimes what patients report as their pain is largely attributable to psychosocial or spiritual problems. However, the modifying factors can have an ameliorating effect and lessen pain, and some patients complain of much less pain than might be expected from their medical situation. The final Clinical Pain, incorporating all the modifying effects from the other causes of potential suffering, represents what the patient says it is and what has to be treated.

Factors modifying the perception of pain

Factors that modify the perception of pain are conveniently grouped by the different causes of potential suffering (Figures 5.1 and 5.2), although there is considerable overlap and many of the factors are aetiologically interrelated with pain and with each other. It is possible that cycles are created that perpetuate pain; for example, worsening pain may produce anxiety or anger, which in turn will further aggravate pain.

Modifying factors related to pain. Severe or progressive pain, pain at multiple or an increasing number of sites, or pain that causes significant limitation of activity can all aggravate the perception of pain; the opposite situations may lessen it. Adverse experiences with poor prior pain management will aggravate pain. The effect of good management of all chronic pain on the perception of future pain should not be underestimated.

Other physical symptoms. Patients with insomnia, exhaustion or fatigue secondary to unrelieved pain will complain of worse pain compared to patients not suffering these consequences. Persistent cough, repeated vomiting or prolonged hiccups can aggravate pain, particularly bone pain. The presence of any other distressing symptoms such as dyspnoea, diarrhoea, incontinence or haemorrhage will aggravate the perception of pain.

Psychological problems. Psychological problems are by far the most common factors to affect the perception of pain, and a review of published studies showed a significant association between increased pain and increased psychological distress.[1] The possible causes of psychological distress in patients with cancer are legion and are discussed in Chapter 30. Psychological distress is often described simply in terms of anxiety and depression, but in practice a wide range of psychological reactions and physical symptoms may be manifest, all representing underlying psychological distress. Unrecognized or untreated psychological distress will aggravate pain; its absence or successful resolution may greatly improve it.

Social difficulties. Patients with cancer do not exist in social isolation; usually they have family and friends as well as social and financial responsibilities. Cancer frequently has devastating effects on these relationships, leading to a range of social problems that are likely to worsen as the disease progresses (see Chapter 31). Increased pain is associated with decreased social activities and social support.[1] Social difficulties are likely to aggravate pain; their successful resolution may greatly improve it.

Cultural issues. Different cultural groups vary greatly in their attitude to disease, suffering and death, which may greatly influence the perception of pain. Some cultural groups are more stoic in their response to pain. Language barriers, which make communication about pain and its treatment difficult, can exacerbate pain. Culturally appropriate management and the circumvention of language barriers may lessen pain. Cultural issues are discussed in Chapter 32.

Spiritual concerns. Spiritual concerns and problems related to existential distress occur frequently in patients with cancer, especially those with advanced disease (see Chapter 33).

Spiritual or existential problems can have a profound effect on the perception of pain and can be responsible for severe pain that responds poorly to analgesics. Resolution of spiritual or religious problems can greatly aid pain control.

Figure 5.2 Clinical Pain

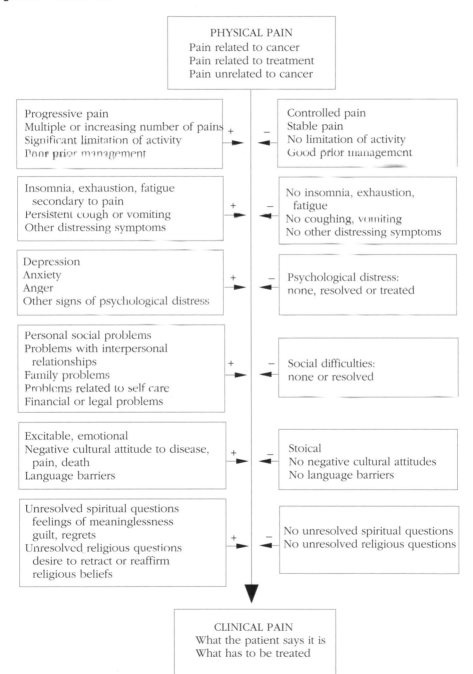

Clinical Pain: implications for assessment and treatment

The concept of Clinical Pain portrays the dynamic interaction between the various causes of suffering and the perception of pain. The important clinical corollary is that problems related to other causes of suffering that may modify the perception of pain must be assessed and treated if pain control is to be successful (Table 5.1). This in turn requires a holistic and multiprofessional approach to the assessment and treatment of pain.[2–4]

Table 5.1 Multiprofessional pain management

Pain	Treatment
	Analgesics, plus
Physical pain	treatment of physical disease
+ factors related to pain	+ factors related to pain
+ factors due to physical symptoms	+ factors due to physical symptoms
+ factors due to psychological problems	+ factors due to psychological problems
+ factors due to social difficulties	+ factors due to social difficulties
+ factors due to cultural issues	+ factors due to cultural issues
+ factors due to spiritual concerns	+ factors due to spiritual concerns
= Clinical pain	**= Multiprofessional pain management**

References

1   Zaza, C. and Baine, N. (2002). Cancer pain and psychosocial factors. A critical review of the literature. *Journal of Pain and Symptom Management* 24, 526–42.
2   Twycross, R. (1994). *Pain Relief in Advanced Cancer*. Edinburgh, Churchill Livingstone.
3   Turk, D.C. and Okifuji, A. (1999). Assessment of patients' reporting of pain: an integrated perspective. *Lancet* 353, 1784–8.
4   Foley, K.M. (2001). Management of Cancer Pain. In *Cancer. Principles and Practice of Oncology. 6th edition* (ed. V.T. De Vita, S. Hellman and S.A. Rosenberg). Philadelphia, Lippincott Williams Wilkins.

6

Assessment of pain

Clinical assessment

Thorough clinical assessment is fundamental to the successful treatment of pain. The important principles are listed in Table 6.1.

Table 6.1 Principles for the assessment of pain

Accept the patient's description
Careful assessment of the pain—history, examination, investigation
Assess each pain
Assess the extent of the patient's disease
Assess the other factors that may influence pain   physical, psychological, social, cultural, spiritual
Reassessment

Accept the patient's description. The patient's description of the type and severity of pain must be accepted as true. Pain is always subjective and patients' pain is what they say it is and not what others think it ought to be. This is necessary if there is to be trust in the doctor–patient relationship; if the doctor is disbelieving or disinterested the patient may compensate by not reporting pain or by exaggerating it.

Careful assessment of the pain. Patients are asked to describe their pain, in their own words, and in their own way. Much information can be gained by observing how they describe their pain, what language they use, what emotions they express, and the accompanying body language. The information given will need to be supplemented with specific questions (Table 6.2) until all the features of the pain are defined. It is important to know the doses of drugs previously taken, what effect they had, and what side effects occurred. Information from family members may be helpful in assessing the severity of pain and its effect on lifestyle.

The results of physical examination, including neurological assessment, are recorded verbally and pictorially on a body chart (Figure 6.1). The site of the responsible lesion can often be defined using the anatomical correlates described below in the section on neurological examination. Further investigations may be required but should be limited to those that are necessary and likely to have a significant bearing on treatment decisions.

Assess each pain. Most cancer patients have more than one pain and each requires assessment.

Evaluate the extent of the patient's disease. As cancer is the most frequent cause of pain, new or worsening pain requires that the extent of the patient's cancer be re-evaluated. This also ensures that any treatment given is appropriate to the stage of the patient's disease.

Assess other factors that may influence pain. The assessment of pain in patients with cancer should proceed on the assumption that physical factors are mainly responsible for the pain. However, as discussed in Chapter 5, assessment needs to include the other factors that may modify the perception of pain.[1] The patient's perception of the significance of a pain, particularly if it is thought to herald recurrence or progression of the disease, may have profound psychological effects. Patients who respond poorly to apparently appropriate analgesic therapy should be assessed for psychosocial or spiritual problems that are not immediately apparent.

Table 6.2 Assessment of pain

The pain	
site	where is it?
radiation	does it spread anywhere else?
present since	how long have you had it?
progressive	has it got worse?
severity	how bad is it?
quality	what is it like?
frequency	how often do you get it?
duration	how long does it last?
precipitating factors	what brings it on?
aggravating factors	what makes it worse?
relieving factors	what helps the pain?
impact on – activity	does it stop you doing things?
– sleep	does it stop you sleeping?
– mood	does it make you unhappy or depressed?
Effect of previous medication	
medication	what did you take?
dose	how much?
route	by mouth?
frequency	how often?
duration	for how long?
effect	did it help?
adverse effects	did it upset you?
Other factors	
patient's perception of the meaning of pain	
psychological, social, cultural, spiritual influences or consequences	

Figure 6.1 Pictorial record. The patient may be requested to mark or indicate the site of the pain, or it may be completed by the examining doctor or nurse.

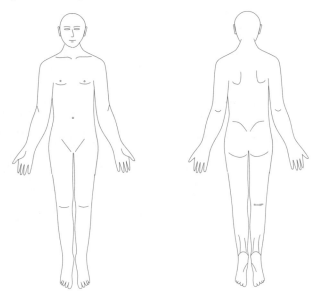

The need to assess psychosocial and spiritual factors that may cause or aggravate pain is emphasized by the use of terms such as 'total body pain' and 'monster pain' to describe pain that is associated with overwhelming emotional distress. Whilst it is permissible for a patient to say that they feel pain everywhere, the medical use of these terms should be discouraged as they are a distraction from the task of unravelling and treating the various factors causing distress, be they physical, psychological, social, cultural or spiritual.

Reassessment. Repeated reviews of a patient's pain are as important as the initial assessment. Pain not responding satisfactorily to treatment may indicate the diagnosis was incorrect or that other factors, such as depression, require therapy. As cancer is a progressive disease, new or more extensive pain can be anticipated, emphasizing the need for continuing reassessment.

Table 6.3 Myotomes. The segmental nerve supply of some basic muscle groups

Upper limb			Lower limb		
shoulder	abduction	C5,6	hip	flexion	L3,4
	adduction	C6,7		extension	L5,S1
elbow	flexion	C5,6	knee	flexion	L5,S1
	extension	C7,8		extension	L3,4
wrist	flexion	C7,8	ankle	dorsiflexion	L4,5
	extension	C6,7		plantar flexion	S1,2
fingers	flexion	C7,8	toes	flexion	L5,S1
	extension	C7,8		extension	L5,S1
	abduction, adduction	T1			

Figure 6.2 Dermatomes

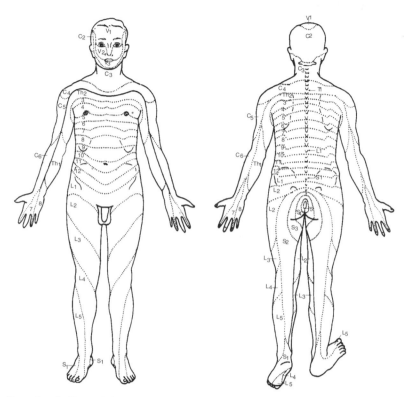

Reproduced with permission from Bonica JJ *The Management of Pain*. Philadelphia, Lea and Febiger, 1990.

Table 6.4 Examples of referred pain

Organ	Innervation	Location of pain
oesophagus	T2–T8	retrosternal, interscapular, neck; left or both arms
diaphragm	C3–C4	root of neck and shoulder
stomach, duodenum	T6–T9	epigastrium, right or left upper quadrant; back
liver, biliary tree	T6–T9	right upper quadrant, right scapula or shoulder
pancreas	T6–T10	upper abdominal; lower thoracic region
small intestine	T8–T12	periumbilical; occasionally suprapubic
colon	T10–L2	periumbilical, right or left abdominal
kidney	T10–L1	back and flank
pelvi-ureteric junction	T10–L2	loin, flank; ± ipsilateral testicle or ovary
terminal ureter	T12–L2	loin and suprapubic region; scrotal or labial skin
bladder	T12–L2	male: lower abdomen; urethra and penis female: lower abdomen; urethra, perimeatal skin

Neurological examination

Neurological examination of the patient with pain often allows some anatomical localization of the cause, especially when there is involvement of the spinal cord or nerve roots. The distribution of the pain or sensory changes may correlate with dermatomes as illustrated in Figure 6.2. Muscular weakness and loss of reflexes (Table 6.3) and the pattern of referred visceral pain (Table 6.4) may also be correlated with spinal segments.

Measurement of pain

As pain is a subjective phenomenon, objective measurement is not possible. However, there are a number of reasons to recommend the routine use of pain measurement tools. First, routine assessment is required to document the incidence of unrelieved pain and the need for better treatment.[2] Second, documented pain scores will help initiate discussions about pain between patient and staff. Third, there can be considerable differences regarding the severity of pain between the patient and the treatment team, which will be made obvious by the use of pain scores; agreement between staff and patients fell from 78% when the pain was mild to 20% when the pain was severe.[3] Fourth, routine documentation of pain scores should alert clinicians and lead to both improved treatment for individual patients as well as better institutional policies for the management of pain.[4, 5] However, routine use of pain scores will not result in changes in practice or improved pain control unless they are introduced as part of an educational and quality improvement package.[6–8]

Pain intensity measurement tools

Pain intensity scales are suitable for routine clinical practice and are useful for measuring pain and pain relief. They include visual analogue scales (VAS), numerical rating scales (NRS) and verbal descriptor scales (VDS) (Figure 6.3).[9, 10]

Figure 6.3   Self-report measures for pain severity

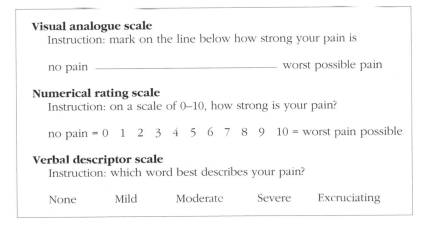

Visual analogue scale
    Instruction: mark on the line below how strong your pain is

    no pain ————————————————— worst possible pain

Numerical rating scale
    Instruction: on a scale of 0–10, how strong is your pain?

    no pain = 0   1   2   3   4   5   6   7   8   9   10 = worst pain possible

Verbal descriptor scale
    Instruction: which word best describes your pain?

    None   Mild   Moderate   Severe   Excruciating

Multidimensional pain measurement tools

Several instruments have been developed to measure pain and the associated affective and functional changes.

Figure 6.4 Memorial Pain Assessment Card. The card is folded along the dotted lines and each measure is presented to the patient separately, in the numbered order.

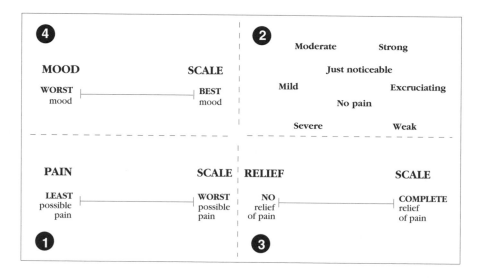

Reproduced from Fisherman B et al.: The Memorial Pain Assessment Card: A valid instrument for the evaluation of cancer pain. Cancer 1987; 60 : 1151–58.

The Memorial Pain Assessment Card (MPAC) combines VAS for pain and for pain relief, a VDS, and a VAS for mood (Figure 6.4).[11] The mood VAS has been shown to represent a global assessment of psychological distress rather than specific pain-related changes in affect.[12] It has been validated and is simple for patients to use.

The Brief Pain Inventory (BPI) is a self-administered questionnaire that provides information about pain history, intensity, location and quality.[13] Least, worst, average and present pain intensities are recorded on numerical rating scales. A percentage scale measures the effect of current therapy on pain. Seven questions assess the effect of pain on mood, function and quality of life. It is a suitable tool for research but may be difficult for patients with advanced cancer.[10, 14]

The McGill Pain Questionnaire (MPQ) is a self-administered questionnaire that provides information about the sensory, affective and evaluative dimensions of pain.[15, 16] Patients choose adjectives or descriptors to describe their pain, which presumes the necessary linguistic skills. Location and intensity of pain are assessed, but not the effect on function. The MPQ has been used in oncology and palliative care,[17, 18] but is best reserved for research projects and may be too demanding for patients with advanced disease.[10]

Pain assessment in the cognitively impaired

Patients with mild cognitive impairment may be able to complete simple pain intensity measurements with assistance. Contrary to expectation, they report more intense pain compared to their caregivers.[19] For patients with more severe impairment, the observations of staff or caregivers can provide useful information. Facial expression and vocalization are reliable means for assessing the presence of pain but not its intensity.[20] The response to a trial dose of an analgesic will usually indicate whether or not a patient has pain.

References

1   Turk, D.C. and Okifuji, A. (1999). Assessment of patients' reporting of pain: an integrated perspective. *Lancet* 353, 1784–8.

2   Bernabei, R., et al. (1998). Management of pain in elderly patients with cancer. SAGE Study Group. Systematic Assessment of Geriatric Drug Use via Epidemiology. *Journal of the American Medical Association* 279, 1877–82.

3   Grossman, S.A., et al. (1991). Correlation of patient and caregiver ratings of cancer pain. *Journal of Pain and Symptom Management* 6, 53–7.

4   American Pain Society Quality of Care Committee (1995). Quality improvement guidelines for the treatment of acute pain and cancer pain. *Journal of the American Medical Association* 274, 1874–80.

5   Chang, V.T., Hwang, S.S. and Kasimis, B. (2002). Longitudinal documentation of cancer pain management outcomes. A pilot study at a VA medical center. *Journal of Pain and Symptom Management* 24, 494–505.

6   Au, E., et al. (1994). Regular use of a verbal pain scale improves the understanding of oncology inpatient pain intensity. *Journal of Clinical Oncology* 12, 2751–5.

7   Du Pen, S.L., et al. (1999). Implementing guidelines for cancer pain management: results of a randomized controlled clinical trial. *Journal of Clinical Oncology* 17, 361–70.

8   Rhodes, D.J., et al. (2001). Feasibility of quantitative pain assessment in outpatient oncology practice. *Journal of Clinical Oncology* 19, 501–8.

9   De Conno, F., et al. (1994). Pain measurement in cancer patients: comparison of six methods. *Pain* 57, 161–6.

10 Caraceni, A., et al. (2002). Pain measurement tools and methods in clinical research in palliative care: recommendations of an Expert Working Group of the European Association of Palliative Care. *Journal of Pain and Symptom Management* 23, 239–55.

11 Fishman, B., et al. (1987). The Memorial Pain Assessment Card. A valid instrument for the evaluation of cancer pain. *Cancer* 60, 1151–8.

12 Foley, K.M. (2001). Management of Cancer Pain. In *Cancer. Principles and Practice of Oncology. 6th edition* (ed. V.T. De Vita, S. Hellman and S.A. Rosenberg). Philadelphia, Lippincott Williams Wilkins.

13 Daut, R.L., Cleeland, C.S. and Flanery, R.C. (1983). Development of the Wisconsin Brief Pain Questionnaire to assess pain in cancer and other diseases. *Pain* 17, 197–210.

14 Twycross, R., Harcourt, J. and Bergl, S. (1996). A survey of pain in patients with advanced cancer. *Journal of Pain and Symptom Management* 12, 273–82.

15 Melzack, R. (1975). The McGill Pain Questionnaire: major properties and scoring methods. *Pain* 1, 277–99.

16 Melzack, R. (1987). The short-form McGill Pain Questionnaire. *Pain* 30, 191–7.

17 Graham, C., et al. (1980). Use of the McGill pain questionnaire in the assessment of cancer pain: replicability and consistency. *Pain* 8, 377–87.

18 Dudgeon, D., Raubertas, R.F. and Rosenthal, S.N. (1993). The short-form McGill Pain Questionnaire in chronic cancer pain. *Journal of Pain and Symptom Management* 8, 191–5.

19 Allen, R.S., et al. (2002). Pain reports by older hospice cancer patients and family caregivers: the role of cognitive functioning. *Gerontologist* 42, 507–14.

20 Manfredi, P.L., et al. (2003). Pain assessment in elderly patients with severe dementia. *Journal of Pain and Symptom Management* 25, 48–52.

7

Principles of treatment

General principles

Acute pain

For patients with cancer, the management of acute pain caused by surgery, fractures or painful procedures is the same as for patients without cancer. Patients with cancer may recover more slowly and require analgesia for longer periods if their general condition is poor. Psychological factors will further complicate the situation if the acute episode is a manifestation of progressive disease.

Incident pain

Incident pain occurs only in certain circumstances, such as pain that occurs after a particular movement or on standing. Where possible, incident pain should be treated with local measures including treatment of the cancer (radiotherapy) and physical therapy (surgery, supports). Analgesics may be used if the pain is mild and the adverse effects of constant administration are tolerable. If the pain is severe, modification of the patient's activity may be preferable to taking strong opioid analgesics on a regular basis for pain that occurs infrequently.

Chronic pain

The treatment of chronic pain due to cancer requires a different approach to that for acute pain or other chronic non-malignant pain.[1-3] The aim of treatment is the relief and prevention of pain. The principles involved are listed in Table 7.1.

Thorough clinical assessment, as described in Chapter 6, is fundamental to successful treatment. Assessment of the type of pain (e.g. neuropathic, bone) will assist in deciding which modalities of therapy or which analgesics are appropriate. Assessment of the stage of a patient's disease may provide information about the cause of pain and indicate which ther-

Table 7.1 Principles of treating chronic pain due to cancer

General principles
    thorough assessment
    good communication
    reassure about pain relief
    discourage acceptance of pain
    encourage patient participation

Principles of treatment
    integrated part of an interdisciplinary plan of care
    should be appropriate to the stage of the disease
    use the appropriate treatment modality
    use multiple treatment modalities
    must be consistent, not variable
    requires continuity of care
    involves repeated reassessment

apeutic modalities are likely to be of benefit; it also ensures that treatment will be appropriate to the stage of the patient's disease and prognosis.

Good communication is essential for good pain control. The doctor needs to listen carefully to the patient's description and in turn provide clear explanation of the cause of the pain, the treatment options, and their relative merits and potential toxicities. Good communication with other members of the treatment team will ensure a co-ordinated approach to pain control.

Many patients believe cancer is inevitably associated with severe pain and that the pain is unrelievable. Patients should be reassured that their pain can be relieved, both immediately and on a continuing basis, and a positive attitude encouraged. Acceptance of pain by patients should be actively discouraged. Allowing patients to participate in the management of their pain builds trust and improves co-operation and compliance with treatment.

Treatment of pain should be an integrated part of an overall plan of total care. Other psychosocial and spiritual aspects of suffering that cause or aggravate pain need to be assessed and treated, and an multidisciplinary approach to the management of chronic pain is therefore a clinical necessity (see Chapter 5). The treatment of pain should always be appropriate to the stage of the patient's disease and treatment for an ambulant patient will differ from that for one who is bed-bound.

Treatment should be consistent and not variable. The patient needs a clear picture of the planned therapy, including the likelihood of any necessary changes; unexpected or sudden changes cause anxiety. Continuity of care is similarly important. Repeated reassessment is necessary to monitor both the efficacy and any adverse effects of the treatment given.

Modalities of therapy

There are a variety of treatment modalities available for chronic pain due to cancer (Table 7.2). Different types of pain respond better to particular treatments, as is the case with radiotherapy for bone pain and the use of anticonvulsants for neuropathic pain. In practice, combinations of different modalities are often used. When feasible, modification of the underlying pathology causing pain, by treatment of the cancer itself, is an effective means of pain control.

Table 7.2 Modalities of treatment

Treatment of underlying cancer

Analgesics

Adjuvant analgesics

Neurostimulatory treatment

Anaesthetic, neurolytic and neurosurgical procedures

Physical therapy

Psychological therapy

Lifestyle modification

Treatment of other aspects of suffering that cause or aggravate pain
    physical, psychological, social, cultural, spiritual

Principles of using analgesics

The use of analgesics for the treatment of acute pain in patients with cancer is the same as for those not suffering from cancer. It is the treatment of chronic pain that is often poorly managed and requires a different approach. The principles of analgesic use for the treatment of chronic cancer-related pain are shown in Table 7.3.

Table 7.3 The use of analgesics for chronic cancer pain

Choice of drug
    appropriate drug for type of pain
    appropriate drug for severity of pain
    use combinations of drugs, not combined drugs
    follow the analgesic ladder
    use adjuvant analgesics
    never use placebo

Administration
    give in adequate dosage
    titrate the dose for each individual patient
    schedule administration according to drug pharmacology
    strict scheduling to prevent pain, not PRN
    give written instructions for patients on multiple drugs
    give instructions for treatment of breakthrough pain
    warn of, and give treatment to prevent, adverse effects
    keep the analgesic programme as simple as possible
    use the oral route wherever possible

Review and reassess

Choice of drug

The choice of which drug or drugs to use depends upon the type and severity of the pain. Different types of pain respond to different analgesics (Table 7.4).[3–5] Somatic pain responds satisfactorily to non-opioid and opioid drugs; if opioids are required, the non-opioid should

Table 7.4 Type of pain: implications for treatment

Nociceptive		
bone, soft tissue	mild, moderate	non-opioid (opioid if required)
	severe	opioid + non-opioid
visceral	mild	non-opioid (opioid if required)
	moderate, severe	opioid ± non-opioid
Neuropathic		
nerve compression		corticosteroid ± opioid
deafferentation		antidepressant
		or anticonvulsant
		or oral local anaesthetic drug
Other		
raised intracranial pressure		corticosteroid
muscle spasm		muscle relaxant

be continued as it has a different mechanism of action and may have an opioid-sparing effect. Neuropathic pain is usually treated with one of the adjuvant analgesics.[6] Neuropathic pain may respond well to non-opioid and opioid drugs, but the general consensus is that it is less sensitive to opioid drugs and that adequate pain control often requires doses that cause unacceptable adverse effects.[7–9] Assessment is complicated by the fact that many patients have pain with both neuropathic and nociceptive features. Pain caused by nerve compression should be treated with corticosteroids. Sympathetic-type pain responds to a sympathetic nerve block.

As it is important that pain be brought under control as quickly as possible, it is preferable to start with a stronger analgesic and subsequently wean the patient to a weaker drug.

When prescribing for patients with chronic pain, it is commonplace to use more than one drug. Different drugs should be given independently and compound preparations avoided because, if it is necessary to escalate the dose of one of the drugs in a combination, the dose of the second drug will also be increased and may cause unwanted toxicity.

If the prescribed analgesia is insufficient, or if the patient's disease progresses, analgesia is escalated in an orderly manner from non-opioid to weak opioid to strong opioid, as illustrated in the World Health Organization's 'Analgesic Ladder' (Table 7.5). 'Weak' opioids are better described as 'opioids for mild to moderate pain' and 'strong' ones as 'opioids for moderate and severe pain'. Non-opioid analgesics should be continued when opioid drugs are commenced,

Table 7.5 The WHO analgesic ladder for cancer pain management

		Analgesics	Examples
Step 1	pain	non-opioid ± adjuvant	aspirin, NSAIDs, paracetamol
Step 2	pain persists or increases	weak opioid ± non-opioid ± adjuvant	codeine, oxycodone, tramadol
Step 3	pain persists or increases	strong opioid ± non-opioid ± adjuvant	morphine, hydromorphone, methadone, oxycodone, fentanyl

From: Cancer Pain Relief. WHO, Geneva, 1986

as their action can be complementary and allow lesser doses of opioids to be used. Adjuvant analgesics should be used whenever indicated.

There is no place for the use of placebo medications in the treatment of chronic pain due to cancer. It is unethical, will lead to distrust if discovered by the patient, and whether or not a response occurs provides no useful information.

Administration

The selected drug or drugs are prescribed in a dose adequate to relieve the pain. A common failing is to give appropriate drugs but in inadequate doses (Figure 7.1a). 'Standard' doses that are appropriate for acute pain have no place in the treatment of chronic cancer-related pain and the dose needs to be titrated against the pain for each individual patient. This individual titration of doses is necessary because there is a wide range of optimal doses resulting from differences in pain sensitivity between individuals and the considerable variation in the analgesic sensitivity of different pains.

The scheduling of drugs is according to pharmacological properties and duration of clinical action. It is important that drugs are given according to a strict schedule, determined by the duration of clinical action, in order to prevent the recurrence of pain (Figure 7.1c). Preventing recurrent pain is important and it is easier to prevent pain than it is to relieve it once it has recurred. Patients given doses that are too small or too infrequent may behave in a manner suggestive of psychological dependence, manipulating the staff for extra doses of medication; this has been termed 'iatrogenic pseudo-addiction' and is resolved by the prescription of doses adequate in amount or frequency to provide continuous pain relief.

There is no place in the treatment of chronic pain due to cancer for giving analgesics on an 'as required' basis or *pro re nata* (PRN). As required or PRN orders invite inadequate treatment: staff may not enquire about pain and patients may not realize they have to ask for analgesics; staff or patients may minimize the number of doses for fear of addiction; or staff may be too busy to tend to requests—all of which result in unrelieved or recurrent pain.

Figure 7.1 Scheduling of drug administration for the treatment of chronic pain. (a) Medication given in inadequate dosage or (b) too infrequently will result in unrelieved pain. (c) The regular scheduling of medication according to the duration of analgesic action will maintain therapeutic drug levels and prevent the recurrence of pain

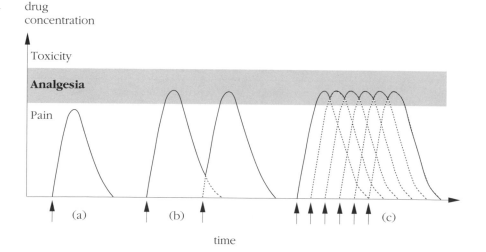

Patients taking a number of different medications should be given written instructions to use at home. These should include the drug names, what each is for, which are to be taken regularly and which are to be taken for a particular indication such as nausea.

It is essential to give the patient instructions for the treatment of breakthrough pain.[10] This is reassuring, avoids the despair that occurs if an analgesic programme is ineffective, and helps the patient feel in control of the situation.

Patients need to be warned of potential adverse effects of the treatment prescribed. For example, unless a patient is warned of the sedation that occurs transiently during the first few days of opioid therapy, the medication may not be taken. Similarly, treatment should be given to avoid preventable adverse effects, such as the prescription of laxatives to prevent constipation when commencing opioids. Fears about dependence and addiction may need to be discussed, although they are never reason to withhold opioid therapy (see Chapter 9).

A patient's analgesic programme should be kept as simple as possible. Too many patients are taking multiple mild analgesics as well as multiple opioid drugs. It is usually possible to simplify the analgesic programme, even for patients with severe pain.

The oral route should be used wherever possible. It has been repeatedly demonstrated that even severe pain can be well controlled with oral medication. Parenteral medication should only be used if the patient is unable to take or retain oral medication or if severe pain has failed to respond satisfactorily.

Continued reassessment is necessary and a number of dose modifications are often required before optimal pain control is achieved. The inevitable progression of the disease also necessitates repeated reassessment and treatment alterations.

Multimodality and multidisciplinary treatment of pain

Analgesics are the cornerstone of the treatment of pain although optimal therapy frequently employs more than one therapeutic modality. The WHO 'Analgesic Ladder' (Table 7.5) does

Figure 7.2 An Inclusive schema for the treatment of pain, including the use of analgesics

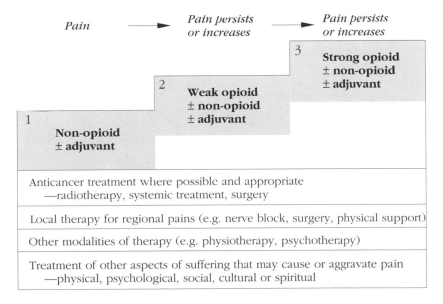

not emphasize the importance of other modalities of pain control and a more inclusive schema is shown in Figure 7.2. The treatment of pain should be part of a multidisciplinary approach to care that includes the assessment and treatment of other aspects of suffering that may cause or aggravate pain.

Barriers to good pain control

Whilst it has been demonstrated that pain can be adequately controlled for the great majority of patients with advanced cancer, using drugs and other treatments that are readily available,[11–13] surveys indicate that up to half of patients still suffer significant pain.[14, 15] Unrelieved pain is more frequent in certain patient groups—female, minorities and the elderly.[12, 16–18] Some of the possible reasons for unrelieved pain are summarized in Table 7.6.

Patients may under report pain for a variety of reasons including concern about adverse effects and dependence.[14, 19, 20] Some patients prefer to put up with their pain.[14] Patient non-compliance may also be significant.[21] It is documented that the pain severity is under-rated by the treatment team compared to the patient's own scoring, and this is more marked when the pain is severe.[22]

Table 7.6 Reasons for unrelieved pain

Related to patient
    failure to report pain or failure to take medication (non-compliance)
        belief that pain is inevitable, belief that pain is untreatable
        putting on a brave face, not wanting to bother the doctor
        adverse effects or fear of them
        fear of tolerance, having nothing in reserve for more severe pain
        fear of dependence, addiction
        physically cannot take the medications prescribed

Related to treatment team
    disbelieve the patient
    inaccurate assessment of the pain severity
    inaccurate assessment of the type and cause of pain
    poor choice of treatment modality, failure to use multiple modalities
    poor use of analgesics
        wrong strength or type of analgesic
        wrong dosage—inadequate, infrequent or PRN
        lack of treatment for incident pain
        lack of provision for breakthrough pain
        failure to warn of, or give treatment to prevent, adverse effects
        failure to use adjuvant analgesics
        withhold opioid analgesics for terminal care or for fear of tolerance, dependence
    failure to both relieve chronic pain and prevent its recurrence
    failure to communicate with and involve the patient in treatment
    failure to provide continuity of care
    failure to assess and treat other aspects of suffering that modify pain
    failure to reassess

Other
    opioid availability
    access to treatment

Table 7.7   RCTs of initiatives to improve pain control

Author	n	Intervention	Outcome
Interventions directed at patients			
de Wit[31]	313	verbal, written, audiotape instruction vs standard care	↓ pain intensity (pS)
Clotfelter[32]	36	video, booklet on pain control vs standard care	↓ pain severity (pS)
Oliver[33]	67	individualized education and coaching vs standard care	↓ average pain severity (pS)
Interventions directed at professionals			
Kravitz[34]	78	visual display of pain intensity at bedside vs no display	no beneficial effect on pain control
Elliott[35]	6	community pain education program vs no program	↓ pain prevalence (pNS) ↑ pain severity (pNS)
Trowbridge[36]	320	patient self-report pain scores sent to oncologist	↓ incidence pain (pS); no ↓ in numbers undertreated
du Pen[30]	81	cancer pain treatment algorithm vs no algorithm	↓ usual pain intensity (pS)

Whilst multidisciplinary palliative care has been shown to improve pain control,[23] there are other studies that document the prescription of inadequate medication.[16] [18,24] This may reflect doctors' lack of knowledge or fears about opioid use. There is a major discrepancy between actual and perceived knowledge with regard to the treatment of cancer pain, even amongst doctors working in a cancer centre.[24]

Incident pain occurs only in certain circumstances, such as the pain that occurs after a particular movement or after certain procedures like the changing of dressings. Incident pain can be very distressing for patients and it should be possible to prevent it by giving appropriate analgesia beforehand.

Breakthrough pain is a transitory increase in pain, increasing to moderate or severe intensity, at a time when chronic pain is well controlled. It occurs in up to 90% of patients with advanced cancer [10,25] and is a significant cause of unrelieved pain. The provision of adequate treatment for breakthrough pain is an important aspect of patient care.[25–27]

A considerable number of educational initiatives designed to improve knowledge about the treatment of cancer pain have been reported. Unfortunately, improvements in knowledge have not translated into improved pain control for patients.[28,29] A number of RCTs have been performed in an attempt to improve pain control (Table 7.7), but with one exception [30] the results show that the interventions have been of limited benefit. In addition to improvements in knowledge, methods are needed to improve the documentation of unrelieved pain, and to ensure that it is promptly assessed and treated.

References

1   Twycross, R. (1994). *Pain Relief in Advanced Cancer*. Edinburgh, Churchill Livingstone.
2   Portenoy, R.K. and Lesage, P. (1999). Management of cancer pain. *Lancet* 353, 1695–700.

3   Foley, K.M. (2001). Management of Cancer Pain. In *Cancer. Principles and Practice of Oncology. 6th edition* (ed. V.T. De Vita, S. Hellman and S.A. Rosenberg). Philadelphia, Lippincott Williams Wilkins.

4   Levy, M.H. (1996). Pharmacologic treatment of cancer pain. *New England Journal of Medicine* 335, 1124–32.

5   Cleary, J.F. (2000). Cancer pain management. *Cancer Control* 7, 120–31.

6   Hewitt, D.J. and Portenoy, R. (1998). Adjuvant drugs for neuropathic cancer pain. In *Topics in Palliative Care. Volume 2* (ed. E. Bruera and R. Portenoy). New York, Oxford University Press.

7   Jadad, A.R. (1998). Opioids in the treatment of neuropathic pain: a systematic review of controlled clinical trials. In *Topics in Palliative Care. Volume 2* (ed. E. Bruera and R. Portenoy). New York, Oxford University Press.

8   Grond, S., et al. (1999). Assessment and treatment of neuropathic cancer pain following WHO guidelines. *Pain* 79, 15–20.

9   Moulin, D.E. (1998). Neuropathic cancer pain: syndromes and clinical controversies. In *Topics in Palliative Care. Volume 2* (ed. E. Bruera and R. Portenoy). New York, Oxford University Press.

10   Zeppetella, G., O'Doherty, C.A. and Collins, S. (2000). Prevalence and characteristics of breakthrough pain in cancer patients admitted to a hospice. *Journal of Pain and Symptom Management* 20, 87–92.

11   Grond, S., et al. (1991). Validation of World Health Organization guidelines for cancer pain relief during the last days and hours of life. *Journal of Pain and Symptom Management* 6, 411–22.

12   Goudas, L., et al. (2001). *Management of cancer pain*. Rockville, MD: Agency for Healthcare Research and Quality. <www.ahrq.gov>

13   Chang, V.T., Hwang, S.S. and Kasimis, B. (2002). Longitudinal documentation of cancer pain management outcomes. A pilot study at a VA medical center. *Journal of Pain and Symptom Management* 24, 494–505.

14   Weiss, S.C., et al. (2001). Understanding the experience of pain in terminally ill patients. *Lancet* 357, 1311–15.

15   Yates, P.M., et al. (2002). Barriers to effective cancer pain management: a survey of hospitalized cancer patients in Australia. *Journal of Pain and Symptom Management* 23, 393–405.

16   Cleeland, C.S., et al. (1997). Pain and treatment of pain in minority patients with cancer. The Eastern Cooperative Oncology Group Minority Outpatient Pain Study. *Annals of Internal Medicine* 127, 813–16.

17   Bernabei, R., et al. (1998). Management of pain in elderly patients with cancer. SAGE Study Group. Systematic Assessment of Geriatric Drug Use via Epidemiology. *Journal of the American Medical Association* 279, 1877–82.

18   Anderson, K.O., et al. (2000). Minority cancer patients and their providers: pain management attitudes and practice. *Cancer* 88, 1929–38.

19   Ward, S.E., et al. (1993). Patient-related barriers to management of cancer pain. *Pain* 52, 319–24.

20   Thomason, T.E., et al. (1998). Cancer pain survey: patient-centered issues in control. *Journal of Pain and Symptom Management* 15, 275–84.

21   Miaskowski, C., et al. (2001). Lack of adherence with the analgesic regimen: a significant barrier to effective cancer pain management. *Journal of Clinical Oncology* 19, 4275–9.

22   Grossman, S.A., et al. (1991). Correlation of patient and caregiver ratings of cancer pain. *Journal of Pain and Symptom Management* 6, 53–7.

23   Higginson, I.J. and Hearn, J. (1997). A multicenter evaluation of cancer pain control by palliative care teams. *Journal of Pain and Symptom Management* 14, 29–35.

24   Cherny, N.I. and Catane, R. (1995). Professional negligence in the management of cancer pain. A case for urgent reforms. *Cancer* 76, 2181–5.

25   Portenoy, R.K. (1997). Treatment of temporal variations in chronic cancer pain. *Seminars in Oncology* 24, S16: 7–12.

26 Cleary, J.F. (1997). Pharmacokinetic and pharmacodynamic issues in the treatment of break-through pain. *Seminars in Oncology* 24, S16: 13–9.

27 Hwang, S.S., Chang, V.T. and Kasimis, B. (2003). Cancer breakthrough pain characteristics and responses to treatment at a VA medical center. *Pain* 101, 55–64.

28 Pargeon, K.L. and Hailey, B.J. (1999). Barriers to effective cancer pain management: a review of the literature. *Journal of Pain and Symptom Management* 18, 358–68.

29 Allard, P., et al. (2001). Educational interventions to improve cancer pain control: a systematic review. *Journal of Palliative Medicine* 4, 191–203.

30 Du Pen, S.L., et al. (1999). Implementing guidelines for cancer pain management: results of a ran-domized controlled clinical trial. *Journal of Clinical Oncology* 17, 361–70.

31 de Wit, R., et al. (1997). A pain education program for chronic cancer pain patients: follow-up results from a randomized controlled trial. *Pain* 73, 55–69.

32 Clotfelter, C.E. (1999). The effect of an educational intervention on decreasing pain intensity in elderly people with cancer. *Oncology Nursing Forum* 26, 27–33.

33 Oliver, J.W., et al. (2001). Individualized patient education and coaching to improve pain control among cancer outpatients. *Journal of Clinical Oncology* 19, 2206–12.

34 Kravitz, R.L., et al. (1996). Bedside charting of pain levels in hospitalized patients with cancer: a randomized controlled trial. *Journal of Pain and Symptom Management* 11, 81–7.

35 Elliott, T.E., et al. (1997). Improving cancer pain management in communities: main results from a randomized controlled trial. *Journal of Pain and Symptom Management* 13, 191–203.

36 Trowbridge, R., et al. (1997). Determining the effectiveness of a clinical-practice intervention in improving the control of pain in outpatients with cancer. *Academic Medicine* 72, 798–800.

8

Non-opioid analgesics

Non-selective COX inhibitors
Selective COX-2 inhibitors
Paracetamol (Acetaminophen)

Non-steroidal anti-inflammatory drugs (NSAIDs)

The non-steroidal anti-inflammatory drugs (NSAIDs) are a structurally diverse group of medications (Table 8.1) that share the ability to inhibit prostaglandin synthetase or cyclo-oxygenase (COX).[1–4]

Table 8.1   NSAIDs

Non-selective COX-1 and COX-2 inhibitors
    salicylates
        aspirin, diflunisal, choline magnesium trisalicylate
    traditional NSAIDs
        acetates: diclofenac, indomethacin, sulindac
        propionates: flurbiprofen, ibuprofen, ketoprofen, ketorolac, naproxen
        oxicams: piroxicam, tenoxicam

Slightly selective COX-2 inhibitors
    meloxicam, nimesulide

Highly selective COX-2 inhibitors (COX-2 specific inhibitors; coxibs)
    celecoxib, rofecoxib, valdecoxib

Centrally acting COX inhibitor
    paracetamol (acetaminophen)

COX inhibition

There are two isoforms of the COX enzyme: COX-1 and COX-2.[5] COX-1 is constitutively expressed in most normal tissues and is responsible for production of prostaglandins necessary for protective and regulatory functions, including maintenance of the gastric mucosa, normal renal function, and platelet aggregation. COX-2 is induced by inflammation, producing the prostaglandins involved in the generation of pain, but is also constitutively expressed in the kidney, brain and premenopausal uterus. Inhibition of COX-2 is responsible for the analgesic and anti-inflammatory properties of NSAIDs, whilst inhibition of COX-1 produces the clinically troublesome adverse effects including gastrointestinal toxicity. The recently introduced COX-2 specific inhibitors (Table 8.1) have been shown to be effective in the treatment of osteoarthritis and rheumatoid arthritis and cause less gastrointestinal toxicity; renal toxicity may be the same as with traditional NSAIDs.

Non-selective COX inhibitors

The actions of non-selective NSAIDs are mediated by the inhibition of both COX-1 and COX-2 in peripheral tissues, reducing the production of prostaglandins. They also act on the cell membrane of neutrophils and macrophages to limit the release of inflammatory mediators. They also have central effects within the central nervous system. NSAIDs reduce central prostaglandin synthesis, are involved in the activation of the central serotonergic pathways, and may act as N-methyl-D-aspartate (NMDA) inhibitors to reduce NMDA-mediated hyperalgesia.[6] In the case of paracetamol, all the effects may be centrally mediated.

Efficacy

NSAIDs are effective analgesics in cancer pain and have analgesic efficacy equivalent to 5–10mg of intramuscular morphine (Table 8.2).[7, 8] They all have a ceiling effect to their analgesic action, but not to their adverse effects. There is considerable variation in both efficacy and toxicity between individual patients and if one NSAID is ineffective or causes unacceptable adverse effects, prescription of another NSAID of differing chemical class (Table 8.1) may be successful. The dose needs to be individually titrated and in all cases the lowest effective dose should be used. Treatment for several days is required to achieve stable plasma levels and maximal effect.

Table 8.2 NSAIDs and cancer pain: RCTs[7, 8]

No. of studies	No. of patients	Results
Comparisons of NSAID with another NSAID or with placebo		
18	1302	NSAIDs significantly more effective than placebo
		No significant differences in efficacy between NSAIDs
Comparisons of NSAID with opioid or of NSAID with NSAID + weak opioid		
25	1563	No significant differences between NSAIDs and NSAID + weak opioid
		NSAIDs equivalent in analgesic efficacy to 5–10mg IM morphine

Pain due to bone metastases has been said to be particularly responsive to NSAIDs. There is no doubt that bone pain responds to NSAIDs,[2, 4, 9] but whether they are superior to other analgesics has not been established. Two RCTs of NSAIDs compared to placebo failed to show a significant benefit; a third trial of patients with bone pain taking oxycodone/acetaminophen showed significant improvement with the addition of ibuprofen (Table 8.4). Continuous intravenous infusion of ketorolac has been reported to relieve intractable bone pain.[10]

NSAIDs may have a role in the treatment of neuropathic pain by virtue of their action at the NMDA receptor. A trial of naproxen and slow release morphine in patients with malignant nerve pain showed that naproxen produced significant pain relief, but not significantly

Table 8.3 General features of non-selective COX inhibitors

Actions	anti-inflammatory, analgesic, antipyretic
Mechanism	inhibition of COX-1 and COX-2 antipyretic action is central
Pharmacology	well absorbed PO, some effective PR considerable pharmacokinetic variation between different drugs metabolized by a variety of pathways, mainly in the liver
Indications	mild to moderate pain disease-related fever
Contraindications	history of hypersensitivity or allergy to NSAIDs or aspirin
Cautions	patients with history of peptic ulcer, erosions thrombocytopenia or other bleeding diathesis patients with asthma, nasal polyps, allergic predisposition
Consider dose reduction	hypoalbuminaemia severe hepatic or renal dysfunction elderly or frail patients
Adverse effects	
gastrointestinal	dyspepsia, erosion, ulceration, bleeding, perforation constipation
haemostasis	inhibition of platelet aggregation (not reversible with aspirin)
renal	fluid retention, renal impairment
hepatic	elevated enzyme levels
neurological	headache, dizziness
skin	rashes
salicylism (aspirin)	nausea, vomiting, dizziness, headaches, tinnitus, deafness
hypersensitivity	allergic reactions

different to morphine; this study has been criticized because the morphine dose was fixed rather than optimized. Ibuprofen was ineffective for the treatment of postherpetic neuralgia (Table 8.5). Continuous subcutaneous infusion of ketorolac has been reported to relieve severe neuropathic pain unresponsive to other therapy.[14]

The use of NSAIDs in conjunction with opioids is logical and may control pain more effectively, given the different mechanisms of action of the two groups of drugs. In addition, there may be an opioid-sparing effect, leading to less opioid-related adverse effects. Several RCTs have reported benefit from combined therapy (Table 8.6), but questions about methodology and the small size of the trials have been raised.[2, 3]

Table 8.4 NSAIDs and bone pain due to cancer: RCTs

Author	n	Intervention	Outcome
Lomen[11]	26	flurbiprofen vs placebo	↓ pain with flurbiprofen (pNS)
Stambaugh[12]	30	oxycodone/acetaminophen + ibuprofen or placebo	↓ pain and other analgesic use with ibuprofen (pS)
Johnson[13]	26	choline magnesium trisalicylate vs placebo	↓ pain with CMT (pNS)

Table 8.5 NSAIDs and neuropathic pain related to cancer: RCTs

Author	n	Intervention	Outcome
Max[15]	20	single dose ibuprofen 800mg vs placebo	ibuprofen ineffective
Dellemijn[16]	16	naproxen 1500mg/d vs morphine SR 60mg/d	↓ pain on naproxen (pS); better pain relief than morphine (pNS)

Table 8.6 NSAIDs and opioids in cancer pain: RCTs

Author	n	Intervention	Outcome
Weingart[17]	14	opioid + ibuprofen or placebo	↓ pain with ibuprofen (pS)
Lomen[11]	26	opioid + flurbiprofen or placebo	↓ pain with flurbiprofen (pNS)
Stambaugh[12]	30	oxycodone/acetaminophen + ibuprofen or placebo	↓ pain and ↓ opioid use with ibuprofen (pS)
Bjorkman[18]	16	morphine + diclofenac or placebo	↓ pain (pNS) and ↓ morphine use (pS) with diclofenac
Mercadante[19]	47	morphine ± ketorolac	↓ pain (pS) and ↓ need for increased morphine (pNS) with ketorolac

Adverse effects

Adverse effects of NSAIDs occur frequently. Each drug has a slightly different toxicity profile.

Gastrointestinal. Gastrointestinal ulceration is the most serious side effect of NSAIDs.[20, 21] NSAIDs produce gastric toxicity by direct local irritation and by inhibition of prostaglandin synthesis, which leads to secretion of more acid and less cytoprotective mucous; this latter mechanism explains the gastric toxicity that occurs after rectal or systemic administration. The prevalence of ulceration in chronic NSAID users is 20–30%, with the great majority involving the stomach; ulceration occurs less frequently in the oesophagus and the small and large bowel. Dyspepsia is reported by about 20% of patients taking NSAIDs, but this does not correlate with gastrointestinal pathology. At least 50% of patients with dyspepsia have no significant mucosal abnormality, and the majority of patients presenting with haemorrhage or perforation have no preceding symptoms.

The risk factors for NSAID-related ulceration are listed in Table 8.7. Patients with advanced cancer are at increased risk for multiple reasons, particularly the co-prescription of corticosteroids.[22] Some NSAIDs are more likely to cause ulceration than others: ibuprofen and diclofenac were associated with lowest risk; indomethacin, naproxen and aspirin were intermediate; and azapropazone, tolmetin, ketoprofen, and piroxicam ranked highest.[23]

All patients with advanced cancer taking NSAIDs should be considered for prophylactic therapy, particularly if they have additional risk factors such as treatment with corticosteroids. The results of a large number of RCTs are analysed in a Cochrane review.[24] Antacids and sucralfate may reduce symptoms but do not protect against ulceration. H_2-receptor antagonists reduce the incidence of duodenal and oesophageal ulceration but do not protect the stomach. Proton pump inhibitors and the prostaglandin analogue, misoprostol, are effective in preventing NSAID-induced gastrointestinal ulceration, but misoprostol causes diarrhoea

Table 8.7 Risk factors for NSAID-associated peptic ulcer[20, 21]

Advanced age (linear increase in risk)
History of peptic ulcer
Higher doses of NSAID, more than one NSAID
Serious systemic disorder

Co-prescription of
    corticosteroids
    anticoagulants
    aspirin (including low dose aspirin)

in up to 40% of patients. Proton pump inhibitors such as lansoprazole are as effective as misoprostol and are better tolerated.[25] Patients requiring continued therapy with NSAIDs should be treated with a proton pump inhibitor such as omeprazole or lansoprazole, which are superior to H_2-receptor antagonists and misoprostol in preventing and healing NSAID-induced lesions and are better tolerated.[25–27]

Haemostasis. NSAIDs cause loss of platelet aggregation by inhibition of COX in platelets. In the case of aspirin, inhibition is irreversible and a single dose may cause prolongation of the clinical bleeding time for 4 to 7 days, until significant numbers of new platelets appear in the circulation. Platelet dysfunction caused by other NSAIDs is reversible and resolves within a day or two of stopping the drug. NSAID-induced platelet dysfunction can cause a significant bleeding tendency in patients with thrombocytopenia or other bleeding diathesis. Patients at risk and those who develop abnormal bleeding should be treated with a non-opioid drug that does not affect platelet function, such as paracetamol or choline magnesium trisalicylate.

Renal. NSAIDs can cause renal impairment in patients with reduced effective circulating volume, who rely on prostaglandin-mediated renal vasodilatation to maintain their renal blood flow. NSAIDs may cause sodium and fluid retention with the development of oedema. Interstitial nephritis is reported, usually after prolonged use.

Hypersensitivity reactions. Hypersensitivity or allergic reactions occur rarely but may be severe and even life threatening. Clinical features include rhinorrhoea, urticaria, angioedema, bronchospasm, and anaphylaxis. Patients at risk include those with a history of sensitivity to aspirin or any other NSAID, asthmatics, and patients with an atopic (allergic) predisposition.

Preparation and dose

A large number of different preparations are available. Some drugs are available in a sustained release formulation that allows once or twice daily administration. Others are available as rectal suppositories for patients unable to take oral medication. If aspirin is used, the enteric-coated form should be employed as it has a lower risk of gastrointestinal toxicity, and the speed of absorption is not important if adequate doses are being given on a regular schedule.

Parenteral NSAIDs

A number of NSAIDs including diclofenac, ketoprofen and ketorolac are available as parenteral preparations. They are useful for the short-term treatment of pain in patients unable to take oral medication. The manufacturer recommends that ketorolac therapy (10–30mg IM q4–6h, up to a maximum of 90mg/d) should not exceed two days because of the risk of gastrointestinal toxicity. Acute renal failure is also reported,[28] although a Cochrane review of the perioperative use of NSAIDs concluded that renal impairment was transient and not clinically important.[29] A review of published case reports of cancer pain treated with ketorolac by subcutaneous infusion identified 88 patients who were treated with 60–150mg/d for a period of 3–185 days.[3] Improvement in pain control was reported in 50–100% of patients, allowing a 5–100% reduction in opioid dose. Gastrointestinal toxicity occurred in 8–14% of patients despite prophylactic treatment with misoprostol or omeprazole. There were no reports of renal impairment.

Intramuscular diclofenac and ketoprofen are effective in the treatment of biliary[30, 31] and ureteric[32] colic.

Topical NSAIDs

Topically applied NSAIDs are effective for both acute and chronic pain associated with non-malignant conditions,[6] but their role in the treatment of pain associated with cancer is not defined. Although only small amounts of drug are systemically absorbed, serious side effects including gastrointestinal bleeding can occur in susceptible individuals.[33]

Selective COX-2 inhibitors

The selective COX-2 inhibitors (coxibs) were developed to provide the analgesic and anti-inflammatory properties of non-selective NSAIDs, whilst minimizing adverse events mediated

Table 8.8 General features of selective COX-2 inhibitors: celecoxib and rofecoxib

Actions	anti-inflammatory, analgesic, antipyretic
Mechanism	inhibition of COX-2
Pharmacology	well absorbed PO plasma half-life: celecoxib 11h, rofecoxib 17h metabolized in the liver
Indications	mild/moderate pain in patients unable to take non-selective NSAID thrombocytopenia or other bleeding diathesis
Dose	celecoxib 100–200mg q12h; rofecoxib 12.5–25mg daily
Duration of action	celecoxib:12–24h; rofecoxib >24h
Contraindications	celecoxib: urticaria or angioedema with NSAIDs or aspirin celecoxib: allergy to sulfonamides
Cautions	patients with history of peptic ulcer, erosions renal impairment, hypertension, hypovolaemia cardiac failure severe hepatic or renal dysfunction elderly or frail patients
Adverse effects gastrointestinal renal hepatic neurological skin hypersensitivity	 nausea, dyspepsia, erosion, ulceration, bleeding, perforation renal impairment, fluid retention, oedema elevated enzyme levels headache, dizziness rashes allergic reactions

by COX-1.[34] Meloxicam, a non-selective NSAID that affects both COX enzymes, is slightly COX-2 selective. Celecoxib and rofecoxib are highly COX-2 selective and show no clinically relevant inhibition of COX-1 at normal doses.[35] The second generation of COX-2 inhibitors includes valdecoxib, parecoxib, etoricoxib and lumaricoxib; parecoxib is an inactive prodrug, which is hydrolysed to valdecoxib after injection.[36]

Celecoxib and rofecoxib have analgesic activity equivalent to traditional non-selective NSAIDs, both for acute pain and for the chronic pain associated with osteoarthritis and rheumatoid arthritis (Table 8.8).[35] These drugs have been used primarily in the treatment of arthritis and their role in the management of pain associated with cancer remains to be defined.[37]

Adverse effects. The selective COX-2 inhibitors are associated with significantly fewer gastrointestinal symptoms, ulcers and ulcer complications than non-selective NSAIDs.[38–40] They have no effect on platelet function. The renal effects are the same as for non-selective NSAIDs;[41, 42] patients with renal impairment, hypertension, or hypovolaemia are at increased risk. Acute neuropsychiatric events including confusion, somnolence, hallucinations and depression have been reported.[43, 44] Celecoxib and rofecoxib do not induce bronchospasm in patients with aspirin- or NSAID-induced asthma.[45, 46] Aspirin- or NSAID-induced urticaria or angioedema is reported to occur in one-third of patients given celecoxib, but rarely with rofecoxib.[47, 48] Celecoxib is contraindicated in patients allergic to sulfonamides, although this cross-reactivity has been questioned.[49] Rare fatal reactions have been reported.[50, 51]

Table 8.9 Paracetamol (Acetaminophen)

Actions	analgesic, antipyretic
Mechanism of action	inhibition of prostaglandin synthesis in the CNS
Pharmacology	well absorbed from small intestine, rectum plasma half-life 2–4h conjugated in liver, excreted in urine
Indications	mild to moderate skeletal and soft tissue pain fever hypersensitivity to aspirin, NSAIDs peptic ulceration or gastric intolerance of aspirin, NSAIDs significant thrombocytopenia or bleeding diathesis
Dose	500–1000 mg q4–6h (maximum 4g/d)
Duration of action	4–6h
Contraindications	allergy to paracetamol (rare)
Cautions	severe hepatic dysfunction elderly or frail patients alcoholic liver disease
Adverse effects	allergic rash (rare) hepatic dysfunction constipation (mild)
Drug interactions	potentiates warfarin[53]
Preparations	tablets, capsules, suspension, suppositories

Paracetamol (Acetaminophen)

Paracetamol is a synthetic derivative of acetanilide and is widely used in oncology and palliative care (Table 8.9). It has little affinity for either COX-1 or COX-2 in peripheral tissues and is thought to act by inhibition of prostaglandin synthesis in the central nervous system (CNS).[52] It has analgesic and antipyretic effects but virtually no anti-inflammatory action.

The standard adult dose is 500–1000 mg, 4- to 6-hourly, with a recommended maximum of 4g per day. The oral and rectal doses are the same, although rectal absorption may be slower and less complete.

Adverse effects. At normal therapeutic doses, the side effects of paracetamol are few and it does not interfere with platelet function or cause gastric irritation or bleeding. Warfarin therapy should be carefully monitored.[53]

Hepatic toxicity. In overdosage (of the order of 15g for a 60kg person), saturation of the metabolic pathways leads to the accumulation of a toxic metabolite that causes hepatocellular necrosis and liver failure. Taken with therapeutic intent, chronic ingestion of more than 4g per day may predispose to hepatic toxicity in patients with reduced glutathione stores, including the elderly and those with a poor nutritional status.[52] Alcohol increases the production of the hepatotoxic metabolite of paracetamol[54] and hepatic toxicity may occur more frequently in regular users of alcohol.[55] Patients with alcoholic liver disease did not show adverse effects from paracetamol 4g per day, given at a time when they were abstinent.[56]

References

1   Pace, V. (1995). Use of nonsteroidal anti-inflammatory drugs in cancer. *Palliative Medicine* 9, 273–86.

2   Jenkins, C.A. and Bruera, E. (1999). Nonsteroidal anti-inflammatory drugs as adjuvant analgesics in cancer patients. *Palliative Medicine* 13, 183–96.

3   Shah, S. and Hardy, J. (2001). Non-steroidal anti-inflammatory drugs in cancer pain: a review of the literature as relevant to palliative care. *Progress in Palliative Care* 9, 3–7.

4   Wallenstein, D.J. and Portenoy, R.K. (2002). Nonopioid and adjuvant analgesics. In *Principles and Practice of Palliative Care and Supportive Oncology* (ed. A.M. Berger, R.K. Portenoy and D.E. Weissman). Philadelphia, Lippincott, Williams and Wilkins.

5   Hawkey, C.J. (1999). COX-2 inhibitors. *Lancet* 353, 307–14.

6   McQuay, H.J. and Moore, R.A. (1998). *An evidence-based resource for pain relief.* Oxford, Oxford University Press.

7   Goudas, L., et al. (2001). *Management of cancer pain.* Rockville, MD: Agency for Healthcare Research and Quality. <www.ahrq.gov>

8   Carr, D., et al. (2002). *Management of Cancer Symptoms: Pain, Depression, and Fatigue. Evidence Report/Technology Assessment No. 61.* Rockville, MD: Agency for Healthcare Research and Quality. <www.ahrq.gov>

9   Mercadante, S., et al. (1999). Analgesic effects of nonsteroidal anti-inflammatory drugs in cancer pain due to somatic or visceral mechanisms. *Journal of Pain and Symptom Management* 17, 351–6.

10 Gordon, R.L. (1998). Prolonged central intravenous ketorolac continuous infusion in a cancer patient with intractable bone pain. *Annals of Pharmacotherapy* 32, 193–6.

11 Lomen, P.L., et al. (1986). Flurbiprofen for the treatment of bone pain in patients with metastatic breast cancer. *American Journal of Medicine* 80, 83–7.

12 Stambaugh, J.E., Jr. and Drew, J. (1988). The combination of ibuprofen and oxycodone/acetaminophen in the management of chronic cancer pain. *Clinical Pharmacology and Therapeutics* 44, 665–9.

13 Johnson, J.R. and Miller, A.J. (1994). The efficacy of choline magnesium trisalicylate (CMT) in the management of metastatic bone pain: a pilot study. *Palliative Medicine* 8, 129–35.

14 Ripamonti, C., et al. (1996). Continuous subcutaneous infusion of ketorolac in cancer neuro-pathic pain unresponsive to opioid and adjuvant drugs. A case report. *Tumori* 82, 413–15.

15 Max, M.B., et al. (1988). Association of pain relief with drug side effects in postherpetic neuralgia: a single-dose study of clonidine, codeine, ibuprofen, and placebo. *Clinical Pharmacology and Therapeutics* 43, 363–71.

16 Dellemijn, P.L., et al. (1994). Medical therapy of malignant nerve pain. A randomised double-blind explanatory trial with naproxen versus slow-release morphine. *European Journal of Cancer* 30A, 1244–50.

17 Weingart, W.A., Sorkness, C.A. and Earhart, R.H. (1985). Analgesia with oral narcotics and added ibuprofen in cancer patients. *Clinical Pharmacy* 4, 53–8.

18 Bjorkman, R., Ullman, A. and Hedner, J. (1993). Morphine-sparing effect of diclofenac in cancer pain. *European Journal of Clinical Pharmacology* 44, 1–5.

19 Mercadante, S., Fulfaro, F. and Casuccio, A. (2002). A randomised controlled study on the use of anti-inflammatory drugs in patients with cancer pain on morphine therapy: effects on dose-escalation and a pharmacoeconomic analysis. *European Journal of Cancer* 38, 1358–63.

20 Wolfe, M.M., Lichtenstein, D.R. and Singh, G. (1999). Gastrointestinal toxicity of nonsteroidal antiinflammatory drugs. *New England Journal of Medicine* 340, 1888–99.

21 Hawkins, C. and Hanks, G.W. (2000). The gastroduodenal toxicity of nonsteroidal anti-inflammatory drugs: a review of the literature. *Journal of Pain and Symptom Management* 20, 140–51.

22 Hawkins, C. (1998). Audit and use of NSAIDs. *Lancet* 352, 658.

23 Henry, D., et al. (1996). Variability in risk of gastrointestinal complications with individual non-steroidal anti-inflammatory drugs: results of a collaborative meta-analysis. *British Medical Journal* 312, 1563–6.

24 Rostom, A., et al. (2002). Prevention of NSAID-induced gastroduodenal ulcers (Cochrane Review). *Cochrane Database of Systematic Reviews* CD002296.

25 Graham, D.Y., et al. (2002). Ulcer prevention in long-term users of nonsteroidal anti-inflammatory drugs: results of a double-blind, randomized, multicenter, active- and placebo-controlled study of misoprostol vs lansoprazole. *Archives of Internal Medicine* 162, 169–75.

26 Hawkey, C.J., et al. (1998). Omeprazole compared with misoprostol for ulcers associated with nonsteroidal antiinflammatory drugs. Omeprazole versus Misoprostol for NSAID-induced Ulcer Management (OMNIUM) Study Group. *New England Journal of Medicine* 338, 727–34.

27 Yeomans, N.D., et al. (1998). A comparison of omeprazole with ranitidine for ulcers associated with nonsteroidal antiinflammatory drugs. Acid Suppression Trial: Ranitidine versus Omeprazole for NSAID-associated Ulcer Treatment (ASTRONAUT) Study Group. *New England Journal of Medicine* 338, 719–26.

28 Feldman, H.I., et al. (1997). Parenteral ketorolac: the risk for acute renal failure. *Annals Internal Medicine* 126, 193–9.

29 Lee, A., et al. (2001). Effects of nonsteroidal anti-inflammatory drugs on post-operative renal function in normal adults (Cochrane Review). *Cochrane Database of Systematic Reviews* CD002765.

30 Akriviadis, E.A., et al. (1997). Treatment of biliary colic with diclofenac: a randomized, double-blind, placebo-controlled study. *Gastroenterology* 113, 225–31.

31 Dula, D.J., Anderson, R. and Wood, G.C. (2001). A prospective study comparing i.m. ketorolac with i.m. meperidine in the treatment of acute biliary colic. *Journal of Emergency Medicine* 20, 121–4.

32 Collaborative Group of the Spanish Society of Clinical Pharmacology (1991). Comparative study of the efficacy of dipyrone, diclofenac sodium and pethidine in acute renal colic. *European Journal of Clinical Pharmacology* 40, 543–6.

33 Zimmerman, J., Siguencia, J. and Tsvang, E. (1995). Upper gastrointestinal hemorrhage associated with cutaneous application of diclofenac gel. *American Journal of Gastroenterology* 90, 2032–4.

34 FitzGerald, G.A. and Patrono, C. (2001). The coxibs, selective inhibitors of cyclooxygenase-2. *New England Journal of Medicine* 345, 433–42.

35 Shah, S. and Hardy, J. (2001). A review of the COX-2 inhibitors. *Progress in Palliative Care* 9, 47–52.

36 Stichtenoth, D.O. and Frolich, J.C. (2003). The Second Generation of COX-2 Inhibitors: What Advantages Do the Newest Offer? *Drugs* 63, 33–45.

37 Ruoff, G. and Lema, M. (2003). Strategies in Pain Management. New and Potential Indications for COX-2 Specific Inhibitors. *Journal of Pain and Symptom Management* 25, 21–31.

38 Deeks, J.J., Smith, L.A. and Bradley, M.D. (2002). Efficacy, tolerability, and upper gastrointestinal safety of celecoxib for treatment of osteoarthritis and rheumatoid arthritis: systematic review of randomised controlled trials. *British Medical Journal* 325, 619.

39 Mamdani, M., et al. (2002). Observational study of upper gastrointestinal haemorrhage in elderly patients given selective cyclo-oxygenase-2 inhibitors or conventional non-steroidal anti-inflammatory drugs. *British Medical Journal* 325, 624.

40 Laine, L. (2003). Gastrointestinal effects of NSAIDs and coxibs. *Journal of Pain and Symptom Management* 25, 32–40.

41 Brater, D.C. (2002). Renal effects of cyclooxygyenase-2-selective inhibitors. *Journal of Pain and Symptom Management* 23, S15–20.

42 DeMaria, A.N. and Weir, M.R. (2003). Coxibs-Beyond the GI Tract. Renal and Cardiovascular Issues. *Journal of Pain and Symptom Management* 25, 41–9.

43 Committee on Safety of Medicines (2000). In Focus: Rofecoxib (Vioxx). *Current Problems in Pharmacovigilance* 26, 13.

44 Adverse Drug Reactions Advisory Committee (2003). Acute neuropsychiatric events with celecoxib and rofecoxib. *Australian Adverse Drug Reactions Bulletin* 22, 3.

45 Stevenson, D.D. and Simon, R.A. (2001). Lack of cross-reactivity between rofecoxib and aspirin in aspirin-sensitive patients with asthma. *Journal of Allergy and Clinical Immunology* 108, 47–51.

46 Woessner, K.M., Simon, R.A. and Stevenson, D.D. (2002). The safety of celecoxib in patients with aspirin-sensitive asthma. *Arthritis and Rheumatism* 46, 2201–6.

47 Sanchez Borges, M., et al. (2001). Tolerability to new COX-2 inhibitors in NSAID-sensitive patients with cutaneous reactions. *Annals of Allergy, Asthma & Immunology* 87, 201–4.

48 Pacor, M.L., et al. (2002). Safety of rofecoxib in subjects with a history of adverse cutaneous reactions to aspirin and/or non-steroidal anti-inflammatory drugs. *Clinical and Experimental Allergy* 32, 397–400.

49 Shapiro, L.E., et al. (2003). Safety of celecoxib in individuals allergic to sulfonamide: a pilot study. *Drug Safety* 26, 187–95.

50 Kumar, N.P., et al. (2002). Fatal haemorrhagic pulmonary oedema and associated angioedema after the ingestion of rofecoxib. *Postgraduate Medical Journal* 78, 439–40.

51 Schneider, F., et al. (2002). Fatal allergic vasculitis associated with celecoxib. *Lancet* 359, 852–3.

52 Twycross, R. (2000). Paracetamol. *Progress in Palliative Care* 8, 198–202.

53 Hylek, E.M., et al. (1998). Acetaminophen and other risk factors for excessive warfarin anticoagulation. *Journal of the American Medical Association* 279, 657–62.

54 Thummel, K.E., et al. (2000). Ethanol and production of the hepatotoxic metabolite of acetaminophen in healthy adults. *Clinical Pharmacology and Therapeutics* 67, 591–9.

55 Zimmerman, H.J. and Maddrey, W.C. (1995). Acetaminophen (paracetamol) hepatotoxicity with regular intake of alcohol: analysis of instances of therapeutic misadventure. *Hepatology* 22, 767–73.

56 Kuffner, E.K., et al. (2001). Effect of maximal daily doses of acetaminophen on the liver of alcoholic patients: a randomized, double-blind, placebo-controlled trial. *Archives of Internal Medicine* 161, 2247–52.

9

Opioid analgesics

Classifications	Opioid substitution
Actions	Adverse effects
Indications	Tolerance, physical and psychological dependence
Contraindications	Opiophobia: the underutilization of opioids

Extracts of the oriental poppy *Papaver somniferum* have been used since antiquity for their analgesic and euphoriant properties. The term opium derives from *opus*, the name applied to poppy juices by the Greek, Theophrastus, in the third century BC. The term morphia derives from *morphium*, the name given to an alkaloid extracted from opium by the German chemist Sertürner in the early 1800s. Since the isolation of morphia, several other substances have been isolated from opium and a number of semisynthetic and synthetic opioid drugs have been developed. The opioid analgesics are defined as drugs having morphine-like effects.

Classifications

Strong and weak opioids

The 'weak' opioids, as might be used in Step 2 of the WHO Analgesic Ladder (Table 7.5), are better termed 'opioids for mild to moderate pain' (Table 9.1). Codeine is the prototype 'weak' opioid; oxycodone used in lower dose or tramadol are alternatives. Morphine is the prototype strong opioid; hydromorphone, fentanyl, oxycodone or methadone are suitable alternatives.

Agonists and antagonists

Knowledge of the actions of the partial agonist and mixed agonist–antagonist drugs is important as their inadvertent use may lead to unanticipated complications.

An *agonist* drug binds to a receptor and produces a physiological effect. The prototype agonist is morphine, which binds to the mu receptor to produce analgesia.

An *antagonist* drug binds to a receptor without producing a physiological effect and can prevent binding of an agonist to, or displace it from, the receptor. Naloxone prevents or reverses the effect of morphine at the mu receptor.

Table 9.1 Classifications of opioid drugs

Class	Weak	Strong
Agonist	codeine dextropropoxyphene dihydrocodeine tramadol	dextromoramide diamorphine (heroin) fentanyl hydromorphone levorphanol methadone morphine oxycodone pethidine (meperidine)
Partial agonist		buprenorphine
Mixed agonist–antagonist		butorphanol nalbuphine pentazocine
Antagonist	naloxone	

A *partial agonist* has less intrinsic activity at the receptor site than a full agonist. It will produce less effect than the full agonist and will exhibit a ceiling effect above which increasing doses produce no extra effect. If the partial agonist has greater affinity for the receptors than the full agonist, it may displace the full agonist. Buprenorphine is the partial agonist used in clinical practice. Given alone, it has an agonist action; given in low dose with an agonist it will have no adverse effect, but given in higher dose it will act as an antagonist and may precipitate pain and withdrawal symptoms.[1]

A *mixed agonist–antagonist* has agonist effects when given alone but can act as an antagonist when given with or after another agonist. Pentazocine is a mixed agonist–antagonist. Given alone, it will have an agonist action at the kappa receptor and a partial agonist action at the mu receptor; given with mu agonist, it may have an antagonist action and precipitate pain and withdrawal symptoms.

Actions

Mechanism of action: the opioid receptors

Morphine and other opioid analgesics act by interaction with the opioid receptors in the brain, spinal cord, and some peripheral tissues.[2] These receptors normally interact with a range of endogenous opioid substances including the endorphins, dynorphins and enkephalins. There are a number of different types of opioid receptors including mu, delta and kappa. Analgesia is primarily mediated by the mu receptor, which is also responsible for the adverse effects of respiratory depression, reduced gastrointestinal motility, miosis, euphoria and physical dependence. The kappa and delta receptors mediate some analgesia as well as sedation, respiratory depression and the dysphoric and psychotomimetic effects.

Clinical effect

The analgesic and adverse effects of individual opioid drugs depend on a number of factors including dose, route of administration, pattern of interaction with the opioid receptors, and whether it is a full or partial agonist. Partial agonists display a ceiling effect to their analgesic action. Pure agonists such as morphine have a wide therapeutic range, producing analgesia in a dose-dependent manner without an apparent ceiling to the effect; the useful dose is limited by adverse side effects.

Opioids act on the opioid receptors in the brain and spinal cord to produce analgesia. The perception of pain is altered both by a direct effect on the spinal cord, modulating peripheral nociceptive input, and by activation of the descending inhibitory systems from the brain stem and basal ganglia. Opioids also act on the limbic system and on higher centres to modify the emotional response to pain.

The systemic effects, including those affecting the gastrointestinal and respiratory tracts, are partly centrally mediated via the autonomic nervous system and may partly be due to a direct effect on opioid receptors in the peripheral tissues.

Indications and uses

Opioids, and morphine in particular, are the drugs of choice for moderate and severe cancer-related pain.

There are no standard doses of opioid drugs for the treatment of chronic pain in patients with cancer. They must be individually titrated for each patient and the correct dose is that which controls the pain whilst causing acceptable adverse effects. The dose required will depend on the severity of the pain, the type of pain, individual pharmacokinetic variations, the development of tolerance, as well as the psychosocial issues that affect the perception of pain.

Opioid-sensitive and opioid-insensitive pain. Opioid analgesics are not equally effective against all types of pain. Neuropathic pain may be less sensitive than somatic and visceral pain. However, because of the wide range of doses that can be employed, the difference between opioid-sensitive and opioid-insensitive pain should be regarded as relative rather than absolute. In the case of neuropathic pain, adequate analgesia may require higher doses of opioids, leading to troublesome adverse effects.[3–5]

Contraindications

Opioids should be given with caution to patients with renal impairment, severe hepatic dysfunction, significant pulmonary disease (including acute or severe bronchial asthma), and CNS depression from any cause. Elderly patients and those who are debilitated or cachectic should initially be treated with reduced doses.

Opioid intolerance and 'allergy'. Patients may present with a history of having been told they were allergic to morphine or another opioid. This frequently relates to nausea or vomiting that occurred after a parenteral opioid injection was given for acute pain to an opioid naive patient. A careful history is required to determine the exact circumstances of the reaction. Given explanation, reassurance, and the cover of antiemetic therapy for the first few days, most of these patients can be commenced on opioids without ill effect.

A small proportion of patients will suffer intolerable sedation or nausea that does not improve after the first few days of therapy and which cannot be attributed to other causes. These patients should be considered intolerant of the drug they are taking and an alternative opioid substituted.

Opioid substitution

With the increasing availability of a range of opioid drugs—morphine, hydromorphone, methadone, oxycodone, and fentanyl—it has become common practice for patients with inadequate analgesia or troublesome adverse effects to be tried on a different drug.[6, 7] This may involve a single substitution or sequential trials with several drugs. Substitution of one opioid drug for another has been termed opioid switching or opioid rotation. Opioid substitution results in improved analgesia and fewer adverse effects for many patients.[8–11]

Opioid substitution is only one means of addressing inadequate analgesia or troublesome adverse effects. If the lack of effect is due to disease progression, use of adjuvant analgesics or radiotherapy may improve pain control; if it is due to the development of significant tolerance, changing to a different drug is likely to be necessary. Some opioid side effects can be adequately palliated with other medications.

Equianalgesic doses

When changing from one opioid drug to another, it is necessary to know the approximate equianalgesic doses of the two drugs (Table 9.2). These conversion factors are approximate and do not take into account individual patient variation. Cross-tolerance may differ at high doses compared to low ones, and may vary according to the direction in which the switch is made.[12–14] In some cases they are derived from studies of single doses rather than

Table 9.2 Approximate equianalgesic doses of opioid analgesics

	Parenteral	Oral
Morphine	10 mg	30 mg
Buprenorphine	0.3 mg	0.4 mg SL
Codeine	–	240 mg
Diamorphine (heroin)	5–8 mg	20 mg
Hydromorphone	1.5 mg	7.5 mg
Levorphanol	2 mg	4 mg
Methadone	10 mg	20 mg
Oxycodone	–	20 mg
Pentazocine	60 mg	180 mg
Pethidine (meperidine)	75 mg	300 mg
Tramadol	80 mg	120 mg
These conversion factors are approximate and do not take into account individual patient variation		

Table 9.3 Guidelines for opioid substitution

Calculate the equianalgesic dose of the new drug

Decrease the dose by 25–50% to accommodate cross-tolerance
 reduce by 75% if changing to methadone
 do not reduce if changing to TD fentanyl

Adjust according to prior pain control
 reduce less if patient in severe pain

Adjust according to the patient's general condition
 reduce more if elderly, frail, or significant organ dysfunction

Give 50–100% of the 4-hourly dose for breakthrough pain

Reassess and titrate new opioid against pain and side effects

continued therapy. Each drug must be titrated against pain and adverse effects for each individual patient.[12–14] General guidelines for substituting one opioid for another are shown in Table 9.3.

Adverse effects

The adverse effects of opioid analgesics are summarized in Table 9.4. There is considerable variation in these effects between individual patients and between different drugs. The common adverse effects in practice are constipation, sedation and nausea.

Table 9.4 Adverse effects of opioids

Central	sedation, cognitive impairment, delirium, narcosis, coma
	dysphoria and psychotomimetic effects
	myoclonus, seizures, hyperalgesia
	miosis
Gastrointestinal	nausea, vomiting, delayed gastric emptying, constipation
	dry mouth
Respiratory	respiratory depression
	suppression of cough reflex
Cardiovascular	postural hypotension
Urinary	urgency, retention
Skin	flushing, sweating, pruritus

There is little evidence that any one opioid agonist has a substantially better adverse effect profile, given the recommendation to avoid pethidine (meperidine) and the mixed agonist–antagonist drugs in palliative care.

The assessment and management of the adverse effects of opioid drugs is summarized in Table 9.5. It is important to consider other possible causes and to employ additional modalities of pain control that may allow reduction of the opioid dose,[15] particularly if the adverse effects develop after a period of stable analgesia. The evidence of benefit for changing the route of administration is weak, with the possible exception of spinal therapy.[16, 17]

Table 9.5 Guidelines for assessment and management of adverse effects of opioid drugs

Consider other causes for the symptoms
    related to underlying disease
    related to other drugs or a drug-opioid interaction

Consider other methods to improve pain control, allowing opioid dose reduction
    adjuvant analgesics, nerve blocks, surgery
    disease modifying: radiotherapy, systemic therapy

Symptomatic management of the adverse effect

Consider changing the route of administration

Opioid substitution

Sedation

Some sedation often occurs with the commencement of opioid therapy. It is usually mild and lasts 2 to 5 days. Patients should be warned of this possibility, reassured that it is likely to improve within a few days and encouraged to persevere with their medication through this period. In a few cases, severe drowsiness and confusion occurs, necessitating dose reduction. Factors predisposing to sedation are listed in Table 9.6.

Table 9.6 Factors predisposing to sedation

Elderly or frail patients

Renal impairment

Other causes of CNS depression, including other medications

Opioid naive patients

Patients with only mild pain

Patients whose pain has been acutely relieved by a procedure such as a nerve block

Persistent sedation requires assessment of renal function, and exclusion of other causes of CNS depression including metabolic disturbances, infection, cerebral metastases, and the effects of other drugs.

Unless there is a readily correctable metabolic cause or other less necessary medication can be withheld, persistent sedation is best treated by substitution of a different opioid, which may

Table 9.7 Methylphenidate for opioid-induced sedation: RCTs

Author	n	Intervention	Outcome
Bruera[19]	28	methylphenidate 10mg mane + 5mg noon vs placebo	methylphenidate: ↓ pain score, ↓ extra doses, ↑ activity, ↓ drowsiness (all pS)
Bruera[20]	20	methylphenidate 10mg mane + 5mg noon vs placebo	methylphenidate: improved cognitive function (pS)
Wilwerding[21]	43	methylphenidate 10mg mane + 5mg noon vs placebo	methylphenidate: ↓ drowsiness (pNS)

lead to significant improvement.[8-11] Methylphenidate is effective in counteracting sedation and may enhance analgesia (Table 9.7); there may be a risk of dysphoric reactions to the stimulant in patients who are elderly or frail. Donepezil, an oral acetylcholinesterase inhibitor, is also reported to be effective for opioid-related sedation.[18]

Driving. Opioid therapy need not necessarily be a contraindication to driving a car. Many patients with advanced cancer are too weak or ill to consider driving, but for others the ability to drive a car constitutes an important part of their personal and social lives. Patients on a stable dose of morphine, without other medical contraindications to driving, should be capable of driving safely.[22] They should be encouraged to assess their ability before venturing on to the open road by having a 'test drive' in quiet surroundings, with someone else in the car, to check they are sufficiently strong and alert, and can react quickly enough, to control the vehicle safely. Patients with advanced cancer who are able to drive safely despite taking morphine should nevertheless be advised to avoid heavy traffic and long journeys.

Narcosis

Severe sedation or narcosis, with respiratory depression and loss of consciousness, can occur if the dose prescribed is too large or if the patient takes an intentional overdose; the latter is likely to be more severe. The risk factors for narcosis are the same as listed above for sedation (Table 9.6).

The treatment of narcosis is with naloxone (Table 9.8) as well as respiratory and circulatory support. The minimum effective dose of naloxone should be used, the aim being to improve respiratory function without reversing analgesia or precipitating physical opioid withdrawal.[23] The recommended method is to dilute one ampoule of naloxone (0.4mg in 1ml) with 9ml of saline or dextrose and give 1–2ml every 3 minutes. This will lessen the chances of the patient suddenly waking up in severe pain and very agitated.

Table 9.8   Naloxone: treatment of narcosis and respiratory depression

Initial therapy
    iatrogenic respiratory depression
        respiration <5/min
            naloxone 0.4mg IV or SC stat
        respiration <8/min, or not rousable, or cyanosed (SaO$_2$ <90%)
            naloxone 0.4mg in 10ml, 1–2ml IV or SC q3min
        respiration >8/min, rousable, not cyanosed (SaO$_2$>90%)
            careful observation
    known or suspected overdose
        naloxone 0.4–2.0 mg IV or SC, q3 min, up to 5 doses
    note
        the minimum effective dose of naloxone should be used.
        if the above doses or a total of 10 mg are ineffective, an opioid effect is unlikely.
        buprenorphine may require larger doses (8–16 mg) to reverse narcosis.

Continued therapy
    repeated injections of the same dose that produced initial response
        as often as required to maintain adequate respiration respiration
    continuous infusion of 2/3 initial successful dose per hour and titrated against effect
    for the duration of action of the responsible drug

Other neuropsychological effects

Cognitive impairment can occur with opioid drugs.[24] It is reported most frequently with morphine, although that may simply reflect the frequency with which the drug is used. Predisposing factors include the dose, and the patient's age, renal function and general frailty. Substitution of an alternative opioid may lead to improvement,[8, 9, 11] although there can be significant differences between patient self-reports and objective assessment of cognitive function.[25]

Psychotomimetic or dysphoric side effects may occur with morphine or other opioid drugs and most frequently manifest as apprehension, confusion, hallucinations or nightmares. If necessary, treatment with a tranquillizer (e.g. haloperidol) may be beneficial; if severe, substituting an alternative opioid should be considered. Psychotomimetic side effects occur in less than 1–2% of patients on morphine but are reported in up to 10% of patients taking pentazocine.

Multifocal myoclonus may occur with high doses of any of the opioid drugs.[26] It may occur with high doses of morphine or hydromorphone, or with normal doses in the terminal phase when there is deterioration of renal function. In terminal care, myoclonus can be palliated with a benzodiazepine; in other situations it is best managed by changing to an alternative opioid, which frequently leads to resolution.[8, 9, 27]

Opioid hyperexcitability and hyperalgesia: opioid-induced pain. Pethidine (meperidine) is not recommended for use in palliative care because of the neurotoxicity related to the accumulation of the metabolite, norpethidine (normeperidine). With continued dosing, the clinical picture progresses from mild nervousness to tremors and twitches, multifocal myoclonus, and generalized seizures; the neurotoxicity correlates with plasma norpethidine levels.[28]

Similar syndromes are reported with high doses of other opioids.[27, 29] Myoclonus and seizures occur, as well as hyperalgesia (manifest as exacerbations of pain), whole-body allodynia (manifest as pain on being touched or at all points of body contact), and delirium.[30] Treatment is by rapid dose reduction and substitution of an alternative opioid such as methadone.[27, 31] Benzodiazepines are given for seizures and myoclonus.

Gastrointestinal

Nausea occurs frequently when opioid therapy is commenced; vomiting is less common.[32] The nausea is usually mild and subsides after a few days. It is due to a direct effect on the chemoreceptor trigger zone in the medulla, compounded by any opioid-related gastric stasis and constipation. Patients should be warned of the possibility of nausea for a few days after starting therapy and given a supply of antiemetics to take if need be. Prophylactic antiemetics should be given if there is a history of nausea and vomiting with previous opioid therapy or if other potential causes of nausea and vomiting are present.

There are no controlled studies comparing the efficacy and tolerability of different antiemetics in the treatment of opioid-induced nausea and vomiting. Knowledge of the neurotransmitters involved at the chemoreceptor trigger zone suggest that antidopaminergic drugs (eg haloperidol, metoclopramide) and $5HT_3$ receptor antagonists will be effective, which is in keeping with clinical observation. However, an RCT comparing ondansetron, metoclopramide and placebo reported the active agents to be no better than placebo in the control of opioid-induced emesis.[33] Opioid substitution may result in significantly less nausea and vomiting.[8–10]

Opioids reduce gastrointestinal secretions and motility, leading to delayed gastric emptying and constipation. Constipation will occur in all patients taking opioids regularly, with

Table 9.9 Opioid antagonists for opioid-induced constipation: RCTs

Author	n	Intervention	Outcome
Sykes[34]	17	naloxone PO (≤ 10% morphine dose) vs placebo	naloxone: no laxative effect, pain, or withdrawal
Sykes[34]	10	naloxone PO (20–80% morphine dose)	naloxone had a laxative effect, but caused pain (1 patient) and withdrawal (2 patients)
Yuan[35]	22	IV methylnaltrexone vs placebo	laxative effect 100%; no withdrawal
Liu[36]	9	naloxone PO 2mg or 4mg tds vs placebo	naloxone had a laxative effect, but caused pain (3 patients), withdrawal (1 patient)

the exception of those with an ileostomy or diarrhoea secondary to malabsorption. Every patient commencing therapy with an opioid requires dietary advice and the prescription of laxatives to *prevent* constipation. Tolerance does not develop to the constipating effects of opioids and dietary and laxative therapy is necessary for the duration of treatment. If refractory to standard measures, substitution of a different opioid should be considered.

Oral naloxone is effective in counteracting opioid-induced constipation, but there is an unacceptable incidence of recurrent pain and symptoms of opioid withdrawal. Methylnaltrexone, an opioid antagonist that does not cross the blood-brain barrier, is effective for methadone-related constipation and does not cause withdrawal symptoms (Table 9.9). It is also effective orally, and trials on cancer patients with pain are awaited. Opioid rotation from morphine to methadone is reported to be associated with less constipation.[10]

Xerostomia occurs in significant proportion of patients on chronic morphine therapy. Treatment is symptomatic. If severe, an assessment for other causes should be made, especially drugs with anticholinergic side effects.

Respiratory

Respiratory depression occurs due to a direct effect on the respiratory centres in the brain stem. There is decreased sensitivity to the circulating carbon dioxide level and reduction in both tidal volume and respiratory rate. Factors predisposing to respiratory depression are listed in Table 9.10.

Patients with cancer and pain are unlikely to develop respiratory depression for several reasons. First, they have pain, which has been described as the physiological antagonist to the

Table 9.10 Factors predisposing to respiratory depression

Patients at risk of respiratory depression for other reasons
Morphine given in excessive dosage and/or too frequently
Renal impairment
Other causes of CNS depression
Opioid naive patients
Patients with only mild pain
Patients whose pain has been acutely relieved by a procedure such as a nerve block

respiratory depressant effect of opioids. Second, most have been taking weak opioids and are not opioid naive. Third, they frequently use oral medication with lower peak concentrations. Fourth, the dose has usually been slowly titrated up against pain. There is no evidence that equianalgesic doses of the various opioid analgesics differ significantly in their potential to cause respiratory depression.

Significant respiratory depression may occur in patients who are at risk of respiratory failure for other reasons. In patients bordering on respiratory failure, opioid analgesics will reduce the response to rising carbon dioxide levels and continued respiration depends on hypoxic drive; administration of oxygen in this situation can be fatal.

In patients with intracranial malignancies, the increased arterial carbon dioxide tension that occurs following opioid administration may cause cerebrovascular dilatation and a paradoxical increase in headache.

Opioid drugs suppress the cough reflex by a direct effect on the cough centre in the brain stem. This may be of benefit for patients with intractable cough but may complicate the treatment of chest infection.

Tolerance, physical dependence and psychological dependence

Lack of understanding about tolerance and dependence is a common cause for the underuse of opioid analgesics for cancer-related pain. Concerns about tolerance, physical dependence or psychological dependence are never a reason to delay treatment with opioid analgesics if they are indicated.

Tolerance

Tolerance is a normal physiological response to chronic opioid therapy in which increasing doses are required to produce the same effect. Experience with cancer patients with chronic pain indicates that significant tolerance is uncommon and the need for increasing doses usually relates to disease progression.[37, 38] Concern regarding tolerance is not a reason for 'saving up' the use of opioid drugs until the terminal phase. Patients concerned that there will be 'nothing left' for more severe pain should be reassured the therapeutic range of morphine is very broad and there is adequate scope to treat more severe pain if it occurs.[39] Cross-tolerance between the various opioid drugs is not complete and an alternative drug can be substituted if the rate of development of tolerance is of concern.

Physical dependence

Physical dependence is a normal physiological response to chronic opioid therapy, which leads to withdrawal symptoms if the drug is abruptly stopped or an antagonist administered. The withdrawal syndrome is characterized by anxiety and agitation, rhinorrhoea and lacrimation, fever and sweating, muscular and abdominal cramps, tremor and other signs of sympathetic overactivity. The time of onset and duration of the withdrawal syndrome depend on the pharmacokinetics of the opioid in use. Withdrawal syndromes are treated by administering 25–50% of the previous daily dose, given in divided doses, 6-hourly. Patients whose pain has been relieved by surgical or other means should have their opioid analgesics reduced by 15–25% per day. Patients need to be reassured that physical dependence does not prevent withdrawal of the medication if their pain is relieved by other means.

Psychological dependence and addiction

Psychological dependence is a condition characterized by abnormal behavioural and other responses that always include a compulsion to take the drug to experience its psychic effects. Drug dependence is a pathological psychological response and not physiological. Several large studies of patients with cancer and pain have shown, that with the exception of a few patients with a past history of psychiatric disturbance or drug dependence, these patients do not become psychologically dependent.[40, 41] Even if it is anticipated that pain will be relieved by other means, opioid analgesics should not be withheld because of any concerns related to psychological dependence, although patients with a history of drug abuse should be managed carefully.

The underutilization of opioids: opiophobia

Morphine and other opioid drugs are underutilized in the treatment of pain associated with cancer, for a variety of reasons. The discussion that follows focuses on morphine, but the issues apply equally to all the strong opioid drugs.

Professional opiophobia

Some of the reasons why doctors underprescribe and nurses underadminister morphine are listed in Table 9.11.[42–46]

Table 9.11 Professional opiophobia

'Morphine should only be used when the patient is dying.'
'Morphine hastens death.'
'Morphine causes respiratory depression.'

'Morphine doesn't work.'
    incorrect administration
    opioid-insensitive pain
    ignoring psychosocial aspects of care

'Morphine causes unacceptable side effects.'   constipation, nausea, somnolence, confusion
Fear of tolerance, physical dependence, psychological dependence

The belief that morphine should be only given when patients are dying is archaic. Morphine may be used for months or years and, correctly administered, is compatible with a normal lifestyle. Used properly, it does not hasten death and respiratory depression should not be a problem. That morphine should be reserved for the 'crescendo of pain' that occasionally occurs before death is incorrect because the broad therapeutic range of morphine allows for increasing doses if required.

Morphine will be ineffective in controlling pain if it is being incorrectly administered, used for morphine-insensitive pain, or if matters of psychosocial concern have not been addressed. The correct dose of morphine is that which relieves the patient's pain whilst causing acceptable adverse effects and must be individually titrated for each patient. Neuropathic pain is relatively opioid-insensitive and may respond better to one of the adjuvant analgesics. Physical pain may be caused or aggravated by psychosocial problems and no amount of well-prescribed analgesia will relieve this pain until the psychological and social concerns are addressed.

Adverse effects should not be severe. In patients with cancer, respiratory depression is very uncommon except in opioid naive patients who are commenced on parenteral therapy. Constipation occurs inevitably and requires explanation and advice about diet and laxative therapy. Patients should be warned of the possibility of somnolence and nausea and reassured that these usually improve after several days.

The most frequent reasons why morphine is withheld relate to misunderstandings about tolerance, physical dependence and psychological dependence. In contrast to intravenous drug users who develop rapid tolerance, patients with cancer rarely develop clinically significant tolerance and frequently require little increase in the dose over weeks or months. Physical dependence requires explanation and patients must be reassured that morphine can be weaned (by 25% a day) if their pain is relieved by other means. Psychological dependence occurs extremely rarely in patients with cancer and pain. Concern about tolerance, physical dependence or psychological dependence is never a reason to delay treatment with morphine if it is indicated.

Patient opiophobia

Patients and their families may also have fears or express concerns about morphine therapy ('Table 9.12').[39, 41]

Table 9.12 Patient opiophobia

'That means I'm going to die soon.'
'There will be nothing left for when the pain gets worse.'
'I'll become an addict.'
'I'm allergic to morphine.'

'The morphine didn't work.'
    incorrect administration
    no instructions for breakthrough pain
    morphine-insensitive pain
    ignoring the psychosocial factors

'I couldn't take the morphine.'   somnolence, confusion, nausea, constipation

Some patients interpret the prescription of morphine as a message that death is imminent. This requires explanation that morphine can be used for months or years and is entirely compatible with a normal lifestyle.

Other patients resist taking morphine for fear there may be nothing in reserve should their pain worsen. This requires reassurance that the therapeutic range of morphine is sufficient to allow escalation of the dose if necessary.

A history of being 'allergic to morphine' usually relates to nausea or vomiting that occurred when parenteral morphine was given to an opioid naive patient for acute pain. Immunological allergy to morphine is rare and given explanation, reassurance and the cover of antiemetics, most patients can be started on morphine without ill effect.

Patients may express concern about addiction. They require explanation about tolerance and physical dependence and reassurance that psychological dependence is not a clinical concern.

If patients claim that morphine did not help their pain it may be that the dose was too low, given too infrequently, or they were not given instructions about what to do for break-through pain. The importance of other aspects of patients' suffering — physical, psychological, social, cultural and spiritual — to their perception of pain cannot be underestimated. Patients given morphine in an apparently appropriate dose but who report no benefit, and especially those who report no benefit after escalation of the dose, nearly always have psychosocial problems compounding their pain.

Given adequate explanation, good prescribing, and individual titration of dosage, most patients will achieve good pain control without suffering unacceptable adverse effects.

References

1   Clark, N.C., Lintzeris, N. and Muhleisen, P.J. (2002). Severe opiate withdrawal in a heroin user precipitated by a massive buprenorphine dose. *Medical Journal of Australia* 176, 166–7.

2   Lipman, A.G. and Gauthier, M.E. (1997). Pharmacology of opioid drugs: basic principles. In *Topics in Palliative Care. Volume 1* (ed. R. Portenoy and E. Bruera). New York, Oxford University Press.

3   Jadad, A.R. (1998). Opioids in the treatment of neuropathic pain: a systematic review of con-trolled clinical trials. In *Topics in Palliative Care. Volume 2* (ed. E. Bruera and R. Portenoy). New York, Oxford University Press.

4   Grond, S., et al. (1999). Assessment and treatment of neuropathic cancer pain following WHO guidelines. *Pain* 79, 15–20.

5   Moulin, D.E. (1998). Neuropathic cancer pain: syndromes and clinical controversies. In *Topics in Palliative Care. Volume 2* (ed. E. Bruera and R. Portenoy). New York, Oxford University Press.

6   Watanabe, S. (1997). Intraindividual variability in opioid response: a role for sequential opioid trial in patient care. In *Topics in Palliative Care. Volume 2* (ed. R. Portenoy and E. Bruera). New York, Oxford University Press.

7   Indelicato, R.A. and Portenoy, R.K. (2002). Opioid rotation in the management of refractory can-cer pain. *Journal of Clinical Oncology* 20, 348–52.

8   de Stoutz, N.D., Bruera, E. and Suarez-Almazor, M. (1995). Opioid rotation for toxicity reduction in terminal cancer patients. *Journal of Pain and Symptom Management* 10, 378–84.

9   Ashby, M.A., Martin, P. and Jackson, K.A. (1999). Opioid substitution to reduce adverse effects in cancer pain management. *Medical Journal of Australia* 170, 68–71.

10 Mercadante, S., et al. (2001). Switching from morphine to methadone to improve analgesia and tolerability in cancer patients: a prospective study. *Journal of Clinical Oncology* 19, 2898–904.

11 McNamara, P. (2002). Opioid switching from morphine to transdermal fentanyl for toxicity reduction in palliative care. *Palliative Medicine* 16, 425–34.

12 Pereira, J., et al. (2001). Equianalgesic dose ratios for opioids. a critical review and proposals for long-term dosing. *Journal of Pain and Symptom Management* 22, 672–87.

13 Lawlor, P., Pereira, J. and Bruera, E. (2001). Dose ratios among different opioids: underlying issues and an update on the use on the equianalgesic table. In *Topics in Palliative Care. Volume 5* (ed. E. Bruera and R. Portenoy). New York, Oxford University Press.

14 Anderson, R., et al. (2001). Accuracy in equianalgesic dosing. conversion dilemmas. *Journal of Pain and Symptom Management* 21, 397–406.

15 Cherny, N., et al. (2001). Strategies to manage the adverse effects of oral morphine: an evidence-based report. *Journal of Clinical Oncology* 19, 2542–54.

16 Goudas, L., et al. (2001). *Management of cancer pain*. Rockville, MD: Agency for Healthcare Research and Quality. <www.ahrq.gov>

17 Carr, D., et al. (2002). *Management of Cancer Symptoms: Pain, Depression, and Fatigue. Evidence Report/Technology Assessment No. 61*. Rockville, MD: Agency for Healthcare Research and Quality. <www.ahrq.gov>

18 Slatkin, N.E., Rhiner, M. and Bolton, T.M. (2001). Donepezil in the treatment of opioid-induced sedation: report of six cases. *Journal of Pain and Symptom Management* 21, 425–38.

19 Bruera, E., et al. (1987). Methylphenidate associated with narcotics for the treatment of cancer pain. *Cancer Treatment Reports* 71, 67–70.

20 Bruera, E., et al. (1992). Neuropsychological effects of methylphenidate in patients receiving a continuous infusion of narcotics for cancer pain. *Pain* 48, 163–6.

21 Wilwerding, M.B., et al. (1995). A randomized, crossover evaluation of methylphenidate in cancer patients receiving strong narcotics. *Supportive Care in Cancer* 3, 135–8.

22 Vainio, A., et al. (1995). Driving ability in cancer patients receiving long-term morphine analgesia. *Lancet* 346, 667–70.

23 Manfredi, P.I., et al. (1996). Inappropriate use of naloxone in cancer patients with pain. *Journal of Pain and Symptom Management* 11, 131–4.

24 Lawlor, P.G. (2002). The panorama of opioid-related cognitive dysfunction in patients with cancer: a critical literature appraisal. *Cancer* 94, 1836–53.

25 Klepstad, P., et al. (2002). Self-reports are not related to objective assessments of cognitive function and sedation in patients with cancer pain admitted to a palliative care unit. *Palliative Medicine* 16, 513–9.

26 Foley, K.M. (2001). Management of Cancer Pain. In *Cancer. Principles and Practice of Oncology. 6th edition* (ed. V.T. De Vita, S. Hellman and S.A. Rosenberg). Philadelphia, Lippincott Williams Wilkins.

27 Hagen, N. and Swanson, R. (1997). Strychnine-like multifocal myoclonus and seizures in extremely high-dose opioid administration: treatment strategies. *Journal of Pain and Symptom Management* 14, 51–8.

28 Kaiko, R.F., et al. (1983). Central nervous system excitatory effects of meperidine in cancer patients. *Annals of Neurology* 13, 180–5.

29 Sjogren, P., et al. (1993). Hyperalgesia and myoclonus in terminal cancer patients treated with continuous intravenous morphine. *Pain* 55, 93–7.

30 Twycross, R. (1998). Re: Opioid-induced myoclonus and seizures. *Journal of Pain and Symptom Management* 15, 143–4.

31 Sjogren, P., Jensen, N.H. and Jensen, T.S. (1994). Disappearance of morphine-induced hyperalgesia after discontinuing or substituting morphine with other opioid agonists. *Pain* 59, 313–6.

32 Campora, E., et al. (1991). The incidence of narcotic-induced emesis. *Journal of Pain and Symptom Management* 6, 428–30.

33 Hardy, J., et al. (2002). A double-blind, randomised, parallel group, multinational, multicentre study comparing a single dose of ondansetron 24 mg p.o. with placebo and metoclopramide 10 mg t.d.s. p.o. in the treatment of opioid-induced nausea and emesis in cancer patients. *Supportive Care in Cancer* 10, 231–6.

34 Sykes, N.P. (1996). An investigation of the ability of oral naloxone to correct opioid-related constipation in patients with advanced cancer. *Palliative Medicine* 10, 135–44.

35 Yuan, C.S., et al. (2000). Methylnaltrexone for reversal of constipation due to chronic methadone use: a randomized controlled trial. *Journal of the American Medical Association* 283, 367–72.

36 Liu, M. and Wittbrodt, E. (2002). Low-dose oral naloxone reverses opioid-induced constipation and analgesia. *Journal of Pain and Symptom Management* 23, 48–53.

37 Mercadante, S. (2001). Problems with opioid dose escalation in cancer pain: differential diagnosis and management strategies. In *Topics in Palliative Care. Volume 5* (ed. E. Bruera and R. Portenoy). New York, Oxford University Press.

38 Nghiemphu, L.P. and Portenoy, R. (2001). Opioid tolerance: a clinical perspective. In *Topics in Palliative Care. Volume 5* (ed. E. Bruera and R. Portenoy). New York, Oxford University Press.

39 Paice, J.A., Toy, C. and Shott, S. (1998). Barriers to cancer pain relief: fear of tolerance and addiction. *Journal of Pain and Symptom Management* 16, 1–9.

40 Schug, S.A., et al. (1992). A long-term survey of morphine in cancer pain patients. *Journal of Pain and Symptom Management* 7, 259–66.

41 Passik, S.D., Kirsh, K.L. and Portenoy, R.K. (2002). Substance abuse issues in palliative care. In *Principles and Practice of Palliative Care and Supportive Oncology* (ed. A.M. Berger, R.K. Portenoy and D.E. Weissman). Philadelphia, Lippincott, Williams and Wilkins.

42 Zenz, M. and Willweber-Strumpf, A. (1993). Opiophobia and cancer pain in Europe. *Lancet* 341, 1075–6.

43 Cherny, N.I. and Catane, R. (1995). Professional negligence in the management of cancer pain. A case for urgent reforms. *Cancer* 76, 2181–5.

44 Zenz, M., et al. (1995). Severe undertreatment of cancer pain: a 3-year survey of the German situation. *Journal of Pain and Symptom Management* 10, 187–91.

45 Merrill, J.M., Dale, A. and Thornby, J.I. (2000). Thanatophobia and opiophobia of hospice nurses compared with that of other caregivers. *American Journal of Hospice and Palliative Care* 17, 15–23.

46 Wells, M., et al. (2001). The knowledge and attitudes of surgical staff towards the use of opioids in cancer pain management: can the Hospital Palliative Care Team make a difference? *European Journal of Cancer Care* 10, 201–11.

10

Morphine

Morphine is the strong opioid drug of choice for the management of patients with cancer who have moderate or severe pain because it has a wide therapeutic range, is effective by many routes of administration, is available in many countries, and is relatively inexpensive.[1]

Pharmacology

Morphine is administered by a number of different routes (Table10.1). It is well absorbed when given orally, with a bioavailability of about one-third compared to parenteral administration. A morphine-chitosan preparation for intranasal use for breakthrough pain has recently been introduced.[2] The plasma half-life of morphine is 2–3 hours and is unaffected by chronic usage. The effective duration of action approximates four hours, a little less after intravenous injection. Morphine is metabolized mainly in the liver, to morphine-3-glucuronide (M3G) and morphine-6-glucuronide (M6G).[3] M6G is a potent opioid receptor agonist and improved pain control is associated with higher morphine plus M6G concentrations;[4] M3G probably has no significant analgesic action.[5] The glucuronide metabolites are excreted in the urine, and renal impairment, including that which occurs normally in old age, may lead to accumulation of M3G and M6G and predispose to adverse effects including cognitive impairment, nausea and vomiting.[6] Liver disease is not reported to alter morphine pharmacokinetics, but care must be taken if there is severe hepatic dysfunction. The increased sedation that may occur when morphine is administered with other drugs that have a CNS depressant action is probably due to an additive effect rather than altered pharmacokinetics.

Actions

Morphine acts on the opioid receptors in the brain and spinal cord to produce analgesia. The perception of pain is altered both by a direct effect on the spinal cord, modulating peripheral

Table 10.1 Morphine

Action	analgesic
Mechanism	interaction with opioid receptors
Administration	effective IV, IM, SC, PO, PR, ED, IT, IN and topical
Pharmacology	plasma half-life 2-3h, unaffected by chronic usage metabolized in the liver to M3G and M6G excreted in urine
Indications	moderate and severe cancer-related pain diarrhoea, cough, dyspnoea
Contraindications	genuine morphine intolerance
Cautions	renal impairment severe hepatic dysfunction significant pulmonary disease CNS depression old age, debility
Dose	no standard dose for chronic pain titrated against pain and adverse effects for each individual patient
Duration of action	3–4h; longer with renal impairment

nociceptive input, and by activating the descending inhibitory systems from the brain stem and basal ganglia. Morphine also acts on the limbic system and on higher centres to modify the emotional response to pain.

The systemic effects, including those affecting the gastrointestinal and respiratory tracts, are partly centrally mediated via the autonomic nervous system and may partly be due to a direct effect on opioid receptors in the peripheral tissues.

Indications

Morphine is the drug of choice for moderate and severe cancer-related pain. It is also used for the treatment of diarrhoea, cough and dyspnoea.

Morphine-sensitive and morphine-insensitive pain. Neuropathic pain may be less sensitive to morphine than somatic and visceral pain. However, because of the wide range of doses that can be employed, the difference between morphine-sensitive and morphine-insensitive pain should be regarded as relative rather than absolute. Neuropathic pain responds to morphine, although adequate analgesia may require higher doses and increase the risk of troublesome adverse effects.[7–9]

Contraindications

Morphine should be given with caution to patients with renal impairment, severe hepatic dysfunction, significant pulmonary disease (including acute or severe bronchial asthma), and CNS depression from any cause. Elderly patients and those who are debilitated or cachectic should initially be treated with reduced doses.

Morphine intolerance and 'allergy'. A small proportion of patients will suffer intolerable sedation or nausea that does not improve after the first few days of therapy and which cannot be attributed to other causes. These patients should be considered intolerant of morphine and changed to an alternative opioid.

Other patients present with a history of having been told they were allergic to morphine. This frequently relates to nausea or vomiting that occurred after a morphine injection was given for acute pain to an opioid-naive patient. A careful history is required to determine the exact circumstances of the reaction. Given explanation, reassurance, and the cover of antiemetic therapy for the first few days, most of these patients can be commenced on morphine without ill effect.

Dose

Morphine has a remarkably wide therapeutic range, producing analgesia in a dose-dependent manner and there appears to be no ceiling effect to the analgesia; the useful dose is limited by adverse effects.

There is no standard dose of morphine for the treatment of chronic pain in patients with cancer. It must be individually titrated for each patient and the correct dose is that which controls the pain whilst causing tolerable side effects. The dose required depends on many factors including the severity of the pain, the type of pain, individual pharmacokinetic variations, the development of tolerance, and the psychosocial issues that affect the perception of pain.

Equianalgesic doses. The approximate equianalgesic doses of different opioid drugs are shown in Table 9.2.

Adverse effects

The adverse effects of morphine are summarized in Table 10.2, and are discussed in Chapter 9. There is considerable variation in these effects between individual patients. The common side effects in practice are constipation, sedation and nausea.

Table 10.2 Adverse effects of morphine

Neuropsychological	sedation, drowsiness, confusion, narcosis, coma dysphoria and psychotomimetic effects myoclonus miosis
Gastrointestinal	nausea, vomiting, delayed gastric emptying, constipation dry mouth biliary colic
Respiratory	respiratory depression suppression of cough reflex
Cardiovascular	postural hypotension
Urological	urgency, retention
Dermatological	flushing, sweating, pruritus

Sedation

Some sedation usually accompanies the commencement of morphine therapy. It is usually mild and lasts 2 to 5 days. Patients should be warned of this possibility, reassured that it is likely to improve within a few days, and encouraged to persevere with their medication through this period. In a few cases, severe drowsiness and confusion occurs, necessitating dose reduction. Factors predisposing to sedation are listed in Table 9.6.

Persistent sedation requires assessment of renal function and exclusion of other causes of CNS depression including metabolic disturbances, infection, cerebral metastases, and the effects of other drugs.

Unless there is a readily correctable metabolic cause or other less necessary medication can be withheld, persistent sedation should be managed by substituting an alternative opioid. The use of stimulants such as amphetamine or methylphenidate is an alternative. They are effective in counteracting sedation but there is a significant risk of dysphoric reactions to the stimulant, particularly in patients who are elderly or frail.

The treatment of severe sedation or narcosis is discussed in Chapter 9. The minimum effective dose of naloxone should be used, the aim being to improve respiratory function without reversing analgesia or precipitating physical withdrawal.

Gastrointestinal

The management of gastrointestinal adverse effects is discussed in Chapter 9. Nausea occurs frequently when therapy with morphine is commenced; vomiting is less common. The nausea is usually mild and subsides after a few days. Patients should be warned of the possibility of nausea for a few days after starting therapy and given a supply of antiemetics to take if need be.

Morphine will cause constipation in all patients except those with an ileostomy or diarrhoea secondary to malabsorption. Every patient commencing therapy with morphine requires dietary advice and the prescription of laxatives to *prevent* constipation. Tolerance does not develop to the constipatory effects and dietary and laxative therapy is necessary for the duration of treatment.

Morphine can cause spasm of the sphincter of Oddi, producing biliary colic. Treatment is with a small dose of naloxone.

Respiratory

Respiratory depression occurs due to a direct effect on the respiratory centres in the brain stem, but significant respiratory depression is unlikely to occur with usual doses of morphine except in patients who are at risk of respiratory failure for other reasons (see Chapter 9, Table 9.10).

Immediate release (IR) oral morphine

An oral morphine preparation is the treatment of choice for patients with moderate or severe pain, providing they are able to take and retain oral medication.

Immediate release tablets

Immediate release (IR) morphine sulfate and hydrochloride tablets are available in a range of strengths. Given the dosage flexibility of morphine mixture and the availability of longer acting oral preparations, IR morphine tablets have no particular advantages in the management of chronic cancer-related pain.

Oral morphine mixture

Morphine sulfate and hydrochloride mixtures are commercially available in a range of strengths between 1 and 20 mg/ml. Morphine mixture is relatively cheap, generally well tolerated, and frequent dose adjustments can be made if necessary. The inclusion of preservatives in commercially available preparations has overcome the earlier problem of a limited shelf life.

Other drugs should not be included in a morphine mixture. Drugs that were included in the past were antiemetics, aspirin, chlorpromazine and cocaine. One of the great advantages of morphine mixture is that the dose can be increased or decreased easily according to need or adverse effects. If the mixture contains other drugs, then the dose of these will also be varied, leading to either an inadequate dose or toxicity. The traditional use of cocaine in Brompton's cocktail is not recommended as it adds nothing to the analgesic properties [10] and may cause confusion, dysphoria and insomnia in the frail and elderly.

Table 10.3   Oral IR morphine mixture

Initial dose
   patients receiving parenteral morphine
      multiply total mg/d IV, IM or SC morphine by 3; divide by 6 for the 4-hourly dose
         e.g. morphine 15mg SC q4h (90mg/d) is 270mg/d PO or 45mg PO q4h
   patients receiving other opioids
      convert to mg/d oral morphine; divide by 6 for the 4-hourly dose
         e.g. codeine 60mg PO q4h (360mg/d) is morphine 45mg/d PO or 7.5mg PO q4h
   patients not previously receiving opioids
      start with 10mg PO q4h
      if frail, elderly or with renal impairment, start with 5mg PO q4-6h

Frequency
   q4h, strictly, except for patients who are frail, elderly or with renal impairment
   2 am dose should be given (**see** text)

Breakthrough pain
   treated with an extra dose, as often as required, of 50-100% of the 4-hourly dose

Incident pain
   treated as for breakthrough pain, 30-60 minutes prior if predictable

Dose adjustment
   if the first dose(s) cause oversedation, reduce the dose by 50% for a trial period
   if the first dose(s) produce inadequate analgesia, increase by 50% for a trial period
   a record of the breakthrough doses required is used to adjust the dose
      breakthrough (mg/d) + scheduled (mg/d), and divide by 6 for the new 4-hourly dose

Guidelines for the use of morphine mixture are shown in Table 10.3. The initial dose is estimated from the amount of opioid drugs the patient is currently taking, although the equianalgesic conversion factors (Table 9.2) are approximate only and do not account for individual patient variation. Breakthrough pain is treated with an extra dose of mixture equivalent to the 4-hourly dose; if the pain is not severe or there is concern about morphine toxicity, 50% of the 4-hourly dose can be used.

Patients taking morphine mixture 4-hourly should receive their 2am dose. Previous recommendations were to give a double dose at 10pm,[11] but an RCT has shown that giving the 2am dose produces better analgesia and fewer adverse effects (Table 10.4).

Table 10.4   Oral morphine: RCTs

Author	n	Intervention	Outcome
2am dose of morphine mixture			
Todd[11]	20	double dose at 10pm vs normal dose at 10pm & 2am	double dose: ↑ breakthrough pain, ↑ morning pain (pS)
Final dose of IR when starting SR morphine			
Hoskin[12]	19	final dose of IR vs placebo with first dose of SR	no differences in pain intensity or pain relief
Dose finding: IR or SR			
Klepstad[13]	40	IR q4h vs SR q24h	equally effective in time to adequate pain relief
8-hourly or 12-hourly treatment			
Mignault[14]	19	12-hourly SR given q8h vs q12h	no differences in pain measures or adverse effects
Comparison of IR with 12-hourly SR preparation			
Goudas[15]	317 (8 RCTs)	SR q12h vs IR q4h	no differences in pain measures or adverse effects
Comparison of 12- and 24-hourly SR preparations			
Goudas[15]	234 (2 RCTs)	12-hourly SR q12h vs 24-hourly SR q24h	no differences in pain measures or adverse effects
Comparison of SR tablet and SR suspension			
Boureau[16]	52	SR tablet q12h vs SR suspension q12h	no differences in pain measures or adverse effects

Sustained release (SR) oral morphine

A number of sustained release (SR) morphine formulations are commercially available including tablets, capsules (containing 'micropellets' or 'microgranules') and suspensions. The commercially available SR suspensions, or one made with the granules from a capsule, are useful for patients with dysphagia and can be administered via a nasogastric or gastrostomy tube.

SR morphine preparations must be swallowed whole. Tablets and the granules or pellets contained in capsules must not be broken, crushed or chewed. Disruption of the tablets or pellets damages the sustained release mechanism and the patient is in effect taking immediate release morphine. This will provide analgesia for only 4 hours but, as the dose is calculated to cover 12 or 24 hours, there is a risk of toxicity if the whole dose is promptly absorbed.

Guidelines for the use of SR morphine preparations are shown in Table 10.5. The frequency of administration varies with different preparations—some are intended for 12-hourly administration, others are given once daily. The initial dose may be estimated from the patient's current opioid medication although the opioid conversion factors shown in Table 9.2 are approximate only and do not account for individual patient variation. The best method of establishing the correct dose of SR morphine is to stabilize the patient on IR oral morphine mixture for one to a few days, although starting patients directly on the SR preparation is reported to be equally effective (Table 10.4). The use of a final 4-hourly dose of IR mixture, given at the same time as the first dose of SR morphine, is reported to be unnecessary (Table10.4).

Breakthrough pain occurring between 12- or 24-hourly doses is treated with IR oral morphine mixture and not by increasing the frequency of the SR preparation. The dose of oral morphine mixture used for breakthrough pain is the same as the 4-hourly dose, equal to one-third of the 12-hourly dose or one-sixth of the 24-hourly dose; if the pain is not severe or there is concern about toxicity, 50% of the 4-hourly dose can be used. Patients requiring substantial doses of SR morphine also require substantial doses of morphine mixture for breakthrough pain and some examples are given in Table 10.5.

The dose of SR morphine is adjusted according to the amount of extra morphine the patient required during the previous 24 hours. If a 12-hourly preparation is used, patients with pain worse at night and those troubled by sedation during the day may benefit from a higher dose in the evening.

A small proportion of patients taking SR morphine consistently develop breakthrough pain, not relieved by increasing the dose, towards the end of each dosing period. For

Table 10.5   Oral sustained release (SR) morphine

Note: 12- and 24-hourly morphine SR preparations
  doses of morphine SR in this table are given in mg/d
    for 12-hourly preparations: give half of the 24h dose, q12h
    for 24-hourly preparations: give whole of the 24h dose, once daily

Initial dose
  patients receiving IR oral morphine mixture
    same dose (mg/d)
      e.g. morphine mixture 50mg q4h → morphine SR 300mg/d
  patients receiving parenteral morphine
    multiply parenteral dose (mg/d) by 3 to get total daily oral dose
      e.g. morphine 20mg SC q4h (120mg/d) → morphine SR 360mg/d
  patients receiving other opioids
    convert to oral morphine (mg/d)
      e.g. codeine 60mg PO q4h is 360mg/d → morphine SR 45mg/d
  patients not receiving opioids
    use IR oral morphine mixture for first 1–3 days

Breakthrough pain
  treated with oral morphine mixture
    equivalent to 4-hourly dose (one-third of the 12h dose, one-sixth of the 24h dose)
      e.g. morphine SR 40mg/d → breakthrough dose of IR morphine is 7mg
      e.g. morphine SR 200mg/d → breakthrough dose of IR morphine is 30mg
      e.g. morphine SR 600mg/d → breakthrough dose of IR morphine is 100mg

Incident pain
  treated as for breakthrough pain, 30–60min prior if predictable

Dose adjustment
  a record of the breakthrough doses required is used to adjust the dose
    breakthrough doses (mg/d) + scheduled doses (mg/d) → new 24h dose

patients taking 12-hourly SR morphine, this problem can be overcome by giving the drug on an 8-hourly schedule; more frequent administration is not recommended. For other patients, there is no benefit in giving the medication 8-hourly (Table10.4). The dose for 8-hourly administration is calculated as shown in Table 10.5 with the 24-hour dose being divided by three.

A number of studies have documented that the efficacy and adverse effects of the SR preparations are essentially the same as IR morphine given 4-hourly, with the exception that the maintenance of analgesia may be smoother (Table 10.4).

Subcutaneous (SC) morphine

Subcutaneous (SC) morphine therapy is effective and safe [17] and particularly useful if parenteral therapy is required in the home setting (Table 10.6). Subcutaneous morphine is indicated for patients unable to take or retain oral medication; in all other circumstances the oral route is to be preferred. Morphine can be given either by 4-hourly injection or by continuous infusion, via a subcutaneous butterfly needle. A continuous subcutaneous infusion (CSCI) using a portable battery-operated syringe driver is the preferred method as it avoids fluctuating blood levels and requires drug preparation only once a day. The frequency with which the needle site needs to be changed depends on how quickly local inflammation develops and varies from daily to 2 or 3 weeks.

Guidelines for the use of subcutaneous morphine are shown in Table 10.7. The initial dose may be calculated from the patient's current opioid therapy, although the opioid conversion factors are approximate only and do not account for individual patient variation. Unrelieved or increased pain at the time of starting subcutaneous morphine will necessitate an increase

---

Table 10.6 Morphine: Continuous subcutaneous infusion (CSCI)

Indications
    relief of pain for patients unable to take or retain oral medication
        nausea and vomiting
        dysphagia, unable to swallow
        sedated, semiconscious or terminal

Advantages
    avoids frequent injections
        patient: less pain and bruising
        family: do not need to be educated to give injections
        nurse: prepares medication once daily
    avoids fluctuating blood levels
        more even analgesia
        less adverse effects
    does not require venous access
    completely portable
    suitable for terminal care at home

Complications
    skin irritation: the injection site should be changed regularly
    fluid leakage from infusion site: unlikely if infusion volume <1–2 ml/h
    requires daily supervision by trained nurse

Table 10.7 Continuous subcutaneous infusion (CSCI) of morphine

Initial dose
    patients receiving IV, IM or intermittent SC morphine
        same total mg/24h
            e.g. morphine 15mg SC or IM q4h (90mg/d) → morphine 90mg/24h CSCI
    patients receiving oral morphine (IR or SR)
        divide total mg/24h by 3
            e.g. morphine SR 60mg PO q12h (120mg/d) → morphine 40mg/24h CSCI
    patients receiving other opioids
        convert to morphine PO mg/d and divide by 3 for the SC dose
            e.g. codeine 60mg PO q4h → morphine 45mg/d PO → morphine 15mg/24h CSCI
    patients not receiving opioids
        start on intermittent SC injections, 4-hourly, to establish the approximate dose

Breakthrough pain
    treated with additional SC morphine
        increasing syringe driver rate
        using 'boost' button available on some syringe drivers (not recommended)
        giving additional SC injection, equivalent to 4h dose or one-sixth of 24h dose

Incident pain
    treated as for breakthrough pain, 20–30 minutes prior if predictable

Dose adjustment
    adjusted according to the need for breakthrough doses
        breakthrough doses (mg/d) + scheduled dose (mg/d) → new 24h dose

in the calculated dose, and a loading dose (IM or SC) equivalent to the 4-hour requirement (one-sixth of 24h dose) can be given at the time of starting the infusion.

Breakthrough pain is treated with extra doses of subcutaneous morphine. This may be done by increasing the syringe driver rate or by giving a separate subcutaneous injection. The dose used for breakthrough pain is the same as the 4-hourly dose, equal to one-sixth of the 24-hourly dose; if the pain is not severe or there is concern about adverse effects, 50% of the 4-hourly dose can be used. Some syringe drivers have a 'boost' button that allows the delivery of a small extra dose, on demand. Use of the 'boost' button is not recommended because the amount of analgesia delivered is completely inadequate when compared to the recommended dose for breakthrough pain.[18]

Solubility and the use of alternative preparations. The dose of morphine that can be delivered by CSCI is limited by the solubility of the drug, and the volume available in the syringe if other drugs are being given at the same time. The maximum concentrations of commercial preparations of morphine sulfate and hydrochloride are 30 mg/ml. If higher doses are required, the syringe may need to be changed each 12 hours, or a more soluble preparation used. Morphine tartrate has a solubility of 80 mg/ml and potency effectively the same as morphine sulfate. Hydromorphone (10mg/ml) is equivalent to 66 mg/ml of morphine. Diamorphine, available only in the UK, is considerably more soluble.

Adding other drugs to the infusion. The use of CSCI of morphine in the terminal care setting has led to other appropriate drugs being given in the infusion. Drugs that are compatible with morphine in this situation are listed in Table 10.8. More detailed information is available elsewhere and on the internet.[18, 19]

Table 10.8 Compatibility of other drugs with morphine given by CSCI

	Compatible	Incompatible
Antiemetics	metoclopramide, cyclizine	prochlorperazine
Tranquillizers	haloperidol	chlorpromazine
Anticonvulsants	midazolam, clonazepam	phenytoin
Sedatives	midazolam, clonazepam	diazepam
Anticholinergic	hyoscine hydrobromide, butylbromide	

Other routes of administration

Intravenous morphine

Single or repeated intravenous injections of morphine are the most efficient means of controlling severe or acute pain. The dose used depends on the patient's previous exposure to opioid drugs and on the effect and adverse reactions. Giving repeated small doses (1.5–2mg) each few minutes usually leads to rapid relief of pain and establishes the appropriate dose for continuing therapy.[20, 21]

Continuous intravenous infusions (CIVI) of morphine may be used where intravenous access has been established for other reasons, as in the postoperative phase or in patients with catheters previously used for chemotherapy.[22] The efficacy of CSCI means it is never necessary to establish intravenous access solely for the purpose of a morphine infusion. Calculation of the dose of morphine for a 24-hour CIVI is the same as given above for CSCI (Table 10.7).

Intravenous infusion may be combined with patient controlled analgesia (PCA), in which the infusion pump includes a device that allows the delivery of an extra small bolus, on demand. PCA is effective in the management of postoperative pain but its role in patients with advanced cancer has not been established.

Intramuscular (IM) morphine

Intramuscular morphine injections are given for the relief of acute or severe pain when intravenous access is not available. Therapy is continued with either oral or subcutaneous morphine when the pain is controlled.

Rectal morphine

Morphine SR suppositories are commercially available in both 12- and 24-hour preparations, and provide an effective alternative for patients unable to take oral medications. The recommended dose is the same as for oral administration. Studies indicate that rectal morphine is equivalent to oral or subcutaneous administration in terms of analgesic efficacy and adverse effects (Table 10.9). Oral SR morphine tablets are effective when given rectally but absorption is slower and less predictable than by the oral route; they can be used to tide a patient over a short period of vomiting, but are not otherwise recommended. Compared to oral absorption, rectal absorption is slower from suppositories but more rapid if a liquid preparation is used. The temporal profile of morphine metabolites also differs following rectal administration, consistent with slower absorption and less first-pass metabolism, although this does not seem to produce any significant clinical differences (Table 10.9).

Table 10.9 Rectal morphine: RCTs

Author	n	Intervention	Outcome
Babul[23]	27	SR tablet PO q12h vs SR supp PR q12h	no diff. in pain measures less nausea with PR (pS)
Moolenaar[24]	25	SR tablet PO q12h vs SR supp PR q12h	no diff. in pain measures or adverse effects
DeConno[25]	34	10mg liquid IR morphine: PO vs PR	PR: more rapid onset, longer pain relief (pS)
Wilkinson[26]	10	oral SR tablet: PO vs PR	no diff. in pain measures or adverse effects
Bruera[27]	6	12-hourly SR supp vs 24-hourly supp	no diff. in pain measures or adverse effects
Bruera[28]	30	SR supp q12h vs SC morphine q4h	no diff. in pain measures or adverse effects

Topical morphine

A number of case reports suggest that the topical application of morphine may provide good pain relief for painful cutaneous ulcers and tumours.[29–32] Two randomized pilot studies reported positive results (Table 10.10).[33, 34] Opioid receptors have been identified in inflamed peripheral tissues, which provide some explanation for these observations. A morphine gel is made with Intrasite or hydrogel (1mg morphine to 1ml gel) and applied topically twice a day.

Table 10.10 Topical opioids for painful ulcers: RCTs

Author	n	Intervention	Outcome
Flock[33]	7	diamorphine gel vs placebo	diamorphine: ↓ pain scores (pS)
Zeppetella[34]	5	morphine gel vs placebo	morphine: ↓ pain scores (pS)

Spinal morphine—see Chapter 12

References

1   Expert Working Group of the European Association for Palliative Care (1996). Morphine in cancer pain: modes of administration. *British Medical Journal* 312, 823–6.

2   Pavis, H., et al. (2002). Pilot study of nasal morphine-chitosan for the relief of breakthrough pain in patients with cancer. *Journal of Pain and Symptom Management* 24, 598–602.

3   Sjogren, P. (1997). Clinical implications of morphine metabolites. In *Topics in Palliative Care. Volume 1* (ed. R. Portenoy and E. Bruera). New York, Oxford University Press.

4   Faura, C.C., et al. (1996). Morphine and morphine-6-glucuronide plasma concentrations and effect in cancer pain. *Journal of Pain and Symptom Management* 11, 95–102.

5   Andersen, G., Christrup, L. and Sjogren, P. (2003). Relationships among morphine metabolism, pain and side effects during long-term treatment. An update. *Journal of Pain and Symptom Management* 25, 74–91.

6   Ashby, M., et al. (1997). Plasma morphine and glucuronide (M3G and M6G) concentrations in hospice inpatients. *Journal of Pain and Symptom Management* 14, 157–67.

7   Jadad, A.R. (1998). Opioids in the treatment of neuropathic pain: a systematic review of controlled clinical trials. In *Topics in Palliative Care. Volume 2* (ed. E. Bruera and R. Portenoy). New York, Oxford University Press.

8   Grond, S., et al. (1999). Assessment and treatment of neuropathic cancer pain following WHO guidelines. *Pain* 79, 15–20.

9   Moulin, D.E. (1998). Neuropathic cancer pain: syndromes and clinical controversies. In *Topics in Palliative Care. Volume 2* (ed. E. Bruera and R. Portenoy). New York, Oxford University Press.

10   Kaiko, R.F., et al. (1987). Cocaine and morphine interaction in acute and chronic cancer pain. *Pain* 31, 35–45.

11   Todd, J., et al. (2002). An assessment of the efficacy and tolerability of a 'double dose' of normal-release morphine sulphate at bedtime. *Palliative Medicine* 16, 507–12.

12   Hoskin, P.J., Poulain, P. and Hanks, G.W. (1989). Controlled-release morphine in cancer pain. Is a loading dose required when the formulation is changed? *Anaesthesia* 44, 897–901.

13   Klepstad, P., et al. (2003). Immediate- or sustained-release morphine for dose finding during start of morphine to cancer patients: a randomized, double-blind trial. *Pain* 101, 193–8.

14   Mignault, G.G., et al. (1995). Control of cancer-related pain with MS Contin: a comparison between 12-hourly and 8-hourly administration. *Journal of Pain and Symptom Management* 10, 416–22.

15   Goudas, L., et al. (2001). *Management of cancer pain*. Rockville, MD: Agency for Healthcare Research and Quality. <www.ahrq.gov>

16   Boureau, F., et al. (1992). A comparative study of controlled-release morphine (CRM) suspension and CRM tablets in chronic cancer pain. *Journal of Pain and Symptom Management* 7, 393–9.

17   Nelson, K.A., et al. (1997). A prospective, within-patient, crossover study of continuous intravenous and subcutaneous morphine for chronic cancer pain. *Journal of Pain and Symptom Management* 13, 262–7.

18   Dickman, A., Littlewood, C. and Varga, J. (2002). *The Syringe Driver*. Oxford, Oxford University Press.

19   Twycross, R., et al. (2002). *Palliative Care Formulary*. Oxford, Radcliffe Medical Press. <www.palliativedrugs.net>

20   Kumar, K.S., Rajagopal, M.R. and Naseema, A.M. (2000). Intravenous morphine for emergency treatment of cancer pain. *Palliative Medicine* 14, 183–8.

21   Mercadante, S., et al. (2002). Rapid titration with intravenous morphine for severe cancer pain and immediate oral conversion. *Cancer* 95, 203–8.

22   Glare, P., et al. (2002). The efficacy and side effects of continuous infusion intravenous morphine (CIVM) for pain and symptoms due to advanced cancer. *American Journal of Hospice and Palliative Care* 19, 343–50.

23   Babul, N., et al. (1998). Comparative efficacy and safety of controlled-release morphine suppositories and tablets in cancer pain. *Journal of Clinical Pharmacology* 38, 74–81.

24   Moolenaar, F., et al. (2000). Clinical efficacy, safety and pharmacokinetics of a newly developed controlled release morphine sulphate suppository in patients with cancer pain. *European Journal of Clinical Pharmacology* 56, 219–23.

25   De Conno, F., et al. (1995). Role of rectal route in treating cancer pain: a randomized crossover clinical trial of oral versus rectal morphine administration in opioid-naive cancer patients with pain. *Journal of Clinical Oncology* 13, 1004–8.

26   Wilkinson, T.J., et al. (1992). Pharmacokinetics and efficacy of rectal versus oral sustained-release morphine in cancer patients. *Cancer Chemotherapy and Pharmacology* 31, 251–4.

27   Bruera, E., et al. (1999). Twice-daily versus once-daily morphine sulphate controlled-release suppositories for the treatment of cancer pain. A randomized controlled trial. *Supportive Care in Cancer* 7, 280–3.

28   Bruera, E., et al. (1995). Clinical efficacy and safety of a novel controlled-release morphine sup-
     pository and subcutaneous morphine in cancer pain: a randomized evaluation. *Journal of Clinical
     Oncology* 13, 1520–7.

29   Back, I.N. and Finlay, I. (1995). Analgesic effect of topical opioids on painful skin ulcers. *Journal
     of Pain and Symptom Management* 10, 493.

30   Krajnik, M. and Zylicz, Z. (1997). Topical morphine for cutaneous cancer pain. *Palliative Medicine*
     11, 325.

31   Krajnik, M., et al. (1999). Potential uses of topical opioids in palliative care—report of 6 cases.
     Pain 80, 121–5.

32   Twillman, R.K., et al. (1999). Treatment of painful skin ulcers with topical opioids. *Journal of Pain
     and Symptom Management* 17, 288–92.

33   Flock, P. (2003). Pilot study to determine the effectiveness of diamorphine gel to control pressure
     ulcer pain. *Journal of Pain and Symptom Management* 25, 547–54.

34   Zeppetella, G., Paul, J. and Ribeiro, M.D. (2003). Analgesic efficacy of morphine applied topically
     to painful ulcers. *Journal of Pain and Symptom Management* 25, 555–8.

11

Other opioid analgesics

Buprenorphine	Hydromorphone
Codeine	Levorphanol
Dextromoramide	Methadone
Dextropropoxyphene	Oxycodone
Diamorphine	Pethidine (Meperidine)
Dihydrocodeine	Tramadol
Fentanyl	Mixed agonist–antagonists

The other opioid drugs have morphine-like effects and act by interaction with the opioid receptors. The approximate equianalgesic doses of different drugs are listed in Table 9.2. Adverse effects are qualitatively similar to morphine (see Table 9.4). The treatment of over-dosage is with naloxone (Table 9.8). As with morphine, there is a tendency to underutilization (see Opiophobia, Chapter 9).

Table 11.1 Buprenorphine

Pharmacology	active SL, IM, SC, TD, and spinal
	metabolized in liver, excreted in bile and urine
	plasma half-life 3h (IV)
	duration of action 6–9h
Indications	moderate to severe pain
Adverse effects	similar to other opioids, possibly more sweating
Drug interactions	patients on buprenorphine
	co-administration of an opioid agonist: reduced or no effect
	patients on agonist drugs
	changing to buprenorphine can produce withdrawal
Dose	0.3–0.6mg IM or 0.4–0.8mg SL, q6–8h
Dose equivalence	0.3mg IM is equivalent to morphine 10mg IM
	0.4mg SL is equivalent to morphine 30mg PO
	52.5µg/h patch is equivalent to fentanyl 25µg/h patch
Preparations	injection, SL tablets, TD patch

Buprenorphine

Buprenorphine is a semisynthetic opioid that is indicated for moderate to severe pain (Table 11.1). It is a partial agonist and has a ceiling effect to its analgesic and respiratory depressant actions. Alternative opioid therapy needs to be given for the first 12 hours after applying a patch. The adverse effects of buprenorphine are qualitatively similar to morphine; more sweating was reported in one study.[1] The strong affinity of buprenorphine for opioid receptors can lead to interactions with other opioid drugs. High doses of buprenorphine may prevent the action of agonist drugs or precipitate physical withdrawal;[2] it is not usually a problem when changing between morphine and buprenorphine at usual doses.

Codeine

Codeine or methylmorphine is a natural alkaloid of opium and is the most commonly used weak opioid drug (Table 11.2). Demethylation in the liver by CYP2D6 produces morphine, and if this enzyme is inhibited by other drugs or genetically absent (as occurs in 7% of Caucasians), codeine is ineffective as an analgesic.[3] At doses above 60 mg 4-hourly, increased toxicity tends to outweigh any improvement in analgesia. The dose-limiting adverse effects are nausea, vomiting and somnolence. The exact dose equivalence between codeine and morphine is uncertain. In RCTs, 12-hourly codeine SR was superior to placebo and equivalent to 6-hourly codeine/acetaminophen tablets.[4, 5]

Table 11.2   Codeine

Pharmacology	well absorbed orally; bioavailability 40%
	metabolized in liver, excreted in urine
	ineffective in the 7% of Caucasians who lack CYP2D6
	plasma half-life 2.5–3h, no accumulation
	duration of action 4–6h
Indications	mild to moderate pain, diarrhoea, cough
Cautions	severe hepatic or renal impairment
	other causes of CNS depression
Adverse effects	qualitatively similar to morphine—generally mild
	more constipating
Dose	analgesic: 30–60mg PO q4–6h
	antitussive: 8–20mg PO q4–6h
Dose equivalence	120mg IM is equivalent to morphine 10mg IM
	240mg PO is equivalent to morphine 30mg PO
Preparations	tablets, SR tablets, syrup, injection
	combined preparations with aspirin or paracetamol

Dextromoramide

Dextromoramide is a strong opioid agonist. It has a short duration of action (2–3h) and is not suitable as a primary analgesic for chronic cancer-related pain.[3] The sublingual tablet has been used for breakthrough pain or painful procedures, but absorption and effect may be unpredictable.[6]

Dextropropoxyphene (Propoxyphene)

Dextropropoxyphene is the dextro-isomer of propoxyphene, which is a synthetic derivative of methadone (Table 11.3). It is indicated for mild to moderate pain. It should be used with caution in patients with significant hepatic or renal impairment and in the elderly, in whom accumulation of the drug or its metabolite, norpropoxyphene, may predispose to toxicity. The adverse effects are similar to other opioid drugs, but usually mild. A small proportion of patients develop light-headedness, dysphoria and confusion at standard doses, necessitating changing to a different drug. In an RCT with opioid-naive patients, dextropropoxyphene produced equivalent analgesia to low dose morphine with significantly fewer adverse effects.[7]

Table 11.3 Dextropropoxyphene

Pharmacology	well absorbed orally; bioavailability 40% metabolized in liver, excreted in urine plasma half-life 6–12h, longer in the elderly duration of action: 4–6h, longer in the elderly
Indications	mild to moderate pain
Cautions	significant hepatic or renal impairment elderly
Adverse effects	as for other opioid analgesics—generally mild occasional light-headedness, dysphoria, confusion CNS depression and seizures in overdose
Drug interactions	potentiates oral anticoagulants predisposes to carbamazepine toxicity
Dose	D. hydrochloride 65mg q4–6h D. napsylate 100mg q4–6h
Preparations	tablets, capsules combined preparations with aspirin or paracetamol

Diamorphine

Diamorphine (diacetylmorphine, heroin) is a strong opioid agonist available for medical use in the United Kingdom (Table 11.4). The analgesic efficacy and adverse effects of oral diamorphine and morphine were equivalent in an RCT.[8] Diamorphine is considerably more soluble than morphine, facilitating the delivery of higher doses by subcutaneous infusion.

Dihydrocodeine

Dihydrocodeine is a synthetic derivative of codeine (Table 11.5). It is a substrate for CYP2D6 but, unlike codeine, inhibition or absence of the enzyme does not reduce the analgesic effect.[3] The adverse effects are similar except dihydrocodeine is less constipating. A sustained release preparation offers the convenience of twice daily administration.

Table 11.4 Diamorphine (heroin)

Pharmacology	active PO, PR, SC, IM, IV, IN, spinal and topical metabolized to 6-acetylmorphine and morphine plasma half-life: several minutes duration of action: 3–4h
Indications	moderate and severe pain
Cautions	severe hepatic or renal dysfunction other causes of severe respiratory impairment other causes of CNS depression
Adverse effects	similar to morphine
Dose	equivalence 4–5mg IM is equivalent to morphine 10mg IM 20mg PO is equivalent to morphine 30mg PO
Preparations	tablet, liquid, injection

Table 11.5 Dihydrocodeine

Pharmacology	not well absorbed: bioavailability 20% PO metabolized in the liver, excreted in the urine plasma half-life 3.5–4.5h duration of action: 4h
Indications	moderate to severe pain antitussive
Cautions	renal impairment other causes of CNS depression
Adverse effects	similar to other opioids; less constipating than codeine dizziness, sedation, hallucinations
Dose equivalence	60mg IM is equivalent to 10mg IM morphine 200mg PO is equivalent to 30mg PO morphine
Dose	analgesia: dihydrocodeine tartrate 20-30mg q4–6h antitussive: dihydrocodeine tartrate 15mg q6–8h
Preparations	tablet, SR tablet, liquid, injection combined preparations with aspirin or paracetamol

Fentanyl

Parenteral

Fentanyl is a synthetic opioid agonist used for perioperative pain (Table 11.6).[9] It has a short duration of action (0.5–1h) and can be used for painful procedures or to prevent incident pain. For patients with inadequate pain control or unacceptable adverse effects with other opioids, fentanyl can be given by continuous intravenous or subcutaneous infusion, although the latter is limited to lower doses because of the volumes required.[10–12] An RCT of fentanyl and morphine given by SC infusion reported no difference in analgesic efficacy or

Table 11.6 Parenteral fentanyl

Pharmacology	active IV, IM, SC and spinal metabolized in liver, excreted in urine plasma half-life 1–2h duration of action 0.5–1h (IV), 1–3h (SC)

Indications
    single dose
    infusion
	moderate and severe pain
	painful procedures, prevention of incident pain
	inadequate pain relief with other opioid
	unacceptable toxicity with other opioid
	renal failure

Adverse effects	qualitatively similar to morphine
Dose equivalence	0.1mg IV equivalent to morphine 10mg IV (but lasts <1h)

adverse effects, except that bowel actions were more frequent with fentanyl (Table 11.7).[13] Fentanyl is not affected by renal function [3,14] and may be of particular benefit in patients suffering toxicity from other opioid drugs caused by renal impairment.

Alfentanil. This is a synthetic derivative of fentanyl that has a more rapid onset of action (<2 min given IV, <5 min IM) and short duration of effect (10 min given IV, 1hour IM).[3] It can be used for short painful procedures, but there is little experience of its use in patients with advanced cancer.

Sufentanil. Another synthetic analogue of fentanyl, sufentanil, has been successfully used for CSCI in palliative care.[11] It is more potent than fentanyl, allowing the use of much smaller volumes.

Table 11.7 Fentanyl: RCTs

Author	n	Intervention	Outcome
CSCI			
Hunt[13]	23	CSCI fentanyl vs CSCI morphine	similar analgesic efficacy and adverse effects; fentanyl: more frequent bowel movements (pS)
Transdermal (TD) fentany			
Ahmedzai[15]	202	TD fentanyl q72h vs morphine SR q12h	similar analgesic efficacy; fentanyl: ↓ sedation, ↓ constipation, ↑ sleep disturbance (all pS)
Wong[16]	40	TD fentanyl q72h vs morphine SR q12h	similar analgesic efficacy and adverse effects
Oral transmucosal fentanyl (OTFC) for breakthrough pain			
Christie[17]	62	OTFC titration vs oral opioid	OTFC successful for 74% patients; OTFC superior to oral opioid (pS)
Farrar[18]	92	OTFC vs placebo	OTFC: ↑ pain relief, ↓ need for rescue doses (pS)
Portenoy[19]	65	OTFC titration vs oral opioid	OTFC safe, successful for 74% patients; OTFC superior to oral opioid (pS)
Coluzzi[20]	134	OTFC vs IR morphine	OTFC: ↓ pain intensity, ↑ pain relief (pS)

Transdermal

Fentanyl patches are available for transdermal use, each patch providing analgesia for 72 hours (Table 11.8). After application of the first patch the plasma concentration of fentanyl rises slowly and other analgesia is required for 12–24 hours. The amount of fentanyl absorbed varies between patients. Care must be taken that the patch area is not heated or tightly covered as this may greatly increase the rate of absorption. Increased body temperature due to environmental factors or illness may also increase the rate of absorption. There will be continued release of drug from the 'reservoir' in the subcutaneous tissues for about 24 hours after the patch is removed. In the event of toxicity, this continued release will require treatment with naloxone for 12–24 hours. The starting dose is calculated from the requirement of oral morphine or equivalent during the previous 24 hours (Table 11.8). Opioid-naive patients can be started on a 25µg/h patch.[21] Oral morphine mixture is provided for breakthrough pain.

Transdermal fentanyl is an effective strong analgesic for patients unable to take oral medication and those with morphine intolerance or significant renal impairment. It produced analgesia equivalent to 12-hourly morphine SR in two RCTs (Table 11.7). It is reported to cause less constipation and daytime sedation than oral morphine, and is suitable for long-term use without evidence of the development of tolerance.[15, 22–25] Up to one-quarter of

Table 11.8 Transdermal fentanyl

Pharmacology	well absorbed: bioavailability 92% onset of action 12–24h continued action after patch removal 12–24h duration of action 72h (<72h in 24% of patients)
Indications	intolerable adverse effects of other opioid unable to take or retain oral analgesia renal failure
Contraindications	severe pain requiring rapid analgesic titration pain unresponsive to morphine or other µ-agonist
Cautions	patients with disease-related fever
Warnings	do not heat the patch area dispose of used patches carefully
Adverse effects	qualitatively similar to morphine—less constipation, sedation skin reactions

Initial dose	patient on strong opioids
	    calculate previous 24h dose as mg/d of PO morphine
	    divide by 3 and choose nearest patch strength in µg/h
	patient on weak opioid or opioid naive
	    start with 25µg/h patch

Titration	each 72h, according to response pain at 48–72h, not relieved by higher dose: change patch q48h
Preparation	25, 50, 75 and 100µg/h fentanyl patches (containing 2.5, 5, 7.5 and 10mg fentanyl)

patients develop pain after 48 hours, that is not relieved by increasing the patch strength, who are best managed by changing patches every 48 hours.[23]

Adverse effects include predictable opioid effects and skin reactions. Overheating of the patch can lead to narcosis.[26] A proportion of patients will suffer symptoms of physical opioid withdrawal for a few days after starting fentanyl, despite having good pain control.[15] This may relate to fentanyl and morphine acting on different subsets of μ-receptors, and is relieved by giving breakthrough doses of oral morphine. Opioid toxicity in a caregiver, presumably related to transdermal absorption, has been reported.[27] The patch preparation is not immune to deliberate abuse.[28]

Transmucosal

Fentanyl solution for injection, given by the sublingual route, provides rapid relief of breakthrough pain.[29] Doses of 25–150μg (0.5–3ml of 50μg/ml solution) reduced pain within 5 to 15 minutes without causing sedation or other adverse effects. Sublingual sufentanil, which is more potent and can be given in smaller volumes, is also reported to provide effective relief of breakthrough pain in doses of 2.5–15μg, without causing any significant adverse effects.[30] Small studies of intranasal fentanyl [31] and sufentanil [32] reported effective control of breakthrough pain without significant adverse effects.

Oral transmucosal fentanyl citrate (OTFC). OTFC is a 'lozenge on a stick' containing fentanyl in a hard sweet matrix (Table 11.9).[3, 33] It is used by placing it against the mucosa of one cheek and constantly moving it up and down, and changing at intervals from one cheek to the other. It provided safe and effective treatment for breakthrough pain in three-quarters of patients studied in RCTs (Table 11.7) and has been used for extended periods without loss of efficacy;[34] one-quarter of patients either do not achieve analgesia with the highest dose (1600μg) or suffer unacceptable adverse effects. There is no relationship between the effective dose of OTFC for breakthrough pain and the dose of opioid being used for background analgesia. Each patient has to be individually titrated to find the appropriate OTFC dose (Table 11.9). OTFC lozenges are expensive.

Table 11.9 Oral transmucosal fentanyl citrate (OTFC)

Pharmacology	bioavailability 50%: half by transmucosal, half by slower GI absorption onset of action 5–10 min plasma half-life 6h duration of action 1–3.5h, longer with higher doses
Indication	breakthrough pain
Adverse effects	somnolence, dizziness, nausea
Dose	OTFC dose not predicted by opioid dose for background pain
Titration	1. patient uses one 200μg lozenge over 15 min ± second 200μg lozenge after 15 min if analgesia inadequate no more than two lozenges per episode of pain 2. repeat this dose for 2–3 episodes of pain effective dose is pain relief with a single lozenge 3. if ineffective, increase to next strength lozenge repeat steps 1 to 3
Preparations	200, 400, 600, 800, 1200, and 1600μg lozenges

Hydromorphone

Hydromorphone is a strong opioid agonist with many pharmacological and clinical similarities to morphine (Table 11.10).[35] A Cochrane review concluded that it is an effective analgesic, with effects that are dose-related, and an adverse effect profile similar to other μ-agonists.[36, 37] The clinical equivalence of various hydromorphone preparations, and their equivalence to morphine and oxycodone, has been demonstrated in RCTs (Table 11.11). A once daily

Table 11.10 Hydromorphone

Pharmacology	active PO, PR, SC, IM, IV and spinal metabolized in liver, excreted in urine plasma half-life 2–3h duration of action 4h
Indications	severe pain morphine intolerance
Contraindications	genuine hydromorphone intolerance
Cautions	renal impairment severe hepatic dysfunction significant pulmonary disease CNS depression old age, debility
Adverse effects	similar to morphine
Dose	no standard dose for chronic pain titrated against pain and adverse effects for each individual patient
Dose equivalence	1.5mg IM is equivalent to morphine 10mg IM 7.5mg PO is equivalent to morphine 30mg PO
Preparations	tablets, capsules, SR capsules, liquid, suppositories, injection

Table 11.11 Hydromorphone (HM) and cancer pain: RCTs

Author	n	Intervention	Outcome
Hays[41]	48	HM SR q12h vs HM IR q4h	no differences in analgesic efficacy or adverse effects
Bruera[42]	95	HM SR q12h vs HM IR q4h	no differences in analgesic efficacy or adverse effects
Moulin[43]	20	HM: CSCI vs CIVI	no differences in analgesic efficacy or adverse effects
Miller[44]	74	HM CSCI vs morphine CSCI	no differences in analgesic efficacy or adverse effects
Moriaty[45]	100	HM SR q12h vs morphine SR q12h	no differences in analgesic efficacy or adverse effects
Hagen[46]	44	HM SR q12h vs oxycodone SR q12h	no differences in analgesic efficacy or adverse effects

SR preparation is also available.[38] There is some uncertainty about the equianalgesic doses and conversion ratios between hydromorphone and morphine.[39, 40] The greater solubility of hydromorphone compared to morphine allows delivery of higher doses by subcutaneous infusion.

Levorphanol

Levorphanol is a synthetic opioid analgesic that may be used for patients suffering unacceptable adverse effects with morphine. It has a long half-life (12–16h) but a short duration of clinical action (4–6h), necessitating careful titration of the dose to avoid sedation and the effects of drug accumulation.

Methadone

Methadone is a strong opioid analgesic that has been used widely for opioid dependence, but more recently it has been shown to be a useful and effective drug for the treatment of cancer-related pain (Table 11.12).[3, 47] It is used for the treatment of severe pain in patients with morphine intolerance or pain poorly responsive to morphine, especially neuropathic pain; the latter effect is attributed to methadone being a potent NMDA receptor antagonist. Methadone

Table 11.12   Methadone

Pharmacology	active PO, PR, IM, IV, SC bioavailability PO 80%, but considerable interindividual variation actions: μ opioid agonist, NMDA receptor antagonist metabolized in liver, mainly excreted by faecal route plasma half-life: 15h initially, 2–3 days with continued use duration of action: 4–6h initially, 8–12h with continued use
Indications	severe pain pain poorly responsive to morphine, especially neuropathic pain intolerance to morphine or other opioid renal failure
Cautions	frail, elderly, confused

Drug interactions	CYP3A4 inhibitors cause increased methadone levels and toxicity
	    e.g. erythromycin, ketoconazole, ciprofloxacin, SSRIs
	CYP3A4 inducers cause decreased methadone levels and effect
	    e.g. phenytoin, carbamazepine, phenobarbital, corticosteroids

Adverse effects	similar to morphine cumulative toxicity heralded by sedation
Dose	calculated from previous therapy, adjusted for effect and toxicity frequency: q4–6h for first 1–3d, then q6–12h
Switching	from morphine to methadone 1. stop morphine 2. give methadone: 1/10 of 24h PO morphine dose (max dose 30mg), q3h PRN 3. day 6: divide total methadone on days 4 + 5 by 4 and give q12h; similar or smaller dose q3h PRN for breakthrough pain
Preparations	tablet, mixture, injection

is not affected by renal function and may be useful in patients with renal impairment. The adverse effects are similar to morphine in addition to which cumulative toxicity may occur with sedation, confusion and narcosis. This is caused by the progressive prolongation of the half-life of the drug with continued therapy, and it is necessary to reduce both the dose and the frequency of administration after the first few days. Sedation may also occur if methadone metabolism is inhibited by a variety of drugs including macrolides (e.g. erythromycin), imidazoles (e.g. fluconazole), quinolones (e.g. ciprofloxacin) and SSRIs.[47, 48] Subcutaneous methadone causes erythema and induration, but CSCIs are feasible provided the needle site is changed as often as required or if dexamethasone 1–2mg/d is added to the infusion.[49]

Methadone and morphine have been shown to produce equivalent analgesia and similar adverse effects in RCTs (Table 11.13). Unrelieved pain or unacceptable adverse effects, or both, in patients taking morphine may be significantly improved by switching to methadone.[50] Switching from morphine to methadone requires careful titration, one method for which is shown in Table 11.12.[51] Patients previously taking methadone for opioid dependence are reported to be relatively refractory to the analgesic effects of other opioids, but can achieve good control of cancer-related pain with increased doses of methadone.[52] Methadone for the treatment of pain needs to be given 6- to 12-hourly, in contrast to the daily dose given to prevent withdrawal in patients with dependence.

Table 11.13 Methadone: RCTs

Author	n	Intervention	Outcome
Ventafridda[53]	66	PO methadone vs PO morphine	no difference in efficacy or adverse effects
Grochow[54]	23	IV methadone vs IV morphine as PCA	no difference in degree or duration of pain relief
Mercadante[55]	40	PO methadone vs morphine SR PO	no difference in efficacy or adverse effects; methadone dose increased less with time

Oxycodone

Oxycodone is a semi-synthetic derivative of codeine and has similar properties (Table 11.14). It has a wider therapeutic range than codeine and may be used in lower doses to treat mild

Table 11.14 Oxycodone

Pharmacology	active PO, PR, SC, IM, IV plasma half-life 3.5h metabolized in liver, excreted in urine duration of action 4–6h (IR), 12h (SR)
Indications	mild to moderate and severe pain
Cautions	renal impairment
Adverse effects	qualitatively similar to morphine
Dose	calculated from previous therapy, adjusted for effect and toxicity
Dose equivalence	20mg PO or PR is equivalent to morphine 30mg PO 7.5mg SC oxycodone is equivalent to morphine 10mg SC
Preparations	tablet, SR tablet, liquid, suppository

to moderate pain (WHO Analgesic Ladder, Step 2), or in higher doses for severe pain (Step 3). The SR preparation, given 12-hourly, produces equivalent analgesia and similar adverse effects to IR oxycodone given 6-hourly (Table 11.15). A longer term study showed a reduction in adverse effects with time.[56] Oxycodone can be given by CSCI although there is limited experience in patients with cancer.[57]

Oxycodone SR gives equivalent analgesia to oral morphine SR and hydromorphone SR (Table 11.15). Oxycodone may be associated with less nausea and vomiting, hallucinations, and pruritus. Significant improvements in confusion, sedation and nausea are reported in patients taking morphine or hydromorphone who are switched to oxycodone.[57–59]

Table 11.15 Oxycodone: RCTs

Author	n	Intervention	Outcome
Kaplan[60]	164	oxycodone SR vs oxycodone IR	no difference in efficacy or adverse effects
Parris[61]	111	oxycodone SR vs oxycodone IR	no difference in efficacy or adverse effects
Salzman[62]	48	oxycodone SR vs oxycodone IR	no difference in efficacy or adverse effects
Stambaugh[63]	30	oxycodone SR vs oxycodone IR	no difference in efficacy or adverse effects
Heiskanen[64]	45	oxycodone SR vs morphine SR	equivalent efficacy; oxycodone more constipation, morphine more vomiting (pS)
Bruera[65]	32	oxycodone SR vs morphine SR	no difference in efficacy or adverse effects
Mucci-LoRusso[66]	100	oxycodone SR vs morphine SR	no difference in efficacy; less pruritus with oxycodone (pS)
Hagen[46]	44	oxycodone SR vs hydromorphone SR	no difference in efficacy or adverse effects

Pethidine (Meperidine)

Pethidine (meperidine) is a synthetic opioid drug used for the treatment of severe acute pain. It has a therapeutic ceiling related to CNS toxicity and should not be used in the management of chronic cancer pain. Accumulation of norpethidine occurs in patients given high or frequent doses and those with significant renal impairment, causing CNS excitation with agitation, tremors, myoclonus and seizures.[67] Sedation and respiratory depression caused by pethidine are reversed by naloxone; the myoclonus and seizures are unresponsive to naloxone and are treated with benzodiazepines and anticonvulsants.

Tramadol

Tramadol is a synthetic opioid analgesic used for moderate to severe cancer pain (Table 11.16).[68] It acts as an opioid agonist and also inhibits presynaptic uptake of noradrenaline and serotonin, which may activate the descending inhibitory pathways. The latter action

Table 11.16 Tramadol

Pharmacology	active PO, PR, SC, IM, IV actions: opioid agonist, monoamine re-uptake inhibitor plasma half-life 6h metabolized in liver, excreted in urine duration of action 4–6h
Indications	moderate pain
Cautions	severe renal or hepatic impairment epilepsy, drugs that reduce seizure threshold e.g. TCAs, SSRIs SSRIs: risk of serotonin syndrome
Adverse effects	similar to other opioids, generally mild less constipating uncommon neuropsychiatric reactions and serotonin syndrome
Dose	50–100mg q4–6h or 100–200mg QD PO q12h
Dose equivalence	80mg IM is equivalent to morphine 10mg IM 120mg PO is equivalent to morphine 30mg PO
Preparations	tablets, capsules, SR capsules, liquid, injection

Table 11.17 Tramadol: RCTs in patients with moderate cancer pain

Author	n	Intervention	Outcome
Tawfik[71]	64	tramadol PO vs morphine SR	morphine more effective in severe pain (pS); less tolerance with tramadol
Wilder-Smith[72]	25	tramadol PO vs morphine IR	equivalent analgesia by day 4; tramadol: less nausea, less constipation (pS)

explains why the effect of tramadol is only partly reversed by naloxone. Tramadol has been compared with morphine for the treatment of cancer pain in two RCTs (Table 11.17). The patients had moderate to severe pain (WHO Analgesic Ladder, Step 2). Tramadol was an effective analgesic and caused less nausea and constipation; sedation was reported to be the same as with morphine. Non-randomized studies reported similar findings.[69, 70]

The adverse effects of tramadol are generally mild and it is reported to be associated with less nausea, constipation, respiratory depression and tolerance than equivalent drugs. Its abuse potential is regarded as low, but physical withdrawal syndromes are well documented.[73, 74] Neuropsychiatric syndromes including confusion and hallucinations can occur.[74, 75] The serotonin syndrome[76] (Table11.18) is also reported with tramadol, typically when it is prescribed for patients taking SSRIs.[74]

Table 11.18 Diagnosis of the serotonin syndrome[76]

1. at least 3 of 10 clinical features

mental state changes	myoclonus	sweating	tremor	incoordination
agitation	hyperreflexia	shivering	diarrhoea	fever

2. coincident with addition of, or increased dose of, a serotonergic drug
   e.g. antidepressants: MAOIs, TCAs, SSRIs; buspirone

Mixed agonist–antagonist opioids

The mixed agonist–antagonist opioid drugs have a high incidence of psychotomimetic effects and may cause withdrawal symptoms when given to patients receiving other opioid agonist drugs. They have no role in the treatment of chronic pain due to cancer.

Butorphanol is administered by injection, 2 mg IM being equivalent to 10 mg IM morphine. It may be of use in the management of acute pain in patients taking no other opioid drugs.

Nalbuphine is administered by injection, 10 mg IM being equivalent to 10 mg IM morphine. It has a lower incidence of psychotomimetic effects than the other mixed agonist–antagonist drugs. It may have a role in the management of acute pain in patients taking no other opioid drugs.

Pentazocine is a synthetic opioid. By injection, pentazocine is rapidly effective; given orally, it is both slower acting and less potent and should be considered only a weak opioid. Psychotomimetic effects occur in up to 10% of patients, and acute physical withdrawal reactions are reported in patients with significant prior exposure to opioids [77].

References

1   De Conno, F., et al. (1991). A clinical study on the use of codeine, oxycodone, dextropropoxyphene, buprenorphine, and pentazocine in cancer pain. *Journal of Pain and Symptom Management* 6, 423–7.

2   Clark, N.C., Lintzeris, N. and Muhleisen, P.J. (2002). Severe opiate withdrawal in a heroin user precipitated by a massive buprenorphine dose. *Medical Journal of Australia* 176, 166–7.

3   Twycross, R., et al. (2002). *Palliative Care Formulary*. Oxford, Radcliffe Medical Press. <www.palliativedrugs.net>

4   Chary, S., et al. (1994). The dose-response relationship of controlled-release codeine (Codeine Contin) in chronic cancer pain. *Journal of Pain and Symptom Management* 9, 363–71.

5   Dhaliwal, H.S., et al. (1995). Randomized evaluation of controlled-release codeine and placebo in chronic cancer pain. *Journal of Pain and Symptom Management* 10, 612–23.

6   Jones, T.E., et al. (1996). Dextromoramide pharmacokinetics following sublingual administration. *Palliative Medicine* 10, 313–17.

7   Mercadante, S., et al. (1998). Dextropropoxyphene versus morphine in opioid-naive cancer patients with pain. *Journal of Pain and Symptom Management* 15, 76–81.

8   Twycross, R.G. (1977). Choice of strong analgesic in terminal cancer: diamorphine or morphine? *Pain* 3, 93–104.

9   Gauthier, M.E. and Fine, P.G. (1997). The emerging role of the fentanyl series in the treatment of chronic cancer pain. In *Topics in Palliative Care. Volume 1* (ed. R. Portenoy and E. Bruera). New York, Oxford University Press.

10   Singer, M. and Noonan, K.R. (1993). Continuous intravenous infusion of fentanyl: case reports of use in patients with advanced cancer and intractable pain. *Journal of Pain and Symptom Management* 8, 215–20.

11   Paix, A., et al. (1995). Subcutaneous fentanyl and sufentanil infusion substitution for morphine intolerance in cancer pain management. *Pain* 63, 263–9.

12   Watanabe, S., et al. (1998). Fentanyl by continuous subcutaneous infusion for the management of cancer pain: a retrospective study. *Journal of Pain and Symptom Management* 16, 323–6.

13   Hunt, R., et al. (1999). A comparison of subcutaneous morphine and fentanyl in hospice cancer patients. *Journal of Pain and Symptom Management* 18, 111–9.

14   Kirkham, S.R. and Pugh, R. (1995). Opioid analgesia in uraemic patients. *Lancet* 345, 1185.

15   Ahmedzai, S. and Brooks, D. (1997). Transdermal fentanyl versus sustained-release oral morphine in cancer pain: preference, efficacy, and quality of life. The TTS-Fentanyl Comparative Trial Group. *Journal of Pain and Symptom Management* 13, 254–61.

16 Wong, J.O., et al. (1997). Comparison of oral controlled-release morphine with transdermal fentanyl in terminal cancer pain. *Acta Anaesthesiologica Sinica*. 35, 25–32.

17 Christie, J.M., et al. (1998). Dose-titration, multicenter study of oral transmucosal fentanyl citrate for the treatment of breakthrough pain in cancer patients using transdermal fentanyl for persistent pain. *Journal of Clinical Oncology* 16, 3238–45.

18 Farrar, J.T., et al. (1998). Oral transmucosal fentanyl citrate: randomized, double-blinded, placebo-controlled trial for treatment of breakthrough pain in cancer patients. *Journal of the National Cancer Institute* 90, 611–6.

19 Portenoy, R.K., et al. (1999). Oral transmucosal fentanyl citrate (OTFC) for the treatment of breakthrough pain in cancer patients: a controlled dose titration study. *Pain* 79, 303–12.

20 Coluzzi, P.H., et al. (2001). Breakthrough cancer pain: a randomized trial comparing oral transmucosal fentanyl citrate (OTFC) and morphine sulfate immediate release (MSIR). *Pain* 91, 123–30.

21 Vielvoye-Kerkmeer, A.P., Mattern, C. and Uitendaal, M.P. (2000). Transdermal fentanyl in opioid-naive cancer pain patients: an open trial using transdermal fentanyl for the treatment of chronic cancer pain in opioid-naive patients and a group using codeine. *Journal of Pain and Symptom Management* 19, 185–92.

22 Grond, S., et al. (1997). Transdermal fentanyl in the long-term treatment of cancer pain: a prospective study of 50 patients with advanced cancer of the gastrointestinal tract or the head and neck region. *Pain* 69, 191–8.

23 Donner, B., et al. (1998). Long-term treatment of cancer pain with transdermal fentanyl. *Journal of Pain and Symptom Management* 15, 168–75.

24 Nugent, M., et al. (2001). Long-term observations of patients receiving transdermal fentanyl after a randomized trial. *Journal of Pain and Symptom Management* 21, 385–91.

25 Radbruch, L., et al. (2001). Transdermal fentanyl for the management of cancer pain: a survey of 1005 patients. *Palliative Medicine* 15, 309–21.

26 Newshan, G. (1998). Heat-related toxicity with the fentanyl transdermal patch. *Journal of Pain and Symptom Management* 16, 277–8.

27 Gardner-Nix, J. (2001). Caregiver toxicity from transdermal fentanyl. *Journal of Pain and Symptom Management* 21, 447–8.

28 Reeves, M.D. and Ginifer, C.J. (2002). Fatal intravenous misuse of transdermal fentanyl. *Medical Journal of Australia* 177, 552–3.

29 Zeppetella, G. (2001). Sublingual fentanyl citrate for cancer-related breakthrough pain: a pilot study. *Palliative Medicine* 15, 323–8.

30 Gardner-Nix, J. (2001). Oral transmucosal fentanyl and sufentanil for incident pain. *Journal of Pain and Symptom Management* 22, 627–30.

31 Zeppetella, G. (2000). An assessment of the safety, efficacy, and acceptability of intranasal fentanyl citrate in the management of cancer-related breakthrough pain: a pilot study. *Journal of Pain and Symptom Management* 20, 253–8.

32 Jackson, K., Ashby, M. and Keech, J. (2002). Pilot dose finding study of intranasal sufentanil for breakthrough and incident cancer-associated pain. *Journal of Pain and Symptom Management* 23, 450–2.

33 Fine, P.G. and Streisand, J.B. (1998). A review of oral transmucosal fentanyl citrate: potent, rapid, and noninvasive opioid analgesia. *Journal of Palliative Medicine* 1, 55–63.

34 Payne, R., et al. (2001). Long-term safety of oral transmucosal fentanyl citrate for breakthrough cancer pain. *Journal of Pain and Symptom Management* 22, 575–83.

35 Sarhill, N., Walsh, D. and Nelson, K.A. (2001). Hydromorphone: pharmacology and clinical applications in cancer patients. *Supportive Care in Cancer* 9, 84–96.

36 Quigley, C. (2002). Hydromorphone for acute and chronic pain (Cochrane Review). *Cochrane Database of Systematic Reviews* CD003447.

37 Quigley, C. (2003). A systematic review of hydromorphone in acute and chronic pain. *Journal of Pain and Symptom Management* 25, 169–78.

38 Palangio, M., et al. (2002). Dose conversion and titration with a novel, once-daily, OROS osmotic technology, extended-release hydromorphone formulation in the treatment of chronic malignant or nonmalignant pain. *Journal of Pain and Symptom Management* 23, 355–68.

39 Anderson, R., et al. (2001). Accuracy in equianalgesic dosing. Conversion dilemmas. *Journal of Pain and Symptom Management* 21, 397–406.

40 Pereira, J., et al. (2001). Equianalgesic dose ratios for opioids. a critical review and proposals for long-term dosing. *Journal of Pain and Symptom Management* 22, 672–87.

41 Hays, H., et al. (1994). Comparative clinical efficacy and safety of immediate release and controlled release hydromorphone for chronic severe cancer pain. *Cancer* 74, 1808–16.

42 Bruera, E., et al. (1996). A randomized, double-blind, double-dummy, crossover trial comparing the safety and efficacy of oral sustained-release hydromorphone with immediate-release hydromorphone in patients with cancer pain. Canadian Palliative Care Clinical Trials Group. *Journal of Clinical Oncology* 14, 1713–7.

43 Moulin, D.E., et al. (1991). Comparison of continuous subcutaneous and intravenous hydromorphone infusions for management of cancer pain. *Lancet* 337, 465–8.

44 Miller, M.G., et al. (1999). Continuous subcutaneous infusion of morphine vs. hydromorphone: a controlled trial. *Journal of Pain and Symptom Management* 18, 9–16.

45 Moriarty, M. (1999). A randomised crossover comparison of controlled release hydromorphone tablets with controlled release morphine tablets in patients with pain. *Journal of Clinical Research* 2, 1–8.

46 Hagen, N.A. and Babul, N. (1997). Comparative clinical efficacy and safety of a novel controlled-release oxycodone formulation and controlled-release hydromorphone in the treatment of cancer pain. *Cancer* 79, 1428–37.

47 Bruera, E. and Sweeney, C. (2002). Methadone use in cancer patients with pain: a review. *Journal of Palliative Medicine* 5, 127–38.

48 Bernard, S.A. and Bruera, E. (2000). Drug interactions in palliative care. *Journal of Clinical Oncology* 18, 1780–99.

49 Mathew, P. and Storey, P. (1999). Subcutaneous methadone in terminally ill patients: manageable local toxicity. *Journal of Pain and Symptom Management* 18, 49–52.

50 Mercadante, S., et al. (2001). Switching from morphine to methadone to improve analgesia and tolerability in cancer patients: a prospective study. *Journal of Clinical Oncology* 19, 2898–904.

51 Morley, J. and Makin, M. (1998). The use of methadone in cancer pain poorly responsive to other opioids. *Pain Reviews* 5, 51–58.

52 Manfredi, P.L., et al. (2001). Methadone analgesia in cancer pain patients on chronic methadone maintenance therapy. *Journal of Pain and Symptom Management* 21, 169–74.

53 Ventafridda, V., et al. (1986). A randomized study on oral administration of morphine and methadone in the treatment of cancer pain. *Journal of Pain and Symptom Management* 1, 203–7.

54 Grochow, L., et al. (1989). Does intravenous methadone provide longer lasting analgesia than intravenous morphine? A randomized, double-blind study. *Pain* 38, 151–7.

55 Mercadante, S., et al. (1998). Morphine versus methadone in the pain treatment of advanced-cancer patients followed up at home. *Journal of Clinical Oncology* 16, 3656–61.

56 Citron, M.L., et al. (1998). Long-term administration of controlled-release oxycodone tablets for the treatment of cancer pain. *Cancer Investigation* 16, 562–71.

57 Maddocks, I., et al. (1996). Attenuation of morphine-induced delirium in palliative care by substitution with infusion of oxycodone. *Journal of Pain and Symptom Management* 12, 182–9.

58 Ashby, M.A., Martin, P. and Jackson, K.A. (1999). Opioid substitution to reduce adverse effects in cancer pain management. *Medical Journal of Australia* 170, 68–71.

59 Gagnon, B., et al. (1999). The use of intermittent subcutaneous injections of oxycodone for opioid rotation in patients with cancer pain. *Supportive Care in Cancer* 7, 265–70.

60 Kaplan, R., et al. (1998). Comparison of controlled-release and immediate-release oxycodone tablets in patients with cancer pain. *Journal of Clinical Oncology* 16, 3230–7.

61 Parris, W.C., et al. (1998). The use of controlled-release oxycodone for the treatment of chronic cancer pain: a randomized, double-blind study. *Journal of Pain and Symptom Management* 16, 205–11.

62 Salzman, R.T., et al. (1999). Can a controlled-release oral dose form of oxycodone be used as readily as an immediate-release form for the purpose of titrating to stable pain control? *Journal of Pain and Symptom Management* 18, 271–9.

63 Stambaugh, J.E., et al. (2001). Double-blind, randomized comparison of the analgesic and pharmacokinetic profiles of controlled- and immediate-release oral oxycodone in cancer pain patients. *Journal of Clinical Pharmacology* 41, 500–6.

64 Heiskanen, T. and Kalso, E. (1997). Controlled-release oxycodone and morphine in cancer related pain. *Pain* 73, 37–45.

65 Bruera, E., et al. (1998). Randomized, double-blind, cross-over trial comparing safety and efficacy of oral controlled-release oxycodone with controlled-release morphine in patients with cancer pain. *Journal of Clinical Oncology* 16, 3222–9.

66 Mucci-LoRusso, P., et al. (1998). Controlled-release oxycodone compared with controlled-release morphine in the treatment of cancer pain: a randomized, double-blind, parallel-group study. *European Journal of Pain* 2, 239–49.

67 Foley, K.M. (2001). Management of Cancer Pain. In *Cancer. Principles and Practice of Oncology. 6th edition* (ed. V.T. De Vita, S. Hellman and S.A. Rosenberg). Philadelphia, Lippincott Williams Wilkins.

68 Bamigbade, T.A. and Langford, R.M. (1998). The clinical use of tramadol hydrochloride. *Pain Reviews* 5, 155–82.

69 Grond, S., et al. (1999). High-dose tramadol in comparison to low-dose morphine for cancer pain relief. *Journal of Pain and Symptom Management* 18, 174–9.

70 Petzke, F., et al. (2001). Slow-release tramadol for treatment of chronic malignant pain—an open multicenter trial. *Supportive Care in Cancer* 9, 48–54.

71 Tawfik, M.O., Elborolossy, K. and Nasr, F. (1990). Tramadol hydrochloride in the relief of cancer pain. A double blind comparison against sustained release morphine. *Pain* 55, S377.

72 Wilder-Smith, C.H., et al. (1994). Oral tramadol, a mu-opioid agonist and monoamine reuptake-blocker, and morphine for strong cancer-related pain. *Annals of Oncology* 5, 141–6.

73 Freye, E. and Levy, J. (2000). Acute abstinence syndrome following abrupt cessation of long-term use of tramadol (Ultram): a case study. *European Journal of Pain* 4, 307–11.

74 Adverse Drug Reactions Advisory Committee (2003). Tramadol— four years' experience. *Australian Adverse Drug Reactions Bulletin* 22, 2.

75 Keeley, P.W., Foster, G. and Whitelaw, L. (2000). Hear my song: auditory hallucinations with tramadol hydrochloride. *British Medical Journal* 321, 1608.

76 Sternbach, H. (1991). The serotonin syndrome. *American Journal of Psychiatry* 148, 705–13.

77 Beaver, W.T., et al. (1966). A comparison of the analgesic effects of pentazocine and morphine in patients with cancer. *Clinical Pharmacology and Therapeutics* 7, 740–51.

12

Neuroaxial opioid therapy

Intraspinal
Intraventricular

Since its introduction in the 1970s, intraspinal opioid therapy has been used increasingly to treat the small proportion of patients with advanced cancer for whom systemic therapy provides inadequate pain relief or causes unacceptable adverse effects. More recently, the use of direct intraventricular opioid therapy has been explored for the treatment of intractable pain in patients with cancer.

Intraspinal therapy

The literature on the use of intraspinal therapy for patients with cancer has been reviewed.[1-3] It comprises a large number of case reports and retrospective studies and very few RCTs. Intraspinal therapy undoubtedly provides improved pain control for some patients with cancer, but the indications for its use and the optimal mode of administration remain to be defined.

Morphine injected into the subarachnoid space, or diffusing into the subarachnoid space after epidural injection, will diffuse into the dorsal horn of the spinal cord and produce analgesia by interaction with opioid receptors. The theoretic advantages of spinal morphine are listed in Table 12.1. However, after epidural injection only 10–20% of the morphine diffuses into the subarachnoid space and there is significant systemic absorption from the epidural space. Plasma levels may be equivalent to those following systemic administration, accounting for the central and systemic adverse effects. At the same time, the drug concentration in the cerebrospinal fluid (CSF) is much higher than after systemic administration, producing

Table 12.1   Theoretic advantages of intraspinal morphine

Use of much smaller doses of morphine

Delivered close to site of action (the spinal opioid receptors)

Less central adverse effects

Less systemic adverse effects

No neurological deficits as occur with anaesthetic blocks or neurosurgical procedures superior analgesia. There will be some rostral diffusion of morphine injected or diffusing into the subarachnoid space, predisposing to central adverse effects.

Indications

The indications and contraindications for spinal morphine are listed in Table 12.2. Spinal morphine is most likely to be successful with deep somatic and visceral pain. Neuropathic pain is less sensitive although good results are achieved for some patients. Spinal metastases need not be a contraindication but the catheter should be sited away from known tumour and better results are likely if it is rostral to the tumour.

Table 12.2 Spinal morphine

Indications	pain not controlled by optimal systemic opioid therapy
	intolerable adverse effects from systemic treatment
Contraindications	raised intracranial pressure
	significant bleeding tendency or anticoagulation
	infection in the region of catheter site
	septicaemia or significant risk of septicaemia

Administration

Intraspinal therapy is administered by injection into the epidural (EP) or subarachnoid space (intrathecal, IT). The spinal catheter may be connected to a subcutaneously implanted reservoir or brought out through the skin for intermittent injection or attachment to an external pumping device. Epidural catheters cause fibrosis, which may lead to blockage. Direct intrathecal therapy is safe and is said to be associated with better pain relief and patient satisfaction, fewer complications, and improved sleeping and walking patterns.[1] In addition, intrathecal therapy employs smaller doses, and as there is less systemic absorption than after epidural injection, there may be less systemic toxicity. In the palliative care setting where life expectancy is limited, an externalized catheter allows for more flexible therapy and avoids the expense of an implanted reservoir and pump. Intrathecal therapy may have a slightly higher risk of meningitis.

Treatment is given by bolus injection each 6–12 hours or by continuous infusion. A comparison of the two methods using the epidural route showed no difference in pain relief, although the need for dose escalation was more with the infusion (Table 12.4). Adverse effects, particularly sensorimotor disturbances related to local anaesthetics, are reportedly less with continuous infusions.

Medications

A variety of drugs may be used in addition to opioids, including local anaesthetics, α-adrenergic agonists, and NMDA receptor antagonists, although the indications for their use are not clearly defined.[4] Drugs used for spinal therapy should be preservative free.

Opioids. Morphine is the drug that has been used most. The dose of morphine used for spinal therapy depends on the route of administration and the patient's current opioid therapy (Table 12.3). The dose is then adjusted according to effect and toxicity. Loss of analgesic efficacy of intrathecal morphine analgesia is associated with high levels of the excitatory amino acids, glutamate and aspartate, in the CSF.[5] Other opioids that have been used include hydromorphone, fentanyl, sufentanil, and methadone.[1, 6]

Table 12.3 Spinal morphine: dose

Epidural (EP)
    10% of previous systemic dose (mg/24h SC)
        e.g. morphine 200mg/24h CSCI → 20mg/24h EP as continuous infusion
        or 5mg q6h EP by bolus injection

Subarachnoid/ Intrathecal (IT)
    1% of previous systemic dose (mg/24h SC)
        e.g. morphine 200mg/24h CSCI → 2mg/24h IT as continuous infusion
        or 0.5mg q6h IT by bolus injection

Local anaesthetics. Addition of bupivacaine appears to act synergistically with the opioid, resulting in better pain relief and sometimes allowing lower doses of opioids to be used (Table 12.4).[1,4] The addition of bupivacaine reduced the need for increasing morphine doses in an RCT (Table 12.4).

Adrenergic agonists. Addition of the α-adrenergic agonist, clonidine, improved pain control in an RCT, and the effect was most noticeable for neuropathic pain (Table 12.4). Adverse effects include dose-dependent bradycardia and hypotension. Tizanidine is under investigation for intrathecal therapy.

NMDA receptor antagonist. A single small trial of morphine, with or without ketamine, reported better pain control with the combination (Table 12.4).

Table 12.4 Intrathecal (IT) and epidural (EP) therapy: RCTs

Author	n	Intervention	Outcome
Gourlay[7]	29	EP morphine: bolus vs infusion	no difference in pain control; more dose escalation required with infusion (pS)
Van Dongen[8]	12	IT morphine ± bupivacaine	less ↑ in morphine dose with combination (pS)
Eisenach[9]	85	EP morphine + clonidine vs placebo	better pain control with clonidine (pS); most marked for neuropathic pain
Yang[10]	20	IT morphine ± ketamine	better pain control with ketamine (pS)
Kalso[11]	10	morphine EP vs SC	EP and SC equivalent; both superior to PO
Smith[12]	202	standard therapy ± IT therapy	+ IT: greater ↓ in pain (pNS), greater ↓ fatigue, sedation (pS)

Adverse effects

The adverse effects of spinal therapy are listed in Table 12.5. The most important is infection and the development of any symptoms or signs that suggest infection must be treated promptly with antibiotics and removal of the catheter. Bacterial filters should be used routinely if the catheter is externalized. Catheter-related problems are uncommon but often require surgical replacement. Radicular pain occurring after bolus epidural injection, due to the proximity of the catheter tip to the nerve root, may respond to corticosteroid injection or require re-siting.

Table 12.5 Adverse effects of spinal therapy

Procedure related
    anaesthesia, haemorrhage, infection, nerve damage
    cost of implanted catheters, reservoirs, pumps

Morphine related
    central side effects: respiratory depression, sedation, vomiting
    systemic side effects: constipation, urinary retention
    pruritus
    dysaesthesia, myoclonus

Catheter related
    obstruction: blockage, kinking, epidural fibrosis
    dislodgement, migration, disconnection
    infection: meningitis, epidural abscess, catheter site, pump pocket
    CSF leak (subarachnoid)
    radicular pain (epidural)

Spinal morphine is not without central side effects and respiratory depression, sedation, dysphoria, nausea and vomiting are all reported. However, the incidence is less in cancer patients who are not opioid-naive. If severe, treatment is with small doses of naloxone. Occasionally, physical withdrawal symptoms occur if systemic opioid therapy is stopped after commencement of spinal therapy; in the absence of signs of respiratory depression, the previous systemic therapy should be weaned over several days.

Systemic side effects including urinary retention and constipation can occur but are less common and less severe in cancer patients who are not opioid-naïve. Pruritus, if severe, can be treated with ondansetron or subhypnotic doses of propofol. Reduction in libido and testosterone levels is reported with spinal therapy.[13]

Tolerance will develop with continued spinal therapy, necessitating dose increments. It is difficult to determine how much of the increased dose relates to disease progression and how much to pharmacological tolerance.[14] There is no evidence that tolerance is particularly more or less likely to develop than with systemic therapy.

Role in palliative care

Decisions concerning spinal therapy for palliative care patients with limited life expectancy need to be individualized. Spinal therapy has been shown to be as effective as subcutaneous opioids in one study, and superior to standard management (without intrathecal therapy) in another (Table 12.4). The latter, industry-sponsored, study [12] concludes that the implantation of a certain device for intrathecal therapy was associated with improved pain control, reduced drug toxicities, and improved survival in patients with refractory cancer pain. The study was not stratified by prognostic factors in order to assess survival, and the reduction in pain was not statistically significant in the intrathecal group compared to the controls. The improvements in sedation and fatigue were significant, suggesting that intrathecal therapy may improve quality of life for patients with advanced cancer.

Spinal therapy should certainly be considered for patients with advanced cancer for whom systemic therapy provides inadequate pain relief or unacceptable toxicity. Intrathecal therapy is probably preferable to epidural, and treatment should be given by infusion rather than bolus injections. Externalization of the catheter allows flexibility with medications and avoids the expense of implantable pumps. Subcutaneous tunnelling helps secure the catheter in place and may reduce the risk of infection. Bacterial filters should be used and changes of tubing minimized.

Intraventricular therapy

Direct injection of morphine into the lateral cerebral ventricle is reported to be effective for the majority of patients with severe pain refractory to other treatment, including pain related to advanced head and neck cancer, pain that is midline, bilateral or diffuse, and neuropathic pain.[15]

Administration is by daily injection into an Ommaya reservoir, which requires a strict aseptic technique. Opioid tolerance is rare. Transient adverse effects, such as nausea and respiratory depression, may be more frequent than with spinal therapy. Persistent problems like urinary retention and nausea occur more frequently with spinal therapy.[16]

Catheter infection and meningitis are the most serious complications, but occur infrequently. Catheter blockage or dislodgement can occur.

Measurement of the levels of morphine and its metabolites in the CSF provides some insight into the action of morphine, including the control of recalcitrant neuropathic pain. Before intraventricular therapy, patients receiving high doses of systemic morphine have elevated CSF levels of morphine and M3G. After initiation of intraventricular therapy, the CSF morphine is increased 50-fold and the M3G level reduced by a factor of 10 to 15.[15, 17] This indicates that high CSF morphine levels are unlikely to be the cause of the development of tolerance or the neuroexcitatory effects such as hyperalgesia, myoclonus and seizures.

The role of intraventricular therapy remains to be defined, but there is sufficient evidence for it to be considered for patients with pain refractory to other treatment.

References

1   Bennett, G., et al. (2000). Evidence-based review of the literature on intrathecal delivery of pain medication. *Journal of Pain and Symptom Management* 20, S12–36.

2   Du Pen, S.L. and Du Pen, A.R. (2000). Intraspinal analgesic therapy in palliative care: evolving perspective. In *Topics in Palliative Care. Volume 4* (ed. R. Portenoy and E. Bruera). New York, Oxford University Press.

3   Sjoberg, M. and Rawal, N. (2001). Intraspinal pain therapy in palliative care. In *Topics in Palliative Care. Volume 5* (ed. E. Bruera and R. Portenoy). New York, Oxford University Press.

4   Bennett, G., et al. (2000). Clinical guidelines for intraspinal infusion: report of an expert panel. PolyAnalgesic Consensus Conference 2000. *Journal of Pain and Symptom Management* 20, S37–43.

5   Wong, C.S., et al. (2002). Loss of intrathecal morphine analgesia in terminal cancer patients is associated with high levels of excitatory amino acids in the CSF. *Canadian Journal of Anaesthesia* 49, 561–5.

6   Shir, Y., et al. (1991). Continuous epidural methadone treatment for cancer pain. *Clinical Journal of Pain* 7, 339–41.

7   Gourlay, G.K., et al. (1991). Comparison of intermittent bolus with continuous infusion of epidural morphine in the treatment of severe cancer pain. *Pain* 47, 135–40.

8   van Dongen, R.T., Crul, B.J. and van Egmond, J. (1999). Intrathecal coadministration of bupivacaine diminishes morphine dose progression during long-term intrathecal infusion in cancer patients. *Clinical Journal of Pain* 15, 166–72.

9   Eisenach, J.C., et al. (1995). Epidural clonidine analgesia for intractable cancer pain. The Epidural Clonidine Study Group. *Pain* 61, 391–9.

10 Yang, C.Y., et al. (1996). Intrathecal ketamine reduces morphine requirements in patients with terminal cancer pain. *Canadian Journal of Anaesthesia* 43, 379–83.

11   Kalso, E., et al. (1996). Epidural and subcutaneous morphine in the management of cancer pain: a double-blind cross-over study. *Pain* 67, 443–9.

12   Smith, T.J., et al. (2002). Randomized clinical trial of an implantable drug delivery system compared with comprehensive medical management for refractory cancer pain: impact on pain, drug-related toxicity, and survival. *Journal of Clinical Oncology* 20, 4040–9.

13   Paice, J.A., Penn, R.D. and Ryan, W.G. (1994). Altered sexual function and decreased testosterone in patients receiving intraspinal opioids. *Journal of Pain and Symptom Management* 9, 126–31.

14   Sallerin-Caute, B., et al. (1998). Does intrathecal morphine in the treatment of cancer pain induce the development of tolerance? *Neurosurgery* 42, 44–9.

15   Cramond, T. (1998). Invasive techniques for neuropathic pain in cancer. In *Topics in Palliative Care. Volume 2* (ed. E. Bruera and R. Portenoy). New York, Oxford University Press.

16   Ballantyne, J.C., et al. (1996). Comparative efficacy of epidural, subarachnoid, and intracerebroventricular opioids in patients with pain due to cancer. *Regional Anesthesia* 21, 542–56.

17   Smith, M.T., et al. (1999). Cerebrospinal fluid and plasma concentrations of morphine, morphine-3-glucuronide, and morphine-6-glucuronide in patients before and after initiation of intracerebroventricular morphine for cancer pain management. *Anesthesia and Analgesia* 88, 109–16.

13

Adjuvant analgesics

Corticosteroids
Neuropathic pain
    antidepressants
    anticonvulsants
    local anaesthetics
    NMDA antagonists
Psychotropics
    neuroleptics
    anxiolytics
    psychostimulants

Muscle relaxants
Bone pain
    bisphosphonates
    radioisotopes
Antibiotics

The adjuvant analgesics or co-analgesics are a diverse group of drugs that were developed for other indications, but which may contribute substantially to pain relief when used either alone or in combination with analgesics. They may enhance the effects of analgesics, and can have an analgesic-sparing effect that results in fewer adverse effects. They are effective in treating certain types of pain, particularly neuropathic pain.

Corticosteroids

Corticosteroids inhibit prostaglandin production with reduction of inflammation and oedema associated with tumour deposits, leading to reduced pain stimulation and nerve compression. They also have a central action, evidenced by their effect on mood and appetite, which may augment analgesia. In patients with lymphoproliferative disorders, and a few with breast and prostate cancers, there is also an antitumour effect.

Indications. The indications for corticosteroid therapy are summarized in Table 13.1. They are particularly useful for pain associated with neurological complications of cancer. In patients with haematological malignancies, corticosteroids are frequently effective in relieving generalized bone pain and that due to hepatosplenomegaly or lymphadenopathy. There are no absolute contraindications to corticosteroid therapy, but the presence or severity of some adverse effects may limit the dose.

Analgesic effect. Two RCTs of treatment with methylprednisolone reported significant improvement in pain (Table 13.2). In the first study, methylprednisolone was reported to be

Table 13.1 Indications for corticosteroids as adjuvant analgesics

Neurological
    raised intracranial pressure
    spinal cord compression
    nerve compression or infiltration

Bone metastases

Capsular stretching
    liver metastases, other visceral metastases

Soft tissue infiltration
    head and neck tumours, abdominal and pelvic tumours

Vascular obstruction
    vena caval obstruction, lymphoedema

Metastases to joints (intra-articular injection)

Tenesmus (rectal suppository or enema)

To reduce effects of haematological malignancies

effective for neuropathic, bone and visceral pain.[1] Improvement in bone pain was reported in 38% of patients with advanced prostate cancer treated with prednisolone and the effect correlated with suppression of adrenal androgens;[2] the analgesic effect was less noticeable in a subsequent RCT.[3] A prospective study of corticosteroid use in palliative care reported reduced pain scores.[4]

Table 13.2 Analgesic effect of corticosteroids: RCTs

Author	n	Intervention	Outcome
Bruera[1]	40	methylprednisolone vs placebo	↓ pain scores (pS)
Della Cuna[5]	403	methylprednisolone vs placebo	↓ pain scores (pS)

Choice of preparation. The commonly used preparations are prednisolone, dexamethasone and hydrocortisone (Table 13.3). If parenteral therapy is required, dexamethasone is cheaper than hydrocortisone and has less mineralocorticoid effects. If continued oral therapy is anticipated, especially at moderate or high dosage, dexamethasone is preferable to prednisolone because of the lesser mineralocorticoid effect.

Table 13.3 Corticosteroid preparations

	Hydrocortisone	Prednisolone	Dexamethasone
Equivalent dose (glucocorticoid effect)	100mg	25mg	4mg
Mineralocorticoid effect	++	+	—

Dose. Acute neurological problems, including spinal cord compression and raised intracranial pressure, are treated with dexamethasone 16–24 mg/day. The dose is weaned as soon as clinically feasible. For patients unable to take oral medications, dexamethasone can be given by continuous subcutaneous infusion.

For other indications, dexamethasone 2–4 mg/d or prednisolone 15–30 mg/d are frequently effective; however, treatment can be initiated at a higher dose, in order not to miss a treatment effect, and the dose then weaned.

Adverse effects. The adverse effects of corticosteroids (Table 13.4) relate to both the dose employed and the duration of treatment. For patients with cancer, the clinical importance of these effects depends very much on their anticipated life expectancy.

Table 13.4 Adverse effects of corticosteroids

General	Cushingoid facies: moonface, hirsuitism body habitus: truncal obesity, interscapular hump
Gastrointestinal	gastric erosion, ulceration, bleeding increased appetite, weight gain
Metabolic	hyperglycaemia, diabetes sodium and fluid retention hypokalaemia and muscle weakness hypoadrenalism (with sudden withdrawal)
Cardiovascular	oedema, hypertension thrombosis
Musculoskeletal	improved muscle strength proximal myopathy arthralgia (with dose reduction) osteoporosis, aseptic necrosis
Infection	predisposition to infection, oral candidiasis, acneiform rash
Psychological	improved sense of well-being, euphoria emotional lability, agitation, dysphoria, hypomania depression, steroid psychosis
Dermatological	impaired wound healing, skin atrophy and thinning easy bruising, purpura, striae
Ophthalmological	cataracts
Haematological	neutrophilia, lymphopenia

The common adverse effects in clinical practice are oropharyngeal candidiasis and proximal myopathy. Dyspepsia occurs relatively frequently, particularly in patients taking NSAIDs, and treatment with a proton pump inhibitor should be considered. There may be subjective improvement in muscle strength, which is often transient. Chronic administration leads to proximal myopathy and weakness that can be debilitating. Fluid retention and oedema are not usually troublesome except with high doses but care must be taken in patients with hypertension and cardiac or renal disease. Abrupt withdrawal can produce hypoadrenalism and some patients suffer severe arthralgia.

The neuropsychological adverse effects of corticosteroids are variable. There is frequently an improved sense of well being, although many patients also suffer insomnia. Less frequently, patients develop more serious side effects including agitation, dysphoria, hypomania, depression, or even frank psychosis.

Adjuvant drugs for neuropathic pain

Antidepressants

Antidepressants block the presynaptic re-uptake of serotonin and noradrenaline in the central nervous system, enhancing the action of the descending inhibitory pathways. The tricyclic antidepressants (TCAs; e.g. amitriptyline), the serotonin noradrenaline re-uptake inhibitors (SNRIs; e.g. venlafaxine), and the noradrenergic and specific serotoninergic antidepressants (NSSAs, e.g. mirtazepine) affect both monoamine systems, whilst selective serotonin re-uptake inhibitors (SSRIs; e.g. fluoxetine, paroxetine) affect only serotonin. Drugs affecting both systems have a greater analgesic effect.[6–9]

Antidepressants are indicated for the treatment of neuropathic pain, based on their efficacy in non-malignant conditions.[6, 9–12] They are also useful for pain complicated by insomnia or depression. There is no evidence that the character of the neuropathic pain determines whether a response will occur, or that antidepressants are more effective than other agents for the burning dysaesthetic type of pain.[6, 7, 13]

The analgesic effect of TCAs is usually seen with doses lower than required for the treatment of depression (50–100 mg/d amitriptyline), occurs more quickly (response should be evident within 5 days) than the antidepressant effect, and has been documented in patients with no features of depression. A TCA (amitriptyline, imipramine or doxepin) is started at a dose of 10–25 mg at night, increasing to 50–100 mg; if there is no benefit in one week the drug is stopped. There is considerable individual variation in patients' responses to different drugs, and a trial of a second antidepressant is sometimes successful. TCAs are probably more effective at relieving neuropathic pain than the newer antidepressants, but have double the rate of adverse effects.[6, 7, 9] Three small RCTs of antidepressant therapy for cancer-related neuropathic pain report limited effectiveness, and further larger studies are needed (Table 13.5). Topical application of doxepin is reported to relieve neuropathic pain.[14]

The adverse effects of TCAs (sedation, anticholinergic effects and postural hypotension) are usually mild when used in low dose for neuropathic pain, but may nevertheless be troublesome in palliative care patients.

Table 13.5 Antidepressants for cancer-related neuropathic pain: RCTs

Author	n	Intervention	Outcome
Mercadante[15]	16	amitriptyline vs placebo	no change in global pain score; ↓ worst pain intensity (pS)
Tasmuth[16]	13	venlafaxine vs placebo	no change in average pain intensity; ↓ worst pain intensity (pS)
Theobald[17]	36	mirtazepine 15 vs 30mg	slight ↓ pain with either dose (pNS)

Anticonvulsants

The mechanisms by which anticonvulsants affect neuropathic pain remain uncertain. They suppress the spontaneous neuronal discharges and neuronal hyperexcitability that occur after nerve injury and may also have a central effect.

The use of anticonvulsants in cancer-related neuropathic pain is based on their widespread use in the treatment of chronic nonmalignant neuropathic conditions.[7, 18, 19] There is no evidence that anticonvulsants are more effective than other drugs for the shooting lancinating type of pain.

Gabapentin was reported to be effective in 20 of 22 patients with neuropathic pain incompletely controlled with opioids, including both burning and lancinating pain and allodynia.[20] Less than half of patients responded to gabapentin in another study.[21] A study of valproate reported a 57% response rate.[22] Gabapentin may be no more effective than carbamazepine, but causes less troublesome adverse effects.[19]

The anticonvulsant drugs used frequently in the treatment of neuropathic pain are gabapentin, carbamazepine, sodium valproate and clonazepam. The dose and the initial titration are the same as for anticonvulsant therapy, although there is no data relating blood levels and analgesic activity. The dose is increased step-wise until a response occurs or toxicity ensues. Serum levels can be checked and the drug should be stopped if there is no response when the levels are in the therapeutic range for anticonvulsant therapy. There is considerable lack of cross-resistance between the drugs and treatment with a second anticonvulsant is sometimes successful.

The adverse effects of the different anticonvulsants are similar, with gastric intolerance (nausea and vomiting), sedation, ataxia, dizziness and confusion being the most common. Carbamazepine can cause leucopenia and the white blood cell count should be checked periodically.

Local anaesthetics

Local anaesthetic agents act by neuronal membrane stabilization by sodium channel blockade, probably at both peripheral and central sites. They are used for neuropathic pain refractory to other therapy.

Lignocaine (lidocaine) infusions (2–5mg/kg IV over 30 minutes) can relieve pain due to peripheral nerve injury, including dysaesthesia and allodynia.[7, 23] Lignocaine is substantially more effective against pain caused by peripheral nerve injury than pain due to central nervous system damage.[24] Response to intravenous lignocaine can be used to predict whether there will be a response to mexiletine,[25] and may be useful for rapidly controlling severe neuropathic pain unresponsive to other measures. However, the RCTs in patients with cancer-related neuropathic pain showed no effect (Table 13.6). Successful subcutaneous infusion of lignocaine has been reported in patients with terminal cancer and refractory pain.[26]

Table 13.6 Lignocaine infusions for neuropathic cancer pain: RCTs

Author	n	Intervention	Outcome
Ellemann[29]	10	IV lidocaine 5mg/kg vs placebo	no significant differences
Bruera[30]	10	IV lidocaine 5mg/kg vs placebo	no significant differences

Mexiletine is the preferred oral local anaesthetic-type drug; flecainide and tocainide have been associated with cardiac and haematological toxicity, respectively. Mexiletine is commenced at a dose of 150 mg/d and increased by the same amount each few days up to a maximum of 750 mg/d. The dose and blood levels of mexiletine do not correlate with pain relief. Mexiletine must be given with particular caution to patients with ischaemic heart disease or cardiac arrhythmias. There are case reports of the successful use of mexiletine in patients with cancer-related neuropathic pain,[27] but it was effective in only two of eight patients in a pilot study.[28]

The adverse effects of mexiletine include dizziness, sedation, tremor, and unsteady gait; nausea and indigestion can be lessened by taking the medication with food. There are no serious adverse effects of lignocaine infusions.

NMDA receptor antagonists

The NMDA (N-methyl D-aspartate) receptors in the spinal cord are activated by continuing stimuli in nociceptive afferents, leading to sensitization of the dorsal horn cells and causing perpetuation of the sensation of pain and reduced opioid sensitivity.[31, 32] This mechanism is believed to underlie opioid tolerance and the relative opioid-insensitivity of neuropathic pain. The NMDA receptor antagonists, including ketamine, dextromethorphan and methadone, inhibit this process. Low magnesium levels predispose to NMDA activity, and administration of intravenous magnesium has been reported to relieve refractory neuropathic pain.[33]

NMDA receptor antagonists are indicated for the treatment of refractory neuropathic pain and other severe pain when opioid tolerance is a concern.

Ketamine. Ketamine is a dissociative anaesthetic used for short surgical procedures (Table 13.7). Administration of subanaesthetic doses has been shown to improve the effect of opioids in relieving refractory neuropathic pain or other opioid-insensitive pain in patients with cancer. It can be given orally,[34] intravenously,[35] or as a 3–5 day 'burst' therapy subcutaneously.[36] There are two RCTs of ketamine therapy in patients with advanced cancer (Table 13.8) that have been assessed in a Cochrane review.[37] Psychotomimetic effects are common and may be treated or prevented by the co-administration of a benzodiazepine or haloperidol.

Table 13.7 Ketamine

Action	anaesthetic, analgesic
Mechanism	NMDA receptor antagonist (subanaesthetic doses)
Pharmacology	active PO, SC, IV, IT plasma half-life 3h plasma half-life active metabolite (norketamine) 12h PO doses yield higher norketamine levels
Indications	refractory neuropathic pain or other opioid-insensitive pain
Cautions	hypertension, cardiac failure, cerebrovascular disease
Dose	reported doses vary widely PO: 25mg q6h, increase by 25–50mg/d CSCI: 0.1–0.5mg/kg/h; 100–200mg/d, increase by 50–100mg/d
Adverse effects neurological	sedation, drowsiness nightmares, hallucinations, dysphoria, delirium
cardiovascular	hypertension, tachycardia
gastrointestinal	nausea, vomiting, anorexia

Dextromethorphan. The antitussive, dextromethorphan, also has activity as an NMDA receptor antagonist and potentiates the action of opioids against diabetic neuropathy but not postherpetic neuralgia. An RCT of cancer patients requiring escalation of their analgesia reported dextromethorphan to be ineffective in allaying the need for increased doses (Table 13.8). Phantom limb pain is reported to respond to dextromethorphan.[41, 42]

Table 13.8 NMDA receptor antagonists: RCTs

Author	n	Intervention	Outcome
Ketamine			
Yang[38]	20	IT morphine ± IT ketamine	ketamine: ↓ pain scores, ↓ morphine requirements (both pS)
Mercadante[35]	10	morphine + ketamine or saline	ketamine: ↓ pain scores (pS)
Dextromethorphan (DM)			
Mercadante[39]	60	standard analgesia requiring escalation: DM or escalation	no improvement with DM
Katz[40]	321	morphine vs morphine/DM	mixture: ↑ duration of action, ↓ morphine dose (both pS)

Recent experience with a 1:1 combination of morphine and dextromethorphan (MorphiDex) showed that the combined preparation was associated with more rapid onset and longer duration of analgesia, and that analgesia was maintained with significantly lower daily doses of morphine.[40,43] A large RCT included patients with cancer-related pain (Table 13.8). The role of combined morphine and dextromethorphan in neuropathic pain remains to be defined.

Other drugs for neuropathic pain

Alpha-2 adrenergic agonists. The alpha-2 adrenergic agonists, clonidine and tizanidine, are effective for some types of non-malignant neuropathic pain.[44] Patients with neuropathic pain refractory to other measures can be given a trial of clonidine (0.1mg/d PO), the dose being increased gradually to a maximum of 0.3 mg/day. The adverse effects are hypotension and sedation that may be dose-limiting. In patients with cancer, epidural clonidine has been shown to be effective for some patients with refractory pain, particularly those with neuropathic pain.[45]

GABA agonist. The gamma-aminobutyric acid (GABA) agonist, baclofen, is effective in the treatment of trigeminal neuralgia and may be of benefit for patients with the lancinating type of neuropathic pain.[46] The usual dose is 5 mg, 8-hourly and titrated against effect up to a maximum of 100 mg/d. Side effects, which are frequently dose-limiting, are sedation and gastrointestinal disturbances. There are no trials of its use in patients with cancer. The drug must be discontinued gradually to prevent withdrawal reactions.

Calcium channel antagonists. Two RCTs of the calcium channel antagonist, nimodipine, used as an adjuvant to morphine for the treatment of cancer pain, reported differing results (Table13.9). Adverse effects include postural hypotension.

Capsaicin. Topical capsaicin is effective in some patients with postherpetic and other neuropathic pain,[14] and an RCT has shown it to be effective for postsurgical neuropathic pain in patients with cancer.[47] It is claimed to cause depletion of the neurotransmitter, sub-

Table 13.9 Calcium channel antagonists: RCTs

Author	n	Intervention	Outcome
Roca[50]	32	morphine + nimodipine or placebo	no differences
Santillan[51]	54	morphine + nimodipine or placebo	nimodipine: ↓ daily morphine dose (pNS), fewer patients required ↑ morphine dose (pS)

stance P, from neurons in the treated area, leading to less nociceptive stimulation in the dorsal horn of the spinal cord. Capsaicin cream needs to be applied at least 3 or 4 times a day and, at least initially, causes transient stinging or burning.

Topical lidocaine. Topical lidocaine patches are reported to be effective for postherpetic neuralgia and other neuropathic pain.[48, 49]

Psychotropic drugs

Neuroleptics

The neuroleptic drugs such as chlorpromazine and haloperidol have no analgesic action but are of benefit in treating patients with pain by reducing anxiety and improving night-time sedation.[52] Olanzapine is reported to be effective for the management of uncontrolled pain in patients with cognitive impairment or anxiety.[53] However, unless specifically indicated for the treatment of delirium or nausea, the same benefits can be obtained with a benzodiazepine without the potentially troublesome anticholinergic and extrapyramidal side effects of neuroleptic drugs.

Levopromazine (methotrimeprazine) is a phenothiazine that has been demonstrated to have analgesic activity in an RCT, 20 mg by injection being equivalent to 10 mg of morphine.[54] The mechanism of action is uncertain and it is not reversed by naloxone. It may be useful for treating very distressed patients for whom a further increase in opioid analgesics is undesirable. Its clinical use is limited by its propensity to cause sedation and postural hypotension.

Anxiolytic drugs

Benzodiazepine drugs do not have independent analgesic action but are of benefit in treating patients with pain by virtue of their anxiolytic effect.[55] Diazepam is of particular use in patients with muscle spasm or acute musculoskeletal pain. Adverse effects include drowsiness, weakness and postural hypotension.

The antihistamine, hydroxyzine, was reported to have analgesic action in an RCT of patients with advanced cancer.[56] Diphenhydramine has been reported to be a useful adjuvant in patients with intractable pain.[57] The opioid-sparing effect probably relates to the sedative anxiolytic action of the drugs.

Psychostimulants

Cocaine. An RCT showed no additional analgesic effect when cocaine was given with morphine (Table 13.10). In elderly or debilitated patients cocaine can cause agitation and confusion.

Cannabinoids. Cannabinoids produce analgesia in animals, but whether or not they do in humans has not been resolved.[58] In RCTs in patients with cancer, tetrahydrocannabinol (THC) produced dose-related analgesia, but also unacceptable adverse effects of sedation and cognitive impairment (Table 13.10). Analgesia produced by the cannabinoid analogue nabilone is not mediated by opioid receptors.[59]

Amphetamine. Amphetamine augments postoperative pain control by opioids but does not have an established role in the treatment of cancer-related pain.[60] It will counteract sedation caused by opioids, but tolerance and dependence to amphetamine may develop quickly. Elderly patients are prone to the dysphoric effects.

Methylphenidate. Methylphenidate has no independent analgesic action and is effective in reducing sedation related to opioids;[61–63] one RCT reported improved pain scores and reduced opioid requirements (Table 13.10). It has the same limitations as amphetamine if used to counteract opioid-induced sedation.

Caffeine. An RCT of caffeine reported a significant reduction in pain intensity, although this was not significant when compared with placebo (Table 13.10).

Table 13.10 Psychostimulants: RCTs

Author	n	Intervention	Outcome
Cannabinoids			
Noyes[64]	9	THC 5, 10, 15, 20mg vs placebo	THC 15 & 20mg: analgesia and unacceptable adverse effects
Noyes[65]	34	THC vs codeine vs placebo	THC 10 & 20mg: equivalent to codeine 60 & 120mg; unacceptable toxicity
Methylphenidate			
Bruera[66]	28	methylphenidate 10mg mane + 5mg noon vs placebo	methylphenidate: ↓ pain score, ↓ extra doses, ↑ activity, ↓ drowsiness (all pS)
Cocaine			
Kaiko[67]	17	morphine vs cocaine vs placebo vs morphine + cocaine	no analgesic effect of cocaine
Caffeine			
Mercadante[68]	10	morphine + IV caffeine or placebo	caffeine: ↓ pain intensity (pS), but pNS when compared with placebo

Muscle relaxants

Pain due to muscle spasm may respond to local measures and physiotherapy. Treatment with a benzodiazepine usually relieves spasm, although sedation may be troublesome. Non-benzodiazepine skeletal muscle relaxants similarly cause weakness and sedation. Baclofen, which acts at a spinal level, is started at a low dose (5 mg three times a day) and cautiously increased up to a maximum of 100 mg/d. The drug must be weaned slowly in order to avoid a withdrawal syndrome and seizures. Dantrolene, which acts directly on muscle, is commenced at 25 mg/d and titrated against effect up to a maximum of 400 mg/d. It is hepatotoxic and liver function should be monitored regularly.

Adjuvant drugs for bone pain

Bisphosphonates

The bisphosphonate compounds are chemical analogues of pyrophosphate that inhibit bone resorption. They are effective in the treatment of hypercalcaemia associated with cancer and have been shown to reduce pain and skeletal events in patients with bone metastases.[69–73] They act by inhibiting osteoclast activity, blocking mineral dissolution, and may have antitumour action.[74] The more recently introduced nitrogen-containing bisphosphonates (pamidronate, ibandronate, olpadronate and zoledronic acid) are more potent than the non-nitrogen-containing compounds etidronate and clodronate.

Systematic and Cochrane reviews of the many RCTs of bisphosphonate therapy indicate that there is improvement in the pain related to bone disease that occurs over time.[69–73]

There is insufficient evidence to recommend bisphosphonates for immediate analgesia, but they should be considered if analgesics and radiotherapy provide inadequate control. Recent trials of zoledronic acid[75–77] and olpadronate [78] report similar results; a study of ibandronate (6mg each 4 weeks) in prostate cancer reported improved pain control, but an RCT of a lower dose (2mg each 4 weeks) had no effect on pain in myeloma.[79, 80] Bisphosphonate therapy is discussed further in Chapter 23.

Radioisotopes

The systemic administration of bone-seeking radioisotopes is effective in controlling pain related to bone metastases.[81, 82] Various isotopes have been used including [89]Strontium, [153]Samarium and [186]Rhenium (see Chapter 23, Table 23.7). The isotopes are preferentially taken up in metastases that have osteoblastic activity, as evidenced by increased uptake on bone scan; they may have more activity in metastases that have markedly increased osteoblastic activity, with sclerotic changes on x-ray, as are seen with prostate and some breast cancers.

Improved pain control is reported in up to 80% of patients, with a small proportion getting complete relief.[81, 82] Responses are usually evident 2 to 3 weeks after treatment and last for 3 to 6 months; the onset of pain relief is reported to occur more quickly with [186]Rhenium.[83] The degree and duration of analgesia after radioisotope therapy is equivalent to local or hemibody irradiation.[84] They are of benefit when used in addition to local radiotherapy; compared to local radiotherapy, they reduce the number of new pain sites for about four months following treatment.[85] The best results are seen in patients with less extensive metastases, suggesting that radioisotope therapy should be considered earlier; response to re-treatment is usually inferior to the initial therapy.[86] Combined modality therapy with [89]Strontium and cisplatin produced significantly better results than [89]Strontium alone.[87] Peripheral blood stem cell support has been used with high dose radioisotope therapy in an attempt to increase the radiation delivered to bone metastases.[88]

Radioisotope therapy is well tolerated and the main adverse effect is myelosuppression, which is usually mild and not clinically significant. There must be adequate haematological reserve before treatment is given. About 10% of patients suffer a transient flare reaction with increased pain following treatment; this settles spontaneously and does not predict response.[86] Compared to radiotherapy, radioisotope treatment produces equivalent results, but has less acute toxicity and is easier to administer. The disadvantage of the radioisotopes is their considerable cost.

Antibiotics

The pain of cellulitis, mucositis and fungating tumours is often compounded by secondary infection. The use of appropriate antibiotic or antifungal agents can improve pain control. Systemic infections may also result in pain, and appropriate treatment of the infection may relieve it. The use of antiviral agents can lessen the pain of acute herpetic neuralgia.

References

1   Bruera, E., et al. (1985). Action of oral methylprednisolone in terminal cancer patients: a prospective randomized double-blind study. *Cancer Treatment Reports* 69, 751–4.
2   Tannock, I., et al. (1989). Treatment of metastatic prostatic cancer with low-dose prednisone: evaluation of pain and quality of life as pragmatic indices of response. *Journal of Clinical Oncology* 7, 590–7.

3   Tannock, I.F., et al. (1996). Chemotherapy with mitoxantrone plus prednisone or prednisone alone for symptomatic hormone-resistant prostate cancer: a Canadian randomized trial with palliative end points. *Journal of Clinical Oncology* 14, 1756–64.

4   Hardy, J.R., et al. (2001). A prospective survey of the use of dexamethasone on a palliative care unit. *Palliative Medicine* 15, 3–8.

5   Della Cuna, G.R., Pellegrini, A. and Piazzi, M. (1989). Effect of methylprednisolone sodium succinate on quality of life in preterminal cancer patients: a placebo-controlled, multicenter study. The Methylprednisolone Preterminal Cancer Study Group. *European Journal of Cancer and Clinical Oncology* 25, 1817–21.

6   McQuay, H.J., et al. (1996). A systematic review of antidepressants in neuropathic pain. *Pain* 68, 217–27.

7   McQuay, H.J. and Moore, R.A. (1998). *An evidence-based resource for pain relief.* Oxford, Oxford University Press.

8   Sindrup, S.H. and Jensen, T.S. (1999). Efficacy of pharmacological treatments of neuropathic pain: an update and effect related to mechanism of drug action. *Pain* 83, 389–400.

9   Fishbain, D. (2000). Evidence-based data on pain relief with antidepressants. *Annals of Medicine* 32, 305–16.

10   Kingery, W.S. (1997). A critical review of controlled clinical trials for peripheral neuropathic pain and complex regional pain syndromes. *Pain* 73, 123–39.

11   Collins, S.L., et al. (2000). Antidepressants and anticonvulsants for diabetic neuropathy and posttherpetic neuralgia: a quantitative systematic review. *Journal of Pain and Symptom Management* 20, 449–58.

12   Sindrup, S.H. and Jensen, T.S. (2000). Pharmacologic treatment of pain in polyneuropathy. *Neurology* 55, 915–20.

13   Max, M.B., et al. (1992). Effects of desipramine, amitriptyline, and fluoxetine on pain in diabetic neuropathy. *New England Journal of Medicine* 326, 1250–6.

14   McCleane, G. (2000). Topical application of doxepin hydrochloride, capsaicin and a combination of both produces analgesia in chronic human neuropathic pain: a randomized, double-blind, placebo-controlled study. *British Journal of Clinical Pharmacology* 49, 574–9.

15   Mercadante, S., et al. (2002). Amitriptyline in neuropathic cancer pain in patients on morphine therapy: a randomized placebo-controlled, double-blind crossover study. *Tumori* 88, 239–42.

16   Tasmuth, T., Hartel, B. and Kalso, E. (2002). Venlafaxine in neuropathic pain following treatment of breast cancer. *European Journal of Pain* 6, 17–24.

17   Theobald, D.E., et al. (2002). An open-label, crossover trial of mirtazapine (15 and 30 mg) in cancer patients with pain and other distressing symptoms. *Journal of Pain and Symptom Management* 23, 442–7.

18   McQuay, H., et al. (1995). Anticonvulsant drugs for management of pain: a systematic review. *British Medical Journal* 311, 1047–52.

19   Wiffen, P., et al. (2000). Anticonvulsant drugs for acute and chronic pain (Cochrane Review). *Cochrane Database of Systematic Reviews* CD001133.

20   Caraceni, A., et al. (1999). Gabapentin as an adjuvant to opioid analgesia for neuropathic cancer pain. *Journal of Pain and Symptom Management* 17, 441–5.

21   Chandler, A. and Williams, J.E. (2000). Gabapentin, an adjuvant treatment for neuropathic pain in a cancer hospital. *Journal of Pain and Symptom Management* 20, 82–6.

22   Hardy, J.R., et al. (2001). A phase II study to establish the efficacy and toxicity of sodium valproate in patients with cancer-related neuropathic pain. *Journal of Pain and Symptom Management* 21, 204–9.

23   Kalso, E., et al. (1998). Systemic local-anaesthetic-type drugs in chronic pain: a systematic review. *European Journal of Pain* 2, 3–14.

24   Galer, B.S., Miller, K.V. and Rowbotham, M.C. (1993). Response to intravenous lidocaine infusion differs based on clinical diagnosis and site of nervous system injury. *Neurology* 43, 1233–5.

25 Galer, B.S., Harle, J. and Rowbotham, M.C. (1996). Response to intravenous lidocaine infusion predicts subsequent response to oral mexiletine: a prospective study. *Journal of Pain and Symptom Management* 12, 161–7.

26 Brose, W.G. and Cousins, M.J. (1991). Subcutaneous lidocaine for treatment of neuropathic cancer pain. *Pain* 45, 145–8.

27 Sloan, P., et al. (1999). Mexiletine as an adjuvant analgesic for the management of neuropathic cancer pain. *Anesthesia and Analgesia* 89, 760–1.

28 Chong, S.F., et al. (1997). Pilot study evaluating local anesthetics administered systemically for treatment of pain in patients with advanced cancer. *Journal of Pain and Symptom Management* 13, 112–17.

29 Ellemann, K., et al. (1989). Trial of intravenous lidocaine on painful neuropathy in cancer patients. *Clinical Journal of Pain* 5, 291–4.

30 Bruera, E., et al. (1992). A randomized double-blind crossover trial of intravenous lidocaine in the treatment of neuropathic cancer pain. *Journal of Pain and Symptom Management* 7, 138–40.

31 Bennett, G.J. (2000). Update on the neurophysiology of pain transmission and modulation: focus on the NMDA-receptor. *Journal of Pain and Symptom Management* 19, S2–6.

32 Price, D.D., et al. (2000). NMDA-receptor antagonists and opioid receptor interactions as related to analgesia and tolerance. *Journal of Pain and Symptom Management* 19, S7–11.

33 Crosby, V., Wilcock, A. and Corcoran, R. (2000). The safety and efficacy of a single dose (500 mg or 1 g) of intravenous magnesium sulfate in neuropathic pain poorly responsive to strong opioid analgesics in patients with cancer. *Journal of Pain and Symptom Management* 19, 35–9.

34 Kannan, T.R., et al. (2002). Oral ketamine as an adjuvant to oral morphine for neuropathic pain in cancer patients. *Journal of Pain and Symptom Management* 23, 60–5.

35 Mercadante, S., et al. (2000). Analgesic effect of intravenous ketamine in cancer patients on morphine therapy: a randomized, controlled, double-blind, crossover, double-dose study. *Journal of Pain and Symptom Management* 20, 246–52.

36 Jackson, K., et al. (2001). 'Burst' ketamine for refractory cancer pain: an open-label audit of 39 patients. *Journal of Pain and Symptom Management* 22, 834–42.

37 Bell, R., Eccleston, C. and Kalso, E. (2003). Ketamine as an adjuvant to opioids for cancer pain (Cochrane Review). *Cochrane Database of Systematic Reviews* CD003351.

38 Yang, C.Y., et al. (1996). Intrathecal ketamine reduces morphine requirements in patients with terminal cancer pain. *Canadian Journal of Anaesthesia* 43, 379–83.

39 Mercadante, S., Casuccio, A. and Genovese, G. (1998). Ineffectiveness of dextromethorphan in cancer pain. *Journal of Pain and Symptom Management* 16, 317–22.

40 Katz, N.P. (2000). MorphiDex (MS:DM) double-blind, multiple-dose studies in chronic pain patients. *Journal of Pain and Symptom Management* 19, S37–41.

41 Ben Abraham, R., et al. (2002). Dextromethorphan for phantom pain attenuation in cancer amputees: a double-blind crossover trial involving three patients. *Clinical Journal of Pain* 18, 282–5.

42 Ben Abraham, R., Marouani, N. and Weinbroum, A.A. (2003). Dextromethorphan mitigates phantom pain in cancer amputees. *Annals of Surgical Oncology* 10, 268–74.

43 Caruso, F.S. (2000). MorphiDex pharmacokinetic studies and single-dose analgesic efficacy studies in patients with postoperative pain. *Journal of Pain and Symptom Management* 19, S31–6.

44 Wallenstein, D.J. and Portenoy, R.K. (2002). Nonopioid and adjuvant analgesics. In *Principles and Practice of Palliative Care and Supportive Oncology* (ed. A.M. Berger, R.K. Portenoy and D.E. Weissman). Philadelphia, Lippincott, Williams and Wilkins.

45 Eisenach, J.C., et al. (1995). Epidural clonidine analgesia for intractable cancer pain. The Epidural Clonidine Study Group. *Pain* 61, 391–9.

46 Fromm, G.H. (1994). Baclofen as an adjuvant analgesic. *Journal of Pain and Symptom Management* 9, 500–9.

47 Ellison, N., et al. (1997). Phase III placebo-controlled trial of capsaicin cream in the management of surgical neuropathic pain in cancer patients. *Journal of Clinical Oncology* 15, 2974–80.

48 Galer, B.S., et al. (1999). Topical lidocaine patch relieves postherpetic neuralgia more effectively than a vehicle topical patch: results of an enriched enrollment study. *Pain* 80, 533–8.

49 Devers, A. and Galer, B.S. (2000). Topical lidocaine patch relieves a variety of neuropathic pain conditions: an open-label study. *Clinical Journal of Pain* 16, 205–8.

50 Roca, G., et al. (1996). Nimodipine fails to enhance the analgesic effect of slow release morphine in the early phases of cancer pain treatment. *Pain* 68, 239–43.

51 Santillan, R., et al. (1998). Nimodipine-enhanced opiate analgesia in cancer patients requiring morphine dose escalation: a double-blind, placebo-controlled study. *Pain* 76, 17–26.

52 Patt, R.B., Proper, G. and Reddy, S. (1994). The neuroleptics as adjuvant analgesics. *Journal of Pain and Symptom Management* 9, 446–53.

53 Khojainova, N., et al. (2002). Olanzapine in the management of cancer pain. *Journal of Pain and Symptom Management* 23, 346–50.

54 Beaver, W.T., et al. (1966). A comparison of the analgesic effects of methotrimeprazine and morphine in patients with cancer. *Clinical Pharmacology and Therapeutics* 7, 436–46.

55 Reddy, S. and Patt, R.B. (1994). The benzodiazepines as adjuvant analgesics. *Journal of Pain and Symptom Management* 9, 510–14.

56 Stambaugh, J.E., Jr. and Lane, C. (1983). Analgesic efficacy and pharmacokinetic evaluation of meperidine and hydroxyzine, alone and in combination. *Cancer Investigation* 1, 111–17.

57 Santiago-Palma, J., et al. (2001). Diphenhydramine as an analgesic adjuvant in refractory cancer pain. *Journal of Pain and Symptom Management* 22, 699–703.

58 Campbell, F.A., et al. (2001). Are cannabinoids an effective and safe treatment option in the management of pain? A qualitative systematic review. *British Medical Journal* 323, 13–16.

59 Hamann, W. and di Vadi, P.P. (1999). Analgesic effect of the cannabinoid analogue nabilone is not mediated by opioid receptors. *Lancet* 353, 560.

60 Dalal, S. and Melzack, R. (1998). Potentiation of opioid analgesia by psychostimulant drugs: a review. *Journal of Pain and Symptom Management* 16, 245–53.

61 Bruera, E., et al. (1992). Neuropsychological effects of methylphenidate in patients receiving a continuous infusion of narcotics for cancer pain. *Pain* 48, 163–6.

62 Yee, J.D. and Berde, C.B. (1994). Dextroamphetamine or methylphenidate as adjuvants to opioid analgesia for adolescents with cancer. *Journal of Pain and Symptom Management* 9, 122–5.

63 Wilwerding, M.B., et al. (1995). A randomized, crossover evaluation of methylphenidate in cancer patients receiving strong narcotics. *Supportive Care in Cancer* 3, 135–8.

64 Noyes, R., Jr., et al. (1975). Analgesic effect of delta-9-tetrahydrocannabinol. *Journal of Clinical Pharmacology* 15, 139–43.

65 Noyes, R., Jr., et al. (1975). The analgesic properties of delta-9-tetrahydrocannabinol and codeine. *Clinical Pharmacology and Therapeutics* 18, 84–9.

66 Bruera, E., et al. (1987). Methylphenidate associated with narcotics for the treatment of cancer pain. *Cancer Treatment Reports* 71, 67–70.

67 Kaiko, R.F., et al. (1987). Cocaine and morphine interaction in acute and chronic cancer pain. *Pain* 31, 35–45.

68 Mercadante, S., Serretta, R. and Casuccio, A. (2001). Effects of caffeine as an adjuvant to morphine in advanced cancer patients. A randomized, double-blind, placebo-controlled, crossover study. *Journal of Pain and Symptom Management* 21, 369–72.

69 Bloomfield, D.J. (1998). Should bisphosphonates be part of the standard therapy of patients with multiple myeloma or bone metastases from other cancers? An evidence-based review. *Journal of Clinical Oncology* 16, 1218–25.

70 Goudas, L., et al. (2001). *Management of cancer pain*. Rockville, MD: Agency for Healthcare Research and Quality. <www.ahrq.gov>

71 Carr, D., et al. (2002). *Management of Cancer Symptoms: Pain, Depression, and Fatigue. Evidence Report/Technology Assessment No. 61*. Rockville, MD: Agency for Healthcare Research and Quality. <www.ahrq.gov>

72 Djulbegovic, B., et al. (2002). Bisphosphonates in multiple myeloma (Cochrane Review). *Cochrane Database of Systematic Reviews* CD003188.

73 Wong, R. and Wiffen, P.J. (2002). Bisphosphonates for the relief of pain secondary to bone metastases (Cochrane Review). *Cochrane Database of Systematic Reviews* CD002068.

74 Green, J.R. (2003). Antitumor effects of bisphosphonates. *Cancer* 97, 840–7.

75 Berenson, J.R. (2001). Zoledronic acid in cancer patients with bone metastases: results of Phase I and II trials. *Seminars in Oncology* 28, 25–34.

76 Rosen, L.S., et al. (2001). Zoledronic acid versus pamidronate in the treatment of skeletal metastases in patients with breast cancer or osteolytic lesions of multiple myeloma: a phase III, double-blind, comparative trial. *Cancer Journal* 7, 377–87.

77 Saad, F., et al. (2002). A randomized, placebo-controlled trial of zoledronic acid in patients with hormone-refractory metastatic prostate carcinoma. *Journal of the National Cancer Institute* 94, 1458–68.

78 Pelger, R.C., et al. (1998). Effects of the bisphosphonate olpadronate in patients with carcinoma of the prostate metastatic to the skeleton. *Bone* 22, 403–8.

79 Heidenreich, A., Elert, A. and Hofmann, R. (2002). Ibandronate in the treatment of prostate cancer associated painful osseous metastases. *Prostate Cancer and Prostatic Diseases* 5, 231–5.

80 Menssen, H.D., et al. (2002). Effects of long-term intravenous ibandronate therapy on skeletal-related events, survival, and bone resorption markers in patients with advanced multiple myeloma. *Journal of Clinical Oncology* 20, 2353–9.

81 Robinson, R.G., et al. (1995). Strontium 89 therapy for the palliation of pain due to osseous metastases. *Journal of the American Medical Association* 274, 420–4.

82 Berger, A.M. and Koprowski, C. (2002). Bone pain:assessment and management. In *Principles and Practice of Palliative Care and Supportive Oncology* (ed. A.M. Berger, R.K. Portenoy and D.E. Weissman). Philadelphia, Lippincott, Williams and Wilkins.

83 Sciuto, R., et al. (2001). Metastatic bone pain palliation with 89-Sr and 186-Re-HEDP in breast cancer patients. *Breast Cancer Research and Treatment* 66, 101–9.

84 Quilty, P.M., et al. (1994). A comparison of the palliative effects of strontium-89 and external beam radiotherapy in metastatic prostate cancer. *Radiotherapy and Oncology* 31, 33–40.

85 Porter, A.T., et al. (1993). Results of a randomized phase-III trial to evaluate the efficacy of strontium 89 adjuvant to local field external beam irradiation in the management of endocrine resistant metastatic prostate cancer. *International Journal of Radiation Oncology, Biology, Physics.* 25, 805–13.

86 Dafermou, A., et al. (2001). A multicentre observational study of radionuclide therapy in patients with painful bone metastases of prostate cancer. *European Journal of Nuclear Medicine* 28, 788–98.

87 Sciuto, R., et al. (2002). Effects of low-dose cisplatin on 89Sr therapy for painful bone metastases from prostate cancer: a randomized clinical trial. *Journal of Nuclear Medicine* 43, 79–86.

88 Anderson, P.M., et al. (2002). High-dose samarium-153 ethylene diamine tetramethylene phosphonate: low toxicity of skeletal irradiation in patients with osteosarcoma and bone metastases. *Journal of Clinical Oncology* 20, 189–96.

14

Anaesthetic, neurolytic and neurosurgical procedures

Local infiltration	Spinal blocks
Nerve blocks	Neurosurgical procedures

Neural blockade, including nerve blocks and neurosurgical procedures, can be used to block or modify the sensation of pain as it is transmitted from the source to the central nervous system (Table 14.1). Neural blockade is most suited for treating well-defined localized pain and is more effective against somatic and visceral pain than neuropathic pain. Recent refinements in the use of spinal opioids have greatly reduced the need for some neural blockade procedures, particularly the neurosurgical operations.

Table 14.1 Anaesthetic, neurolytic and neurosurgical procedures

Local infiltration of anaesthetic	Intraspinal nerve blocks
painful bone metastases	local anaesthetic
myofascial pain: trigger point injection	neurolytic
neuromas	Neurosurgical procedures
Peripheral nerve blocks	peripheral nerve
spinal nerves	spinal cord
cranial nerves	brain
autonomic nerves	

Local anaesthetic agents. Local anaesthetics are used for local infiltration of painful lesions, to perform diagnostic and prognostic nerve blocks before any neurolytic procedures, and for epidural spinal blocks. The two commonly used agents are lignocaine (lidocaine) and bupivacaine. Bupivacaine has a longer duration of action (8–12h) than lignocaine (1–2h). The lowest effective dose should be used.

Toxic effects can occur with excessive dosage, inadvertent intravenous injection, or if there is impaired metabolism or excretion. Hypotension, bradycardia and CNS excitation can occur; in severe cases, there may be CNS depression and cardiovascular collapse. Hypotension and bradycardia also occur after extradural or subarachnoid injection. The inadvertent subarachnoid injection of a larger dose planned for extradural administration can cause cardiovascular collapse with CNS and respiratory depression. Preservative-free local anaesthetics are used for epidural and spinal anaesthesia to avoid chemical meningitis.

Neurolytic agents and instruments. Therapeutic nerve blocks are performed by a variety of methods (Table 14.2). All produce severe neuronal damage with wallerian degeneration, although the persistence of the basal lamina around the schwann cell tube allows the nerve fibres to regenerate and avoids the formation of painful neuromas.

Table 14.2 Therapeutic nerve blocks

Local anaesthetic	Cryotherapy
Chemical neurolysis	Thermocoagulation
laser therapy	Laser therapy
radiofrequency lesions	Radiofrequency lesions

Local infiltration

Pain due to rib metastases may be treated by local infiltration with local anaesthetic and the addition of corticosteroid may prolong the effect. Painful metastases in other parts of the skeleton where the lesion is palpable may be treated similarly.

Neuromas following surgery or amputation may be treated by injection of local anaesthetic. The duration of effect is significantly prolonged by the addition of a long-acting corticosteroid preparation.

Myofascial pain is characterized by local pain and tenderness in muscles, associated with pain radiating in a non-dermatomal distribution. There are local trigger points, palpation of which produce or aggravate the symptoms. Injection of the trigger point with local anaesthetic, with or without corticosteroid, usually produces complete relief.

Nerve blocks

A *diagnostic* nerve block is performed to determine which nerve or nerves are responsible for a patient's pain. A *prognostic* nerve block is performed to assess the adequacy of analgesia, to allow the patient to experience the sensory loss that would be produced by a neurolytic block, and to assess any motor or sphincteric disturbance. *Therapeutic* nerve blocks may be temporary, prophylactic or permanent. Temporary therapeutic nerve blocks with local anaesthetic are used for the short term relief of severe pain whilst other treatment is instituted. Prophylactic nerve blocks are used where predictable local progression of cancer is likely to produce severe pain; for example, intercostal nerve blocks can be performed at the time of surgery where there is extensive chest wall infiltration. Permanent nerve blocks will provide pain relief for weeks or months but are only suitable for purely sensory nerves or in those areas where the loss of motor and other sensory functions will not interfere with the patient's performance status.

Spinal nerve blocks

The only block performed frequently is that of intercostal nerves for chest and abdominal wall pain. Severe limb pain, which in the past may have been treated with plexus blocks, can now be treated with measures that are more selective for sensory nerves (epidural local anaesthetic) and pain (spinal opioids).

Cranial nerve blocks

A trigeminal or gasserian ganglion block may be performed in patients with severe pain in the anterior two-thirds of the head. This results in good analgesia lasting several months for 80% of patients. Complications include keratitis and corneal ulceration.

Autonomic nerve blocks

Sympathetic nerve damage produces burning pain, often with allodynia. It is usually associated with vasomotor and sudomotor changes (vasoconstriction, coldness, increased sweating) of the affected part. Sympathetic-type pain responds poorly to non-opioid and opioid analgesics but resolves with local sympathetic nerve block. Post-amputation phantom limb pain and stump pain have similar qualities and are relieved by local sympathetic nerve block.

Stellate ganglion block. Block of the lower cervical and upper thoracic sympathetic chain (referred to as a 'stellate ganglion block') may be considered for visceral pain associated with intrathoracic disease, sympathetic pain involving the head and neck or upper limb, and for sympathetic-type pain associated with upper limb amputation. Complications include damage to local tissues, vessels and other nerves; Horner's syndrome normally develops.

Coeliac plexus block. A coeliac plexus block is indicated for severe pain from disease in upper abdominal viscera and will provide immediate relief of pain for about 80–90% of patients, the relief lasting a number of months for most.[1] Five RCTs of coeliac plexus block are reported.[2] The only trial that was double-blinded compared intraoperative coeliac plexus blocks performed with alcohol or saline and showed lasting benefit in the alcohol group (Table 14.3).[3] Orthostatic hypotension and diarrhoea are the only frequent adverse effects and usually settle within a few days. Other complications include damage to local tissues, vessels and other nerves, and there are rare reports of paraplegia.

Table 14.3   Coeliac plexus block: RCT

Author	n	Intervention	Outcome
Lillemoe[3]	139	intraoperative coeliac plexus block: alcohol vs saline	alcohol: ↓ pain at 2,4,6 mo. in patients with and without preoperative pain (pS)

Lumbar sympathetic block. Lumbar sympathetic block may be considered for pelvic visceral pain, sympathetic pain involving the pelvis or lower limb, and for sympathetic-type pain associated with lower limb amputation. Complications include hypotension (because of splanchnic and lower limb vasodilatation) and unintentional lumbosacral plexus block causing weakness and numbness of the leg.

Hypogastric plexus block. Neurolytic blockade of the superior hypogastric plexus is of benefit to patients with pelvic visceral pain.

Spinal blocks

Local anaesthetic blocks

Injection of local anaesthetic into the epidural space will provide excellent analgesia over several spinal segments. This can be performed either by a single injection or by the temporary or permanent placement of a catheter in the epidural space at the desired level. For example, injection in the region of the cervico-thoracic junction will provide analgesia in both arms; at the mid-thoracic spine level, the lower chest and upper abdomen; at the thoraco-lumbar junction, the lower abdomen and upper thighs; at the lumbo-sacral junction, both legs; and in the mid-sacral region, the perineum. The anaesthetic diffuses through the epidural space, affecting the dorsal nerve root, usually with minimal motor or autonomic effect. The epidural catheter can be tunnelled subcutaneously and connected to a reservoir or to a continuous infusion pump. Tolerance will develop after a number of days or weeks and epidural blocks are particularly useful for temporary pain relief, whilst other therapy is instituted. The complications of spinal catheters are listed in Table 12.5.

Neurolytic blocks

Intraspinal neurolytic blocks involve the injection of alcohol or phenol into the epidural or subarachnoid space to block the dorsal nerve roots. The risks of the procedure are that motor and autonomic nerves may also be damaged, causing limb weakness or paralysis, and bladder or bowel dysfunction. Neurolytic blocks have been largely superseded by the use of epidural local anaesthetics and intraspinal opioids, which often produce the same benefit without the attendant risks.

Neurosurgical procedures

Neurosurgical procedures are now required infrequently for patients with advanced cancer, due mainly to the development of spinal therapy with opioids and other drugs. They can be considered in the rare situation of pain refractory to all other measures.

Operations on the peripheral nerve. Surgical neurotomy or peripheral nerve section will produce anaesthesia, but only for a limited period of time, and regeneration may be associated with a painful neuroma. Dorsal rhizotomy, or the surgical section of the sensory nerve roots where they enter the spinal cord, may be useful in patients with severe pain limited to a few spinal segments in the trunk; it is not indicated for limb pain, as the sensory loss would produce a useless limb.

Operations on the spinal cord. Operations including dorsal entry zone lesions, anterolateral cordotomy and commissural myelotomy are specialized procedures reported to be of benefit in carefully selected patients with intractable pain. All are associated with complications, some of them severe. The role of these procedures in patients with cancer and chronic pain is not clearly established.

Operations on the brain. Specialized neurosurgical procedures have been reported to benefit small numbers of highly selected patients with intractable pain related to cancer. As all require craniotomy they have very limited application to patients with advanced cancer. The indications for such procedures remain to be established.

References

1   Eisenberg, E., Carr, D.B. and Chalmers, T.C. (1995). Neurolytic celiac plexus block for treatment of cancer pain: a meta-analysis. *Anesthesia and Analgesia* 80, 290–5.
2   Goudas, L., et al. (2001). *Management of cancer pain*. Rockville, MD: Agency for Healthcare Research and Quality. <www.ahrq.gov>
3   Lillemoe, K.D., et al. (1993). Chemical splanchnicectomy in patients with unresectable pancreatic cancer. A prospective randomized trial. *Annals of Surgery* 217, 447–55.

15

Physical therapies

Surgery	Topical counter-irritants
Heat therapy	Acupuncture
Cold therapy	Mechanical therapy
Electrical therapy	

Surgery

Surgery is most frequently required for orthopaedic complications and visceral obstruction. Ablative endocrine surgery for hormone-sensitive tumours has been largely replaced by hormonal and pharmacological therapies.

Internal surgical fixation is indicated for pathological fractures of long bones and should be considered in situations where there is a high risk of fracture (Table 15.1).[1] Internal fixation will provide prompt pain control and will allow more rapid mobilization and rehabilitation of the patient. Where the responsible metastases are adjacent to a joint, such as the hip joint, replacement arthroplasty may be required for pain control. Internal fixation may be followed by radiotherapy.

Table 15.1 Palliative surgery for pain relief

Surgical internal fixation for metastases to long bones	
pathological fractures	
medullary lesions	>50% diameter of bone
cortical lesions	with >50%cortical width eroded
	with axial length > diameter of bone
	>2-3 cm
lesions causing persisting pain after radiotherapy	
Visceral obstruction	
oesophageal	laser resection, celestin tube, stent
intestinal	bypass surgery, stent
colonic	bypass surgery, defunctioning colostomy, laser resection, stent
biliary	bypass surgery, stent
ureteric	ureteric stenting, percutaneous nephrostomy

Pain secondary to gastrointestinal, biliary or urinary obstruction can be relieved by various surgical procedures (Table 15.1).

Heat therapy

Heat has been used to treat pain since ancient times. Heat relieves pain as a counter-irritant and by direct effect on the tissues treated. In the first situation, the sensation of heat acts to reduce the transmission of pain signals in the dorsal horn of the spinal cord and may also induce inhibitory stimuli from the brain stem. The local effects of heat include muscle relaxation, increased blood flow and tissue compliance.

Superficial heating of tissue is achieved with hot packs, hot water bottles, electric heating pads, radiant heat lamps (white and infrared) and hydrotherapy. Heating of deeper tissues may be achieved with ultrasound, short wave diathermy and microwave treatment, in which electromagnetic energy is converted into heat in the tissues. They should not be used near metal or plastic prostheses or areas where bone cement has been used.

Heat therapy is of particular benefit in the treatment of muscle spasm, myofascial pain, and the general musculoskeletal discomforts associated with immobility and debility.

Heat treatment can cause tissue damage and should not be used (or used with caution) in areas where there is diminished sensation or paralysis and where tissues are ischaemic. It should not be used where there is infection or directly over tumour tissue.

Cold therapy

Cryotherapy has the same local effects as heat in relation to local pain, pain due to muscle spasm and myofascial pain.[2] The analgesic effects of cold last longer than heat. The more frequent use of heat probably relates to patient comfort and preference.

Cold therapy may be performed with ice massage, cold packs or vapo-coolant sprays such as ethylchloride. Cold therapy should not be used in areas where there is diminished sensation or vascular insufficiency or in patients with Raynaud's syndrome or other cold hypersensitivity.

Electrical therapy

Transcutaneous electrical nerve stimulation (TENS) involves the electrical stimulation of nerves, using electrodes applied to the skin, for the purposes of pain control. TENS causes electrical activity in the large afferent fibres (mainly mechanoreceptive) that takes precedence over pain signals in the dorsal horn of the spinal cord. Electrode placement and the choice of frequency and intensity of stimulation should be performed by an experienced operator and the optimal settings are different for each patient. When operating, TENS produces paraesthesiae in the painful area. A more intensive form of TENS using stronger electrical stimulation, with or without needle electrodes (acupuncture-like TENS), may be advocated if conventional TENS fails.

TENS can be effective in treating pain of mild to moderate severity due to musculoskeletal disorders and neuralgia; it is ineffective against visceral pain. TENS is contraindicated in patients with a cardiac pacemaker. TENS causes skin irritation (mild burns, chemical irritation) and must not be used on ulcerated or hyperaesthetic skin.

Therapy with TENS results in a high initial response rate (70–80%), although only 15–20% of patients will obtain long term benefit and it is of limited use in the treatment of chronic cancer-related pain. However, if successful, it will reduce the requirement for systemic analgesics and it has the advantages of being cheap, easy to use, and relatively free of complications. A Cochrane review of TENS for chronic pain identified only one RCT involving patients with cancer, which reported no benefit, underlining the need for properly controlled trials for cancer pain.[3]

Topical counter-irritants

Heat and cold therapy and massage relieve pain by counter-irritation, stimulating neuronal activity that inhibits the passage of pain signals in the dorsal horn of the spinal cord. Commercially available analgesic ointments work in the same way. Capsaicin cream causes transient burning or stinging and may act partly by counter-irritation.

Acupuncture

Acupuncture involves needle insertion at classical acupuncture points, with or without electrical stimulation, or in painful areas. Its role in the treatment of pain related to cancer is not defined and there have been no RCTs. Good response rates of more than 50% have been reported with classical[4, 5] and auricular acupuncture,[6] but there is no information about the duration of response. The highest response rate was for myofascial pain, and pain due to tumour was less responsive than pain related to treatment. Acupuncture is relatively cheap and safe and, if successful, will reduce the requirement for systemic analgesics.

Mechanical therapies

Massage. Massage can relieve pain due to muscle spasm, myofascial syndromes, or the general musculoskeletal discomfort associated with immobility and debility, and may be seen as a way of communicating empathy and concern.[7, 8] Improvements in pain scores occur after foot massage.[9] Massage will also help relieve the pain of lymphoedema (see Chapter 21).

Exercise. Programs of physiotherapy, physical exercise and rehabilitation can improve pain control. Hydrotherapy is particularly useful for patients with pain related to weight bearing. Passive and active exercise may lessen or relieve the general musculoskeletal discomfort associated with inactivity or debility.

Manipulation. Physical manipulation by chiropractors, osteopaths and physiotherapists is the most commonly practised treatment for non-malignant back pain. Patients with cancer often seek such treatment but manipulation is contraindicated, or must be performed with great care, in the presence of vertebral metastases.

Orthotic devices. Braces and supporting devices will relieve and prevent pain by stabilizing or immobilizing painful tissues and are of particular benefit for pain related to movement and weight bearing. Orthotic devices include braces, corsets, collars, splints, callipers, bandages, and slings.

Mobility aids. Walking sticks, crutches, and walking frames are of value in preventing pain associated with movement and walking. As with orthotic devices, the aim is to minimize incident pain and at the same time maximize function.

Immobilization. Patients suffering severe pain despite the use of optimal analgesia and the physical supports described above may be forced to accept the use of a wheelchair or bed rest. This is often distressing for patients as it is an acknowledgement of the progression of their disease, but the relief of pain may be dramatic.

References

1   Brown, H.K. and Healey, J.H. (2001). Metastatic cancer to the bone. In *Cancer. Principles and Practice of Oncology. 6th edition* (ed. V.T. De Vita, S. Hellman and S.A. Rosenberg). Philadelphia, Lippincott Williams Wilkins.

2   Ernst, E. and Fialka, V. (1994). Ice freezes pain? A review of the clinical effectiveness of analgesic cold therapy. *Journal of Pain and Symptom Management* 9, 56–9.

3   Carroll, D., et al. (2001). Transcutaneous electrical nerve stimulation (TENS) for chronic pain (Cochrane Review). *Cochrane Database of Systematic Reviews* CD003222.

4   Leng, G. (1999). A year of acupuncture in palliative care. *Palliative Medicine* 13, 163–4.

5   Johnstone, P.A., et al. (2002). Integration of acupuncture into the oncology clinic. *Palliative Medicine* 16, 235–9.

6   Alimi, D., et al. (2000). Analgesic effects of auricular acupuncture for cancer pain. *Journal of Pain and Symptom Management* 19, 81–2.

7   Ferrell-Torry, A.T. and Glick, O.J. (1993). The use of therapeutic massage as a nursing intervention to modify anxiety and the perception of cancer pain. *Cancer Nursing* 16, 93–101.

8   Wilkie, D.J., et al. (2000). Effects of massage on pain intensity, analgesics and quality of life in patients with cancer pain: a pilot study of a randomized clinical trial conducted within hospice care delivery. *Hospice Journal* 15, 31–53.

9   Grealish, L., Lomasney, A. and Whiteman, B. (2000). Foot massage. A nursing intervention to modify the distressing symptoms of pain and nausea in patients hospitalized with cancer. *Cancer Nursing* 23, 237–43.

16

Psychological and psychosocial aspects of pain control

Social, cultural and spiritual issues
Psychological therapies

Psychological, social, cultural and spiritual issues can play a major role in the aggravation or amelioration of pain, as described in Chapter 5. Adequate evaluation of pain includes an assessment of these factors; pain unrelieved by apparently appropriate therapy should prompt a search for unrecognized psychological or psychosocial problems. Treatment of these issues is necessary for pain control to be successful and is an integral part of the management of pain. Unresolved or undetected psychosocial problems are a frequent cause of unrelieved pain.

Social, cultural and spiritual issues

Problems related to the social, cultural and spiritual aspects of suffering are discussed in Chapters 31–33. They may cause or aggravate pain and their successful treatment may have a profound effect. Pain may also be lessened by cultural and spiritual attitudes, particularly those related to certain Eastern religions. Identification of social, cultural and spiritual issues is part of the general palliative care assessment and is particularly important in the evaluation of pain. Treatment of these issues is essential in the management of pain, which in turn is an integrated part of a co-ordinated plan of overall patient care.

Psychological therapies

Psychological factors have profound effects on the perception of pain. Anxiety and depression are discussed further in Chapter 26 and other psychological issues in Chapter 30. As described in Chapter 5, the management of pain includes the assessment and treatment of psychological issues, and there are a number of psychological approaches to the treatment of pain (Table 16.1). These treatments evolved in the therapy of non-malignant pain and the efficacy of some of the techniques in the treatment of chronic pain related to cancer is still to be defined. Relaxation, simple behavioural training, and basic cognitive therapy are more appropriate for patients with advanced cancer and whether or not the more complex therapies provide additional benefit has not been determined.

Table 16.1 Psychological approaches to the treatment of pain

General psychological supportive care	Cognitive therapies
Behavioural therapies	distraction
relaxation	art, music, hobbies
deep breathing	occupational therapy, socialization
progressive muscular relaxation	psychological
autogenic relaxation	imagery, meditation, hypnosis
biofeedback	cognitive
operant conditioning	coping skills training
cognitive-behavioural therapy	stress management techniques
	Psychotherapy
	anxiolytics, antidepressants
	supportive psychotherapy

The psychological therapies for pain are non-invasive, should be less threatening to patients, and are essentially free of adverse effects. They are therapist-intensive, at least initially. All require active patient participation, which will enhance patients' feelings of being involved in their treatment.

General psychosocial supportive care

All patients with cancer deserve general psychological and psychosocial supportive care (Table 16.2). This basic care is important in pain control; without it, patients are more likely to complain of pain and may be less likely to respond well to treatment for it.

Table 16.2 General psychosocial supportive care

General	caring, considerate, unhurried approach
	good listening
	good communication
	supportive companionship
	reassurance about continuing care
	respect for person and individuality
	involvement in treatment and care, maintain sense of control
	allow discussion of fears regarding future suffering, life expectancy
Social	address social issues
	encourage available social supports
	facilitate use of social services
	assist with financial, legal issues
	provide support for family and carers
Cultural	respect cultural differences
	use interpreters for language barriers
	involve ethnic support services
Spiritual	address religious or spiritual concerns

Relaxation therapy

Relaxation therapy makes a significant contribution to pain control for patients with cancer (Table 16.3). [1–3] It will produce general calming and help treat exacerbations of pain related to anxiety or emotional stress as well as the anxiety associated with increased pain. Muscle relaxation techniques can help the musculoskeletal discomfort related to physical inactivity and debility.

A number of different techniques of varying complexity are used. The simplest is deep breathing and control of respiration. Progressive muscular relaxation, with or without imagery, involves the sequential tensing and relaxing of specific muscle groups, moving progressively across the body. Autogenic relaxation involves the sequential relaxation of each area of the body whilst focusing on a feeling of warmth and heaviness. With imagery a patient either concentrates on a comfortable situation or focuses on the pain. Meditation is a state of detached observation during which a patient either concentrates on a comfortable situation or focuses on the pain, and by assessing different sensations as they occur, develops insight. Meditation with imagery is considered by some to be akin to self-hypnosis. Relaxation therapy is performed initially with a therapist and then continued by the patient alone.

Table 16.3 Relaxation therapy for cancer pain: RCTs

Author	n	Intervention	Outcome
Arathuzik[1]	24	relaxation & visualization training vs no training	no difference in pain intensity; training: ↑ ability to decrease pain (pS)
Sloman[2]	67	relaxation training vs no training	training: ↓ pain scores and ↓ breakthrough analgesics (both pS)

Biofeedback therapy

Biofeedback therapy employs electronic devices to measure various biological responses such as muscle tension and convert them into signals understood by the patient. The patient is then trained to reduce muscular tension or other responses that may produce or aggravate pain. The role of biofeedback therapy in cancer-related pain remains to be established and well-taught relaxation therapy probably produces equivalent results.

Distraction

Distraction strategies help some patients with cancer cope with their pain. These include personal actions (like focusing hard on something particular—an object, a thought, some music—to allow an exacerbation of pain to pass) or activities that provide some external stimulation including music, art, craft, television and even just socializing with other patients.[4] Music therapy is being explored in palliative care for the treatment of both physical and psychosocial aspects of suffering.[5–7]

Hypnosis

Hypnosis is effective for controlling procedure-related pain,[8–10] but its effect on chronic tumour-related pain is less well documented. Successful hypnosis requires that the patient has good hypnotic susceptibility, is willing to undergo hypnosis, and has confidence in the therapist. Hypnosis may relieve anxiety and reduce anxiety-related pain; it may also produce elevation of mood and reduce feelings of helplessness.

Various strategies of hypnotic suggestion are used including a hallucination of anaesthesia with direct blocking of pain from awareness. Other techniques include diminution of pain by increasing pain tolerance, sensory substitution (involving substitution of another sensation for pain), pain displacement (moving the pain to a smaller or less important part of the body), and disassociation, in which the painful part of the body is disassociated from the patient's awareness.

Cognitive therapies

Teaching patients coping skills and stress management techniques will help them deal with their pain. Cognitive therapy directed at thought and affect control will help them manage pain crises. Whether cognitive training adds significantly to relaxation and imagery is uncertain.[1, 11] Operant conditioning, which is designed to modify pain behaviours, has no established role in the treatment of patients with advanced cancer.

Psychotherapy

Patients with severe pain who suffer a lot of emotional distress, anxiety or depression may benefit from supportive psychotherapy as well as the appropriate use of antidepressant and anxiolytic drugs (see Chapter 26).

References

1   Arathuzik, D. (1994). Effects of cognitive-behavioral strategies on pain in cancer patients. *Cancer Nursing* 17, 207–14.

2   Sloman, R., et al. (1994). The use of relaxation for the promotion of comfort and pain relief in persons with advanced cancer. *Contemporary Nurse* 3, 6–12.

3   Carroll, D. and Seers, K. (1998). Relaxation for the relief of chronic pain: a systematic review. *Journal of Advanced Nursing* 27, 476–87.

4   Trauger-Querry, B. and Haghighi, K.R. (1999). Balancing the focus: art and music therapy for pain control and symptom management in hospice care. *Hospice Journal* 14, 25–38.

5   Gallagher, L.M., et al. (2001). Music therapy in palliative medicine. *Supportive Care in Cancer* 9, 156–61.

6   Magill, L. (2001). The use of music therapy to address the suffering in advanced cancer pain. *Journal of Palliative Care* 17, 167–72.

7   Hogan, B.E. (2002). Music therapy in palliative care: a state of the art. *Progress in Palliative Care* 10, 108–12.

8   Sellick, S.M. and Zaza, C. (1998). Critical review of 5 nonpharmacologic strategies for managing cancer pain. *Cancer Prevention and Control* 2, 7–14.

9   Lang, E.V., et al. (2000). Adjunctive non-pharmacological analgesia for invasive medical procedures: a randomised trial. *Lancet* 355, 1486–90.

10 Goudas, L., et al. (2001). *Management of cancer pain*. Rockville, MD: Agency for Healthcare Research and Quality. <www.ahrq.gov>

11 Syrjala, K.L., et al. (1995). Relaxation and imagery and cognitive-behavioral training reduce pain during cancer treatment: a controlled clinical trial. *Pain* 63, 189–98.

17

Anticancer therapy

Radiotherapy
Chemotherapy
Hormonal therapy

The appropriate and judicious use of anticancer therapy is sometimes the most effective means of controlling pain, even for patients with very advanced disease. Anticancer treatment should be considered for all patients with pain and may lead to a significant reduction in the need for analgesics. Radiotherapy is the modality most frequently used but chemotherapy, hormonal therapy and surgery are also useful in certain clinical situations. In each case an assessment must be made of the potential benefits and toxicity, and treatment must be appropriate to the stage of the patient's disease and the prognosis.

Radiotherapy

Radiotherapy is a most effective means of controlling pain due to local tumour infiltration. The potential benefits must be weighed against the possible adverse effects, as well as the inconvenience of transporting the patient to and from a radiotherapy facility. The rationale for the use of radiotherapy is that it causes death of some tumour cells, leading to a reduction of pain or other symptoms caused by tumour infiltration or pressure.

The response to radiotherapy depends on factors related to both the tumour and the radiation. More rapidly growing tumours (with a high rate of cell division) and those with good vascular supply (in which the cells are well oxygenated) are likely to be more sensitive to radiotherapy. Tumours also vary in their inherent radiosensitivity, but this classification and the concept of 'radioresistant tumours' relate to radiocurability of the cancer and not to palliative radiotherapy. In palliative care, tumour shrinkage is not necessarily the major determinant of pain relief, and local pain due to tumour infiltration is usually responsive to local radiotherapy, irrespective of the histological type or tissue of origin of the tumour.

Adverse effects

The adverse effects of radiotherapy (Table 17.1) depend primarily on the volume of tissue irradiated and the effects of irradiation on normal tissues within the treatment field. Treatment of larger volumes will cause more adverse effects and will involve more normal tissues. The acute

Table 17.1 Determinants of the adverse effects of radiotherapy

Treatment factors	Patient factors
volume irradiated	general condition
total dose	body site irradiated
dose per fraction	radiosensitivity of adjacent normal tissues
dose rate	other concurrent treatment
energy of the radiation	surgery, chemotherapy

Table 17.2 Acute local adverse effects of radiotherapy

Skin	erythema, alopecia
Mucosa	pharyngitis, oesophagitis, gastritis, enteritis, colitis, proctitis, cystitis, vaginitis
Lung	pneumonitis
Liver	hepatitis
Kidney	nephritis
Brain	encephalitis
Marrow	myelosuppression
Systemic	lethargy, tiredness, nausea, anorexia ('radiation sickness')

local effects of radiotherapy occur within days or weeks of treatment and relate to inflammation, oedema and cell death within the treated field (Table 17.2). Irradiation of the head or abdomen is frequently associated with nausea and vomiting. Patients receiving radiotherapy often develop some 'radiation sickness' with tiredness, fatigue, nausea and anorexia. The adverse effects of radiotherapy are further discussed in Chapter 29.

There may be increased pain for a few days after the commencement of radiotherapy, due to reactive oedema. The patient should be forewarned of this possibility and, if necessary, treated with a corticosteroid or NSAID.

Treatment

Palliative radiotherapy should employ the minimum dose of radiotherapy required to achieve the desired result, given in the minimum number of treatment fractions (Table 17.3). Radiotherapy given in this manner is less likely to produce significant adverse effects, is of less inconvenience to the patient, and produces equivalent results.[1] It produces relief of pain in 50–80% of patients with bone metastases; the response rate is lower for soft tissue infiltration. The duration of response is often several months.

Bone metastases. A considerable number of different radiotherapy schedules has been advocated for the treatment of bone metastases.[2] A number of studies have shown that a

Table 17.3 Principles of palliative radiotherapy for pain relief

Minimum effective dose
Minimum number of treatment sessions (fractions)
Histological type and tissue of origin are not relevant for palliative radiotherapy

Table 17.4   Radiotherapy for bone metastases: RCTs

Author	n	Intervention	Outcome
Single 8Gy fraction vs longer courses			
Price[10]	288	8Gy vs 30Gy	equivalent speed of onset and duration of analgesia
Nielsen[11]	241	8Gy vs 20Gy	equivalent frequency and duration of analgesia
Bone Pain Trial[12]	765	8Gy vs 20Gy or 30Gy	equivalent frequency, speed of onset and duration of analgesia; more retreatments with 8Gy
Steenland[13]	1171	8Gy vs 24Gy	equivalent frequency, speed of onset and duration of analgesia; more retreatments with 8Gy
Single 8Gy fraction vs lower doses			
Hoskin[14]	270	8Gy vs 4Gy	8Gy: 69 vs 44% pain relief at 4w (pS); fewer retreatments (pS)
Jeremic[15]	327	8Gy vs 6Gy vs 4Gy	8Gy: more rapid onset of analgesia (pS); 4Gy: inferior frequency of analgesia (pS)

single dose of 8 Gy produces equivalent results to longer courses of therapy (Table 17.4). Pain relief is reported in 50–80% of patients and lasts a median of 3 months; a significant proportion of patients do not develop recurrent pain at the treated site within 12 months.[3] Retreatment is required more frequently with the 8 Gy dose, but this may reflect a readiness to give further treatment after a single fraction than after a longer course. A single dose of 4 Gy produced fewer responses, but the duration of pain relief was similar. The response to radiotherapy is usually manifest within 2 to 4 weeks of starting treatment. It may occur more rapidly, even within a day or two, with higher dose fractions.

Patients with widespread bone metastases may be considered for hemibody irradiation or the systemic administration of radioisotopes. Hemibody irradiation involves a single treatment to the whole of the upper or lower half of the body and this can be followed, if indicated, with irradiation to the other half of the body four to six weeks later. It produces pain relief in days for 90% of patients.[4, 5] However, the toxicity of hemibody irradiation is considerable and includes nausea, vomiting and diarrhoea, myelosuppression, mucositis, pneumonitis and alopecia. It is therefore not appropriate for patients with significantly reduced blood counts, those in generally poor physical condition, or with a life expectancy of less than a few months.

The systemic administration of bone-seeking radioisotopes is effective in controlling pain related to bone metastases.[6, 7] Various isotopes have been used including 89-Strontium, 153-Samarium and 186-Rhenium (see Chapter 23, Table 23.7). The isotopes are preferentially taken up at sites of osteoblastic activity and cause only mild myelotoxicity. They are used to treat metastases that have increased osteoblastic activity, as evidenced by abnormality on bone scan; they are best for tumours that have markedly increased osteoblastic activity, with sclerotic changes on x-ray, as is seen with prostate and some breast cancers. Improved pain control is reported in up to 80% of patients. Responses are usually evident 2 to 3 weeks after treatment and last for 3 to 6 months. The degree and duration of analgesia after radioisotope therapy is equivalent to local or hemibody irradiation.[8] They are of benefit when used in addition to local radiotherapy; compared to local radiotherapy, they reduce the number of new pain sites for about four months following treatment.[9] Radioisotope therapy is well tolerated and the main adverse effect is myelosuppression, which is usually mild and not clinically significant. The main drawback of radioisotope therapy is the cost.

Thoracic irradiation. Conventional radiotherapy given for tumour control might involve a dose of 30–40 Gy given in 10 to 20 treatment fractions over a period of 2 to 4 weeks. Studies of radiotherapy given for the palliation of inoperable lung cancer have shown that shorter courses of treatment (two fractions of 8.5 Gy, 7 days apart) produce equivalent pain relief compared with longer courses of treatment (Table 17.5).

Table 17.5 Chest radiotherapy: RCTs

Author	n	Intervention	Outcome
MRC[16]	235	8.5Gy x2,7d apart vs single 10Gy	pain relief equivalent
Macbeth[17]	509	8.5Gy x2,7d apart vs 39Gy longer course	pain relief equivalent at 3mo.
Rees[18]	216	8.5Gy x2,7d apart vs 22.5Gy longer course	pain relief equivalent

Skin. Malignant infiltration of the skin or superficial tissues is often painful. Treatment with electron beams, which deliver a high dose to the lesions whilst sparing deeper tissues, is usually effective in relieving pain.

Chemotherapy

Chemotherapy can produce significant relief of pain for patients whose cancers are sensitive to treatment. This has been demonstrated in large studies of patients with prostate[19, 20] and breast cancers,[21, 22] in which the relief of pain was correlated with objective tumour responses.

Decisions to proceed with palliative chemotherapy are based on a number of considerations, the most important of which is the inherent chemosensitivity of the tumour (Table 17.6). Younger patients and those with a good performance status are less likely to suffer troublesome toxicity and are more likely to benefit from treatment, although age is said not to be a prognostic factor provided there are no significant comorbid medical conditions.[23]

Table 17.6 Relative chemosensitivity of different tumours

Chemosensitive	Less Chemosensitive
(>30% response rate)	(<30% response rate)
bladder	gastric
breast	hepatobiliary
colon	kidney
head and neck	melanoma
leukaemia	mesothelioma
lung	prostate
lymphoma	sarcoma
myeloma	thyroid
oesophagus	
ovary	
testicle	
uterus	

Patients need to be adequately informed of their treatment options as well as the possible adverse effects in order to make their own informed decision. However, a large study reported that patients with cancer are more likely to accept toxic therapy with little chance of benefit than are patients without cancer or health professionals.[24]

Chemotherapy given for the palliation of pain should be geared to produce manageable and acceptable toxicity. The use of single agent treatment or combination chemotherapy in reduced doses may be appropriate. The adverse effects of chemotherapy are further discussed in Chapter 29.

Hormonal therapy

Corticosteroids. The use of corticosteroids as adjuvant analgesics is discussed in Chapter 13. In addition, corticosteroids have an antitumour action in patients with lymphoproliferative diseases and a few with breast and prostate cancers, and can be of particular benefit in the palliation of pain.

Sex hormones. A proportion of breast, prostate and endometrial cancers will respond to treatment with sex hormones or to therapy directed at altering the body's normal levels of sex hormones. If a tumour is sensitive to hormonal manipulation, there will be improvement in pain.

References

1   Hosking, P.J. (2003). Radiotherapy in symptom management. In *Oxford Textbook of Palliative Medicine, 3rd edition* (ed. D. Doyle, G. Hanks, N. Cherny and K. Calman). Oxford, Oxford University Press.

2   McQuay, H.J., et al. (2000). Radiotherapy for the palliation of painful bone metastases (Cochrane Review). *Cochrane Database of Systematic Reviews* CD001793.

3   Brown, H.K. and Healey, J.H. (2001). Metastatic cancer to the bone. In *Cancer. Principles and Practice of Oncology. 6th edition* (ed. V.T. De Vita, S. Hellman and S.A. Rosenberg). Philadelphia, Lippincott Williams Wilkins.

4   McSweeney, E.N., et al. (1993). Double hemibody irradiation (DHBI) in the management of relapsed and primary chemoresistant multiple myeloma. *Clinical Oncology* 5, 378–83.

5   Salazar, O.M., et al. (2001). Fractionated half-body irradiation (HBI) for the rapid palliation of widespread, symptomatic, metastatic bone disease: a randomized Phase III trial of the International Atomic Energy Agency (IAEA). *International Journal of Radiation Oncology, Biology, Physics* 50, 765–75.

6   Robinson, R.G., et al. (1995). Strontium 89 therapy for the palliation of pain due to osseous metastases. *Journal of the American Medical Association* 274, 420–4.

7   Berger, A.M. and Koprowski, C. (2002). Bone pain: assessment and management. In *Principles and Practice of Palliative Care and Supportive Oncology* (ed. A.M. Berger, R.K. Portenoy and D.E. Weissman). Philadelphia, Lippincott, Williams and Wilkins.

8   Quilty, P.M., et al. (1994). A comparison of the palliative effects of strontium-89 and external beam radiotherapy in metastatic prostate cancer. *Radiotherapy and Oncology* 31, 33–40.

9   Porter, A.T., et al. (1993). Results of a randomized phase-III trial to evaluate the efficacy of strontium-89 adjuvant to local field external beam irradiation in the management of endocrine resistant metastatic prostate cancer. *International Journal of Radiation Oncology, Biology, Physics* 25, 805–13.

10 Price, P., et al. (1986). Prospective randomised trial of single and multifraction radiotherapy schedules in the treatment of painful bony metastases. *Radiotherapy and Oncology* 6, 247–55.

11 Nielsen, O.S., et al. (1998). Randomized trial of single dose versus fractionated palliative radiotherapy of bone metastases. *Radiotherapy and Oncology* 47, 233–40.

12   Bone Pain Trial Working Party (1999). 8 Gy single fraction radiotherapy for the treatment of metastatic skeletal pain: randomised comparison with a multifraction schedule over 12 months of patient follow-up. *Radiotherapy and Oncology* 52, 111–21.

13   Steenland, E., et al. (1999). The effect of a single fraction compared to multiple fractions on painful bone metastases: a global analysis of the Dutch Bone Metastasis Study. *Radiotherapy and Oncology* 52, 101–9.

14   Hoskin, P.J., et al. (1992). A prospective randomised trial of 4 Gy or 8 Gy single doses in the treatment of metastatic bone pain. *Radiotherapy and Oncology* 23, 74–8.

15   Jeremic, B., et al. (1998). A randomized trial of three single-dose radiation therapy regimens in the treatment of metastatic bone pain. *International Journal of Radiation Oncology, Biology, Physics* 42, 161–7.

16   Medical Research Council Lung Cancer Working Party (1992). A Medical Research Council (MRC) randomised trial of palliative radiotherapy with two fractions or a single fraction in patients with inoperable non-small-cell lung cancer (NSCLC) and poor performance status. *British Journal of Cancer* 65, 934–41.

17   Macbeth, F.R., et al. (1996). Randomized trial of palliative two-fraction versus more intensive 13-fraction radiotherapy for patients with inoperable non-small cell lung cancer and good performance status. Medical Research Council Lung Cancer Working Party. *Clinical Oncology* 8, 167–75.

18   Rees, G.J., et al. (1997). Palliative radiotherapy for lung cancer: two versus five fractions. *Clinical Oncology* 9, 90–5.

19   Tannock, I.F., et al. (1996). Chemotherapy with mitoxantrone plus prednisone or prednisone alone for symptomatic hormone-resistant prostate cancer: a Canadian randomized trial with palliative end points. *Journal of Clinical Oncology* 14, 1756–64.

20   Small, E.J., et al. (2000). Suramin therapy for patients with symptomatic hormone-refractory prostate cancer: results of a randomized phase III trial comparing suramin plus hydrocortisone to placebo plus hydrocortisone. *Journal of Clinical Oncology* 18, 1440–50.

21   Ramirez, A.J., et al. (1998). Do patients with advanced breast cancer benefit from chemotherapy? *British Journal of Cancer* 78, 1488–94.

22   Geels, P., et al. (2000). Palliative effect of chemotherapy: objective tumor response is associated with symptom improvement in patients with metastatic breast cancer. *Journal of Clinical Oncology* 18, 2395–405.

23   Ellison, N.M. and Chevlen, E.M. (2002). Palliative chemotherapy. In *Principles and Practice of Palliative Care and Supportive Oncology* (ed. A.M. Berger, R.K. Portenoy and D.E. Weissman). Philadelphia, Lippincott, Williams and Wilkins.

24   Slevin, M.L., et al. (1990). Attitudes to chemotherapy: comparing views of patients with cancer with those of doctors, nurses, and general public. *British Medical Journal* 300, 1458–60.

Section III

Other physical symptoms and clinical problems

To do away with the suffering of the sick,
to lessen the violence of the disease

Hippocrates (5th Century BC)

It remains that we retard what we cannot repel
and palliate what we cannot cure

Samuel Johnson (1709–84)

Good symptom control is fundamental to the opportunity
to care for the whole person.

Jo Hockley (1993)

18

Respiratory

Primary lung cancer	Pneumonitis
Lung metastases	Pulmonary embolism
Dyspnoea	Pleural effusion
Cough	Tracheostomy
Haemoptysis	Hoarseness
Pneumonia	Terminal respiratory congestion

Primary lung cancer

The symptoms and signs of primary lung cancer are listed in Table 18.1.[1] Dyspnoea is a frequent symptom that may be caused by bronchial obstruction, lymphangitis, pleural effusion, or cardiac involvement; many patients also have dyspnoea related to chronic lung damage from smoking. In addition, fatigue, anorexia and weight loss are common.

Lymphangitis carcinomatosis occurs when cancer involving hilar nodes spreads in a retrograde manner along lymphatic vessels in the lung. It is characterized by dyspnoea, a dry irritating cough, and an x-ray that shows hilar enlargement with linear markings radiating from the involved nodes.

Spread to the mediastinum may lead to compression or obstruction of various structures. Obstruction of the central lymphatics may lead to a chylous pleural effusion. Compression of the recurrent laryngeal and phrenic nerves leads to hoarseness and dyspnoea, respectively. Bronchial aspiration may occur if there is complete oesophageal obstruction, a tracheo-oesophageal fistula, or vocal cord paralysis.

Chest wall infiltration causes pain. A Pancoast tumour is a locally invasive cancer arising in the apex of the lung that spreads to involve the brachial plexus, causing motor and sensory signs in the arm and a Horner's syndrome.

Metastatic disease may occur at any site. The tissues most frequently involved are mediastinum, pleura, liver, bone, adrenal and brain. Non-metastatic paraneoplastic syndromes are common; small cell carcinoma is associated with inappropriate antidiuretic hormone (ADH) secretion, Cushing's syndrome and the neurological paraneoplastic syndromes, whilst hypercalcaemia and hypertrophic osteoarthropathy occur more frequently with non-small cell tumours.

Table 18.1   Clinical features of primary lung cancer

Endobronchial tumour	cough, haemoptysis
	bronchial obstruction
	    wheeze, stridor
	    segmental or lobar collapse
	    predisposition to pneumonia

Hilar involvement	bronchial compression lymphangitis carcinomatosis
Mediastinal involvement	tracheal compression oesophageal obstruction superior vena caval obstruction lymphatic obstruction chylous pleural effusion recurrent laryngeal nerve palsy phrenic nerve palsy
Cardiac involvement	pericardial infiltration, effusion
Pleural involvement	pleural infiltration, effusion
Chest wall involvement	pain, Pancoast syndrome
Distant metastases	
Paraneoplastic syndromes	

Lung metastases

The lung is a frequent site for metastases from tumours developing elsewhere in the body. In clinical practice, the majority of pulmonary metastases originate from the more common cancers including breast, gastrointestinal tract and lung. Some less common cancers have a high incidence of pulmonary metastases, including sarcomas, renal cell carcinoma, and testicular cancer.

Pulmonary metastases vary greatly in size and number. They may be asymptomatic although widespread metastases usually cause dyspnoea (Table 18.2). Metastases usually involve the lung parenchyma itself; endobronchial involvement and haemoptysis are less

Table 18.2   Symptoms and signs of lung metastases

Metastases to lung parenchyma	asymptomatic
	dyspnoea
	extrinsic bronchial
	compression
	    cough, wheeze and stridor
	    segmental or lobar collapse
	    predisposition to infection
	pleural involvement
	pericardial involvement

Hilar, mediastinal involvement	*see* Table 18.1
Endobronchial metastases (uncommon)	cough, haemoptysis bronchial obstruction

common than with primary tumours. Growth of the metastases may lead to extrinsic bronchial compression. Secondary tumours may involve the pleura or pericardium but chest wall invasion is much less common than with primary lung cancer. Involvement of hilar nodes may produce the syndrome of lymphangitis carcinomatosis. Metastases to the mediastinal nodes can cause all of the features described for primary lung tumours (Table 18.1).

Treatment

Patients with sensitive tumours should have a trial of systemic therapy. Radiotherapy is of benefit for haemoptysis or pain secondary to pleural infiltration. Surgery is not indicated in patients with advanced cancer. Treatment is otherwise symptomatic, as outlined in the other sections in this chapter. Patients with widespread metastases or lymphangitis carcinomatosis may benefit from corticosteroids. They should be started on a higher dose (prednisolone 40–60 mg/d) for a few days, and the dose then gradually weaned to the lowest dose that maintains a symptomatic response.

Dyspnoea

Dyspnoea, or breathlessness, is the unpleasant awareness of difficulty in breathing. Like pain, it is subjective and involves both the perception of breathlessness and the reaction of the patient to it. Dyspnoea interferes with both the physical and psychological aspects of quality of life and is associated with increased stress for family members.[2–4] A number of recent reviews of dyspnoea have been published.[5–8]

Normal respiration is directed by centres in the medulla, which control the respiratory muscles—the diaphragm, intercostal and accessory muscles. The medullary centres receive input from peripheral and central chemoreceptors (sensitive to hypoxia, hypercapnia and acidosis), from mechanoreceptors in the respiratory muscles, airways and lung, and from higher cortical centres. This afferent information influences the frequency and depth of ventilation. The sensation of dyspnoea occurs when there is a mismatch between the efferent respiratory motor activity and the afferent feedback from the chemoreceptors and mechanoreceptors. However, the pathophysiological changes that lead to the perception of dyspnoea in individual patients are poorly understood and individuals with similar impairment of lung function may report much more or less dyspnoea.[5, 6]

Dyspnoea is reported to occur in about one half of patients with advanced disease, increasing to about 70% during the last six weeks of life.[5, 6, 9] The incidence is higher in patients with malignant infiltration of the lung and those with anxiety.[10, 11]

There are many possible causes of dyspnoea (Table 18.3). In many patients it is due to a combination of different causes. In others, no specific cause may be identified other than general debility. Some of the causes listed are amenable to relatively simple therapy, underlining the need for careful clinical assessment.

The multidimensional nature of dyspnoea is important and it has been described as resulting from interactions among multiple physiological, psychological, social and environmental factors[5]. The association of anxiety and psychological distress with the occurrence and severity of dyspnoea emphasizes the importance of cognitive and psychological factors.[10–12]

Respiratory muscle weakness has been demonstrated in patients with advanced cancer and may contribute significantly to dyspnoea. Respiratory muscle strength is measured by the maximum inspiratory pressure (MIP) or sniff nasal inspiratory pressure (SNIP). The cause, significance and management of respiratory muscle weakness require further study.[10, 11, 13, 14]

Table 18.3 Causes of dyspnoea

Airway obstruction
    tracheal
        tumour of larynx, thyroid, mediastinum, bronchus
        tracheo-oesophageal fistula
    bronchial
        tumour
        chronic bronchitis
        acute infection, bronchitis
        bronchospasm: bronchitis, asthma, carcinoid syndrome

Reduction in functional lung tissue
    surgical resection: lobectomy, pneumonectomy
    tumour: atelectasis, lymphangitis, multiple metastases
    fibrosis: pre-existing, radiation, chemotherapy
    pleural effusion
    pneumothorax
    infection
    haemorrhage
    pulmonary embolism
    chronic emphysema

Impaired ventilatory movement
    chest wall weakness, motor impairment, general debility
    chest wall pain
    chest wall tumour infiltration
    elevated diaphragm: ascites, hepatomegaly, phrenic nerve lesion

Cardiovascular
    superior vena caval obstruction
    congestive cardiac failure, cardiomyopathy
    pericardial effusion, constrictive pericarditis
    shock, haemorrhage, septicaemia

Other
    anaemia
    anxiety
    fever
    metabolic acidosis

Assessment. Many of the conditions listed in table 18.3 have characteristic clinical features and the results of a history and clinical examination, together with knowledge about pre-existing lung disease, are often sufficient to determine the cause of dyspnoea. Tracheal or bronchial obstruction cause stridor or wheeze and a tracheo-oesophageal fistula will cause acute dyspnoea immediately after swallowing. Dyspnoea due to mediastinal tumours is often associated with dysphagia and signs of superior vena caval obstruction. Purulent sputum and fever suggest infection.

A chest x-ray may confirm a pleural effusion or show cardiomegaly suggestive of pericardial effusion.[13] There may be infiltration by primary or secondary cancer, with or without collapse distal to the bronchial obstruction. Lymphangitis carcinomatosis produces reticular markings radiating from the hilar region. The changes of radiation pneumonitis conform to the radiation field. Widespread or miliary markings are more difficult to interpret and can be due to multiple metastases, infection, haemorrhage or drug toxicity.

Further tests should be considered if the results are likely to significantly affect treatment decisions and provided such further investigations are appropriate to the stage of the patient's disease and prognosis.

Measurement. Dyspnoea is a subjective symptom that cannot be objectively measured. The results of pulmonary function tests may correlate poorly with the degree of dyspnoea reported by the patient.[6, 15] A number of different instruments have been developed for the assessment of dyspnoea in patients with nonmalignant lung disease, which have not been used extensively in patients with cancer.[16] A visual analogue scale (VAS) and verbal rating scale (VRS) for dyspnoea have been validated for patients with advanced cancer.[6, 9, 17] In the palliative care setting, simpler tests such as a VAS, the shuttle walking test,[18] and reading numbers aloud [19] may be more appropriate. A more comprehensive assessment tool, taking account of the multidimensional nature of dyspnoea, may be required for research.[17, 20]

Treatment

Treatment is directed at the specific cause, where possible and appropriate (Table 18.4). Nonmalignant causes of dyspnoea, including chronic lung disease, bronchial asthma, heart failure and anaemia, are treated by standard means. Tracheal and bronchial obstruction can be treated with radiotherapy and, for sensitive tumours, systemic therapy. Tracheal and proximal

Table 18.4   Dyspnoea: treatment of specific causes

Obstruction	endoscopic: laser resection, electrocautery, stenting, brachytherapy external radiotherapy corticosteroids systemic therapy (sensitive tumours)
Effusions	drainage instillation of sclerosants systemic therapy (sensitive tumours)

Metastases
    solitary
    multiple
    lymphangitis
	
	surgery, corticosteroids, radiotherapy, systemic therapy
	corticosteroids, systemic therapy (sensitive tumours)
	corticosteroids, systemic therapy (sensitive tumours)

Pneumonitis
    radiation
    chemotherapy
	
	corticosteroids
	corticosteroids, stop chemotherapy

Pneumonia	antimicrobial therapy
Pulmonary embolism	anticoagulation
Haemorrhage	treatment of systemic bleeding diathesis
Bronchospasm	bronchodilators
SVC obstruction	corticosteroids, radiotherapy, stenting
Oesophageal fistulas	stenting

Treatment must be appropriate to the stage of the patient's disease and prognosis

bronchial lesions can be treated with endoscopic laser resection, electrocautery or stenting, followed by radiotherapy.[21] Endobronchial laser resection provides good relief of obstruction but only treats tumour that is endobronchial and usually needs to be repeated after 6 to 8 weeks. The use of endobronchial irradiation or brachytherapy is also effective. Dyspnoea and cough related to oesophago-respiratory fistulas is treated by stenting (see Cough). Pleural and pericardial effusions and ascites causing dyspnoea can be drained. Dyspnoea due to multiple metastases, lymphangitis carcinomatosis and pneumonitis may improve with prednisolone 40–60 mg/d or dexamethasone 8–12 mg/d; the dose is weaned to the minimum effective dose after a few days.

Radiotherapy, both external beam and brachytherapy, are effective for controlling dyspnoea and other symptoms in patients with advanced lung cancer (Table 18.5). The optimal schedules remain to be defined, but in general shorter courses of radiotherapy produce comparable symptom control for most patients. Brachytherapy is particularly useful where there is obstructing endobronchial tumour, although the use of larger single doses may increase the risk of massive haemoptysis.[22, 23]

Table 18.5 Palliative radiotherapy: RCTs

Author	n	Intervention	Outcome
MRC[24]	369	8.5Gy x 2, 7d apart vs 30Gy in 10 fractions	no significant differences in symptom control or survival
MRC[25]	235	8.5Gy x 2, 7d apart vs 10Gy in a single fraction	no significant differences in symptom control or survival
Macbeth[26]	509	8.5Gy x 2, 7d apart vs 39Gy in 13 fractions	2 fractions: more rapid palliation of symptoms, shorter survival (pS)
Rees[27]	216	8.5Gy x 2, 7d apart vs 22.5Gy in 5 fractions	no significant differences in symptom control or survival
Stout[28]	99	External beam vs brachytherapy	External beam: more durable improvement in symptoms (pS)
Langerdijk[29]	95	External beam ± brachytherapy	Combination: ↑ lung re-expansion, ↓ dyspnoea (both pS)

General symptomatic measures. A number of symptomatic and non-drug measures are available for the treatment of dyspnoea (Table 18.6). The dyspnoeic patient is managed in a calm and reassuring manner, given a gentle and sure explanation about the dyspnoea, and reassured that it can be treated and that they will not die of suffocation. Patients should be allowed to choose the position in which they are most comfortable, even if this means sleeping in a chair. Dyspnoeic patients frequently appreciate fresh cool air from a fan or open window. The use of breathing education, relaxation exercises, and activity pacing, together with an exploration of the meaning of breathlessness to the patient and the development of coping strategies, have been shown to reduce dyspnoea (Table18.7).[30, 31] Patients should be encouraged to exercise to the point of breathlessness to improve their tolerance of dyspnoea and to gain a sense of control. Relaxation training and acupuncture are reported to lessen dyspnoea in patients with chronic lung disease.[32, 33]

Table 18.6 Management of dyspnoea

Calm, reassuring attitude	Activity management
Position of comfort	Energy conservation
Improved air circulation	Encourage exercise to improve tolerance of dyspnoea
Oxygen	Psychosocial support
Breathing control techniques	support development of coping strategies
Relaxation exercises	allow expression of fears, anxieties
Distraction therapy	

Table 18.7 Nursing interventions for dyspnoea: RCTs

Author	n	Intervention	Outcome
Corner[30]	20	non-pharmacological therapies vs best supportive care	Intervention group: ↓ dyspnoea, ↓ distress, ↑ functional capacity (all pS)
Bredin[31]	119	non-pharmacological therapies vs best supportive care	Intervention group: ↓ dyspnoea at best, ↑ performance status, ↓ depression (all pS)

Oxygen. For patients with chronic obstructive pulmonary disease who are hypoxemic ($PaO_2 < 55$mm Hg), oxygen therapy has been shown to reduce mortality and improve quality of life. Oxygen therapy for patients with less severe hypoxemia does not increase survival, but the effects on chronic activity-related dyspnoea and quality of life have not been systematically studied.[5, 34] Studies in patients with chronic lung disease suggest that non-hypoxemic patients may also benefit from oxygen therapy and it is not uncommon to observe improvement in dyspnoea in patients with cancer who are not hypoxemic.[35] This is in keeping with the observation that measurements of hypoxemia (arterial blood gases or pulse oximetry) do not correlate with the severity of dyspnoea reported by the patient, and that such measurements are of no value in assessing dyspnoea or its relief [6]. In palliative care, RCTs of oxygen therapy have shown mixed results (Table 18.8).[36, 37] For individual patients, a trial of multiple blinded cross-overs between oxygen and air will quickly determine which patients benefit from supplemental oxygen.[38]

If dyspnoea occurs only intermittently or on exertion, patients should be encouraged to reserve oxygen therapy for exacerbations and before exercise. Oxygen therapy must be used with caution in patients with chronic lung disease and hypoxia, as some are tolerant of elevated levels of carbon dioxide and depend on hypoxia for their respiratory drive; administration of oxygen in this situation may cause respiratory failure and death. A portable oxygen concentrator is the easiest and most economic means of providing oxygen therapy at home.

Table 18.8 Oxygen therapy for dyspnoea: RCTs

Author	n	Intervention	Outcome
Bruera[36]	14	All hypoxaemic; 5L/min air vs oxygen	less dyspnoea on oxygen (VAS) (pS)
Booth[37]	38	6/38 hypoxaemic; 4L/min air vs oxygen	no difference (VAS, Borg scale)

Opioids. Opioids are the most useful drugs for the treatment of dyspnoea in patients with advanced cancer.[39] Prospective studies showed subcutaneous and intravenous morphine to be effective in reducing dyspnoea;[40, 41] there was no impairment of respiratory function in the study of subcutaneous therapy, but sedation and hypercapnia occurred in the intravenous study which included opioid-naive patients. These findings have been confirmed in RCTs (Table 18.9).[42, 43] A further randomized trial comparing supplemental doses of morphine equivalent to 25% and 50% of the regular 4-hourly dose suggested that the lower dose was adequate and effective in reducing dyspnoea.[44] The recommended starting dose of morphine for the treatment of dyspnoea is 5–10mg PO given 4-hourly, or a 25% increase in the 4-hourly dose for those already taking morphine for pain, and titrated against effect and toxicity.[44] Whether morphine should be administered regularly for dyspnoea or on an as needed basis is unresolved; regular dosing may be associated with increased toxicity, including sedation.[45]

Table 18.9 Systemic opioids for cancer-related dyspnoea: RCTs

Author	n	Intervention	Outcome
Bruera[42]	10	morphine SC (50% higher than regular dose) vs placebo	less dyspnoea (VAS) (pS); no deterioration in respiratory function
Mazzocato[43]	9	morphine SC (5mg or regular dose + 3.75mg) vs placebo	less dyspnoea (VAS, Borg scale) (pS); no deterioration in respiratory function

Nebulized opioids. A number of studies have reported nebulized morphine to be effective in the treatment of dyspnoea in patients with advanced cancer, including some already receiving systemic opioids for analgesia.[46–50] Morphine is presumed to act on opioid receptors in the lung and the advantages of nebulized therapy include more rapid effect and the possibility of fewer systemic side effects. However, a single RCT in which patients were given a single predetermined morphine dose did not show a significant difference between morphine and saline (Table 18.10).[51] Overall, there was a non-significant trend in favour of morphine compared to saline, and there was a trend towards greater improvement in breathlessness with higher doses of morphine. It has been suggested that individual patients have a threshold dose, below which nebulized morphine will not affect dyspnoea;[48] the lower doses included in the RCT may have biased the results and further controlled studies are needed. A systematic review of the use of nebulized morphine for patients with chronic lung disease did not show benefit.[52]

Table 18.10 Nebulized morphine for cancer-related dyspnoea: RCT

Author	n	Intervention	Outcome
Davis[51]	79	nebulized morphine 5-50mg vs placebo	no statistical differences (VAS, Borg) [non-significant trend in favour of morphine]

High response rates have been reported for nebulized fentanyl [53] and morphine 6-glucuronide[54] without significant adverse effects or deterioration in respiratory function.

Nebulized morphine is usually started at a dose of 10–20mg in 5ml of normal saline, given 4-hourly or as required for dyspnoea, and titrated against effect. A small proportion of patients will develop bronchospasm and the initial dose should be given in a situation where appropriate therapy is immediately available. In addition, there is a report of a patient who was already taking oral morphine who developed serious respiratory depression after the initial 4mg dose of nebulized morphine.[55]

Anxiolytics. Benzodiazepines may reduce dyspnoea, probably by an anxiolytic and sedative effect. Diazepam, lorazepam and alprazolam are all effective and are scheduled according to need—either regularly through the 24 hours, only at night, or to counteract anxiety attacks. Buspirone is a non-benzodiazepine anxiolytic that does not cause sedation or respiratory depression, which may be of value in patients with chronic lung disease; its value in palliative care is limited by the fact that it takes 2–4 weeks to be effective.

Bronchodilators. These drugs are useful when there is a reversible element to bronchial obstruction. In the non-acute situation, the usefulness of these drugs should be estimated by measuring peak flows before and after treatment, ensuring that they are used only in situations where they are effective. Bronchodilators in use include β-adrenergic stimulants (e.g. salbutamol, albuterol), anticholinergics (e.g. ipratropium) and the xanthine derivatives, aminophylline and theophylline (Table 18.11). The adverse effects of salbutamol include tremor, tachycardia and headache. The xanthines act by β-adrenergic stimulation and have a respiratory stimulant action in the medulla. They are available in various long acting oral preparations. Adverse effects include cardiac and cerebral stimulation, and a number of drug interactions are documented.

Table 18.11   Dyspnoea: examples of drug therapy*

Opioids
    morphine 5–10mg PO, q4h or 4-hourly PRN, and titrate
    morphine 10–20mg by nebulizer, q4h or 4-hourly PRN, and titrate

Anxiolytics
    diazepam 2mg PO q8h ± 5–10mg nocte
    lorazepam 0.5–1mg SL, q6–8h

Bronchodilators
    salbutamol by metered aerosol or 2.5–5mg by nebulizer, q4–6h
    ipratropium by metered aerosol or 250–500µg by nebulizer, q6h
    aminophylline, theophylline PO

Corticosteroids
    prednisolone 40–60mg/d PO, dexamethasone 8–12mg/d PO

Mucolytics (for sputum retention)
    humidified air (steam, nebulized saline)
    acetylcysteine 10%, 6–10ml by nebulizer, q6–8h

Anticholinergics (for excessive secretions)
    hyoscine hydrobromide 0.4–0.8mg SC q4h; 1.2–2.4 mg/24h CSCI

* Nebulizer therapy for patients with chronic obstructive lung disease who may have hypercapnia should be with air, not oxygen.

Corticosteroids. Corticosteroids are effective bronchodilators and may also improve dyspnoea associated with pulmonary metastases and lymphangitis carcinomatosis.

Other drugs. Dyspnoea aggravated by sputum retention or tenacious sputum can be helped by breathing humidified air (steam, nebulized saline) or by mucolytic agents such as acetylcysteine. Physiotherapy, with deep breathing, posturing and percussion, is important. Anticholinergic drugs are of benefit when excessive secretions contribute to dyspnoea. If dyspnoea is aggravated by coughing, antitussives or nebulized local anaesthetics may be of benefit (see Cough). Nebulized frusemide is reported to relieve dyspnoea in terminally ill cancer patients.[56] Nebulized lignocaine is ineffective.[57]

Terminal care

In the last week or days of life, treatment should be purely symptomatic. Investigations have little place except for the patient who would be made more comfortable by the drainage of a significant pleural effusion. Antibiotic therapy is usually not warranted and may only serve to prolong the dying process. If of benefit, bronchodilator therapy can be continued by mask. Semiconscious or unconscious patients who still appear dyspnoeic should be treated with morphine by CSCI.

Cough

Cough is the physiological reflex employed to clear irritant, foreign or particulate material from the respiratory tract. It is reported to occur in 40 to 80% of patients with advanced cancer and is most frequent in patients with primary or secondary lung cancer. A number of recent reviews of cough have been published.[58–60]

Cough can be caused by physical or chemical stimulation of receptors in both the upper and lower respiratory tract and also in the pleura, pericardium and diaphragm (Table 18.12). Aspiration may be caused by swallowing dysfunction, cranial nerve palsies, cancer therapy, or oesophageal fistulas.[61]

Table 18.12   Causes of cough

Airway irritation
    atmosphere: smoke, fumes, dry atmosphere
    tumour: endobronchial tumour, extrinsic bronchial compression
    aspiration: swallowing dysfunction, vocal cord paralysis, oesophageal fistula
    gastro-oesophageal reflux
    infection/inflammation: post-nasal drip, laryngitis, tracheitis, bronchitis
    increased bronchial reactivity: ACE inhibitors, asthma
    sputum retention
    excess sputum, bronchorrhoea

Lung pathology
    infection
    infiltration: primary or secondary cancer, lymphangitis carcinomatosis
    pneumonitis: radiation, chemotherapy
    pulmonary fibrosis
    chronic obstructive lung disease
    pulmonary oedema: congestive heart failure, pericardial effusion with tamponade

Irritation of other structures associated with the cough reflex
    pleura, pericardium, diaphragm

Cough is most often associated with infection and is not persistent or distressing. Other patients, particularly those with cancer involving the lung, may develop a persistent and troublesome cough. Besides being distressing for the patient and the family, persistent coughing is associated with a number of other complications (Table 18.13).

The clinical history, physical examination and chest x-ray will usually define the cause of cough. Other investigations should be considered if clinically indicated; bronchoscopy may be necessary to document endobronchial tumour.

Table 18.13 Complications of severe or persistent coughing

Cough syncope	Exhaustion
Headache	Insomnia
Retinal and conjunctival haemorrhage	Hoarseness
Pneumothorax	Induction of vomiting
Chest wall and muscular pain	Urinary incontinence
Pathological rib fractures	Aggravation of haemorrhoids

Treatment

Where possible and appropriate, treatment should be directed at the underlying cause as discussed for dyspnoea (Table 18.4). The management of oesophageal fistulas is discussed below. Gastro-oesophageal reflux is treated with an H_2-receptor antagonist or a proton pump inhibitor. Postnasal drip usually responds to antihistamine-decongestant therapy

General symptomatic measures. A number of general measures aid the symptomatic treatment of cough (Table 18.14). Atmospheric irritants should be avoided and smoking discouraged. A dry atmosphere will irritate a dry cough and inhibit expectoration with a productive cough. Atmospheric humidification or humidification of the inspired air can be of significant symptomatic benefit. For the same reason, dehydration should be avoided. The patient with troublesome cough is nursed in the position they find most comfortable, which is usually sitting in a semi-recumbent position.

Protussive therapy. Patients with a productive cough may benefit from measures that aid expectoration (Table 18.14), although this is not indicated for the terminally ill and may be distressing for patients who are weak or debilitated. Physiotherapy and education about effective coughing are important. Nebulized saline reduces the viscosity of secretions and helps expectoration. Steam can be used in the home setting. A variety of inhalations, such as menthol and eucalyptus, are used but there is no evidence of additional benefit. Irritant mucolytics increase the amount of respiratory tract fluid and reduce the viscosity of secretions, aiding expectoration. Ammonium chloride and potassium iodide cause nausea; others, such as guaifenesin, are included in proprietary cough medications. Chemical mucolytic agents reduce the viscosity of pulmonary secretions, aiding expectoration.

Antitussive therapy. Patients with a persistent dry cough are treated by suppression of the cough with antitussive agents (Table 18.14). [62,63] The drugs most frequently used are opioids and opioid analogues. The opioid analogues may be less sedating than opioids and dextromethorphan is reported to have similar antitussive activity to codeine. Dihydrocodeine and hydrocodone are reported to be more effective than codeine, but less antitussive than morphine. Hydromorphone and methadone are reported to be more effective antitussives than morphine, although the pharmacokinetic peculiarities of methadone make it less suitable. Pethidine (meperidine) is not antitussive. The dose and timing of antitussive medication should be tailored to suit the individual patient and is sometimes required only at night.

Table 18.14 Symptomatic treatment of cough

General measures	avoid smoke, fumes
	atmospheric humidification
	position of least discomfort
Protussive therapy	
Humidification	atmospheric humidification
	avoid dehydration
	humidified, nebulized air
Physiotherapy	postural drainage, cough education
Mucolytics	
topical	nebulized saline 2.5ml q4–6h & before physiotherapy
	steam
	inhalations *e.g.* menthol and eucalyptus
irritant	ammonium chloride, potassium iodide, guaifenesin
chemical	acetylcysteine 10%, 6–10ml by nebulizer, q6–8h
	carbocisteine 750mg PO q8h
Bronchodilators	if bronchospasm present
Antibiotics	if infection present
Antitussive therapy	
Opioid analogues	dextromethorphan 10–20mg PO q4–6h
	pholcodine 10–15mg PO q4–6h
Opioids	codeine 8–20mg PO q4–6h
	dihydrocodeine 10–15mg PO q4–6h
	hydrocodone 5–10mg PO q4–6h
	morphine 2.5–5mg PO q4–6h
Local anaesthetics	lidocaine 2%, 5ml by nebulizer q6–8h
	bupivacaine 0.25%, 5ml by nebulizer q6–8h
Other antitussives	benzonatate 100–200mg PO q8h
	levodropropizine 75mg q8h
Bronchodilators	if bronchospasm present
Antibiotics	if infection present
Corticosteroids	pulmonary metastases, lymphangitis carcinomatosis
Anticholinergics	to reduce secretions

Nebulized local anaesthetics may be of benefit in the treatment of intractable cough, although there have been no controlled studies in patients with cancer.[47, 64] Bupivacaine is preferred to lignocaine as it is not associated with a lingering bad taste. A small proportion of patients will develop bronchospasm and the first dose must be given in a situation where appropriate therapy is immediately available. Other side effects include pharyngeal numbness and loss of the gag reflex; patients should be offered a drink immediately before treatment and then made to fast for one to two hours.

Other non-opioid antitussives act on the peripheral cough receptors. Opioid-resistant cough in patients with advanced cancer has been reported to respond to benzonatate.[65] Other drugs reported to be effective are sodium cromoglycate,[66] levodropropizine [62] and baclofen.[67]

Bronchorrhoea. Bronchorrhoea is defined as the production of more than 100ml of sputum per day. It is commonly associated with bronchoalveolar carcinoma, an uncommon form of primary lung cancer, or with metastatic disease that infiltrates the respiratory mucosa. Patients suffer severe dyspnoea and cough, and may be hypoxaemic. Treatment is with antisecretory drugs (hyoscine hydrobromide, glycopyrrolate), corticosteroids (inhaled or high dose systemic therapy),[68] nebulized indomethacin,[69–71] or macrolide antibiotics (erythromycin, clarithromycin).

Cough related to oesophagorespiratory fistulas. Patients with tracheo- and broncho-oesophageal fistulas complain of paroxysmal coughing immediately after swallowing. These fistulas will not close spontaneously, even if effective radiotherapy or systemic therapy is given. Double stenting, with parallel oesophageal and tracheobronchial stents can result in good palliation of both cough and dysphagia.[72, 73]

Terminal care

The treatment of persistent cough is with an opioid drug, which has the added benefit of reducing respiratory secretions. Antibiotics and vigorous physical therapy are inappropriate. The use of sedatives may be of benefit especially at night. Haloperidol, which will dry respiratory secretions by its anticholinergic effect, is preferable to a benzodiazepine. Smoking can be discouraged but, as the respiratory benefits of stopping smoking may take a month to be manifest, forcing terminally ill patients to stop smoking may compound their misery.

Haemoptysis

Haemoptysis is the coughing or expectoration of blood from the lower respiratory tract. Massive haemoptysis is rare and most patients have blood-streaked sputum.[74]

Haemoptysis occurs commonly in patients with advanced cancer and is most frequently due to malignant infiltration or infection (Table 18.15). Haemoptysis occurs in about 40–70% of patients with primary lung cancer [7] and less frequently with pulmonary metastases from other tumours. The incidence of massive haemoptysis is increased in patients treated with large fraction brachytherapy.[22, 23]

Table 18.15 Causes of haemoptysis

Tumour	primary, metastatic
Infection	bronchitis, pneumonia
Pneumonitis	radiation, chemotherapy
Pulmonary embolism	
Cardiac failure	
Bleeding diathesis	thrombocytopenia, coagulopathy, drugs (e.g. aspirin, warfarin)
Trauma	endotracheal tube, bronchoscopy

Haemoptysis should be distinguished from gastrointestinal and nasopharyngeal bleeding. Haemoptysis is preceded by or associated with coughing; the blood is usually bright and frothy and often mixed with phlegm. Haematemesis is associated with vomiting or retching and the blood is usually darker red or brown and can be mixed with recognizable food particles. Bleeding from the nasopharynx or mouth produces bright blood, the cause of which may be visible on clinical examination.

Active management requires determination of the cause and site of bleeding, for which bronchoscopy is often necessary. Bronchoscopy and CT scanning provide complementary information.[7]

Treatment

Haemoptysis frequently provokes considerable anxiety, the fear being that massive haemorrhage may follow smaller haemoptyses. The patient and family should be reassured that massive haemoptysis is very rare, occurring in only about 3% of patients with lung cancer.

Treatment of tumour-related haemoptysis depends on the severity (Table 18.16). For patients with minor haemoptysis, the bleeding may be reduced with antitussive medication or an oral haemostatic drug. Hypofractionated external beam radiotherapy, given as one or two treatment fractions, will control haemoptysis for most patients.[24, 25] Bronchoscopic laser therapy or electrocautery are also effective.[75–77] Endoscopic radiotherapy or brachytherapy effectively controls bleeding from proximal bronchial lesions,[74, 78] although there is evidence that high dose-rate brachytherapy may be associated with an increased incidence of subsequent massive haemoptysis.[22, 23] Haemoptysis not directly related to tumour is treated appropriately.

Massive haemoptysis. Massive haemoptysis is rare, and is frequently associated with a centrally located squamous cell carcinoma that shows evidence of cavitation. It is usually a terminal event and the patient rapidly becomes unconscious as a result of hypoxia and haemorrhage. There is a brief period when patients may experience suffocation, during which time they should never be left unattended. If possible, they are treated promptly with morphine and midazolam by injection to allay anxiety and fear. If a massive haemoptysis is anticipated, morphine and midazolam should be readily available, as well as coloured towels or blankets to cover or mask the blood.

Table 18.16   Treatment options for haemoptysis related to tumour

Mild	reassure tranexamic acid 1g PO q8h *or* ethamsylate 500mg q6h antitussive drugs
Moderate or persistent	radiotherapy endobronchial radiotherapy (brachytherapy) laser coagulation
Massive	morphine and midazolam by injection

Terminal care

Haemoptysis occurring in terminally ill patients should be managed with reassurance and explanation, to both patient and family. Antibiotics are usually inappropriate. Antitussives may reduce the amount of haemoptysis. The management of massive haemorrhage is discussed above.

Pneumonia

Pneumonia occurs frequently in patients with advanced cancer and is a common terminal event.[7] The clinical features are the same as for patients without cancer. A chest x-ray will show a localized or diffuse infiltrate.

Treatment

The management of pneumonia for patients with advanced cancer must be appropriate to the stage of the disease and the prognosis from cancer. Intensive therapy is only appropriate if successful treatment of the chest infection will allow the patient to survive a significant period of time with an acceptable quality of life. Antibiotic therapy should also be considered if there are distressing symptoms (cough, pain, fever) not responding satisfactorily to symptomatic measures. Decisions have to be individualized for each patient, taking into account the wishes of the patient and the family, as well as the benefits and burdens of any anticipated treatment.[7, 79]

If considered appropriate, localized infection is treated with appropriate antimicrobial therapy together with measures to relieve bronchial obstruction (radiotherapy, endobronchial laser therapy, or brachytherapy). Physiotherapy and postural drainage are important. Mucolytic and expectorant therapy may be beneficial and are discussed in the section on Cough.

Pneumonia presenting as a diffuse infiltrate has to be distinguished from drug induced pneumonitis, miliary metastases and lymphangitis carcinomatosis. If clinically appropriate, treatment is started with broad-spectrum antibiotics, modified according to response and the results of cultures. If there is continued lack of improvement and the initial cultures have failed to identify the causative organism, bronchoscopy and bronchoalveolar lavage can be considered or antifungal therapy added empirically. In some cases, open lung biopsy may be the only means to establish the diagnosis and exclude miliary metastases or drug induced pneumonitis.

For patients with a shorter life expectancy, intensive therapy with intravenous antibiotics is usually inappropriate and oral antibiotics should be used.

Terminal care

In the last days or week of life, antibiotic therapy is usually inappropriate and is seldom effective. Dyspnoea, cough, pain and fever are treated symptomatically.

Pneumonitis

Radiation pneumonitis

Acute pneumonitis occurs in 5–15% of patients receiving radiation to the lung.[80] The incidence and severity depend on treatment factors and increase with the volume irradiated, the total dose, and the dose-rate of each fraction; for any given total dose, the toxicity is less if it is divided into more treatment fractions.[81] The incidence does not vary significantly with age, but pneumonitis is likely to be more severe in older patients. Other factors that may predispose to the development of pneumonitis include concurrent chemotherapy and the withdrawal of corticosteroids.

Symptoms of radiation pneumonitis usually occur 2 to 3 months after the completion of treatment, with a range of 1 to 6 months. The main symptom is dyspnoea, which varies from mild to severe and progressive (Table 18.17).[82, 83] There may also be a nonproductive cough. Examination reveals crepitations and rales in the affected area and there may be a pleural friction rub. Chest x-ray shows hazy shadowing or 'ground-glass' opacification in the treated area, with margins conforming to the treatment field. Respiratory function tests may show reduction in lung volumes and compliance, together with a reduction in gas transfer.

Radiation damage to normal lung tissue can result in an immunologically mediated lymphocytic alveolitis affecting non-irradiated areas. Women receiving radiotherapy to the

Table 18.17   RTOG/EORTC radiation pneumonitis grading criteria[82, 83]

Acute

0   no change
1   mild dry cough or dyspnoea on exertion
2   persistent cough requiring antitussives, dyspnoea with minimal effort
3   severe cough unresponsive to opioids, dyspnoea at rest, intermittent oxygen required
4   severe respiratory insufficiency, continuous oxygen or assisted ventilation required

Chronic

0   none
1   asymptomatic or mild symptoms (dry cough); slight x-ray changes
2   moderate symptoms pneumonitis, severe cough; patchy x-ray changes
3   severe symptoms pneumonitis; dense x-ray changes
4   severe respiratory insufficiency, continuous oxygen or assisted ventilation required

breast are reported to have developed migrating pulmonary infiltrates outside the treatment field, biopsy of which showed bronchiolitis obliterans with organising pneumonia (BOOP).[84] Bronchoalveolar lavage studies on these women showed that most had evidence of lymphocytic alveolitis affecting both lungs, although it did not correlate with the development of clinical pneumonitis.[85] This 'out of field pneumonitis' usually responds rapidly to corticosteroid therapy with no evidence of permanent damage. The optimal dose and duration of therapy is uncertain. There is a high recurrence rate when corticosteroid therapy is stopped, indicating that treatment should be withdrawn slowly.

Treatment of acute radiation pneumonitis is with prednisolone 50–100 mg/d, continued for several weeks. The dose is then cautiously reduced over a number of weeks, the rate being determined by the patient's symptoms.

Amifostine reduces the incidence and severity of radiation pneumonitis (Table 18.18).[86, 87] It should be considered for patients at increased risk of developing radiation pneumonitis.

Chronic pneumonitis. Acute pneumonitis may progress to chronic fibrosis over a period of six months to two years. The fibrosis may be asymptomatic or cause dyspnoea that may be mild or severe. Chest x-ray shows fibrotic scarring with shrinkage of the lung in the treated area. Treatment is symptomatic.

Table 18.18   Prevention of radiation pneumonitis with amifostine: RCTs

Author	n	Intervention	Outcome
Antonadou[86]	146	lung cancer 55-60Gy ± amifostine	amifostine: grade ≥2 pneumonitis 9 vs 43%, fibrosis at 6mo 28 vs 53% (both pS)
Komaki[87]	53	lung cancer 69Gy ± amifostine	amifostine: acute pneumonitis 4 vs 23% (pS)

Chemotherapy-related pneumonitis

A number of chemotherapy drugs are reported to cause pneumonitis, including several of the more recently introduced agents (Table 18.19).

Drug induced pneumonitis may occur shortly after administration or may be delayed for a few to many months. Concurrent radiation or oxygen therapy may predispose to the development of pneumonitis.

Table 18.19 Chemotherapy drugs associated with pneumonitis

Busulphan	Mitomycin	Gemcitabine[88]
Cyclophosphamide	Carmustine (BCNU)	Paclitaxel[89]
Chlorambucil	Methotrexate	Docetaxel[90, 91]
Melphalan	Cytosine arabinoside	Irinotecan[92]
Bleomycin	Procarbazine[93]	Temazolamide[94]

Chemotherapy-related pneumonitis causes dyspnoea and a nonproductive cough. The clinical features are variable, ranging from a mild and transient illness to rapidly fatal respiratory failure (Table 18.20). Pneumonitis presenting as a severe acute illness with fever may resemble widespread pneumonia. Examination reveals crepitations and rales, usually more noticeable in the lower zones. The chest x-ray shows a diffuse reticulonodular pattern. Respiratory function tests show a restrictive ventilatory defect with reduced diffusing capacity. The differentiation of drug toxicity from infection or malignant infiltration can be difficult and may require consideration of a lung biopsy.

Treatment. If drug induced pneumonitis is suspected, the offending or suspected agent is stopped. Prednisolone 50–100 mg/d is helpful in some cases. Treatment is otherwise symptomatic.

Table 18.20 NCI Common Toxicity Criteria grading of chemotherapy pneumonitis[95]

0	none
1	x-ray changes and asymptomatic or mild symptoms not requiring sterolds
2	x-ray changes and symptoms requiring steroids or diuretics
3	x-ray changes and symptoms requiring oxygen
4	x-ray changes and symptoms requiring assisted ventilation

Pulmonary embolism

Pulmonary embolism is estimated to occur in about 10% of patients with advanced cancer. A number of recent reviews of pulmonary embolism have been published.[96–98]

The clinical features of pulmonary embolism are listed in Table 18.21. The clinical manifestations depend on the size and number of emboli and the general condition and cardiorespiratory reserve of the patient. Large or multiple emboli may cause acute cardiovascular collapse and sudden death. Alternatively, a small embolus may cause only transient dyspnoea and tachypnoea without other signs. Multiple small emboli may cause progressive dyspnoea without pain, haemoptysis or chest x-ray signs and may only be diagnosed with a lung perfusion scan.

Table 18.21 Clinical features of pulmonary embolism

Dyspnoea	Tachypnoea
Cough	Tachycardia
Haemoptysis	Hypoxaemia
Pleuritic pain	Syncope

Investigation is warranted if active therapy is contemplated and in those patients with otherwise unexplained progressive dyspnoea. A chest x-ray may show a nonspecific infiltrate or a small effusion. The ECG usually shows nonspecific T-wave changes. A negative D-dimer assay is useful in excluding a diagnosis of thrombosis.[99] Perfusion lung scanning is useful if the results are normal or indicate a high probability of pulmonary embolism. Helical computed tomography and magnetic resonance pulmonary angiography will detect most emboli in the proximal pulmonary vasculature,[100–102] but pulmonary angiography is required to assess the peripheral vessels.

Treatment

The immediate treatment of pulmonary embolism includes oxygen for dyspnoea and morphine for pain and anxiety. Decisions regarding anticoagulation for patients with advanced cancer should be individualized, taking into account the potential benefits and complications as well as the stage of the patient's disease and life expectancy. (See also the section on Thrombosis in Chapter 22.)

Initial anticoagulation is with either unfractionated heparin (UH) or a low molecular weight heparin (LMWH) preparation (Table 18.22).[97, 103–105] LMWHs are given by once- or twice-daily subcutaneous injection, do not require laboratory monitoring and are well tolerated, making home therapy feasible. Whilst UH is normally given by intravenous infusion, it can be given by 8- or 12-hourly subcutaneous injection in the home setting, but still requires laboratory monitoring. Heparin prevents further thrombus formation and allows dissolution of some of the clot, and often helps resolve the acute dyspnoea and pleuritic pain. Cochrane reviews indicate that fixed-dose subcutaneous LMWH is as effective as titrated intravenous UH in the initial treatment of venous thromboembolism, is associated with less haemorrhage and recurrent thrombosis, and may be able to be given as a single daily injection.[106–108] LMWHs may be more expensive and less convenient to administer, but are significantly safer and may be more effective in the palliative care population. Initial therapy should not be with warfarin alone as it may cause a paradoxical increase in thrombotic tendency,[96] and because a significant proportion of cancer-associated thromboses are resistant to warfarin. Thrombolytic therapy is generally regarded as contraindicated in patients with advanced cancer because of the risk of major bleeding; this is further discussed in the section on Thrombosis in Chapter 22.

Table 18.22 Active management of pulmonary embolism

Initial anticoagulation	unfractionated heparin (UH) or LMWH
	not warfarin alone
	thrombolysis contraindicated
Continued anticoagulation	warfarin PO
	LMWH SC
Vena caval filters	if anticoagulation contraindicated
	anticoagulation-related bleeding
	recurrent emboli despite anticoagulation

Continued anticoagulation has traditionally been with oral warfarin for 3 to 6 months.[109, 110] However, stable anticoagulation is difficult to achieve in patients with advanced cancer because of physiological changes that occur with disease progression as well as variations in nutritional intake and other drug therapy.[111–113] Patients with cancer are two- to three-times more likely to develop recurrent thrombosis whilst on warfarin therapy compared to patients without cancer;[114–117] some of these develop because the INR is subtherapeutic, but others occur when the INR is in the therapeutic range, indicating 'warfarin resistance'. Cancer patients also have a higher incidence of bleeding,[114] and this is not confined to patients with an abnormally prolonged INR.[118]

Continued therapy with LMWH is at least as effective as warfarin in preventing recurrent thrombosis and is associated with significantly less haemorrhage.[119–121] In patients with cancer, continued therapy with LMWH avoids the difficulties and inadequacies of warfarin therapy.

For patients with advanced cancer and pulmonary embolism who are considered suitable for anticoagulation, the available evidence suggests they are best treated with LMWHs. In the acute phase, LMWHs produce results at least equivalent to standard heparin therapy, with less risk of haemorrhage, and without the need for intravenous lines and laboratory monitoring. For continued therapy, LMWHs appear to be safer and more effective than warfarin, do not require laboratory tests, and are not subject to dietary or drug interactions. The disadvantage of LMWHs is their cost.

Vena caval filters should be considered for patients with contraindications to anticoagulation, those with recurrent emboli despite anticoagulation, and patients in whom anticoagulation has to be withdrawn because of bleeding.[122–124]

Terminal care

Pulmonary embolism is a not uncommon terminal event and is managed by symptomatic treatment of pain and dyspnoea.

Pleural effusion

Almost 50% of patients with disseminated cancer develop a malignant pleural effusion.[125, 126] A number of recent reviews of the management of malignant pleural effusions have been published.[125, 127, 128]

A pleural effusion develops if the normal physiological flow of pleural fluid is disturbed by pleural inflammation (including tumour infiltration) or obstruction of the pulmonary lymphatic or venous channels. The causes are listed in Table 18.23.

Table 18.23 Pleural effusion: aetiology and fluid characteristics

	Transudate/Exudate	Cytology
Inflammation of pleural surface		
infiltration by tumour	E	+*
infection, infarction, irradiation	E	–
Lymphatic obstruction		
peripheral obstruction by tumour	T or E	+/–†
central (mediastinal) obstruction	E (chylous)	–
Raised pulmonary venous pressure		
local venous obstruction by tumour	T or E	+/–†
cardiac failure, pericardial tamponade	T	–
Other oedematous conditions		
hypoproteinaemia, renal or liver failure	T	–

*   positive fluid cytology depends on whether tumour cells are shed into the fluid
†   positive fluid cytology depends on pleural infiltration by tumour in addition to blockage of the veins or lymphatics

Pleural effusions cause dyspnoea, a nonproductive cough and chest pain that may be dull and aching or pleuritic. Dyspnoea varies from mild to severe and depends on both the size and speed of accumulation of the effusion. Small effusions and those occurring in patients who are relatively immobile are unlikely to cause significant symptoms. The characteristic physical signs of a pleural effusion include reduced chest wall expansion, dullness to percussion, reduced air entry and reduced vocal fremitus.

Assessment

Chest x-ray will confirm the presence of an effusion, which is usually unilateral in the case of malignant infiltration. A contrast-enhanced CT scan will distinguish malignant from nonmalignant effusions and will also provide more detail regarding underlying pathology, including the presence of mediastinal disease in patients with a chylous effusion.[129]

Diagnostic pleural aspiration. Malignant pleural effusions are obviously blood-stained in about 50% of cases. Cloudy or turbid fluid may be due to cells and debris or high lipid levels. If chylothorax is present, centrifugation of the fluid yields a turbid supernatant, which on biochemical analysis contains increased concentrations of lipids.

Pleural effusions are customarily classified as transudates or exudates (Table 18.23). Transudates, as occur in cardiac failure and hypoproteinaemia, have lower protein concentrations, lactate dehydrogenase (LDH) levels and blood cell counts; exudates have increased levels. An effusion is classified as an exudate if it meets one or more of the criteria shown in Table 18.24.[130] This distinction between transudate and exudate is of limited value in oncology and palliative care, as the usual diagnostic problem is differentiating between malignancy and infection, both of which produce exudates.

Table 18.24 Criteria distinguishing exudates from transudates

Ratio of pleural fluid protein level to serum protein level >0.5
Ratio of pleural fluid LDH level to serum LDH level >0.6
Pleural fluid LDH level > two-thirds the upper limit of normal for serum LDH level

Malignant cells will be identified on cytological examination in 60–90% of effusions due to pleural infiltration by tumour; the remainder are cytologically negative because cells fail to 'desquamate' from the pleural tumour. Effusions due to local venous or lymphatic obstruction will be cytologically positive if there is also pleural infiltration. Other types of effusions are cytologically negative.

If cytological examination is negative and doubt exists as to the cause of the effusion, biopsy should be considered. Blind pleural biopsy has a relatively poor yield. CT-guided biopsy is useful if there is visible pleural abnormality on scan. Thoracoscopy, which allows visualization of the pleura and direct biopsy of suspicious lesions, gives the best results.

Treatment

The treatment of pleural effusion is palliative and symptomatic. The treatment options and their relative merits are listed in Table 18.25. Selection depends on clinical circumstances and particularly on the patient's general condition and life expectancy. Patients with small or asymptomatic effusions require no therapy.

Pleural aspiration. Repeated pleural aspiration is not recommended as standard therapy as it requires multiple procedures with an increasing risk of infection, pneumothorax and

Table 18.25 Pleural effusion: treatment options

Observation (asymptomatic effusions)

Systemic therapy (sensitive tumours)

Repeated pleural aspiration (thoracocentesis)
    simple procedure
    can involve multiple/repeated procedures
    cumulative protein loss
    increasing risk of infection, pneumothorax, loculation

Pleurodesis at time of pleural aspiration
    simple procedure
    fluid drainage incomplete, lung expansion not verified
    risks creating a loculated effusion

Pleurodesis after tube drainage or at thoracoscopy
    fluid drainage complete, lung expansion verified
    highly effective
    (minor) surgical procedure, longer hospital stay

Pleurodesis at thoracotomy
    highly effective
    only if thoracotomy indicated for other reasons

Pleuroperitoneal shunt, Indwelling pleural catheter
    for recurrent or refractory effusions, 'trapped lung'
    effective, simple, inexpensive

loculation, as well as a cumulative loss of protein. It is suitable if only a limited number of procedures are likely, as with patients whose effusions reaccumulate only very slowly, the terminally ill, and those responding to systemic therapy.

Pleurodesis. The treatment of effusions that are symptomatic or have recurred following aspiration is by pleurodesis. Pleurodesis involves the introduction of a sclerosant substance to obliterate the pleural space and prevent reaccumulation. For pleurodesis to be successful, the pleural fluid should be completely drained and the underlying lung fully expanded, in order to achieve good apposition between the visceral and parietal pleura. Pleurodesis will be unsuccessful if the effusion is not completely drained or if the underlying lung fails to re-expand. Failure of the lung to re-expand occurs if there is extensive pleural tumour infiltration ('trapped lung') or if there is main stem bronchial occlusion by tumour.

Pleurodesis performed at the time of needle aspiration does not allow the adequacy of fluid drainage or lung expansion to be verified. It is less likely to be successful and often results in loculation of the effusion, making definitive therapy more complicated.

Adequate evacuation of pleural fluid can be achieved by either tube drainage or thoracoscopy. Traditionally, larger (24–32 Fr) chest tubes have been used to drain effusions and pleurodesis is performed when the drainage is less than 100–200ml/24h. Equivalent results, in terms of both fluid drainage and successful pleurodesis, have been reported with small-bore catheters (8–16 Fr).[131, 132] Patients with loculated effusions that drain poorly can be treated with intrapleural streptokinase, which is frequently successful in allowing complete drainage.[133]

Pleurodesis is performed by spraying the pleural surface with talc (talc poudrage) at thoracoscopy or by injecting a sclerosing agent (talc slurry, bleomycin or doxycycline) via the thoracostomy tube. The sclerosant is dissolved in 100ml saline and local anaesthetic should be added, particularly if talc is being used; simultaneous parenteral analgesia is recommended. After injection, it used to be customary for the patient's position to be rotated, but RCTs have shown this to be unnecessary (Table 18.26).[134, 135] The tube is left in place until the drainage is less than 100–150ml/d.

Table 18.26 Rotation of the patient after pleurodesis: RCTs

Author	n	Intervention	Outcome
Dryzer[134]	40	tetracycline pleurodesis ± 2 hours patient rotation	no effect on success rate for pleurodesis
Mager[135]	20	talc pleurodesis ± 1 hour patient rotation	no effect on talc dispersion or success rate for pleurodesis

A number of substances have been used as sclerosing agents and the three in common use are talc, bleomycin and doxycycline. Talc produces consistently higher response rates (Table 18.27), although this is not statistically significant in some studies because of their smaller size. Pleurodesis induced by talc is more durable than bleomycin or doxycycline and there are very few recurrent effusions in patients followed for six and twelve months;[136, 137] one study reported 82% of patients had life-long pleurodesis.[138] Talc can be administered by poudrage at thoracoscopy or as a slurry via a thoracostomy tube, but cannot be used if there is pleural infection. The results of the two methods of administration are comparable (Table 18.28). Common side effects of talc include pain and fever; more serious complications are uncommon and include pulmonary oedema (2%) and respiratory failure (1%).[139] Instillation of methylprednisolone has been shown in an RCT to be ineffective for treating pleural effusions.[140]

Table 18.27 Efficacy of agents used for pleurodesis: RCTs

Author	n	Successful pleurodesis
Walter-Renard[141]	424	review: talc 93%, bleomycin 54%, doxycycline 72%
Hartman[142]	124	RCT: talc 97%, bleomycin 64% (pS)
Patz[143]	106	RCT: bleomycin 72%, doxycycline 79% (pNS)
Ong[144]	38	RCT: talc 89%, bleomycin 70% (pNS)
Diacon[136]	32	RCT: talc 87%, bleomycin 59% (pS at 90d)
Zimmer[145]	33	RCT: talc 90%, bleomycin 79% (pNS)

The most effective and economic method of pleurodesis remains to be defined. Talc appears to be the superior sclerosant, although its use is associated with a very low incidence of serious side effects; it is much cheaper than bleomycin. Instillation of talc slurry is associated with less overall cost than thoracoscopic poudrage, and cost-effectiveness is one of the end-points of a current study comparing the two techniques.

Table 18.28 Talc poudrage or slurry: RCT

Author	n	Successful pleurodesis
ATS[5]	646	review: poudrage 91% (of 461), slurry 91% (of 185)
Yim[146]	57	RCT: poudrage 96%, slurry 90% (pNS)

Thoracotomy. Talc poudrage performed at thoracotomy is highly effective in preventing recurrent pleural effusions. It should be reserved for effusions that have recurred despite tube drainage and pleurodesis or if thoracotomy is performed for other indications such as an open lung biopsy or resection of a metastasis.

Pleuroperitoneal shunt. A pleuroperitoneal shunt is used when malignant infiltration prevents lung expansion after pleural aspiration ('trapped lung'), preventing pleurodesis, and for effusions that have proved refractory to thoracostomy and pleurodesis. The catheter is placed in the subcutaneous tissue and has a valved chamber that allows fluid to be manually pumped against the normal pleuroperitoneal pressure gradient. These shunts are reported to provide effective palliation, although the need for regular manual pumping may limit their usefulness.[147, 148] Catheter obstruction is reported in 12% of cases.

Indwelling pleural catheter. An indwelling pleural catheter, tunnelled in the subcutaneous tissue, can be considered for effusions refractory to pleurodesis and those associated with 'trapped lung'.[149, 150] Patients drain the effusion using vacuum bottles every other day or as needed for the relief of dyspnoea. Insertion of the pleural catheter is a relatively simple and safe outpatient procedure. An RCT comparing indwelling pleural catheters with tube thoracostomy and doxycycline pleurodesis showed comparable improvement in dyspnoea and quality of life. Recurrent effusions occurred in 21% of the doxycycline group, whilst 13% of the catheter group developed either recurrent effusion or catheter blockage.[151]

Chylous effusions. Chylous effusions are caused by disruption of the lymphatics in the mediastinum. Repeated pleural aspiration is ineffective and treatment is usually by radiotherapy to the mediastinum. Patients resistant to radiotherapy and chemotherapy may benefit from thoracoscopic talc pleurodesis.[152]

Terminal care

Pleural aspiration in the terminally ill should only be considered if drainage is likely to produce significant symptomatic improvement. For most patients, symptomatic treatment of dyspnoea, pain and cough is all that is required.

Tracheostomy

Patients with cancer of the larynx and pharynx may have a permanent tracheostomy created at the time of their initial treatment. Patients require a special programme of education including the use of humidified air to avoid dryness and crusting, use of a special protective bib when showering, and occluding the stoma to aid defaecation and micturition.

Infection of the stoma is treated with frequent local toilet and antibiotics, the appropriate drug being indicated by the results of cultures.

Stenosis occurring as a result of local trauma or previous radiotherapy can be treated by dilatation, surgical refashioning or stenting. Stenosis caused by local recurrence of tumour may be treated with stenting, local laser resection or external radiotherapy.

Hoarseness

Hoarseness may be caused by local laryngeal pathology or damage to the vagus nerve, particularly the recurrent laryngeal branch (Table 18.29). Neurological damage may be caused by surgery, cancer or radiotherapy.

Recurrent laryngeal nerve palsy causes hoarseness and the characteristic ineffectual 'bovine' cough. Because of the inability to close the cords, the cough is ineffective and does not allow the explosive expiration necessary to clear secretions.

Table 18.29 Hoarseness

Laryngeal disease	Vagus nerve
infection	cancer: intracranial, in neck
voice abuse	surgery to neck
harsh coughing	radiotherapy
radiotherapy	Recurrent laryngeal nerve
endotracheal intubation	surgery to thorax, neck
bronchoscopy	cancer

Laryngoscopy will demonstrate laryngeal disease or, with laryngeal nerve palsy, paralysis of the cord on one side. Clinical examination usually allows localization of a neurological cause: intracranial pathology will be associated with other cranial nerve lesions as well as cerebellar and long tract signs; lesions at the base of the skull cause abnormalities of the IXth, Xth and XIth cranial nerves together (jugular foramen syndrome); lesions lower in the neck and in the thorax cause only laryngeal signs and, in the absence of any palpable mass or recent surgery to the neck, the lesion is likely to be in the mediastinum.

Treatment

Laryngeal disease is treated appropriately. If feasible, nerve lesions causing vocal cord paralysis are treated with radiotherapy. Patients with troublesome symptoms due to vocal cord paralysis may be treated by injection of teflon into the affected cord. This improves both the voice and the quality of the cough, but requires a general anaesthetic.

Terminal respiratory congestion or 'Death Rattle'

'Death rattle' is the commonly used term to describe the rattling, noisy or gurgling respiration of some patients who are dying. It occurs in about 50% of patients and is caused by the accumulation of pharyngeal and pulmonary secretions in patients who are unconscious or semi-conscious and too weak to expectorate.[153, 154]

As most patients with 'death rattle' are no longer aware of their surroundings, therapy is often more for the comfort of the relatives and other patients. Relatives need to be reassured that the noisy breathing is not causing any added suffering for the patient.

Treatment

Patients should be positioned on their side and this may be all that is required. Oropharyngeal suction should be reserved for unconscious patients, as it may be distressing to the patient.

Treatment is with anticholinergic drugs to suppress the production of secretions (Table 18.30).[153, 155–159] It should be started early because it has no effect on secretions already present, but not so early that an alert patient suffers uncomfortable dryness of the mouth. It is likely to be more effective for oropharyngeal than tracheobronchial secretions. Hyoscine hydrobromide, which also has sedative and antiemetic effects, is probably the drug of choice; however, repeated injections occasionally produce paradoxical excitation. Hyoscine hydrobromide and butylbromide may be given as repeated subcutaneous injections or as a continuous infusion. Atropine may cause tachycardia after repeated injections. Transdermal scopolamine patches have the benefit of being effective for 72 hours, but the onset of action is delayed for several hours and other anticholinergic treatment needs to be given during this period.

Table 18.30 Treatment of terminal respiratory congestion

Subcutaneous	hyoscine hydrobromide	0.2–0.4mg SC q2–4h	or 0.6–1.2mg/24h CSCI
	hyoscine butylbromide	20mg SC q2–4h	or 20–60mg/24h CSCI
	glycopyrrolate	0.2–0.4mg SC q2–4h	or 0.6–1.2mg/24h CSCI
	atropine	0.4–0.8mg SC q2–4h	
Transdermal	hyoscine hydrobromide	1.5mg patch q72h	

References

1   Ginsberg, R.J., Vokes, E.E. and Rosenzweig, K. (2001). Non-small cell lung cancer. In *Cancer. Principles and Practice of Oncology. 6th edition* (ed. V.T. De Vita, S. Hellman and S.A. Rosenberg). Philadelphia, Lippincott, Williams and Wilkins.

2   Edmonds, P., et al. (2000). Is the presence of dyspnea a risk factor for morbidity in cancer patients? *Journal of Pain and Symptom Management* 19, 15–22.

3   Smith, E.L., et al. (2001). Dyspnea, anxiety, body consciousness, and quality of life in patients with lung cancer. *Journal of Pain and Symptom Management* 21, 323–9.

4   Tanaka, K., et al. (2002). Prevalence and screening of dyspnea interfering with daily life activities in ambulatory patients with advanced lung cancer. *Journal of Pain and Symptom Management* 23, 484–9.

5   American Thoracic Society (1999). Dyspnea: mechanisms, assessment, and management: a consensus statement. *American Journal of Respiratory and Critical Care Medicine* 159, 321–40.

6   Dudgeon, D.J. and Rosenthal, S. (2000). Pathophysiology and assessment of dyspnea in the patient with cancer. In *Topics in Palliative Care. Volume 4* (ed. R. Portenoy and E. Bruera). New York, Oxford University Press.

7   Ripamonti, C. and Fusco, F. (2002). Respiratory problems in advanced cancer. *Supportive Care in Cancer* 10, 204–16.

8   Bruera, E., Sweeney, C. and Ripamonti, C. (2002). Management of dyspnea. In *Principles and Practice of Palliative Care and Supportive Oncology* (ed. A.M. Berger, R.K. Portenoy and D.E. Weissman). Philadelphia, Lippincott, Williams and Wilkins.

9   Dudgeon, D.J., et al. (2001). Dyspnea in cancer patients: prevalence and associated factors. *Journal of Pain and Symptom Management* 21, 95–102.

10   Bruera, E., et al. (2000). The frequency and correlates of dyspnea in patients with advanced cancer. *Journal of Pain and Symptom Management* 19, 357–62.

11   Dudgeon, D.J., Lertzman, M. and Askew, G.R. (2001). Physiological changes and clinical correlations of dyspnea in cancer outpatients. *Journal of Pain and Symptom Management* 21, 373–9.

12   Tanaka, K., et al. (2002). Factors correlated with dyspnea in advanced lung cancer patients. Organic causes and what else? *Journal of Pain and Symptom Management* 23, 490–500.

13   Dudgeon, D.J. and Lertzman, M. (1998). Dyspnea in the advanced cancer patient. *Journal of Pain and Symptom Management* 16, 212–19.

14 Edgecombe, J., et al. (1999). Re: Dyspnea in the advanced cancer patient. *Journal of Pain and Symptom Management* 18, 313–15.

15 Heyse-Moore, L., Beynon, T. and Ross, V. (2000). Does spirometry predict dyspnoea in advanced cancer? *Palliaitive Medicine* 14, 189–95.

16 Mancini, I. and Body, J.J. (1999). Assessment of dyspnea in advanced cancer patients. *Supportive Care in Cancer* 7, 229–32.

17 Dudgeon, D.J. (2003). Multidimensional assessment of dyspnea. In *Issues in Palliative Care Research* (ed. R. Portenoy and E. Bruera). New York, Oxford University Press.

18 Booth, S. and Adams, L. (2001). The shuttle walking test: a reproducible method for evaluating the impact of shortness of breath on functional capacity in patients with advanced cancer. *Thorax* 56, 146–50.

19 Wilcock, A., et al. (1999). Reading numbers aloud: a measure of the limiting effect of breathlessness in patients with cancer. *Thorax* 54, 1099–103.

20 Corner, J. and O'Driscoll, M. (1999). Development of a breathlessness assessment guide for use in palliative care. *Palliative Medicine* 13, 375–84.

21 Seijo, L.M. and Sterman, D.H. (2001). Interventional pulmonology. *New England Journal of Medicine* 344, 740–9.

22 Hennequin, C., et al. (1998). Predictive factors for late toxicity after endobronchial brachytherapy: a multivariate analysis. *International Journal of Radiation Oncology, Biology, Physics* 42, 21–7.

23 Langendijk, J.A., et al. (1998). Massive haemoptysis after radiotherapy in inoperable non-small cell lung carcinoma: is endobronchial brachytherapy really a risk factor? *Radiotherapy and Oncology* 49, 175–83.

24 Medical Research Council Lung Cancer Working Party (1991). Inoperable non-small-cell lung cancer (NSCLC): a Medical Research Council randomised trial of palliative radiotherapy with two fractions or ten fractions. *British Journal of Cancer* 63, 265–70.

25 Medical Research Council Lung Cancer Working Party (1992). A Medical Research Council (MRC) randomised trial of palliative radiotherapy with two fractions or a single fraction in patients with inoperable non-small-cell lung cancer (NSCLC) and poor performance status. *British Journal of Cancer* 65, 934–41.

26 Macbeth, F.R., et al. (1996). Randomized trial of palliative two-fraction versus more intensive 13-fraction radiotherapy for patients with inoperable non-small cell lung cancer and good performance status. Medical Research Council Lung Cancer Working Party. *Clinical Oncology* 8, 167–75.

27 Rees, G.J., et al. (1997). Palliative radiotherapy for lung cancer: two versus five fractions. *Clinical Oncology* 9, 90–5.

28 Stout, R., et al. (2000). Clinical and quality of life outcomes in the first United Kingdom randomized trial of endobronchial brachytherapy (intraluminal radiotherapy) vs. external beam radiotherapy in the palliative treatment of inoperable non-small cell lung cancer. *Radiotherapy and Oncology* 56, 323–7.

29 Langendijk, H., et al. (2001). External irradiation versus external irradiation plus endobronchial brachytherapy in inoperable non-small cell lung cancer: a prospective randomized study. *Radiotherapy and Oncology* 58, 257–68.

30 Corner, J., et al. (1996). Non-pharmacological intervention for breathlessness in lung cancer. *Palliative Medicine* 10, 299–305.

31 Bredin, M., et al. (1999). Multicentre randomised controlled trial of nursing intervention for breathlessness in patients with lung cancer. *British Medical Journal* 318, 901–4.

32 Filshie, J., et al. (1996). Acupuncture for the relief of cancer-related breathlessness. *Palliative Medicine* 10, 145–50.

33 Pan, C.X., et al. (2000). Complementary and alternative medicine in the management of pain, dyspnea, and nausea and vomiting near the end of life. A systematic review. *Journal of Pain and Symptom Management* 20, 374–87.

34 Barnes, P.J. (2000). Chronic obstructive pulmonary disease. *New England Journal of Medicine* 343, 269–80.

35   Watanabe, S. (2000). The role of oxygen in cancer-related dyspnoea. In *Topics in Palliative Care. Volume 4* (ed. R. Portenoy and E. Bruera). New York, Oxford University Press.

36   Bruera, E., et al. (1993). Effects of oxygen on dyspnoea in hypoxaemic terminal-cancer patients. *Lancet* 342, 13–14.

37   Booth, S., et al. (1996). Does oxygen help dyspnea in patients with cancer? *American Journal of Respiratory and Critical Care Medicine* 153, 1515–18.

38   Bruera, E., Schoeller, T. and MacEachern, T. (1992). Symptomatic benefit of supplemental oxygen in hypoxemic patients with terminal cancer: the use of the N of 1 randomized controlled trial. *Journal of Pain and Symptom Management* 7, 365–8.

39   Jennings, A.L., et al. (2001). Opioids for the palliation of breathlessness in terminal illness (Cochrane Review). *Cochrane Database of Systematic Reviews* CD002066.

40   Bruera, E., et al. (1990). Effects of morphine on the dyspnea of terminal cancer patients. *Journal of Pain and Symptom Management* 5, 341–4.

41   Cohen, M.H., et al. (1991). Continuous intravenous infusion of morphine for severe dyspnea. *Southern Medical Journal* 84, 229–34.

42   Bruera, E., et al. (1993). Subcutaneous morphine for dyspnea in cancer patients. *Annals of Internal Medicine* 119, 906–7.

43   Mazzocato, C., Buclin, T. and Rapin, C.H. (1999). The effects of morphine on dyspnea and ventilatory function in elderly patients with advanced cancer: a randomized double-blind controlled trial. *Annals of Oncology* 10, 1511–14.

44   Allard, P., et al. (1999). How effective are supplementary doses of opioids for dyspnea in terminally ill cancer patients? A randomized continuous sequential clinical trial. *Journal of Pain and Symptom Management* 17, 256–65.

45   Boyd, K.J. and Kelly, M. (1997). Oral morphine as symptomatic treatment of dyspnoea in patients with advanced cancer. *Palliative Medicine* 11, 277–81.

46   Farncombe, M., Chater, S. and Gillin, A. (1994). The use of nebulized opioids for breathlessness: a chart review. *Palliative Medicine* 8, 306–12.

47   Davis, C.L. (1995). The role of nebulised drugs in palliating respiratory symptoms of malignant disease. *European Journal of Palliative Care* 2, 9–15.

48   Quelch, P.C., Faulkner, D.E. and Yun, J.W. (1997). Nebulized opioids in the treatment of dyspnea. *Journal of Palliative Care* 13, 48–52.

49   Zeppetella, G. (1997). Nebulized morphine in the palliation of dyspnoea. *Palliative Medicine* 11, 267–75.

50   Tanaka, K., et al. (1999). Effect of nebulized morphine in cancer patients with dyspnea: a pilot study. *Japanese Journal of Clinical Oncology* 29, 600–3.

51   Davis, C.L., et al. (1996). Single dose randomised controlled triall of nebulised morphine in patients with cancer related breathlessness. *Palliative Medicine* 10, 64–5.

52   Jennings, A.L., et al. (2002). A systematic review of the use of opioids in the management of dyspnoea. *Thorax* 57, 939–44.

53   Coyne, P.J., Viswanathan, R. and Smith, T.J. (2002). Nebulized fentanyl citrate improves patients' perception of breathing, respiratory rate, and oxygen saturation in dyspnea. *Journal of Pain and Symptom Management* 23, 157–60.

54   Quigley, C., et al. (2002). A phase I/II study of nebulized morphine-6-glucuronide in patients with cancer-related breathlessness. *Journal of Pain and Symptom Management* 23, 7–9.

55   Lang, E. and Jedeikin, R. (1998). Acute respiratory depression as a complication of nebulised morphine. *Canadian Journal of Anaesthesia* 45, 60–2.

56   Shimoyama, N. and Shimoyama, M. (2002). Nebulized furosemide as a novel treatment for dyspnea in terminal cancer patients. *Journal of Pain and Symptom Management* 23, 73–6.

57   Wilcock, A., Corcoran, R. and Tattersfield, A.E. (1994). Safety and efficacy of nebulized lignocaine in patients with cancer and breathlessness. *Palliative Medicine* 8, 35–8.

58   Cowcher, K. and Hanks, G.W. (1990). Long-term management of respiratory symptoms in advanced cancer. *Journal of Pain and Symptom Management* 5, 320–30.

59 Irwin, R.S. and Madison, J.M. (2000). The diagnosis and treatment of cough. *New England Journal of Medicine* 343, 1715–21.

60 Irwin, R.S., et al. (1998). Manging cough as a defense mechanism and as a symptom. A consensus panel report of the American College of Chest Physicians. *Chest* 114, 133s–81s.

61 Eisbruch, A., et al. (2002). Objective assessment of swallowing dysfunction and aspiration after radiation concurrent with chemotherapy for head-and-neck cancer. *International Journal of Radiation Oncology, Biology and Physics* 53, 23–8.

62 Luporini, G., et al. (1998). Efficacy and safety of levodropropizine and dihydrocodeine on non-productive cough in primary and metastatic lung cancer. *European Respiratory Journal* 12, 97–101.

63 Homsi, J., Walsh, D. and Nelson, K.A. (2001). Important drugs for cough in advanced cancer. *Supportive Care in Cancer* 9, 565–74.

64 Udezue, E. (2001). Lidocaine inhalation for cough suppression. *American Journal of Emergency Medicine* 19, 206–7.

65 Doona, M. and Walsh, D. (1998). Benzonatate for opioid-resistant cough in advanced cancer. *Palliative Medicine* 12, 55–8.

66 Moroni, M., et al. (1996). Inhaled sodium cromoglycate to treat cough in advanced lung cancer patients. *British Journal of Cancer* 74, 309–11.

67 Dicpinigaitis, P.V. and Rauf, K. (1998). Treatment of chronic, refractory cough with baclofen. *Respiration* 65, 86–8.

68 Nakajima, T., et al. (2002). Treatment of bronchorrhea by corticosteroids in a case of bronchioloalveolar carcinoma producing CA19–9. *Internal Medicine* 41, 225–8.

69 Homma, S., et al. (1999). Successful treatment of refractory bronchorrhea by inhaled indomethacin in two patients with bronchioloalveolar carcinoma. *Chest* 115, 1465–8.

70 Tamaoki, J., et al. (2000). Inhaled indomethacin in bronchorrhea in bronchioloalveolar carcinoma: role of cyclooxygenase. *Chest* 117, 1213–14.

71 Hiratsuka, T., et al. (1998). [Severe bronchorrhea accompanying alveolar cell carcinoma: treatment with clarithromycin and inhaled beclomethasone (English abstract only)]. *Nihon Kokyuki Gakkai Zasshi* 36, 482–7.

72 van den Bongard, H.J., et al. (2002). The role of parallel stent insertion in patients with esophagorespiratory fistulas. *Gastrointestinal Endoscopy* 55, 110–15.

73 Yamamoto, R., et al. (2002). Double stent for malignant combined esophago-airway lesions. *Japanese Journal of Thoracic and Cardiovascular Surgery* 50, 1–5.

74 Lipchik, R.J. (2002). Hemoptysis. In *Principles and Practice of Palliative Care and Supportive Oncology* (ed. A.M. Berger, R.K. Portenoy and D.E. Weissman). Philadelphia, Lippincott, Williams and Wilkins.

75 Lee, P., Kupeli, E. and Mehta, A.C. (2002). Therapeutic bronchoscopy in lung cancer. Laser therapy, electrocautery, brachytherapy, stents, and photodynamic therapy. *Clinics in Chest Medicine* 23, 241–56.

76 Morice, R.C., et al. (2001). Endobronchial argon plasma coagulation for treatment of hemoptysis and neoplastic airway obstruction. *Chest* 119, 781–7.

77 Sheski, F.D. and Mathur, P.N. (1999). Cryotherapy, electrocautery, and brachytherapy. *Clinics in Chest Medicine* 20, 123–38.

78 Muto, P., et al. (2000). High-dose rate brachytherapy of bronchial cancer: treatment optimization using three schemes of therapy. *Oncologist* 5, 209–14.

79 Pereira, J., Watanabe, S. and Wolch, G. (1998). A retrospective review of the frequency of infections and patterns of antibiotic utilization on a palliative care unit. *Journal of Pain and Symptom Management* 16, 374–81.

80 Stover, D.E. and Kaner, R.J. (2001). Pulmonary toxicity. In *Cancer. Principles and Practice of Oncology. 6th edition* (ed. V.T. De Vita, S. Hellman and S.A. Rosenberg). Philadelphia, Lippincott, Williams and Wilkins.

81 Hernando, M.L., et al. (2001). Radiation-induced pulmonary toxicity: a dose-volume histogram analysis in 201 patients with lung cancer. *International Journal of Radiation Oncology, Biology, Physics* 51, 650–9.

82 Radiation Therapy Oncology Group (RTOG) (2000). Acute Radiation Morbidity Scoring Criteria. <www.rtog.org/members/toxicity/acute.html>

83 Radiation Therapy Oncology Group (RTOG)/European Organisation for Research and Treatment of Cancer (EORTC) (2000). RTOG/EORTC Late Radiation Morbidity Scoring Schema. <www.rtog.org/members/toxicity/late.html>

84 Arbetter, K.R., et al. (1999). Radiation-induced pneumonitis in the 'nonirradiated' lung. *Mayo Clinic Proceedings* 74, 27–36.

85 Martin, C., et al. (1999). Bilateral lymphocytic alveolitis: a common reaction after unilateral thoracic irradiation. *European Respiratory Journal* 13, 727–32.

86 Antonadou, D., et al. (2001). Randomized phase III trial of radiation treatment +/– amifostine in patients with advanced-stage lung cancer. *International Journal of Radiation Oncology, Biology, Physics* 51, 915–22.

87 Komaki, R., et al. (2002). Randomized phase III study of chemoradiation with or without amifostine for patients with favorable performance status inoperable stage II-III non-small cell lung cancer: preliminary results. *Seminars in Radiation Oncology* 12, 46–9.

88 Vander Els, N.J. and Miller, V. (1998). Successful treatment of gemcitabine toxicity with a brief course of oral corticosteroid therapy. *Chest* 114, 1779–81.

89 Ramanathan, R.K., et al. (1996). Pulmonary infiltrates following administration of paclitaxel. *Chest* 110, 289–92.

90 Wang, G.S., Yang, K.Y. and Perng, R.P. (2001). Life-threatening hypersensitivity pneumonitis induced by docetaxel (taxotere). *British Journal of Cancer* 85, 1247–50.

91 Read, W.L., Mortimer, J.E. and Picus, J. (2002). Severe interstitial pneumonitis associated with docetaxel administration. *Cancer* 94, 847–53.

92 Madarnas, Y., et al. (2000). Irinotecan-associated pulmonary toxicity. *Anticancer Drugs* 11, 709–13.

93 Mahmood, T. and Mudad, R. (2002). Pulmonary toxicity secondary to procarbazine. *American Journal of Clinical Oncology* 25, 187–8.

94 Abrey, L.E., et al. (2001). A phase II trial of temozolomide for patients with recurrent or progressive brain metastases. *Journal of Neurooncology* 53, 259–65.

95 National Cancer Institute Cancer Therapy Evaluation Program (1998). Common Toxicity Criteria, version 2.0. <http://ctep.cancer.gov/reporting/ctc.html>

96 Goldhaber, S.Z. (1998). Pulmonary embolism. *New England Journal of Medicine* 339, 93–104.

97 Hyers, T.M., et al. (2001). Antithrombotic therapy for venous thromboembolic disease. *Chest* 119, 176S–93S.

98 Levine, M.N. (2001). Management of thromboembolic disease in cancer patients. *Haemostasis* 31, 68–9.

99 ten Wolde, M., et al. (2002). The clinical usefulness of D-dimer testing in cancer patients with suspected deep venous thrombosis. *Archives of Internal Medicine* 162, 1880–4.

100 Meaney, J.F., et al. (1997). Diagnosis of pulmonary embolism with magnetic resonance angiography. *New England Journal of Medicine* 336, 1422–7.

101 Bates, S.M. and Ginsberg, J.S. (2000). Helical computed tomography and the diagnosis of pulmonary embolism. *Annals of Internal Medicine* 132, 240–2.

102 Oudkerk, M., et al. (2002). Comparison of contrast-enhanced magnetic resonance angiography and conventional pulmonary angiography for the diagnosis of pulmonary embolism: a prospective study. *Lancet* 359, 1643–7.

103 Weitz, J.I. (1997). Low-molecular-weight heparins. *New England Journal of Medicine* 337, 688–98.

104 Breddin, H.K., et al. (2001). Effects of a low-molecular-weight heparin on thrombus regression and recurrent thromboembolism in patients with deep-vein thrombosis. *New England Journal of Medicine* 344, 626–31.

105 Hirsh, J., et al. (2001). Heparin and low-molecular-weight heparin: mechanisms of action, pharmacokinetics, dosing, monitoring, efficacy, and safety. *Chest* 119, 64S–94S.

106 Siragusa, S., et al. (1996). Low-molecular-weight heparins and unfractionated heparin in the treatment of patients with acute venous thromboembolism: results of a meta-analysis. *American Journal of Medicine* 100, 269–77.

107 van Den Belt, A.G., et al. (2000). Fixed dose subcutaneous low molecular weight heparins versus adjusted dose unfractionated heparin for venous thromboembolism (Cochrane Review). *Cochrane Database of Systematic Reviews* CD001100.

108 van Dongen, C.J., Mac Gillavry, M.R. and Prins, M.H. (2003). Once versus twice daily LMWH for the initial treatment of venous thromboembolism (Cochrane Review). *Cochrane Database of Systematic Reviews* CD003074.

109 Gage, B.F., Fihn, S.D. and White, R.H. (2000). Management and dosing of warfarin therapy. *American Journal of Medicine* 109, 481–8.

110 Ansell, J., et al. (2001). Managing oral anticoagulant therapy. *Chest* 119, 22S–38S.

111 Johnson, M.J. (1997). Problems of anticoagulation within a palliative care setting: an audit of hospice patients taking warfarin. *Palliative Medicine* 11, 306–12.

112 Johnson, M.J. and Sherry, K. (1997). How do palliative physicians manage venous thromboembolism? *Palliative Medicine* 11, 462–8.

113 Bauer, K.A. (2000). Venous thromboembolism in malignancy. *Journal of Clinical Oncology* 18, 3065–7.

114 Hutten, B.A., et al. (2000). Incidence of recurrent thromboembolic and bleeding complications among patients with venous thromboembolism in relation to both malignancy and achieved international normalized ratio: a retrospective analysis. *Journal of Clinical Oncology* 18, 3078–83.

115 Douketis, J.D., et al. (2000). Clinical risk factors and timing of recurrent venous thromboembolism during the initial 3 months of anticoagulant therapy. *Archives of Internal Medicine* 160, 3431–6.

116 Luk, C., et al. (2001). Extended outpatient therapy with low molecular weight heparin for the treatment of recurrent venous thromboembolism despite warfarin therapy. *American Journal of Medicine* 111, 270–3.

117 Rickles, F.R. and Levine, M.N. (2001). Epidemiology of thrombosis in cancer. *Acta Haematologica* 106, 6–12.

118 Palareti, G., et al. (2000). A comparison of the safety and efficacy of oral anticoagulation for the treatment of venous thromboembolic disease in patients with or without malignancy. *Thrombosis and Haemostasis* 84, 805–10.

119 Gonzalez-Fajardo, J.A., et al. (1999). Venographic comparison of subcutaneous low-molecular weight heparin with oral anticoagulant therapy in the long-term treatment of deep venous thrombosis. *Journal of Vascular Surgery* 30, 283–92.

120 Lopaciuk, S., et al. (1999). Low molecular weight heparin versus acenocoumarol in the secondary prophylaxis of deep vein thrombosis. *Thrombosis and Haemostasis* 81, 26–31.

121 Meyer, G., et al. (2002). Comparison of low-molecular-weight heparin and warfarin for the secondary prevention of venous thromboembolism in patients with cancer: a randomized controlled study. *Archives of Internal Medicine* 162, 1729–35.

122 Schwarz, R.E., et al. (1996). Inferior vena cava filters in cancer patients: indications and outcome. *Journal of Clinical Oncology* 14, 652–7.

123 Jarrett, B.P., Dougherty, M.J. and Calligaro, K.D. (2002). Inferior vena cava filters in malignant disease. *Journal of Vascular Surgery* 36, 704–7.

124 Marcy, P.Y., et al. (2002). Cost-benefit assessment of inferior vena cava filter placement in advanced cancer patients. *Supportive Care in Cancer* 10, 76–80.

125 Schrump, D.S. and Nguyen, D.M. (2001). Malignant pleural and pericardial effusions. In *Cancer. Principles and Practice of Oncology. 6th edition* (ed. V.T. De Vita, S. Hellman and S.A. Rosenberg). Philadelphia, Lippincott, Williams and Wilkins.

126 Ruckdeschel, J.C. and Robinson, L.A. (2002). Management of pleural and pericardial effusions. In *Principles and Practice of Palliative Care and Supportive Oncology* (ed. A.M. Berger, R.K. Portenoy and D.E. Weissman). Philadelphia, Lippincott, Williams and Wilkins.

127 American Thoracic Society (2000). Management of malignant pleural effusions. *American Journal of Respiratory and Critical Care Medicine* 162, 1987–2001.

128 Antunes, G. and Neville, E. (2000). Management of malignant pleural effusions. *Thorax* 55, 981–3.

129 Traill, Z.C., Davies, R.J. and Gleeson, F.V. (2001). Thoracic computed tomography in patients with suspected malignant pleural effusions. *Clinical Radiology* 56, 193–6.

130 Light, R.W. (2002). Clinical practice. Pleural effusion. *New England Journal of Medicine* 346, 1971–7.

131 Parulekar, W., et al. (2001). Use of small-bore vs large-bore chest tubes for treatment of malignant pleural effusions. *Chest* 120, 19–25.

132 Chen, Y.M., et al. (2000). Usefulness of pig-tail catheter for palliative drainage of malignant pleural effusions in cancer patients. *Supportive Care in Cancer* 8, 423–6.

133 Davies, C.W., et al. (1999). Intrapleural streptokinase in the management of malignant multiloculated pleural effusions. *Chest* 115, 729–33.

134 Dryzer, S.R., et al. (1993). A comparison of rotation and nonrotation in tetracycline pleurodesis. *Chest* 104, 1763–6.

135 Mager, H.J., et al. (2002). Distribution of talc suspension during treatment of malignant pleural effusion with talc pleurodesis. *Lung Cancer* 36, 77–81.

136 Diacon, A.H., et al. (2000). Prospective randomized comparison of thoracoscopic talc poudrage under local anesthesia versus bleomycin instillation for pleurodesis in malignant pleural effusions. *American Journal of Respiratory and Critical Care Medicine* 162, 1445–9.

137 Prevost, A., et al. (2001). Long-term effect and tolerance of talc slurry for control of malignant pleural effusions. *Oncology Reports* 8, 1327–31.

138 Viallat, J.R., et al. (1996). Thoracoscopic talc poudrage pleurodesis for malignant effusions. A review of 360 cases. *Chest* 110, 1387–93.

139 de Campos, J.R., et al. (2001). Thoracoscopy talc poudrage : a 15-year experience. *Chest* 119, 801–6.

140 North, S.A., et al. (2003). A randomized, phase III, double-blind, placebo-controlled trial of intrapleural instillation of methylprednisolone acetate in the management of malignant pleural effusion. *Chest* 123, 822–7.

141 Walker-Renard, P.B., Vaughan, L.M. and Sahn, S.A. (1994). Chemical pleurodesis for malignant pleural effusions. *Annals of Internal Medicine* 120, 56–64.

142 Hartman, D.L., et al. (1993). Comparison of insufflated talc under thoracoscopic guidance with standard tetracycline and bleomycin pleurodesis for control of malignant pleural effusions. *Journal of Thoracic and Cardiovascular Surgery* 105, 743–7.

143 Patz, E.F., Jr., et al. (1998). Sclerotherapy for malignant pleural effusions: a prospective randomized trial of bleomycin vs doxycycline with small-bore catheter drainage. *Chest* 113, 1305–11.

144 Ong, K.C., et al. (2000). A comparative study of pleurodesis using talc slurry and bleomycin in the management of malignant pleural effusions. *Respirology* 5, 99–103.

145 Zimmer, P.W., et al. (1997). Prospective randomized trial of talc slurry vs bleomycin in pleurodesis for symptomatic malignant pleural effusions. *Chest* 112, 430–4.

146 Yim, A.P., et al. (1996). Thoracoscopic talc insufflation versus talc slurry for symptomatic malignant pleural effusion. *Annals of Thoracic Surgery* 62, 1655–8.

147 Petrou, M., Kaplan, D. and Goldstraw, P. (1995). Management of recurrent malignant pleural effusions. The complementary role talc pleurodesis and pleuroperitoneal shunting. *Cancer* 75, 801–5.

148 Genc, O., et al. (2000). The long-term morbidity of pleuroperitoneal shunts in the management of recurrent malignant effusions. *European Journal of Cardiothoracic Surgery* 18, 143–6.

149 Pien, G.W., et al. (2001). Use of an implantable pleural catheter for trapped lung syndrome in patients with malignant pleural effusion. *Chest* 119, 1641–6.

150 Pollak, J.S., et al. (2001). Treatment of malignant pleural effusions with tunneled long-term drainage catheters. *Journal of Vascular and Interventional Radiology* 12, 201–8.

151 Putnam, J.B., Jr., et al. (1999). A randomized comparison of indwelling pleural catheter and doxycycline pleurodesis in the management of malignant pleural effusions. *Cancer* 86, 1992–9.

152 Mares, D.C. and Mathur, P.N. (1998). Medical thoracoscopic talc pleurodesis for chylothorax due to lymphoma: a case series. *Chest* 114, 731–5.

153 Bennett, M.I. (1996). Death rattle: an audit of hyoscine (scopolamine) use and review of management. *Journal of Pain and Symptom Management* 12, 229–33.

154 Watts, T., Jenkins, K. and Back, I. (1997). Problem and management of noisy rattling breathing in dying patients. *International Journal of Palliative Nursing* 3, 245–52.

155 Hughes, A., Wilcock, A. and Corcoran, R. (1997). Management of 'death rattle'. *Palliative Medicine* 11, 80–1.

156 Hughes, A., et al. (2000). Audit of three antimuscarinic drugs for managing retained secretions. *Palliative Medicine* 14, 221–2.

157 Back, I.N., et al. (2001). A study comparing hyoscine hydrobromide and glycopyrrolate in the treatment of death rattle. *Palliative Medicine* 15, 329–36.

158 Bennett, M., et al. (2002). Using anti-muscarinic drugs in the management of death rattle: evidence-based guidelines for palliative care. *Palliative Medicine* 16, 369–74.

159 Wildiers, H. and Menten, J. (2002). Death rattle: prevalence, prevention and treatment. *Journal of Pain and Symptom Management* 23, 310–17.

19

Gastrointestinal

Xerostomia	Faecal incontinence
Stomatitis	Perianal and vulval pruritus
Nausea and vomiting	Flatulence
Hiccups	Stomas
Dysphagia	Fistulas
Oesophagitis	Lower GI bleeding
Upper GI bleeding	Ascites
Indigestion	Liver metastases
Bowel obstruction	Hepatic failure, encephalopathy
Constipation	Biliary tract obstruction
Diarrhoea	

Xerostomia (dry mouth)

Xerostomia or dryness of the mouth is reported in 75–90% of patients with advanced cancer and may be associated with significant distress.[1, 2] A number of recent reviews of xerostomia have been published.[3–7]

Table 19.1   Causes of xerostomia

Decreased production of saliva	Extensive mucosal damage
dehydration	erosion
salivary gland disorder	infiltration
radiotherapy	infection
radical surgery	radiotherapy
malignant infiltration	neutropenic mucositis
sialadenitis	Increased evaporation
infective, obstructive	mouth breathing
xerostomia of age	hyperventilation
anxiety	smoking
drugs	dry atmosphere
diuretics, anticholinergics, opioids	oxygen therapy
tranquillizers, antidepressants	

Xerostomia results from decreased production of saliva, widespread damage to the buccal mucosa, or excessive evaporation of saliva from the mouth (Table 19.1). The most frequent cause of xerostomia in palliative care is drug therapy; severe xerostomia is usually due to irradiation of the salivary glands. Lack of saliva impairs stimulation of taste receptors that are responsible for reflex salivation, and there may be diminished or no response to visual or olfactory stimuli. Some xerostomia occurs with increasing age and older patients are more likely to suffer from dryness of the mouth from any cause.

Xerostomia causes discomfort and predisposes to a number of consequences including depression (Table 19.2). Examination shows a dry smooth mucosa with only a small amount of ropy or tenacious saliva. The tongue is smooth and red and the lips are dry and cracked. Secondary infection, particularly with candida, is common. Palpation of the salivary glands will be painful if there is sialadenitis. After radiotherapy the saliva is more viscous and a less efficient lubricant, and reduction of the normally alkaline pH predisposes to stomatitis and dental caries. Xerostomia is associated with significant psychosocial effects that may lead to feelings of isolation.[8]

Table 19.2   Consequences of xerostomia

Discomfort and pain
Thirst
Alteration of taste

Difficulty chewing, swallowing, talking, retaining dentures
    poor nutrition
    inability to take medications
    psychosocial effects

Infection: stomatitis, sialadenitis
Dental caries
Halitosis

Xerostomia related to radiotherapy may be graded according to the RTOG/EORTC criteria (Table 19.3).[9] A Xerostomia Inventory (XI) has been developed and validated for use in clinical studies.[10]

Table 19.3   RTOG/EORTC grading of salivary gland dysfunction caused by radiotherapy[9]

0	none
1	slight dryness of mouth; good response to stimulation
2	moderate dryness of mouth; poor response to stimulation
3	complete dryness of mouth; no response to stimulation
4	salivary gland fibrosis

Treatment

Preventive. The incidence and severity of radiation-induced xerostomia is related to the radiation dose to the salivary glands, and can be reduced using intensity-modulated radiation therapy.[11] Use of the cytoprotective agent, amifostine, reduces the incidence of xerostomia in patients with head and neck cancer treated with radiotherapy (Table19.4).[12] It is given by intravenous or subcutaneous injection immediately before each radiation treatment.[13] Adverse effects are uncommon and include nausea and vomiting, transient mild hypotension, and allergic reactions.[14] There is a single report of life-threatening anaphylaxis with amifostine.[15] Administration of pilocarpine during radiotherapy does not influence the incidence of xerostomia.[16]

Table 19.4 Prevention of xerostomia by amifostine: RCTs

Author	n	Intervention	Outcome
Buntzel[17]	39	Radiation + chemotherapy ± amifostine	Amifostine: grade 2 xerostomia at 12 mo: 17 vs 55% (pS)
Brizel[14]	315	Radiation ± amifostine	Amifostine: grade ≥2 xerostomia at 12 mo: 34 vs 57% (pS)
Antonadou[18]	50	Radiation + chemotherapy ± amifostine	Amifostine: grade 2 xerostomia at 18 mo: 4.5 vs 30% (pS)

Symptomatic. The treatment of xerostomia includes avoidance of any causative or aggravating factors, attention to oral hygiene, and various means of stimulating salivary flow (Table 19.5). The patient's drug therapy should be reviewed. Regular mouthwashing is encouraged to keep the mucosa moist and reduce the incidence of stomatitis; commercially available mouthwashes that contain alcohol are avoided as they may have a drying effect. Patients are advised to use fluoride toothpaste and to apply fluoride gel regularly.[4] Food should be soft, moist and appetizing. Dietary salivary stimulants may be helpful. Commercially available salivary substitutes, moisturising agents and chewing gum have been shown to reduce dryness and improve eating and swallowing.[19-22] Salivary substitutes contain a lubricant (such as mucin or carboxymethyl cellulose), sugar (sorbitol, xylitol), ions to preserve tooth mineralization, flavouring and preservatives.

Table 19.5 Treatment of xerostomia

Treat or avoid aggravating factors
    drugs, dehydration, dry atmosphere, smoking, anxiety

Oral hygiene
    mouth washing, lip care, dental hygiene, denture care
    fluoride gels

Frequent fluids

Dietary advice
    soft moist foods, appetizing (visually appealing), nutritionally adequate

Artificial saliva, moisturizing agents

Stimulation of saliva
    dietary: sucking ice cubes, frozen tonic water, citrus drinks, pineapple, ascorbic acid lozenges, sugarless gum, slowly dissolving sweets
    sialogogues: pilocarpine 5mg PO q8h, bethanechol 10mg PO q8h
    acupuncture

Salivary stimulants. RCTs (Table 19.6) and a prospective study [23] have shown that pilocarpine improves symptoms and salivary flow in patients with radiation-induced xerostomia.[24, 25] Continued use is reported to be effective and safe.[26] The increased salivary flow is attributed to stimulation of the mucosal and minor salivary glands and not the parotids.[23, 27] Adverse effects including sweating, urinary frequency and intestinal colic are described as mild, although up to one-quarter of patients withdrew from therapy in some studies. Pilocarpine is contraindicated in patients with narrow-angle glaucoma or uncontrolled asthma and chronic obstructive lung disease; it should be used with caution in patients with intestinal or urinary obstruction. The optimal dose is 5mg three times a day; a few patients may benefit from a higher dose. Pilocarpine may also be of benefit in patients with xerostomia due to causes other than radiation, including opioid drugs.[28, 29]

Acupuncture is reported to benefit some patients with xerostomia, including those resistant to pilocarpine.[30, 31]

Table 19.6 Pilocarpine for postirradiation xerostomia: RCTs

Author	n	Intervention	Outcome for pilocarpine
Johnson[32]	207	pilocarpine 5 or 10mg tds vs placebo	increased salivary flow (pS); improved symptoms (pS)
LeVeque[33]	162	pilocarpine 2.5, 5 or 10mg tds vs placebo	increased salivary flow (pS) for >2.5mg; improved symptoms (pS) for >2.5mg
Davies[34]	20	pilocarpine 5mg tds mouthwash vs placebo	improved symptoms (pS)
Rieke[35]	162	pilocarpine 2.5, 5, or 10mg (dose titration) vs placebo	increased salivary flow (pS); improved symptoms (pS)
Rieke[35]	207	pilocarpine 5 or 10mg tds (fixed dose) vs placebo	increased salivary flow (pS); improved symptoms (pS)
Hamlar[36]	40	pilocarpine pastille vs placebo	improved symptoms (pS); no increased salivary flow

Terminal care

Mouth care is important during the terminal phase. Keeping the oral mucosa moist and clean will relieve discomfort, prevent stomatitis, and overcome any sensation of thirst caused by dehydration. This can be achieved by regular mouthwashes and the use of sprays or atomizers.

Stomatitis

Stomatitis is inflammation, infection or ulceration of the mouth. It is frequently due to a combination of causes (Table 19.7). A number of recent reviews of stomatitis have been published.[4–6]

The main symptom of stomatitis is pain (Table 19.8). If severe, it may prevent eating, drinking and taking oral medications. In immunosuppressed patients, stomatitis may be the focus for the development of systemic infection. Patients with severe stomatitis may become withdrawn and depressed.[37]

Table 19.7 Stomatitis: causative and predisposing factors

Chemotherapy	direct mucosal damage, neutropenic mucositis, neutropenic sepsis
Radiotherapy	direct mucosal damage, xerostomia
Xerostomia	diminished amount of less alkaline saliva
Poor oral hygiene	gingivitis, dental caries, poorly fitting dentures
Malnutrition	thin atrophic mucous membranes
Infection	fungal, viral, bacterial, aphthous ulcers
Drugs	steroids, antibiotics predispose to fungal infection
Allogeneic BMT	chronic GVH disease

Table 19.8 Consequences of stomatitis

Pain	Bleeding
Inanition, dehydration, malnourishment	Loss of taste
Inability to take oral medications	Halitosis
Systemic infection	Depression

Examination shows varying degrees of erythema, excoriation, ulceration and mucosal bleeding (Table 19.9). Fungal, viral or bacterial infection may be present although it may be difficult to distinguish between them and appropriate microbiological studies should be performed. Infection with candida typically manifests as small white plaques on inflamed mucosa and in severe cases the tongue is coated. Candidiasis may also present as diffuse erythema of the mucosa or angular stomatitis, without any white patches. Bacterial stomatitis, often caused by gram-negative organisms, produces localized grey or brown lesions with pseudomembrane formation. Stomatitis due to herpes simplex is extremely painful and causes varying degrees of vesiculation and ulceration with a yellowish pseudomembrane; vesiculation may be seen on the lips and perioral area. The grading system for therapy-related stomatitis is shown in Table 19.9.[38]

Table 19.9 NCI Common Toxicity Criteria grading of therapy-related stomatitis[38]

Chemotherapy

0	none
1	painless ulcers, erythema, or mild soreness in the absence of lesions
2	painful erythema, oedema, or ulcers, but can eat or swallow
3	painful erythema, oedema, or ulcers requiring iv hydration
4	severe ulceration or requires parenteral or enteral nutritional support

Radiotherapy

0	none
1	erythema of the mucosa
2	patchy pseudomembranous reaction: patches ≤1.5cm in diameter and non-contiguous
3	confluent pseudomembranous reaction: contiguous patches >1.5cm in diameter
4	necrosis or deep ulceration; may include bleeding not induced by minor trauma

Treatment

All patients with advanced cancer, particularly those receiving chemotherapy or radiotherapy, require a program of regular mouth care to prevent stomatitis (Table 19.10). The mainstay of therapy is regular mouth washing to clean away debris and to keep the mucous membranes moist. Normal saline mouthwash can be made by adding a teaspoon of salt to a litre of warm water; an alternative is a saline and soda solution made by adding one teaspoon each of salt and sodium bicarbonate to a litre of water. Commercial mouthwashes containing alcohol or phenol should be avoided as they may cause pain and further damage.

Table 19.10 Preventive mouth care

Examination	pretreatment dental examination
Observation	regular program of daily inspection
Regular washing	saline, saline/soda, or commercial mouthwash
Dental hygiene	regular brushing with soft brush
Denture care	dentures cleaned after each meal, stored overnight in weak antiseptic
Lip care	vaseline, petroleum jelly
Dietary advice	avoidance of very hot or very hard food

Preventive. A considerable number of different agents have been employed to prevent or ameliorate the mucositis and stomatitis caused by radiation and chemotherapy (Table 19.11).[4, 5, 39] Details of the RCTs of more recently introduced treatments are shown in Table 19.12.

A variety of antimicrobial therapies have been advocated to prevent mucositis. There have been a number of RCTs of topical chlorhexidine therapy, most of which showed no benefit for patients treated with either radiation or chemotherapy.[40, 41] Povidone-iodine mouthwash was shown to reduce mucositis for patients receiving chemoradiotheapy.[42] An antibiotic lozenge containing polymyxin, tobramycin and amphotericin was reported to be

Table 19.11 Prevention of treatment-related mucositis: RCTs

	Effective	Not effective
Antimicrobials	povidone-iodine[42] polymyxin/tobramycin/amphotericin[44-46] bacitracin/clotrimazole/gentamicin[47]	chlorhexidene[40, 41]
Cytoprotectants	amifostine (see Table 19.12)	sucralfate[50, 51]
Growth factors	G-CSF, GM-CSF (SC) (see Table 19.12)	GM-CSF (MW)[52, 53]
NSAID	benzydamine[54]	
Miscellaneous	cryotherapy[55, 56] laser therapy (see Table 19.12) glutamine[59] melatonin[61] homeopathic Traumeel S[60]	prostaglandin E[62] pilocarpine[16] allopurinol[63] silver nitrate[66] chamomile[64]

of benefit for patients treated with radiation in most trials.[43–46] A similar antibiotic lozenge containing bacitracin, clotrimazole and gentamicin did not reduce the incidence of radiation-related mucositis.[47]

The antioxidants azelasine [48] and β-carotene [49] are reported to reduce the incidence of mucositis. The cytoprotective agent, amifostine, has been shown to reduce the incidence and severity of mucositis associated with both radiation and chemotherapy (Table19.12). Prophylactic use of sucralfate did not reduce the incidence of mucositis for patients treated with either chemotherapy or radiation.[50, 51]

Treatment with the haematopoietic growth factors G-CSF (granulocyte colony stimulating factor) and GM-CSF (granulocyte-macrophage colony stimulating factor), given subcutaneously, reduced the incidence of mucositis in most studies of chemotherapy, but not radiotherapy (Table19.12). This difference may relate to the greater incidence of neutropenia after

Table 19.12 Therapy to prevent treatment-related mucositis: selected RCTs

Author	n	Intervention	Outcome
Growth factors			
Pettengell[67]	80	chemotherapy ± G-CSF	no differences
Chi[68]	20	chemotherapy ± GM-CSF	GM-CSF: ↓ incidence, severity, and duration of mucositis (pS)
Nemunaitis[69]	100	chemotherapy ± GM-CSF	GM-CSF: ↓ grade 3/4 mucositis (pS)
Welte[70]	34	chemotherapy ± G-CSF	G-CSF: ↓ grade 3/4 mucositis (pNS)
Makkonen[71]	40	radiation ± GM-CSF	no differences
Amifostine			
Buntzel[17]	39	radiation, chemotherapy ± amifostine	amifostine: ↓ grade 3/4 mucositis (pS)
Brizel[14]	315	radiation ± amifostine	no differences
Koukourakis[72]	40	radiation ± SC amifostine	amifostine: ↓ mucositis (pS)
Hartmann[73]	40	chemotherapy + G-CSF ± amifostine	amifostine: grade 3/4 stomatitis 0 vs 25% (pS)
Antonadou[18]	50	radiation, chemotherapy ± amifostine	amifostine: grade 4 mucositis at 5 weeks: 4.5 vs 52% (pS)
Laser therapy			
Barasch[57]	20	chemotherapy ± He-Ne laser	laser: ↓ mucositis (pS)
Bensadoun[58]	30	radiation ± He-Ne laser	laser: grade 3 mucositis 8% vs 35% (pS)

chemotherapy, prevention or amelioration of which may reduce the incidence of mucositis. RCTs of GM-CSF used as a mouthwash showed no benefit.[52, 53]

Benzydamine mouthwash has been shown to be beneficial for radiotherapy patients [54]. Other agents reported to be effective in preventing mucositis include oral cryotherapy (sucking ice chips for 30 minutes, starting 5 minutes before chemotherapy), [55, 56] low energy laser therapy,[57, 58] glutamine [59], the homeopathic medication Traumeel S,[60] and melatonin.[61] Medications reported to be ineffective include prostaglandin E,[62] pilocarpine,[16] allopurinol,[63] and chamomile.[64] Pretreatment of the mucosa with silver nitrate reduced the incidence of mucositis in a trial of accelerated radiation therapy,[65] but not with standard radiation dose intensity.[66]

A Cochrane review of interventions to prevent chemotherapy-related mucositis indicated that oral cryotherapy was the only therapy that was effective.[74] This review excluded patients with head and neck cancer, and did not include treatment with laser therapy, melatonin, amifostine, or systemic administration of haematopoietic growth factors.

Active treatment. A Cochrane review reported that treatments with allopurinol or Vitamin E were the only effective therapies for mucositis in patients receiving cancer treatment, although the evidence was weak and unreliable.[75] Medications shown to be effective in RCTs include topical vitamin E,[76] topical sodium alginate,[4] and oral glutamine.[77] Topical sucralfate is ineffective.[78, 79]

Treatment of pain. Mild to moderate pain can usually be managed using mouthwashes containing local anaesthetics, topical analgesics and coating agents (Table 19.13). In some centres, these are mixed together, such as the National Cancer Institute (USA) stomatitis cocktail of lignocaine, diphenhydramine and simethicone. The coating agents help the anaesthetic and analgesic medications adhere to the mucosa. Sucralfate is not effective in preventing mucositis, but may reduce the associated pain. With local anaesthetic preparations, care is required not to anaesthetize the pharynx before eating or drinking. Overuse of

Table 19.13 Stomatitis: some analgesic and anaesthetic preparations

Local anaesthetics	
lignocaine (lidocaine)	viscous 2%: 15ml q3–4h, rinse and expel
	spray 10%: 4–8 sprays q2–4h
benzocaine	solution 20%: 10–15ml q4h, rinse and expel
	gel: apply with gentle massage q4–6h
dyclonine	solution 0.5 or 1%: 5–10ml q4h, rinse and expel
	lozenge 3mg: one to suck q2–4h
cocaine	solution 0.5%: 10ml q4h, rinse and expel
Topical analgesics	
benzydamine	solution 0.15%: 15ml q2–4h, rinse and expel
	lozenge 3mg: one to suck q2h
diphenhydramine	solution 12.5mg/5ml: 5ml q4h, rinse and expel
choline salicylate	gel: apply with gentle massage q3–4h
Coating agents	
sucralfate	mouthwash (1g tab dissolved in 10ml) q4h
kaopectate	
sodium alginate	

local anaesthetics, or excessive absorption because of ulceration, can cause cardiac or other systemic effects. A doxepin mouth rinse has been reported to be effective and acceptable.[80] A mouthwash containing morphine was superior to a combined anaesthetic/analgesic mouthwash in reducing both the severity and duration of the pain associated with severe mucositis caused by chemoradiotherapy.[81]

Systemic analgesics are often required for the pain associated with mucositis. A randomized comparison of morphine and a tricyclic antidepressant for mucositis pain reported the opioid to be significantly more effective, although some patients were adequately managed with the antidepressant alone.[82] Patients who have severe pain and are unable to take oral medication should be treated with parenteral opioid analgesics.

Treatment of infection. Specific antimicrobial therapy is given if the causative organism is known. If it is uncertain, mouth washing with povidone-iodine solution is recommended, as it has activity against bacteria, fungi and viruses.

Bacterial stomatitis is treated with antibiotics, selected on the basis of culture results, and which should cover gram-negative organisms. The role of antibacterial therapy in the prevention of mucositis is controversial, but it is customary to treat patients who are immunosuppressed or significantly neutropenic with prophylactic antibacterial therapy such as povidone-iodine.

Oral candidiasis has traditionally been treated with topical nystatin or amphotericin, and clinical experience suggests that this is effective for most palliative care patients (Table 19.14). However, recent Cochrane reviews report that topical nystatin is ineffective for the prevention or treatment of candidiasis for patients significantly immunodepressed or receiving cancer therapy.[83, 84] In these situations, treatment should be with an agent that is partially (miconazole, clotrimazole) or completely absorbed (ketoconazole, fluconazole, itraconazole). Ketoconazole may be hepatotoxic and cause drug interactions; fluconazole does not have these adverse effects but is more expensive.

Table 19.14 Stomatitis: candidiasis

Nystatin	suspension (100 000 units/ml) 1–2ml q4–6h pastilles (100 000 units) q4–6h
Amphotericin	lozenge 10mg q4–6h
Miconazole	oral gel q6h
Clotrimazole	troche or solution 10mg q6h
Ketoconazole	200mg/d PO for 7–14 days
Fluconazole	50–100mg/d PO for 7–14 days

Herpetic gingivostomatitis is treated with povidone-iodine mouthwash and oral aciclovir or valaciclovir (Table 19.15). Herpes labialis is treated with topical aciclovir ointment and is most effective if used frequently during the prodrome.

Aphthous ulceration is treated with topical tetracycline, topical steroid in orabase, or a steroid mouthwash (Table 19.16). Thalidomide is effective in the short-term treatment of aphthous ulcers for patients with HIV infection but may cause somnolence, rash and peripheral neuropathy.[85]

Table 19.15   Stomatitis: herpetic infection

Labialis	aciclovir 5% cream, q4h
	povidone-iodine 10% ointment, q6h
Gingivostomatitis	povidone-iodine mouthwash, q4–6
	aciclovir 200mg PO, 5 times daily, for 5–10d
	or valaciclovir 500mg PO q12h for 5–10d

Table 19.16   Stomatitis: aphthous ulceration

Tetracycline 250mg as a mouthwash, q6h
Triamcinolone 0.1% in orabase, applied topically q6h
Thalidomide 100-200mg/d PO

Terminal care

Continued mouth care is important in maintaining comfort. Severe pain should be managed with parenteral opioid analgesics.

Alteration of taste

Many patients with cancer suffer some alteration of taste. Taste may be reduced (hypogeusia), lost (ageusia) or distorted (dysgeusia) and the disturbance may be general or specifically affect a particular taste.[86] Disturbances of taste often come to notice when patients are questioned about eating poorly. Taste is important for both nutrition and digestion as it stimulates salivation as well as gastrointestinal motility and secretion. Loss of taste may lead to both poor intake and poor digestion.

The common causes of altered taste include oral pathology and the effects of drugs (Table 19.17). Besides cancer chemotherapy drugs, alteration in taste may be caused by hormones, drugs that cause xerostomia, and a range of other medications.[87] Oral candidiasis is a common cause in palliative care patients. A small number of patients with cancer have altered taste that cannot be explained by anything other than the presence of cancer and which may improve with tumour control.

Table 19.17   Causes of altered taste

Reduced number of taste buds	surgery, radiotherapy, chemotherapy, old age
Impaired taste bud cell renewal	chemotherapy, radiotherapy, poor nutritional state
Impaired taste bud stimulation	poor oral hygiene, necrotic tumour, stomatitis, xerostomia
Cranial nerve, brain stem lesions	
Drugs	chemotherapy, hormones
	drugs causing xerostomia
	other medication e.g. phenytoin
Metabolic disturbances	hypoadrenalism, diabetes, renal failure
Cancer *per se*	

Treatment

The management of altered taste includes treatment of the cause, care in the preparation and presentation of food, and the use of appetite stimulants (Table 19.18). The choice and presentation of food is the mainstay of treatment and involving a dietician is helpful. Corticosteroids and alcohol are of benefit for some patients, probably due to improvement in appetite and mood (see Anorexia, Chapter 28).

Table 19.18 Management of alteration of taste

Treatment of cause	general oral hygiene
	treat stomatitis, xerostomia
	consider medication changes
Presentation of food	discuss choice with patient and dietician
	food: hot, strong aromas, strong and tart tastes
	visually appealing
	eat in a room free of odours, noxious smells
Appetite stimulants	corticosteroids, alcohol, progestogens, dronabinol
Zinc supplements	

Zinc supplements have been reported to lessen the degree of taste disturbance associated with radiotherapy for head and neck cancer (Table 19.19).

Table 19.19 Zinc supplements during radiotherapy: RCTs

Author	n	Intervention	Outcome
Silverman[88]	19	radiation + zinc vs placebo	Zn: 64 vs 22% had improved taste 3 weeks after treatment
Ripamonti[80]	18	radiation + zinc sulfate vs placebo	Zn: less disturbance of taste during therapy, more rapid recovery after treatment (pS)

Terminal care

Abnormalities of taste are usually of little concern during the terminal phase. If the patient is still eating, they should be encouraged to request what they fancy. Caregivers need to understand that nutritional considerations are not relevant.

Nausea and vomiting

The majority of patients with advanced cancer will suffer nausea and vomiting at some stage of their illness, particularly those treated with chemotherapy or radiation. A number of recent reviews of this topic have been published.[90–93]

Nausea is an unpleasant feeling of the need to vomit. Other autonomic symptoms may accompany severe nausea or precede vomiting, including pallor, sweating, salivation and tachycardia. Retching consists of rhythmic, laboured, spasmodic movement of the diaphragm and abdominal muscles, facilitating regurgitation into the oesophagus. Vomiting

Table 19.20   Consequences of nausea and vomiting

Metabolic	Psychological
metabolic alkalosis and hypokalaemia	misery, depression
dehydration	poor morale: relatives, nursing staff
aggravation of uraemia, hypercalcaemia	Interference with treatment
malnutrition and weight loss	drugs not absorbed
Physical	drugs stopped (non-compliance)
exhaustion, weakness	withdrawal from chemo-, radiotherapy
Mallory-Weiss tears	
fractured ribs	
aspiration pneumonia	

is the expulsion of the gastric contents through the mouth, caused by forceful and sustained contraction of the abdominal muscles and diaphragm. The clinical consequences of nausea and vomiting are listed in Table 19.20.

Physiology. The vomiting centre (VC), located in the brainstem, coordinates the processes involved in emesis. It may be activated by stimuli from the chemoreceptor trigger zone (CTZ), the upper gastrointestinal tract and pharynx, the vestibular apparatus, and higher cortical centres (Figure 19.1). The CTZ is located in the area postrema in the floor of the fourth ventricle where it is exposed to both blood and cerebrospinal fluid. It is sensitive to chemical stimuli, both endogenous (e.g. uraemia) and exogenous (e.g. chemotherapy drugs).

The vomiting centre coordinates the act of vomiting via autonomic efferents to the gastrointestinal tract. Interaction with other brain stem centres produces the other autonomic features including sweating, pallor, salivation and tachycardia. Coordination with the respi-

Figure 19.1   Diagrammatic representation of the mechanism of vomiting

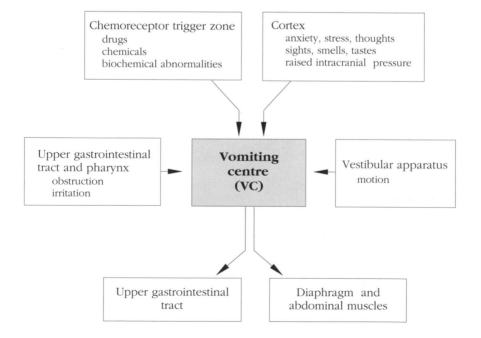

ratory centre facilitates breath holding and the contraction of the respiratory muscles that causes vomiting.

Neuropharmacology. A number of different types of neuroreceptors are present in the various neural pathways involved in emesis.[90] Knowledge of the pathways and receptors involved allows selection of a pharmacologically appropriate antiemetic (Table 19.21), although in practice there is significant overlap between the classes of drugs (see Table19.26). In addition, the neurotransmitter substance P is involved in the emetic pathway at or near the vomiting centre. It acts via the neurokinin-1 receptor and the recently introduced selective neurokinin-1 receptor antagonists are reported to be effective against the acute and delayed emesis caused by chemotherapy.[94–96]

Table 19.21 Neuroreceptors involved in emesis

Receptors	Antiemetics Class	Example
Vomiting centre (VC)		
acetylcholine	anticholinergic	hyoscine hydrobromide
histamine (H$_1$)	antihistamine	cyclizine
serotonin (5HT$_2$)	5HT$_2$ antagonist	levomepromazine
Chemoreceptor trigger zone (CTZ)		
dopamine (D$_2$)	antidopaminergic	
	phenothiazine	prochlorperazine
	orthopromide	metoclopramide
	butyrophenone	haloperidol
serotonin (5HT$_3$)	5HT$_3$ antagonist	ondansetron
Gastrointestinal tract		
serotonin (5HT$_3$)	5HT$_3$ antagonist	ondansetron
Vestibular apparatus		
histamine (H$_1$)	antihistamine	cyclizine
acetylcholine	anticholinergic	hyoscine hydrobromide

Cause. In patients with advanced cancer, nausea and vomiting are frequently due to a combination of causes (Table 19.22).

Assessment. A careful history will often indicate the likely cause of nausea and vomiting. The onset, duration, severity, frequency, and any aggravating or relieving factors should be documented. Evidence of constipation, bowel obstruction, renal failure, or raised intracranial pressure should be sought. The patient's medications should be reviewed. Interference with nutrition, hydration, and taking medications should be assessed. The character of the vomiting may suggest the cause; for example, infrequent large volume vomiting suggests gastric outlet obstruction, and projectile vomiting with relatively little nausea suggests intracranial pathology.

Measurement. Nausea is a subjective symptom and its expression varies from patient to patient and will depend on a range of other physical and psychosocial influences. Visual analogue scales (VAS) and numerical rating scales can be used for comparison over time or to measure the effect of therapy.[92] Comprehensive assessment of nausea and vomiting requires a multidimensional approach employing one of the validated tools that measure symptom distress and functional impairment such as the Functional Assessment of Cancer Therapy

Table 19.22 Causes of nausea and vomiting

Via peripheral afferent	Via chemoreceptor trigger zone
irritation, obstruction of the GI tract	biochemical abnormalities
(including pharynx, hepatobiliary system)	hypercalcaemia
cancer	hyponatraemia
chronic cough	liver failure, renal failure
oesophagitis	sepsis
gastritis	drugs
peptic ulceration	chemotherapy
gastric distension	opioids
gastric compression	digoxin, antibiotics, other
delayed gastric emptying	Via vestibular system
bowel obstruction	malignant vestibular infiltration
constipation	drugs: aspirin, platinum
hepatitis	Via cortical centres
biliary obstruction	psychological factors, anxiety
chemotherapy	sights, smells, tastes
radiotherapy	conditioned vomiting
	raised intracranial pressure

(FACT) or Functional Living Index-Cancer (FLIC). An Index of Nausea, Vomiting and Retching (INVR) has been proposed.[97] The grading system for vomiting caused by chemotherapy is shown in Table 19.23.

Table 19.23 NCI Common Toxicity Criteria grading of vomiting caused by chemotherapy[38]

0	none
1	1 episode in 24h over pretreatment
2	2–5 episodes in 24h over pretreatment
3	≥6 episodes in 24h over pretreatment; or need for IV fluids
4	requiring parenteral nutrition, intensive care; haemodynamic collapse

Treatment

The principles of treatment are outlined in Table 19.24. An underlying cause is sought and treated where possible and clinically appropriate; in patients with cancer, there are often multiple causes. Antiemetics are discussed below.

General measures that can be employed include fasting if vomiting is frequent, rest to avoid vestibular stimulation, and avoidance of noxious or suggestive stimuli (smells, odours). Liquid and soft foods, selected by the patient, are taken in small meals, eaten slowly. Fatty, sweet or spicy foods are best avoided. Relaxation techniques may be helpful.

Nasogastric intubation and intravenous hydration should be avoided in patients whose symptoms can be controlled by other means, and in the terminally ill.

Non-drug measures. Acupressure and acupuncture are reported to reduce nausea and vomiting associated with chemotherapy (Table 19.25).[98, 99] Acupressure wristbands are advocated although their efficacy has not been demonstrated in controlled studies.[100] Progressive muscle relaxation is also reported to reduce nausea and vomiting associated with chemotherapy (Table 19.25).[101] For cancer patients not receiving chemotherapy, the role of these non-drug measures has not been investigated.

Table 19.24 Nausea and vomiting: principles of treatment

Assess for and treat underlying cause

General and dietary measures

Non-drug measures

Use of antiemetics
    drug selected on basis of presumed causative mechanism
    commence before vomiting starts if possible
    in adequate doses
    in combination if necessary
    by parenteral or rectal route if necessary

If unresponsive
    assess for psychological factors
    reassess for missed physical causes
    try different antiemetics and/or combinations

Table 19.25 Non-drug measures for nausea and vomiting: RCTs

Author	n	Intervention	Outcome
Dibble[98]	17	chemotherapy, antiemetics ± finger acupressure	acupressure: ↓ nausea experience and intensity (pS)
Shen[99]	104	chemotherapy, antiemetics + electroacupuncture vs sham vs none	acupuncture: ↓ vomiting episodes (pS)
Molassiokis[101]	71	chemotherapy, antiemetics ± progressive muscle relaxation	PMR: ↓ nausea, vomiting, mood disturbance on days 1-4 (pS)

Antiemetic drugs

The antiemetic drugs in clinical use are described in Table 19.26. Where possible, antiemetics are selected for use on the basis of the presumed causative mechanism for the nausea and vomiting; the receptor site affinities of some commonly used antiemetics are summarized in Table 19.27. Ideally, antiemetics are given prophylactically, before vomiting starts. The drugs need to be given in adequate doses and scheduled according to the clinical duration of action. If patients are vomiting, treatment should be initiated by injection or with rectal suppositories.

Phenothiazines. The phenothiazines act primarily on the CTZ and the antiemetic effect is proportional to the antidopaminergic activity. Chlorpromazine has modest antiemetic activity and a relatively high incidence of sedation, postural hypotension and anticholinergic adverse effects. The piperazine derivatives (including prochlorperazine, perphenazine and thiethylperazine) are stronger antiemetics and cause less sedation and hypotension but more extrapyramidal adverse effects. The extrapyramidal and anticholinergic adverse effects may be dose-limiting (Tables 19.28 and 19.29). Levomepromazine has a broader spectrum of antiemetic activity and is a potent $5HT_2$ receptor antagonist, but is more likely to cause sedation and hypotension.[102]

Butyrophenones. Haloperidol and other butyrophenones are potent dopamine antagonists that act on the CTZ. They are effective antiemetics but sedation and extrapyramidal side effects are relatively common.[103]

Table 19.26   The antiemetic agents

Phenothiazines	*e.g.* prochlorperazine, levomepromazine
action	antidopaminergic effect at the CTZ
adverse effects	EP (prochlorperazine), sedation and hypotension (levomepromazine)
Butyrophenone	*e.g.* haloperidol
action	antidopaminergic effect at the CTZ
adverse effects	sedation and EP (see Table 19.28)
Orthopromides	*e.g.* metoclopramide, domperidone
actions	antidopaminergic effect at the CTZ, direct gastrokinetic effect
precaution	may aggravate high small bowel obstruction
adverse effects	sedation and EP (metoclopramide)
Anticholinergics	*e.g.* hyoscine hydrobromide
action	anticholinergic effect at VC, reduces GI secretions and motility
adverse effects	whole spectrum of anticholinergic effects (see Table 19.29)
Antihistamines	*e.g.* cyclizine, diphenhydramine, dimenhydrinate
action	anticholinergic and antihistaminic effect at VC
use	potentiates effect of a dopamine antagonist and prevents EP
adverse effects	sedation, dryness of the mouth
Cannabinoids	*e.g.* nabilone, dronabinol
action	at a cortical level: antiemetic effect parallels the euphoric period
adverse effects	dizziness, dysphoria, depression, hallucinations, paranoia
Corticosteroids	*e.g.* prednisolone, dexamethasone, hydrocortisone
action	undefined mechanism
use	particular value for vomiting caused by raised intracranial pressure
adverse effects	see Table 13.4
Benzodiazepines	*e.g.* diazepam, lorazepam
action	at a cortical level
use	anxiety, patients receiving chemotherapy
adverse	effects sedation
$5HT_3$ antagonists	*e.g.* ondansetron, granisetron, tropisetron
action	prevent vagal stimulation in GI tract; also at CTZ
use	vomiting associated with chemotherapy, radiotherapy
adverse effects	constipation, headache
Prokinetic agent	*e.g.* cisapride
action	acetylcholine release in the myenteric plexus increases GI motility
adverse effects	colic, diarrhoea, cardiac arrhythmias

CTZ—chemoreceptor trigger zone; EP—extrapyramidal side effects (see Table 19.28); VC—vomiting centre

Orthopromides. Metoclopramide acts both on the CTZ and the gastrointestinal tract. The gastrokinetic effect is effective for gastric stasis but can aggravate the symptoms of high small bowel obstruction. Adverse effects include sedation, dizziness and extrapyramidal effects. Domperidone has central and peripheral antiemetic actions similar to metoclopramide but does not cause sedation or extrapyramidal adverse effects.

Antihistamines. Antihistamines are used in the treatment of motion sickness and vestibular disorders but have little antiemetic effect when given alone in other situations.

Table 19.27 Receptor site affinities of commonly used antiemetics

	Dopamine antagonist	Histamine antagonist	Acetylcholine antagonist	5HT$_2$ antagonist	5HT$_3$ antagonist	5HT$_4$ agonist
Prochlorperazine	++	+	0	0	0	0
Chlorpromazine	++	++	+	0	0	0
Levomepromazine	++	+++	++	+++	0	0
Haloperidol	+++	0	0	0	0	0
Metoclopramide	++	0	0	0	(+)	++
Domperidone	++	0	0	0	0	++
Hyoscine hydrobromide	0	0	+++	0	0	0
Cyclizine	0	++	++	0	0	0
Ondansetron	0	0	0	0	+++	0
Cisapride	0	0	0	0	0	+++

0 none or insignificant, + slight, ++ moderate, +++marked

Table 19.28 Extrapyramidal reactions

Acute dystonic reactions	
onset	within days of starting oral therapy, within minutes of IV injection
features	trismus, torticollis, facial spasm, oculogyric crisis, opisthotonos, anxiety
treatment	benztropine 1–2mg IV/IM or diphenhydramine 25–50mg IV/IM
Akathisia	
onset	within weeks of starting oral therapy, within minutes of IV injection
features	motor restlessness, compulsive moving, anxiety
treatment	as for acute dystonic reactions
Parkinsonism	
onset	usually after several weeks of therapy
features	intention tremor, muscular rigidity, bradykinesia
treatment	discontinue causative agent; benztropine or procyclidine
Tardive dyskinesia	
onset	usually after months of treatment
features	involuntary chewing movements, vermicular movements of tongue
treatment	discontinue causative agent

However, given in conjunction with a dopamine antagonist, they may potentiate the antiemetic effect and prevent extrapyramidal reactions. Common adverse effects are sedation and dryness of the mouth.

Anticholinergics. Hyoscine (scopolamine) acts at or near the VC and also reduces gastrointestinal motility and secretions. It is useful, in conjunction with other antiemetics, in the treatment of troublesome vomiting associated with chronic gastrointestinal obstruction. The adverse effects of hyoscine include drowsiness and the whole spectrum of anticholinergic symptoms (Table 19.29).

Table 19.29 Anticholinergic adverse effects

Dry mouth (xerostomia)

Blurred vision (mydriasis and loss of accommodation)

Difficulty with micturition, retention

Constipation

Reflux oesophagitis

Tachycardia, palpitations

Anhidrosis, fever

Acute confusion or delirium

Cannabinoids. Dronabinol (tetrahydrocannabinol), the active constituent of marijuana, is an effective antiemetic. Its action is probably cortical as the antiemetic effect parallels the euphoric period. Adverse effects are frequent, especially in older patients, and include dizziness, sedation, dysphoria or depression, hallucinations, paranoia, and hypotension.[104, 105] The water-soluble analogue, nabilone, causes less neuropsychological toxicity.

Corticosteroids. Corticosteroids have an antiemetic effect when used alone and provide additional benefit when used in combination with standard antiemetics. The mechanism of this action is unknown. Corticosteroids are of particular value in the treatment of nausea and vomiting associated with raised intracranial pressure and with chemotherapy.[106] The adverse effects of corticosteroids are detailed elsewhere (Table 13.4).

Benzodiazepines. Diazepam and lorazepam are useful adjuncts in antiemetic therapy for patients receiving chemotherapy. It is presumed that they act at a cortical level. Lorazepam may cause amnesia, which may be desirable in the treatment of conditioned or anticipatory vomiting.

5-HT$_3$ receptor antagonists. These agents act by preventing the binding of serotonin to the 5-HT$_3$ receptor in the gastrointestinal tract and the CTZ in the brainstem. Ondansetron was the first of these drugs to be used widely and proved very effective for nausea and vomiting associated with chemotherapy or radiotherapy. Tropisetron and granisetron have the advantage of once daily administration. The drugs are metabolized by cytochrome P-450 enzymes CYP2D6, and increased metabolism caused by other drugs or genetic factors may cause lower blood levels and loss of clinical effect.[107] Adverse effects are uncommon except for constipation and mild headache.

Cisapride. This gastrointestinal prokinetic agent is a potent 5HT$_4$ receptor agonist, which leads to release of acetylcholine in the myenteric plexus. It increases lower oesophageal sphincter tone and improves both gastric and intestinal peristalsis. It is effective for patients with gastric stasis or compression. Gastrointestinal adverse effects include colic and diarrhoea. Rare cases of serious (occasionally fatal) cardiac arrhythmias associated with prolongation of the QT interval have been reported in patients taking cisapride in conjunction with imidazole antifungal agents (fluconazole, itraconazole, ketoconazole, miconazole) or macrolide antibiotics (erythromycin, clarithromycin). Cisapride is contraindicated in patients who have, or may have, prolongation of the QT interval.

Neurokinin-1 receptor antagonists. This new class of antiemetic agent, which prevents the binding of substance P to the neurokinin-1 receptors in the VC, is under clinical evaluation.[94–96]

Olanzapine. This atypical antipsychotic drug is a potent dopamine and $5HT_2$ receptor antagonist and also has antihistaminic and anticholinergic activity. This profile suggests it should be a potent antiemetic. A pilot study showed it was effective and well tolerated in patients with nausea related to opioid therapy.[108] It may also be of use in treating delayed emesis following chemotherapy.[109] The common adverse effects are sedation and weight gain.

Nausea and vomiting associated with chemotherapy

The American Society of Clinical Oncology (ASCO) has published evidence-based guidelines for the use of antiemetic therapy with chemotherapy (Table 19.30).[110] The use of antiemetics is determined by individual patient circumstances, but they are probably used more liberally in practice, given that vomiting is such an undesirable adverse effect of treatment.

Table 19.30   ASCO guidelines for antiemetic therapy for chemotherapy[110]

Chemotherapy with high emetic risk (e.g. cisplatin, carboplatin, doxorubicin)
prevention acute emesis	$5HT_3$ antagonist + corticosteroid (dexamethasone 20mg)
prevention delayed emesis	corticosteroid ± $5HT_3$ antagonist or metoclopramide

Chemotherapy with intermediate emetic risk (e.g. irinotecan, paclitaxel, mitoxantrone)
prevention acute emesis	corticosteroid (dexamethasone 4-8mg)

Chemotherapy with low emetic risk (e.g. fluorouracil, vinorelbine)
prevention acute emesis	no routine pretreatment antiemetics

Nausea and vomiting associated with radiotherapy

A large Italian study of patients treated with radiotherapy reported that 37% suffered nausea and 17% vomiting.[111] Radiation to the upper abdomen and larger treatment field sizes were the major risk factors for nausea and vomiting. $5HT_3$ antagonists and dexamethasone are effective in reducing the nausea and vomiting associated with radiotherapy (Table19.31). A systematic review of the $5HT_3$ antagonists reported that they were of benefit for a proportion of patients.[112]

Table 19.31   Prevention of emesis related to radiotherapy (RT): RCTs

Author	n	Intervention	Outcome
Bey[113]	50	abdominal RT + dolasetron vs placebo	dolasetron: ↓ nausea and emesis (both pS)
Franzen[114]	111	abdominal RT + ondansetron vs placebo	ondansetron: ↓ emesis (pS)
Sykes[115]	66	abdominal RT + chlorpromazine/ dexamethasone vs ondansetron	ondansetron: ↓ nausea and emesis (both pS)
Kirkbride[116]	150	abdominal RT + dexamethasone vs placebo	dexamethasone: ↓ emesis (pS)

The American Society of Clinical Oncology (ASCO) evidence-based guidelines for the use of antiemetics with radiation therapy are shown in Table 19.32.[110] In practice, the use of antiemetics is determined by individual patient circumstances.

Table 19.32   ASCO guidelines for antiemetic therapy for radiotherapy[110]

High risk: total body irradiation
   5HT$_3$ antagonist ± corticosteroid

Intermediate risk: hemibody, abdomen, mantle, craniospinal, cranial radiosurgery
   5HT$_3$ antagonist or dopamine antagonist before each fraction

Low risk: cranium, breast, head and neck, extremities, pelvis, thorax
   5HT$_3$ antagonist or dopamine antagonist on an as-needed basis

Nausea and vomiting in palliative care

Nausea and vomiting occur frequently in palliative care patients who are not receiving radiation or chemotherapy, but few trials have been performed.[117] Where possible and appropriate, the cause is defined and treated. Antiemetic drugs should be selected according to the putative cause (see above). Gastric stasis and compression may respond to the gastrokinetic effect of metoclopramide, domperidone or cisapride. Cortical causes of nausea and vomiting may respond to anxiolytic drugs. Metoclopramide is effective for nausea associated with advanced cancer.[118] The role of 5HT$_3$ antagonists in palliative care remains to be defined.[119, 120] There are only two RCTs of 5HT$_3$ therapy: in one tropisetron or tropisetron-containing combinations were superior to other antiemetics;[121] in the other ondansetron was no better than metoclopramide or placebo for nausea related to opioid therapy.[122] In practice, a trial of a 5HT$_3$ antagonist is warranted if other antiemetics are ineffective and in patients with abdominal disease or bowel obstruction.

Terminal care

During the last days or week of life, treatment directed at an underlying cause may be inappropriate. Symptomatic treatment with antiemetics is continued and the use of drugs with sedative effects may be valuable. Many antiemetic drugs can be given by CSCI and metoclopramide, haloperidol, cyclizine and hyoscine hydrobromide can be included in syringe drivers with morphine. Nasogastric intubation should be avoided.

Hiccups

Hiccups are due to involuntary contraction of the diaphragm causing sudden inspiration associated with abrupt closure of the glottis.

Table 19.33   Causes of hiccups

Diaphragmatic irritation
   malignant infiltration
   inflammation or infection: empyema, chemical pleurodesis, subphrenic abscess
   marked hepatomegaly, ascites

Gastric distension: obstruction, overload, gastric tumour

Oesophagitis

Phrenic nerve irritation: mediastinal tumour

Intracranial disease: cerebral or medullary tumour

Metabolic: uraemia

Hiccups are most frequently caused by diaphragmatic irritation or gastric distension (Table 19.33). A patient with protracted or distressing hiccups should have a chest x-ray and a serum creatinine estimation performed.

Treatment

If hiccups occur only intermittently or for short periods, no treatment may be necessary except perhaps for one of the 'home cures' (Table 19.34). These work by vagal stimulation or by raising the carbon dioxide tension in the blood. Alternatively, direct nasopharyngeal stimulation will abort most attacks.

Table 19.34 Management of hiccups

To abort an attack	
vagal stimulation	pharyngeal stimulation: swab, nasogastric tube
elevation of pCO_2	breath holding, rebreathing into paper bag
reduction of gastric distension	aerated drink, peppermint water
	metoclopramide
	nasogastric tube
pharmacological	chlorpromazine 25mg PO
	baclofen 5mg PO
	nifedipine 10mg PO or SL
	midazolam 2mg SC and titrate
To prevent further attacks	
treat underlying cause	
prevent gastric distension	antiflatulent e.g. simethicone
	gastrokinetic agent e.g. metoclopramide
prevent gastro-oesophageal reflux	proton pump inhibitor e.g. omeprazole
	gastrokinetic agent e.g. metoclopramide
hiccups due to intracranial disease	anticonvulsant e.g. sodium valproate
other causes	baclofen
	nifedipine
	haloperidol, chlorpromazine
	midazolam

Protracted hiccups that fail to respond to simple measures are treated with a muscle relaxant (baclofen, nifedipine), a neuroleptic drug that inhibits the hiccup reflex centrally (haloperidol, chlorpromazine), or by sedation with midazolam for the terminally ill.[123–126] If baclofen is used on a regular basis, it should not be abruptly discontinued but weaned slowly. Hiccups due to intracranial disease may respond to an anticonvulsant such as sodium valproate

Prevention of further attacks requires that the underlying cause be treated, where possible and clinically appropriate (Table 19.34). If hiccups persist and the underlying cause cannot be palliated, continued drug therapy may be necessary.

Terminal care

Troublesome hiccups during the terminal phase should be treated with chlorpromazine or a subcutaneous infusion of midazolam. Treatment of an underlying cause is only considered when it may improve the patient's comfort, as with the relief of gastric distension.

Dysphagia

Dysphagia is difficulty with swallowing. Swallowing (deglutition) is accomplished in three stages. In the first or buccal phase, food and fluid are voluntarily pushed to the back of the throat by the action of the tongue and palate. During the second or pharyngeal phase the swallowing reflex is initiated, including glottic closure to prevent inhalation. In the third or oesophageal phase, food passes down the oesophagus by reflex peristalsis.

The causes of dysphagia are outlined in Table 19.35. At each level, dysphagia may be caused by inflammation, an obstructing lesion, or by neuromuscular dysfunction. Neuromuscular incoordination may be due to either local factors (physical defects or local nerve damage due to infiltration or surgery) or cranial nerve and brain stem lesions. There is a high incidence of incoordination of swallowing in patients treated with chemoradiotherapy for oropharyngeal cancer, which predisposes these patients to aspiration.[127]

Table 19.35 Causes of dysphagia

Buccal phase: food voluntarily pushed backward by the tongue and palate	
tumour	intrinsic obstruction, functional deficit
stomatitis	infection, radiation, chemotherapy
xerostomia	
neuromuscular	surgery
	cranial nerve dysfunction
	cerebral or brain stem lesions
	general weakness and debility
Pharyngeal phase: swallowing reflex initiated, including glottic closure	
tumour	intrinsic obstruction, extrinsic compression
pharyngitis	infection, radiation
neuromuscular	surgery
	cranial nerve dysfunction
	cerebral or brain stem lesions
	general weakness and debility
	radiation fibrosis or stricture
Oesophageal phase: food passed down the oesophagus by reflex peristalsis	
tumour	intrinsic obstruction, extrinsic compression
oesophagitis	infection, radiation, reflux
tube	dislodgement of endo-oesophageal tube
neuromuscular	surgery
	mural plexus infiltration
	radiation fibrosis or stricture
	anxiety

Clinical features. With abnormalities of the buccal phase, food stays in the mouth and there is often drooling. With pharyngeal dysphagia, food sticks in the throat and attempts at swallowing cause gagging, coughing and regurgitation of food through the nose. Patients with oesophageal disorders complain that food sticks somewhere behind the sternum. Pain associated with dysphagia (odynophagia) suggests inflammation or infection but may occur with malignant infiltration.

Obstruction caused by tumour usually causes dysphagia that is initially more marked for solids than liquids; dysphagia due to neuromuscular pathology affects solids and fluids to much the same extent.

Assessment. Examination includes testing cranial nerve function and inspection of the oropharynx for evidence of tumour or infection. A test swallow of water will often allow patients to be more specific about their symptoms. Swallowing may be assessed radiologically using a dilute barium solution. Patients with oesophageal dysphagia require a chest x-ray or CT scan to assess mediastinal disease and endoscopy is used to differentiate intrinsic pathology and extrinsic pressure.

Measurement. A grading system or dysphagia score can be used to quantify severity and monitor the results of therapy (Table 19.36).

Table 19.36 Dysphagia score

0	no dysphagia
1	able to eat solids
2	semisolid foods only
3	liquids only
4	complete dysphagia

Treatment

Treatment depends on the site and cause of the obstruction as well as the stage of the patient's disease. The options are set out in Table 19.37.

Table 19.37 Dysphagia: some treatment options

Buccal and pharyngeal	
stomatitis, pharyngitis, xerostomia	standard therapy (see Tables 19.5, 19.13)
obstructing tumour	surgery, laser resection, radiotherapy
extrinsic compression	corticosteroids, radiotherapy
neuromuscular incoordination	corticosteroids, radiotherapy
general	feeding education, dietary advice, enteral nutrition
Oesophageal	
oesophagitis	standard therapy (see Table 19.41)
chronic stricture	dilatation
neuromuscular incoordination	dietary advice, corticosteroids
extrinsic compression	corticosteroids, radiotherapy, systemic therapy
intrinsic tumour	endo-oesophageal tube, stent
	radiotherapy, systemic therapy
	endoscopic laser resection, photodynamic therapy
	endoscopic radiotherapy (brachytherapy)

Treatment must be appropriate to the stage of the patient's disease and prognosis

Oropharyngeal dysphagia. Patients with oropharyngeal dysphagia require a programme of feeding education that includes assistance with positioning to make swallowing easier and dietary advice about small meals and soft moist food. Corticosteroids are of value in treating dysphagia due to extrinsic compression, local nerve infiltration or cranial nerve dysfunction.

The accumulation of saliva in patients with complete obstruction will cause drooling and may lead to aspiration; treatment is with an anticholinergic drug to reduce salivary flow.

Enteral nutrition. Patients with severe oropharyngeal dysphagia may require feeding by an alternative route. Long-term nasogastric intubation should be avoided and placement of a percutaneous endoscopic gastrostomy (PEG) tube under local anaesthetic is preferred. Compared to nasogastric tubes, there are less mechanical failures, less aspiration pneumonia, and a better cosmetic result with PEG tubes.[128, 129] They are not suitable for patients with ascites, peptic ulceration or a bleeding diathesis.

Oesophageal obstruction. Oesophageal obstruction due to tumour can be managed by endo-oesophageal laser therapy, radiotherapy, the placement of an endo-oesophageal tube or stent, or by a combination of them.

Laser therapy can be used for either thermal ablation of tumour or photodynamic therapy following the administration of a photosensitizer. The response to photodynamic therapy may be more durable and is associated with fewer complications.[130, 131] Both treatments require the availability of specialized expertise and equipment. Laser therapy for thermal ablation usually needs to be repeated every 6 to 8 weeks. Addition of endoscopic radiotherapy (brachytherapy) or external beam radiation increases the dysphagia-free interval, but may also increase the complication rate.[132–134]

Brachytherapy used alone is effective treatment, although the optimum treatment schedule remains to be defined.[135] It is usually performed in two or three sessions and patients may suffer odynophagia for several weeks. A small but significant number of patients will develop fistulas or strictures.

Traditional plastic endo-oesophageal tubes (e.g. Celestin, Atkinson) are being replaced by the use of self-expanding metal stents. These are easily introduced without need for a general anaesthetic, and the procedural complication rate is much lower than with plastic tubes. The first generation of stents was subject to blockage by tumour in-growth through the mesh. This was overcome by using a covered stent with a membrane covering the outside of the mesh, but these were prone to migration.[136] The development of an internally covered stent, with the membrane applied to the inside of the mesh, prevents tumour in-growth and is less prone to migration. An anti-reflux valve can be used to prevent problems related to gastro-oesophageal reflux, particularly if the stent is sited across the gastro-oesophageal junction.[137, 138] If tumour obstructs one end of the stent, a second stent can be placed inside the first, but protruding to cover the new growth. Self-expanding metal stents are considerably more expensive than plastic tubes, but are associated with a much lower complication rate and shorter hospital stay. Plastic self-expanding stents, currently under development, may be less expensive.[139]

RCTs comparing self-expanding metal stents with plastic tubes consistently report lower rates of procedural complications and shorter hospital stays with metal stents, with at least equivalent improvement in the dysphagia score.[140–144] RCTs comparing self-expanding metal stents with endoscopic laser therapy, one of which included external beam radiation, have reported mixed results (Table 19.38). Continuing improvements in stent technology suggest that stent placement will become the preferred procedure for palliation in the future.

Patients with endo-oesophageal tubes or stents require dietary advice. They are advised to take multiple small meals accompanied by an aerated drink. Foods that are likely to cause obstruction of the tube, such as lumpy or stringy foods and fresh bread, are avoided. If blockage occurs, the patient can try to clear the tube with an aerated drink or with physical movement. Endoscopic clearance is sometimes necessary.

Table 19.38 Self-expanding metal stents (SEMS) and endoscopic laser therapy: RCTs

Author	n	Intervention	Outcome
Mason[145]	474	SEMS vs laser	SEMS: single procedure, more improvement in dysphagia
Adam[146]	60	SEMS vs laser	SEMS: single procedure, more improvement in dysphagia
Konigsrainer[147]	39	SEMS vs laser + RT	SEMS: single procedure, ↓ local complications, ↓ cost, shorter stay; equivalent survival and relief of dysphagia
Dallal[148]	65	SEMS vs laser	SEMS: single procedure, ↓ cost, shorter stay; equivalent relief of dysphagia; more pain, shorter survival

Terminal care

Patients with oropharyngeal dysphagia should be managed conservatively with dietary manipulation. An endo-oesophageal tube or stent should be considered for complete oesophageal obstruction, as insertion causes little distress and it may greatly improve the quality of life if it allows saliva to be swallowed.

Oesophagitis

The common causes of oesophagitis in patients with advanced cancer are listed in Table 19.39. Oesophagitis causes pain on swallowing (odynophagia), some degree of difficulty with swallowing (dysphagia) and may produce angina-like mediastinal pain. Severe oesophagitis may result in blood stained vomitus or melaena. Reflux oesophagitis characteristically causes burning retrosternal discomfort ('heartburn') associated with regurgitation of acid-tasting material into the pharynx ('waterbrash').

Table 19.39 Causes of oesophagitis

Tumour infiltration	
Radiation	predisposition to infection, peptic irritation
Chemotherapy	neutropenia
Infection	fungal, bacterial, viral
Reflux oesophagitis	raised intra-abdominal pressure (any cause) endo-oesophageal tubes nasogastric tube prolonged recumbent posture persistent vomiting anticholinergic drugs, anticholinergic side effects of drugs

Examination may show oropharyngeal infection or evidence of raised intra-abdominal pressure. Barium examination will show mucosal irregularity or ulceration. Endoscopy with biopsies and cultures is often required to determine the cause of infective oesophagitis. The grading criteria for radiation oesophagitis are listed in Table 19.40.

Table 19.40 RTOG/EORTC grading criteria for radiation oesophagitis[149]

0	none
1	mild dysphagia, but can eat normal diet
2	dysphagia requiring pureed or liquid diet
3	dysphagia requiring feeding tube, IV hydration or hyperalimentation
4	complete obstruction (cannot swallow saliva); ulceration with bleeding or perforation

Treatment

Therapy is directed at pain relief, prevention and healing of ulceration, control of reflux, treatment of infection and, where possible, treatment of the underlying cause (Table 19.41). There is evidence that that the cytoprotective agent, amifostine, reduces the incidence of radiation oesophagitis (Table19.42)[72, 150]; sucralfate is ineffective.[151]

Table 19.41 Management of oesophagitis

Pain relief
  topical local anaesthetics: oxethazaine, lignocaine, cocaine
  analgesics: oral (mild), parenteral opioids (severe)
  antacids
  dietary advice: liquid or semisolid diet, avoid very hot or cold foods

Prevention and healing of ulceration
  antacids combined with coating agent or alginate
  sucralfate

Reduce gastric acid production
  H_2-receptor antagonist, proton pump inhibitor

Reduce reflux
  reduce increased intra-abdominal pressure
  avoid large meals, carbonated drinks, alcohol
  avoid stooping, lying flat
  increase lower oesophageal sphincter tone: metoclopramide, cisapride

Infection
  specific antimicrobial therapy (see Stomatitis)

Table 19.42 Amifostine and radiation oesophagitis: RCTs

Author	n	Intervention	Outcome
Koukourakis[72]	60	thoracic radiation ± amifostine	amifostine: less oesophagitis (pS)
Antonadou[150]	146	thoracic radiation ± amifostine	amifostine: grade ≥2 oesophagitis 4 vs 42% (pS)

The pain of mild oesophagitis usually responds well to simple analgesics and local anaesthetics but severe oesophagitis frequently requires systemic opioid drugs. Oxethazaine in combination with antacids (Mucaine) often provides good symptom relief. Topical local anaesthetics such as lignocaine or cocaine may relieve pain but predispose to aspiration if the pharynx is anaesthetized. The use of sucralfate or the reduction of gastric acid by an H_2-receptor antagonist or proton pump inhibitor may significantly aid analgesia.

Terminal care

The treatment of oesophagitis should be purely symptomatic. Elevating the head of the bed, topical anaesthetics, combined antacids and dietary manipulation are helpful. Parenteral opioid analgesics are given for severe pain.

Upper gastrointestinal bleeding

The causes of upper gastrointestinal bleeding in patients with advanced cancer are listed in Table 19.43. Aspirin and NSAIDs are frequent causes of erosion and ulceration, and the risk is increased by older age, serious illness, and the co-prescription of corticosteroids;[152] *Helicobacter pylori* infection also increases the risk of ulcers and bleeding in patients treated with NSAIDs.[153]

Table 19.43   Causes of upper gastrointestinal bleeding

Oesophagus
    oesophagitis
    malignant infiltration
    Mallory Weiss tears
    oesophageal varices/portal hypertension
        cirrhosis, hepatic tumour, portal or hepatic vein thrombosis

Stomach and duodenum
    erosion, ulceration, malignant infiltration

General bleeding diathesis

Upper gastrointestinal haemorrhage may cause the vomiting of blood or 'coffee grounds' and is usually associated with melaena. The observation of bright blood in the vomitus or 'red currant' stools per rectum indicates more rapid bleeding. If the haemorrhage is mild and chronic, there may be no haematemesis or melaena but simply a slowly developing anaemia. Blood staining of vomitus may occur with severe stomatitis and 'coffee grounds' type vomitus may be caused by swallowed blood from chronic nasopharyngeal bleeding.

Assessment of upper gastrointestinal bleeding requires endoscopy, which will determine the cause of bleeding in the majority of patients. However, it has been argued that the results of endoscopy do not greatly affect the immediate management of many patients with advanced cancer. The advantages of endoscopy include visualization of tumour, performance of biopsies and cultures, identification of patients likely to continue to bleed or re-bleed, and identification of more than one site or cause of haemorrhage. Endoscopy also provides the opportunity for topical treatment to stop haemorrhage, including sclerotherapy or electrocoagulation. Thrombocytopenia or other coagulopathy are excluded by appropriate testing.

Treatment

Management includes treatment of the cause, blood transfusion if indicated, and the correction of any bleeding diathesis (Table 19.44). If endoscopy is not performed the patient may be treated symptomatically with transfusion and given empiric therapy for the presumed cause of bleeding.

Table 19.44   Upper gastrointestinal bleeding: treatment options

Erosions and peptic ulceration
   withdraw causative or aggravating agents
   antacids, sucralfate, H₂-receptor antagonist, proton pump inhibitor, misoprostol
   local photocoagulation, electrocoagulation (if vessels visualized)
   therapy for *H. pylori*

Bleeding varices
   endoscopic sclerotherapy or ligation
   octreotide infusion (25μg/h IV)
   balloon tamponade
   propranolol

Bleeding tumours
   laser photocoagulation
   electrocoagulation, sclerotherapy (if vessels visualized)
   surgery, embolization

Treatment of erosions and peptic ulceration includes withdrawal of any causative or aggravating drugs, endoscopic therapy, and treatment to reduce gastric acid production. Octreotide may help control acute haemorrhage.[154] Patients with a better prognosis who have *H. pylori* infection should be considered for eradication therapy. Patients requiring continued therapy with NSAIDs should be treated with a proton pump inhibitor such as omeprazole or lansoprazole, which are superior to H₂-receptor antagonists and misoprostol in preventing and healing NSAID-induced lesions and are better tolerated.[155–157]

For bleeding varices, endoscopic ligation is more effective than sclerotherapy.[158] An octreotide infusion can be used to help control acute haemorrhage. Octreotide causes vasoconstriction of the splanchnic circulation and is preferred to vasopressin, which causes generalized vasoconstriction that may lead to tissue damage. Balloon tamponade with a Sengstaken tube may be considered in the acute situation but would be inappropriate for terminally ill patients. Propranolol reduces the risk of recurrent bleeding in patients with portal hypertension.

Haemorrhage from tumours may be treated with laser photocoagulation or local sclerotherapy if bleeding vessels are visualized, but the incidence of recurrent bleeding is high.[159, 160] Other methods of treatment, if appropriate to the patient's condition and prognosis, include surgery and arterial embolization.

Terminal care

Treatment is symptomatic with antiemetics to reduce vomiting and analgesics for epigastric pain. Antacids and therapy to reduce gastric acid production can be continued if they contribute to pain control and administration does not distress the patient. Patients who suffer massive or repeated haematemesis as a terminal event should be treated with parenteral morphine or midazolam to allay anxiety, and green or dark coloured sheets and towels should be available to camouflage the blood.

Indigestion

The term indigestion is used to describe a variety of symptoms. There is usually fullness, discomfort, or pain in the epigastrium, which may be associated with distention, flatulence, nausea, or symptoms of oesophageal reflux. The common causes of indigestion in patients with advanced cancer are listed in Table 19.45.

The syndromes relating to an effective reduction in stomach size or its inability to expand with feeding are characterized by early satiety and inability to eat large amounts. There is epigastric discomfort often associated with nausea and symptoms of oesophageal reflux. The

Table 19.45   Causes of indigestion

Oesophagus: oesophagitis

Stomach and duodenum
    gastritis: radiotherapy, chemotherapy, alcohol, other drugs (e.g. iron, potassium)
    ulceration and erosions: aspirin, NSAIDs, corticosteroids
    small stomach syndrome: gastrectomy, linitis plastica
    gastric compression syndrome: hepatomegaly, splenomegaly, ascites
    gastric outlet obstruction: tumour, peptic ulceration, opioid drugs
    dumping syndrome: gastrectomy, vagotomy
    aerophagia: anxiety, pharyngeal abnormalities

Pancreas: pancreatitis, pancreatic cancer

Biliary system: cholecystitis, cancer

Table 19.46   Indigestion: medications

Antacids	
action	symptomatic relief by neutralization of gastric acid
adverse effects	aluminium hydroxide: constipation, drug malabsorption
	magnesium salts: diarrhoea, hypermagnesaemia (in renal failure)
	sodium bicarbonate: sodium overload, metabolic alkalosis
	calcium carbonate: constipation, rebound hyperacidity
Combined antacids	
action	with simethicone: facilitates expulsion of wind
	with alginic acid: provides a protective mucosal coating
Mucosal protective agent: sucralfate	
action	forms a protective mucosal coating; aids ulcer healing
given	>30min after antacids, >2h after H_2-receptor antagonists
H_2-receptor antagonists: e.g. cimetidine, ranitidine, famotidine, nizatidine	
action	reduce gastric acid production
adverse effects	increased hepatic enzymes, drug interactions
Proton pump inhibitors: e.g. omeprazole, lansoprazole, esomeprazole	
action	prevents gastric acid secretion
adverse effects	mild nausea and diarrhoea
Prostaglandin analogue: misoprostol	
action	inhibits gastric acid secretion
adverse effects	diarrhoea
Gastrokinetic agents: metoclopramide, cisapride	
action	promote gastric emptying
adverse effects	metoclopramide: sedation, extrapyramidal effects
	cisapride: colic, diarrhoea, cardiac arrhythmias

dumping syndrome, caused by the rapid transit of food out of the stomach in patients who have had a partial gastrectomy or vagotomy, is characterized by epigastric discomfort and fullness associated with nausea, colic and diarrhoea accompanied by vasomotor symptoms of weakness, faintness and sweating.

The characteristics of the pain and associated symptoms often indicate the probable cause. Indigestion occurring during or immediately after eating suggests oesophageal pathology or one of the restrictive gastric syndromes. Indigestion occurring after eating suggests peptic ulceration. Constant pain suggests malignant infiltration. Endoscopy is frequently required for the diagnosis of ulcers, erosions and other mucosal lesions.

Treatment

The management of dyspepsia includes measures to relieve symptoms, withdrawal of offending drugs, and treatment of underlying or predisposing factors. A variety of medications may be employed (Table 19.46).

The treatment of the gastric restriction syndromes is symptomatic (Table 19.47). Gastrokinetic drugs are particularly useful for patients with obstruction caused by other medications that need to be continued, such as opioid analgesics and anticholinergic drugs.

Table 19.47   Indigestion: management

Gastric restriction
    dietary advice: multiple small meals
    antiflatulent: simethicone-containing antacid
    gastrokinetic agent
    stop drugs causing gastric stasis/outlet obstruction, if possible

Erosions and peptic ulceration
    sucralfate, H_2-receptor antagonist, proton pump inhibitor, misoprostol

Terminal care

Antacids can be continued to control symptoms. H_2-receptor antagonists or opioids can be used for pain not relieved by antacids.

Bowel obstruction

Bowel obstruction can be caused by mechanical obstruction or by paralysis of the bowel wall musculature (paralytic ileus) (Table 19.48). Mechanical obstruction is most frequently due to cancer or constipation. Obstruction due to muscular paralysis may occur if there is disruption of the autonomic nerve supply to the bowel. Localized paralysis may occur as a result of radiation fibrosis; 'strictures' caused by radiotherapy are not particularly narrow but are atonic and do not show normal peristaltic movement.

Bowel obstruction occurring in patients with advanced cancer is frequently multifactorial. It is also common for obstruction to occur at multiple sites, particularly in patients with widespread peritoneal infiltration. These two considerations are important in assessment and management.

Clinical features

The classical features of bowel obstruction are abdominal pain and distension, nausea and vomiting, and failure to pass flatus or faeces. The clinical features will depend on whether the

Table 19.48   Causes of bowel obstruction

Mechanical obstruction
    luminal obstruction: cancer, constipation, faecal impaction
    wall infiltration, stricture: cancer, radiation, surgery, benign (e.g. peptic ulcer)
    extrinsic compression: cancer, adhesions (malignant or surgical)

Paralytic obstruction
    disruption of autonomic nerve supply: retroperitoneal infiltration, spinal disease
    drugs: opioids, anticholinergics
    postoperative
    peritonitis
    metabolic: hypokalaemia, hypercalcaemia, hyperglycaemia
    radiation fibrosis
    arterial or venous insufficiency

obstruction is acute or subacute, complete or partial, and which part of the bowel is involved. Acute complete obstruction will cause severe colicky pain with nausea, vomiting and constipation. In patients with advanced cancer the obstruction is more likely to be incomplete and the onset may be insidious and associated with bouts of nausea and colic. Patients with obstruction due to faecal impaction may continue to pass faecal material, which is an overflow phenomenon.

The site of the obstruction is an important determinant of the symptoms and signs. In patients with cancer, about one half of bowel obstructions occur in the small bowel, one third in the large bowel, and both are involved in the remainder. The higher the obstruction, the earlier and more profuse the vomiting; lower obstruction is associated with more abdominal distension.

Physical examination will show a varying degree of distension often without any specific areas of abdominal tenderness. There may be audible borborygmi or high pitched 'tinkling' bowel sounds heard on auscultation. Constipation or faecal impaction will be evident on rectal examination. If bowel necrosis occurs and peritonitis develops, the abdominal pain will become constant and associated with paralytic ileus and tenderness.

Assessment. The clinical investigation of the cause of bowel obstruction depends on what interventions are considered possible and appropriate. Plain abdominal x-rays will show distended bowel with fluid levels on the erect or decubitus view. It is usually possible to determine from the plain film whether the obstruction involves the small or the large bowel: the haustral markings in the large bowel do not completely encircle the bowel. A barium swallow may be ordered if gastric outlet obstruction is suspected. A barium small bowel enema may help differentiate dysfunctional intestine (for which conservative treatment would be appropriate) from obstructed intestine (for which surgery would be indicated), but should be reserved for patients for whom surgery is a realistic possibility.

Treatment

The management of bowel obstruction is traditionally based on surgical intervention but conservative therapy will produce equivalent results for some patients with advanced cancer.[161] The options available are listed in Table 19.49.

Nasogastric drainage with intravenous fluid administration should be used as a temporary measure only. Patients with advanced cancer are more likely to have incomplete and subacute

Table 19.49 Bowel obstruction: treatment options

Nasogastric intubation and intravenous fluids: as a temporary measure only
    preoperative
    pending a decision regarding surgery
    whilst systemic therapy is initiated (sensitive tumours)
    acute phase of recurrent obstruction

Surgery
    resection or bypass of obstruction
    creation of colostomy, ileostomy
    percutaneous gastrostomy
    endoscopic laser resection (colorectal)

Symptomatic
    medications (see Table 19.51)
    relieve and prevent constipation
    small meals with reduced roughage, served when the patient requests

Treatment must be appropriate to the stage of the patient's disease and the prognosis

obstructions, many of which will resolve spontaneously. They should be managed with symptomatic treatment as described below and not with chronic nasogastric intubation.

The clinical features that recommend surgical intervention are listed in Table 19.50. A significant proportion of patients (estimated at between 10 and 30%) will have a benign and correctable cause. A Cochrane review of surgical treatment for bowel obstruction showed considerable variation in the rates of symptom relief and re-obstruction.[162] Whilst some patients may not re-obstruct even though the cancer continues to progress, there is an operative mortality and a few patients will develop post-operative faecal fistulas. Peritonitis is an

Table 19.50 Bowel obstruction: management guidelines

Favour earlier surgical intervention	Favour symptomatic management
Acute ± complete	Subacute ± intermittent ± incomplete
Peritonitis	No focal signs
	Multiple palpable masses
Strangulated hernia	
Gastric outlet obstruction	
First episode of obstruction	Multiple episodes of obstruction
Previous benign obstruction	
Previous radiotherapy	
Previous surgical findings do not preclude successful surgery	Previous surgical findings preclude successful surgery
Younger, fitter patient	Older, more debilitated
Other systemic therapy available	No systemic therapy available
Patient's consent	Patient declines surgery

indication for surgery, except for the terminally ill. Patients with gastric outlet obstruction are less likely to respond to symptomatic management than patients with lower obstruction. Creation of a gastroenterostomy or the use of a percutaneous gastrostomy as a venting procedure should be considered for patients with a high complete obstruction whose nausea and vomiting are otherwise difficult to control.[163]

Colorectal obstruction due to luminal tumour may be treated with endoscopic laser resection or stent insertion.[164] The procedures are well tolerated and preferred to a colostomy. Colorectal stents provide good palliation for the majority of patients.[165]

Symptomatic management. Symptomatic management of nausea, vomiting and pain will benefit many patients with advanced cancer and bowel obstruction for whom surgery is considered inappropriate (Table 19.51).[161] Nausea and vomiting are reduced to a minimum; for some patients with chronic obstruction, vomiting once or twice a day may be 'well tolerated'

Table 19.51 Symptomatic treatment of bowel obstruction

Antiemetics	
metoclopramide	10mg PO, SC q4-6h or 40-60mg/24h CSCI
cyclizine	50mg PO, SC q8h or 150mg/24h CSCI
haloperidol	0.5-1mg PO q6h or 3-5mg/24h CSCI
Analgesics	
morphine	PO, PR or CSCI
Anticholinergics	
hyoscine butylbromide	20mg PO or SC q6h or 60-120mg/24h CSCI
hyoscine hydrobromide	0.4mg SC q6h or 0.6-1.2mg/24h CSCI
Prokinetic agent	
cisapride	10mg PO q6-8h
Somatostatin analogue	
octreotide	0.1mg SC q8h or 0.3-0.5mg/24h CSCI
Corticosteroid	
dexamethasone	8-16mg/d PO or 8-16mg/24h CSCI

Table 19.52 Symptomatic management of bowel obstruction: RCTs

Author	n	Intervention	Outcome
Hardy[169]	35	dexamethasone vs placebo	no conclusion: obstruction resolved on dexamethasone (13) and placebo (8)
Laval[171]	52	methylprednisolone vs placebo	prednisolone: symptom relief 68 vs 33% (pS) in patients without nasogastric tubes
Mercadante[166]	18	octreotide vs hyoscine butylbromide	octreotide: less nausea and vomiting (pS)
Ripamonti[167]	17	octreotide vs hyoscine butylbromide	both reduce secretions and colicky pain; ↓ secretions greater with octreotide (pS)
Mystakidou[168]	68	analgesics, antiemetics ± octreotide	octreotide: less nausea, vomiting, fatigue, anorexia (all pS)

and preferred to a nasogastric tube. The gastrokinetic drugs (metoclopramide, domperidone) are contraindicated for patients with high small bowel obstruction as they may aggravate vomiting. Cisapride has a prokinetic effect on the whole bowel and may be used if there is no physical obstruction or ileus. Anticholinergic drugs reduce gastrointestinal secretions and lessen nausea, vomiting and colic. Octreotide reduces gastrointestinal secretions and motility and can control refractory vomiting in patients with bowel obstruction (Table19.52).[166–168] Corticosteroids are of benefit in some patients with chronic bowel obstruction (Table 19.52).[169–171] Additional measures include the treatment and prevention of constipation and a dietary programme of small meals with reduced roughage. Several small RCTs have been performed regarding symptomatic management of bowel obstruction (Table 19.52).

Terminal care

Treatment is symptomatic with analgesic, antiemetic and anticholinergic drugs. Surgical considerations are usually inappropriate. Nasogastric tubes and intravenous lines are unnecessary and undignified.

Constipation

Constipation is infrequent or difficult defaecation. It is the passage of a reduced number of bowel actions, which may or may not be abnormally hard, with increased difficulty. The term obstipation is sometimes used to refer to extreme constipation or faecal impaction. Constipation implies a significant variation from the normal bowel habit for an individual patient.

Normal defaecation depends on a number of physiological processes, abnormalities of which produce constipation. A large volume of fluid is secreted in the upper gastrointestinal

Table 19.53 Causes of constipation

General	Colorectal
immobility, inactivity	obstruction
muscular weakness, debility	pelvic tumour mass
confusion, sedation	radiation fibrosis, stricture
fear of bedpans	painful anorectal conditions
inability to access or use toilet	Drugs
Nutritional	opioid analgesics
decreased intake	antidiarrhoeals
low residue diet	non-opioid analgesics
poor fluid intake	anticholinergic drugs or side effects
Metabolic	anticholinergics
dehydration	antispasmodics
hypercalcaemia	antidepressants
hypokalaemia	phenothiazines
uraemia	haloperidol
Neurological	antacids
cerebral tumour	antiemetics: 5HT$_3$ antagonists
spinal cord disease	anticancer: vinca alkaloids
sacral nerve root lesion	diuretics
Psychological	iron
depression	barium
fear of diarrhoea, incontinence	

tract, most of which is reabsorbed in the small intestine and most of the remainder in the colon; excessive resorption of fluid or a prolonged intestinal transit time will produce dry hard faeces. Defaecation is initiated by distension of the rectum with faecal material, which leads to reflex contraction of rectal smooth muscle and relaxation of the internal anal sphincter. Defaecation is achieved by contraction of the abdominal muscles and diaphragm and relaxation of the external anal sphincter. Reduced colonic motility or any abnormality of the motor or sensory nerves subserving defaecation will lead to constipation.

Cause. Constipation in patients with cancer is frequently multifactorial and due to two or more of the causes listed in Table 19.53. Many drugs used in palliative care predispose to constipation, especially the opioid analgesics.

Clinical features. Constipation varies from a reduction in the number or frequency of bowel actions in an otherwise asymptomatic patient, to complete cessation of activity with the symptoms and signs of faecal impaction. Stools may be abnormally hard, although constipation may occur with normal or soft stools if there is neurological disability. Patients with faecal impaction or rectal obstruction can present complaining of diarrhoea and continue to pass faecal material either as an overflow phenomenon or due to increased mucous production. Anorexia, nausea and vomiting frequently accompany severe constipation. Urinary retention may occur, especially in males.

Examination of the abdomen may reveal faecal masses in the left iliac fossa or along the whole length of the colon. Faecal masses are usually non-tender, relatively mobile and can be indented with pressure. Rectal examination will reveal any painful rectal condition or local tumour infiltration, whether or not there are faeces in the rectum, and whether they are hard or soft. Patients with spinal cord pathology may have reduced sensation but the anal tone and reflex are usually preserved. Patients with sacral nerve root lesions will have sensory loss over the sacral dermatomes and the anal tone and reflex are reduced or absent.

Assessment. The clinical assessment of constipation is summarized in Table 19.54. Further investigations are seldom necessary except for a plain x-ray to exclude bowel obstruction.

Table 19.54 Assessment of constipation: information required

Pattern of patient's recent bowel movements

Pattern of patient's pre-illness bowel movements
    previous long term use of laxatives

Use of potentially constipating drugs

Use of laxatives and their effect

Patient's food intake and its fibre content

Patient's fluid intake

Presence or absence of faeces in the rectum

Consistency of faeces - soft or hard

Presence of anal tone, reflex

Sacral nerve root sensation

Underlying cause - usually multiple

Stage of patient's disease and prognosis

Treatment

General measures. An adequate fluid intake is important in the prevention and treatment of constipation. Patients are encouraged to take food or fluids that have some laxative properties, such as fruit and prune juice. In the absence of intestinal obstruction, foods with high fibre content are encouraged. Large amounts of fibre are often poorly tolerated by elderly or debilitated patients and the amount should be increased slowly.

Lack of easy access to toilet facilities, or the ready availability of assistance to use them, can cause or aggravate constipation especially for elderly or frail patients. Privacy is important. An elevated toilet seat makes it easier for the patient to get on and off the toilet, and a foot stool facilitates the use of leg and abdominal muscles in the act of defaecation.

Laxatives. Laxatives are the mainstay of the treatment of constipation in palliative care. A range of different laxatives is commercially available and it is important to know what a patient has been taking, successfully or not. There is considerable variation between patients regarding the acceptability of different laxatives including palatability, frequency of cramps or colic, flatulence, and diarrhoea. A patient who has successfully used a particular laxative should have it continued unless there are specific medical reasons to change.

The various laxatives in clinical use are listed in Table 19.55. Bulk laxatives require one to three days to be effective and additional measures may be necessary during this phase. Some bulk forming laxatives are appropriate for long term use and may be preferred to bran or high fibre foods for reasons of palatability and because they do not produce flatulence. Bulk laxatives require the patient to drink extra fluid and are unsuitable for elderly or debilitated patients. Liquid paraffin (mineral oil) causes lipoid pneumonia if aspirated and should not be administered at night or to debilitated patients. It is available as a liquid or an emulsion and in proprietary preparations with phenolphthalein (Agarol) or magnesium hydroxide (Milpar). Most contact (stimulant) laxatives act primarily in the large bowel; docusate and castor oil act on both the small and large intestine. Docusate is one of the most commonly used laxatives and is available either alone or in mixed preparations with other laxatives. Castor oil is not recommended for patients with advanced cancer as it may cause profound diarrhoea. Osmotic laxatives are effective and safe for many patients but should not be given to the elderly or debilitated because of the risk of fluid and electrolyte imbalance.

The optimal laxative preparation for patients with opioid-induced constipation remains to be defined. Lactulose and senna were found to have similar efficacy in an RCT.[172] Another RCT comparing lactulose with a solution of polyethylene glycol with electrolytes (macrogol 3350) in patients taking methadone showed them to be equally effective but the polyethylene glycol had fewer adverse effects and was better tolerated.[173]

The opioid antagonist, naloxone, will prevent or reverse constipation due to opioid drugs,[174–177] but a proportion of patients will suffer symptoms of opioid withdrawal and a few will experience reversal of analgesia. Methylnaltrexone is an opioid antagonist that does not cross the blood-brain barrier and acts as a selective peripheral opioid receptor antagonist.[178] In volunteers and patients on methadone maintenance therapy, it prevents or reverses the effect of opioid drugs on the bowel without causing withdrawal symptoms or loss of analgesia (see Chapter 9, Table 9.8). [179, 180]

Erythromycin exerts a prokinetic effect by interaction with the motilin receptors. It is of benefit in some patients with constipation associated with scleroderma and (neuropathic) chronic intestinal pseudo-obstruction, but the effect may last only a few weeks.[181]

Table 19.55 Laxatives and suppositories

Bulk forming laxatives	
includes	psyllium, ispaghula, sterculia, methylcellulose, dietary fibre supplements
action	retention of intraluminal fluid → softens faeces and stimulates peristalsis
precautions	patients must drink extra fluids; unsuitable for elderly, debilitated
adverse effects	unpalatable, colic, flatulence (considerable individual variation)
Faecal softener and lubricant	
includes	liquid paraffin (mineral oil)
action	faecal softener and lubricant
adverse effects	lipoid pneumonia if aspirated
Faecal softener and stimulant	
includes	docusate, poloxamer
action	faecal softener and stimulant; also promotes secretion of fluid into bowel
Contact (stimulant) laxatives	
includes	polyphenolics: phenolphthalein, bisacodyl
	anthracenes: senna, cascara, danthron
action	promote secretion of fluid → softens faeces and stimulates peristalsis
adverse effects	dehydration and electrolyte imbalance in debilitated patients
Osmotic laxatives	
includes	magnesium salts: sulfate (Epsom salts), hydroxide (milk of magnesia)
	non-absorbable sugars: lactulose, sorbitol, mannitol, polyethylene glycol
action	draws fluid into bowel → softens faeces, stimulates peristalsis
precautions	patient must drink extra fluids; unsuitable for elderly, debilitated
adverse effects	colic, flatulence (considerable individual variation)
	dehydration and electrolyte imbalance in debilitated patients
Rectal suppositories	
includes	glycerin, bisacodyl
action	faecal softener (glycerin), contact or stimulant (bisacodyl)
use	glycerin inserted into faecal matter, bisacodyl against mucosa

Suppositories. Rectally administered laxatives (Table 19.55) are used to initiate evacuation of the lower bowel whilst awaiting the effect of orally administered medications. Regular use should be unnecessary except in patients with a neurogenic bowel.

Enemas. Enemas are used to relieve constipation if suppositories are ineffective. Small volume enemas such as Microlax are less distressing for the patient and easier to use in the home environment. For more difficult constipation, sodium phosphate enemas can be used but may cause fluid and electrolyte imbalance in debilitated or dehydrated patients. Soap and water enemas may cause fluid overload and should be discouraged. For refractory constipation an olive oil retention enema given overnight may be successful.

Prevention of constipation. The factors and situations that predispose to constipation are well known, and preventive treatment should be introduced before clinical problems develop (Table 19.56). This is particularly important for patients taking morphine or other opioid drugs. If treatment is to be for a longer term, every effort should be made to use dietary adjustment or bulk forming laxatives as the only means of treatment.

Treatment of established constipation. The treatment of established constipation requires the use of suppositories and enemas to clear the lower bowel before a normal bowel

Table 19.56 Prevention of constipation

Initial assessment	Laxatives
recent bowel action pattern	docusate 240-480mg nocte
pre-illness bowel action pattern	*or* bisacodyl 10-20mg nocte
recent use and effect of laxatives	± senna 15mg nocte
use of other constipating drugs	± lactulose 30ml nocte
General measures (where feasible)	and titrate against clinical effect
increased food intake	Explanation to patient, family
increased dietary fibre	Treatment of painful rectal conditions
or bulk forming laxative	Ensure access and ability to use toilet
increased fluid intake	Avoid constipating drugs if possible
encourage activity	Keep a record of bowel activity

Table 19.57 Management of constipation

Initial assessment (Table 19.54)

Rectal examination	
absent rectal tone, reflex or sensation: neurogenic bowel (see Table 19.58)	
no neurological abnormality	
faeces in rectum	
hard faeces	glycerin PR, microenema, enema (oil), disimpaction
soft faeces	bisacodyl or docusate PR, microenema, enema, disimpaction
empty rectum → plain x-ray	
no bowel obstruction	bisacodyl or docusate PR, oral medications
bowel obstruction	appropriate treatment

Institute a program of prevention (Table 19.56)

pattern can be established with oral medication (Table 19.57). Patients with faecal impaction may require manual disimpaction, which is only performed under cover of appropriate analgesia and sedation. With the exception of neurogenic constipation, the regular or continued use of suppositories and enemas should not be necessary.

Management of neurogenic bowel. The aim of bowel care is to evacuate the bowel every one or two days (depending on previous bowel habit) and at night or morning depending on what is most convenient for the patient (Table 19.58). With spinal cord lesions there is

Table 19.58 Management of neurogenic bowel

Spinal cord lesion: spastic bowel, hypertonic anal sphincter, sacral reflexes intact
   adequate fluid and fibre intake
   oral laxatives (avoid laxatives which cause excessive softening)
   rectal suppositories or stimulation leads to increased peristalsis and sphincter relaxation

Sacral nerve root lesion: reduced peristalsis, flaccid sphincter, sacral reflexes absent
   adequate fluid and fibre intake
   oral laxatives
   rectal suppositories or stimulation may lead to evacuation
   straining and abdominal massage
   cholinergic drugs (e.g. bethanechol 10mg PO q8h)

often an initial period of paralytic ileus and the programme of bowel care is initiated when bowel sounds return.

A similar programme with regard to diet, fluids and fibre is used for patients with sacral nerve root lesions. If the sacral reflexes are completely absent, rectal stimulation (manually or by suppositories) may be ineffective and evacuation is usually achieved by straining and abdominal massage. Bethanechol (10mg, 8-hourly) or neostigmine (25mg, 8-hourly) are helpful for some patients.

Terminal care

Significant symptoms due to constipation are rare during the last days or week of life. Oral intake of food and fluid is frequently limited and laxatives can usually be discontinued. A suppository or microenema can be used if the patient has pain, feels the urge to defaecate but is unable to do so, or if there is continued faecal incontinence due to impaction.

Diarrhoea

Diarrhoea is an increase in the frequency and fluidity of bowel actions. Diarrhoea implies a significant variation from the normal pattern of bowel movements for a particular patient.

Diarrhoea occurs when there is increased faecal water, caused by either increased secretion or reduced absorption. Osmotic diarrhoea occurs when increased amounts of water are drawn into the bowel by increased solute loads or laxatives. The amount of water is greater than can be absorbed by the bowel distal to the site of production, or the resorptive process is short-circuited by surgical or malignant fistulas. Secretory diarrhoea, with enhanced formation of gastrointestinal secretions, occurs with infection, inflammation and the hormone-related syndromes.

Diarrhoea in patients with advanced cancer is frequently multifactorial and due to two or more of the causes listed in Table 19.59. The hormone-related syndromes are described in Chapter 27.

Table 19.59 Causes of diarrhoea

Dietary	Inflammation
excess roughage, fibre	radiation, drugs
nasogastric, PEG feeding	Steatorrhoea (fat malabsorption)
enteric supplements	pancreatic insufficiency
Drugs	biliary obstruction, exclusion
laxatives	bacterial overgrowth
magnesium antacids	Bile salt malabsorption
misoprostol, cisapride	ileal resection or bypass
antibiotics, cytotoxics, others	bacterial overgrowth
Surgical	Hormonal
gastrectomy, vagotomy	carcinoid
enterocolic anastomosis	Zollinger-Ellison syndrome
Cancer	medullary carcinoma of thyroid
gastrocolic fistula	VIPoma and others
enterocolic fistula	Psychological
Haemorrhage	anxiety
Infection	Obstruction with overflow
pseudomembranous colitis	faecal impaction
blind loops	rectal tumour

Certain clinical features may suggest the cause. Diarrhoea associated with recent dietary alterations or the use of enteric supplements suggests an osmotic cause. Profuse watery diarrhoea unaffected by fasting suggests a hormonal cause. Postprandial diarrhoea associated with sweating and faintness occurs in the dumping syndrome due to vagotomy or partial gastrectomy. The acute onset of copious diarrhoea with mucous and blood occurring during (or up to six weeks after) antibiotic therapy suggests pseudomembranous colitis due to *Clostridium difficile* infection. Tenesmus suggests local rectal pathology.

Examination may show dehydration and anaemia. There may be generalized or local abdominal tenderness. Rectal examination will document the presence of proctitis or other rectal pathology and must be performed if faecal impaction is suspected.

Stool examination. Examination of the stool may be informative. The presence of frank blood indicates colonic or rectal disease although severe diarrhoea may cause minor bleeding from haemorrhoids or the rectum. Melaena indicates higher gastrointestinal bleeding. The bulky, greasy, malodorous stools of steatorrhoea indicate malabsorption. Small stools comprising mainly mucous and pus with very little faecal matter, with or without blood, suggest proctitis. The presence of clear fluid in or with the stool can be due to mucous secretion by a colorectal tumour or secondary to a bowel obstruction. Stool microscopy will show increased numbers of leucocytes in infective and inflammatory colitis but not in osmotic, secretory or malabsorptive diarrhoeas. Microscopy and culture may define the causative organism in infective diarrhoea.

Assessment. The cause is usually evident from the history and clinical assessment, which includes rectal examination and inspection of the stool. Pseudomembranous colitis is confirmed by the sigmoidoscopic appearance and by assay for the *C. difficile* toxin. A plain x-ray is performed if bowel obstruction is suspected. Depending on the patient's general condition and prognosis, other investigations (sigmoidoscopy, radiological examinations and special tests related to malabsorption) are performed if the results will significantly affect treatment. Terminally ill patients should be treated symptomatically and not investigated.

The grading criteria for diarrhoea caused by radiation and chemotherapy are listed in Table 19.60.

Table 19.60 NCI Common Toxicity Criteria grading of treatment-related diarrhoea[38]

0	none
1	increase of <4 stools/d over pretreatment
2	increase of 4-6 stools/d, or nocturnal stools
3	increase of ≥7 stools/d, or incontinence, or need for parenteral hydration
4	physiological consequences requiring intensive care; or haemodynamic collapse

Treatment

The treatment of diarrhoea includes symptomatic measures and therapy directed at the underlying cause (Table 19.61).

General measures. Maintenance of hydration is important except in the terminally ill. Commercially available soft drinks can be used although colas containing caffeine (a bowel stimulant) and diet drinks containing sorbitol (a laxative) are best avoided. Oral rehydration solutions are commercially available. Intravenous rehydration may be necessary if diarrhoea is severe or if there is vomiting. Dietary modification to both reduce diarrhoea and to ensure adequate nutrition are important and the assistance of a dietician is useful. Measures to protect the perianal skin, including the use of zinc creams are important.

Table 19.61 Management of diarrhoea

General measures
    maintenance of hydration
    dietary modification
    skin protection
    pain relief

Treatment of underlying cause (Table 19.62)

Antidiarrhoeal agents (Table 19.63)

Table 19.62 Treatment of selected underlying causes of diarrhoea

Dietary: dietary modification, more dilute enteric feeding

Drugs: adjust, withdraw

Gastrectomy, vagotomy: small frequent meals

Infection
    pseudomembranous colitis: vancomycin 125mg q6h or metronidazole 400mg q8h
    bacterial overgrowth: broad spectrum antibiotic

Radiation: low residue diet, aspirin or NSAID, octreotide

Chemotherapy: loperamide, corticosteroid, octreotide

Steatorrhoea
    obstructive jaundice: appropriate therapy (see Table 19.79)
    ileal resection, bypass: cholestyramine 12-16g/d, low fat diet
    pancreatic insufficiency: enzyme supplements, H_2 receptor antagonist, dietary advice

Hormonal
    Zollinger-Ellison: proton pump inhibitor
    carcinoid: cyproheptadine, octreotide
    VIPoma: octreotide

Treatment of the underlying cause. The underlying cause is treated, where possible (Table 19.62).

Antidiarrhoeal agents. Medications used in the treatment of diarrhoea are listed in Table 19.63. Unless morphine or codeine is being given for analgesia, loperamide is the agent of choice. It is more effective than diphenoxylate or codeine, has few side effects, and does not cause central nervous system depression.

Radiation enteritis. Sucralfate has been recommended for the prevention and amelioration of radiation enteritis, but two RCTs have shown that it does not reduce the incidence or severity of diarrhoea or proctitis and that there may be more rectal bleeding and other gastrointestinal symptoms.[182, 183] Amifostine reduces the incidence and severity of proctitis associated with pelvic radiotherapy (Table 19.64).[72, 184] RCTs with salicylates (5-aminosalicylic acid) have produced mixed results: sulfasalazine reduced the diarrhoea caused by pelvic radiotherapy,[185] mesalazine had no significant effect,[186] and olsalazine increased the severity and duration of diarrhoea.[187] Psyllium (Metamucil) was effective in preventing diarrhoea,[188] but ispaghula was ineffective in treating it.[189] Antibiophilus (*Lactobacillus rhamnosus*) reduced radiation-induced diarrhoea,[190] as did octreotide.[191] A Cochrane

Table 19.63 Antidiarrhoeal agents

Absorbant agents	
include	hydrophilic bulking agents e.g. methylcellulose, ispaghula
action	absorption of excess fluid
Adsorbant agents	
include	kaolin preparations
action	adsorption of bacteria, toxins and excess fluid
Prostaglandin inhibitors	
include	aspirin, NSAIDs (excepting mefenamic acid, indomethacin)
action	reduction in gastrointestinal secretions
use	radiation enteritis
Opioids	
include	loperamide, diphenoxylate (with atropine 25μg) (Lomotil), codeine
action	inhibition of peristalsis
use	loperamide: 4mg initially, 2-4mg q8-12h, up to 16mg/d
	diphenoxylate 5-10mg initially, 2.5-5.0mg q4-8h, up to 20mg/d
	codeine: 15-60mg q4h
adverse effects	loperamide: few significant side effects, no CNS depression
	diphenoxylate: CNS depression may occur at doses >20mg/d
	codeine: nausea, sedation and CNS depression at higher doses

Table 19.64 Radiation-related diarrhoea: RCTs

Author	n	Intervention	Outcome
Koukourakis[72]	40	pelvic radiation ± amifostine	amifostine: less proctitis and bladder toxicity (pS)
Kouvaris[184]	36	pelvic radiation ± amifostine	amifostine: grade ≥1 proctitis in 11 vs 88% (pS)
Martenson[187]	58	pelvic radiation + olsalazine vs placebo	olsalazine: ↑ severity and duration of diarrhoea (pS)
Resbeut[186]	153	pelvic radiation + mesalazine vs placebo	mesalazine: no significant effect
Kilic[185]	87	pelvic radiation + sulfasalazine vs placebo	sulfasalazine: diarrhoea in 55 vs 86% (pS)
Murphy[188]	60	pelvic radiation ± psyllium	psyllium: ↓ incidence and severity of diarrhoea (pS)
Lodge[189]	10	radiation diarrhoea: codeine vs ispaghula	codeine significantly more effective (trial terminated)
Urbancsek[190]	206	radiation diarrhoea: Antibiophilus vs placebo	Antibiophilus: ↓ severity of diarrhoea (pS)
Yavuz[191]	61	radiation diarrhoea: octreotide vs Lomotil	octreotide: resolution of diarrhoea within 3d: 55 vs 14% (pS)

review of therapy for diarrhoea and other symptoms of late radiation proctitis reported that a number of different treatments were used including NSAIDs, sucralfate, metronidazole and corticosteroids, but that the lack of controlled studies did not allow any firm conclusions or recommendations.[192]

Chemotherapy enteritis. Treatment of chemotherapy-induced diarrhoea includes withdrawal of the offending agent, loperamide and general supportive measures. Oral therapy with the topical corticosteroid budesonide[193] and subcutaneous octreotide[194] are both reported to be effective in reducing diarrhoea.

Terminal care

Diarrhoea should be controlled with oral loperamide or, for patients not taking oral medication, subcutaneous morphine. Investigations and energetic rehydration are inappropriate.

Faecal incontinence, rectal discharge

Faecal incontinence may occur with any cause of diarrhoea, especially if the diarrhoea is severe or the patient weak (Table 19.65).

Table 19.65   Causes of faecal incontinence and rectal discharge

Diarrhoea	Rectovesical and rectovaginal fistulas
Faecal impaction with overflow	Neurogenic
Rectal tumours	spinal cord lesions
Proctitis	sacral nerve root lesions
Rectal or pelvic surgery	

The complications of faecal incontinence include anal pain and discomfort, pruritus, and maceration or excoriation of the perianal skin that predisposes to ulceration. It may also cause considerable psychological distress with feelings of shame or disgust caused by loss of control over bowel function and the need for frequent washing and changing.

Clinical assessment usually indicates the cause. Rectal examination will disclose impaction, rectal disease or neurological abnormalities. Further investigations are rarely necessary.

Treatment

Treatment is directed at the cause and to protection of the perianal skin (Table 19.66). Successful treatment of faecal incontinence will do much for patients' physical functioning, self-esteem, dignity, and quality of life. A Cochrane review of therapy for late radiation proctitis reported that a number of different treatments were used including NSAIDs, sucralfate,

Table 19.66   Treatment of faecal incontinence, rectal discharge

Diarrhoea	appropriate therapy (see Diarrhoea)
Faecal impaction	appropriate therapy (see Constipation)
Local tumour	diathermy, laser, radiotherapy, surgery
Proctitis	corticosteroids (PR or PO), antibiotics
Skin care	

metronidazole and corticosteroids, but that the lack of controlled studies did not allow any firm conclusions or recommendations.[192]

Skin care. Whatever the cause of faecal incontinence, the perianal and perineal skin needs to be protected. The perineum is washed using a soft cloth after each bowel action or more frequently if the discharge is considerable. Soaps and abrasive toilet paper are avoided as they aggravate skin irritation. The skin is patted dry with a soft cloth and dusted with zinc stearate or baby powder. If the skin is inflamed, hydrocortisone cream can be used for a few days, but may predispose to maceration and fungal infection. In general, ointments and creams are avoided as they will tend to keep the skin moist. Zinc oxide paste can be used to protect areas of intact skin that are otherwise hard to keep dry. Candida infection is treated with 1% clotrimazole solution. Loose cotton undergarments are worn and need to be changed frequently.

Neurogenic incontinence. For patients with a spinal cord lesion and a reasonable life expectancy, a programme of bowel training is initiated (see Table 19.58). Patients with sacral nerve root damage and those with a short life expectancy, for whom bowel retraining is not feasible, require a different approach. Dietary fibre is reduced and bulk laxatives avoided. Constipation is induced using codeine or loperamide, and regular bowel evacuations are planned once or twice a week using suppositories (if successful) or enemas.

Terminal care

Faecal incontinence should be managed as simply as possible. If present, faecal impaction should be treated. In other situations it is probably best to induce a constipated state. Troublesome rectal discharge due to proctitis is treated with topical corticosteroids.

Perianal and vulval pruritus

The cause of perianal and vulval pruritus (Table 19.67) is usually evident on clinical examination. Microbiological specimens are taken if infection is suspected.

Table 19.67 Causes of perianal and vulval pruritus

Infection
candida, herpes simplex, condyloma acuminatum, bacterial
Irradiation
Malignant infiltration
Poor local hygiene
Incontinence, discharge
rectal, vaginal, urinary
Generalized pruritus, generalized dermatological condition

Treatment

Treatment. Treatment is that of the cause together with scrupulous skin hygiene, as described above for incontinent patients. Ointments and creams are best avoided as they may be allergenic and they will tend to keep the skin moist. Topical hydrocortisone cream can be used for a few days if irritation is severe. Zinc oxide paste will protect intact skin. Antipruritic lotions that may help in severe cases are crotamiton (Eurax) and aluminium acetate (Burow's solution).

Flatulence

Flatulence is the passage of excessive amounts of intestinal gas.

Gastric. Upper gastrointestinal flatulence is due to swallowed air. It is more common in people who are anxious, eat quickly or smoke. Behavioural modifications are usually successful. Other treatments include peppermint water, aerated drinks, or simethicone, a defoaming agent that facilitates bringing up wind.

Intestinal. Intestinal gas is due to swallowed air and the chemical and bacterial degradation of food. Gas production will be increased by the ingestion of high fibre foods and nonabsorbable carbohydrates, or with bacterial overgrowth in the small intestine. Increased intestinal gas production may cause distension, bloating, audible bowel sounds (borborygmi), painful colic and embarrassment at the noise and smell of wind passed. Dietary modifications or the use of an alternative laxative usually alleviate symptoms. Physical exercise, which aids the passage of flatus, should be encouraged. Abdominal massage may help frail and bedbound patients. Activated charcoal can reduce both the amount of flatus passed and the odour. Antispasmodic anticholinergic drugs such as dicyclomine and mebeverine are useful in the treatment of intestinal colic. Patients with small bowel bacterial overgrowth are treated with antibiotics.

Lower gastrointestinal bleeding

The cause of rectal or lower gastrointestinal bleeding (Table 19.68) can usually be determined by rectal examination and sigmoidoscopy.

Table 19.68   Causes of lower gastrointestinal bleeding

Rectal	carcinoma
	proctitis: infection, radiotherapy, chemotherapy
	haemorrhoids
Colonic	carcinoma
	colitis: infection, pseudomembranous colitis, radiotherapy
	diverticular disease
Proximal	massive upper gastrointestinal bleeding
Systemic	thrombocytopenia, coagulopathy

Treatment

The treatment is that of the cause. Unresectable tumours can be treated with diathermy, laser photocoagulation or radiotherapy.[164] The topical application of 1% alum will help control bleeding from rectal tumours. Proctitis and colitis are treated with topical or oral corticosteroids. Pseudomembranous colitis is treated with oral vancomycin or metronidazole. Other infective causes are treated with appropriate antibiotics. Prevention of constipation and diarrhoea will avoid aggravation of haemorrhoids or other rectal conditions.

Terminal care

Simple symptomatic measures are used to stop or control the bleeding, and the patient reassured. Massive rectal haemorrhage in a dying patient should be treated with parenteral morphine and midazolam, given to allay anxiety.

Stomas

A colostomy may be created following bowel resection for cancer, to relieve obstruction, or to relieve the symptoms of a distal fistula. It may be either temporary or permanent. A loop colostomy is usually temporary and is the externalization of a loop of colon. A terminal colostomy is usually permanent, the proximal colon being secured to the surface. A colostomy is usually managed by wearing a drainage bag or appliance.

An ileostomy is created as a permanent procedure after proctocolectomy or where there are multiple sites of malignant obstruction in the distal bowel. An ileostomy will never drain solid faeces and skin problems are more likely because of the fluid nature of the discharge and the content of digestive enzymes.

Appliances. The appliance used for an ileostomy or colostomy is either one- or two-piece. A one-piece appliance is a self-adhesive bag that is applied directly to the skin; these are disposable and relatively easy to handle. A two-piece appliance has an adhesive flange that is attached to the skin, and a bag that separately clips onto the flange. These are better for patients with sore or sensitive skin as the flange can be left in place whilst the bag is changed. The bags used with these appliances are drainable or closed. A drainable bag is used for an ileostomy or colostomy with a fluid output. It should be emptied frequently and changed each two or three days. Flatus filters are not used as fluid faeces will inactivate the charcoal and can leak through the filter. A closed bag, used when faeces are the consistency of normal stool, is changed once or twice a day and flatus filters are used.

Skin care. Skin care is of great importance. Local inflammation and excoriation predispose to the appliance fitting poorly, which in turn leads to leakage and more skin damage. The peristomal skin is cleansed with water and mild soap; detergents, disinfectants and antiseptics should not be used as they may cause irritation and dryness. A variety of preparations are available to protect skin, improve appliance adhesion and to allow healing of sore or broken skin. Severely inflamed peristomal skin can be treated with a corticosteroid cream or, if indicated by laboratory tests, a topical antibiotic. After application of this cream, the area is sealed with Opsite spray or similar sealant and the appliance fitted.

Table 19.69 Treatment of some ostomy-related problems

Diarrhoea		Flatus and odour	
ileostomy	opioid antidiarrhoeal	dietary modification	
colostomy	hydrophilic bulking agent	odour resistant disposable bags	
	stop drugs causing diarrhoea	deodorants added to bag	
	dietary modification	charcoal filters	
Constipation		oral medications *e.g.* charcoal	
colostomy	increase fluid intake		
	increase food, fibre		
	stop constipating drugs		
	laxative ± initial enema		

Other care. All patients who are to have a colostomy or ileostomy created require preoperative counselling and postoperative training by a stomal therapist. The management of diarrhoea, constipation, flatus and odour are outlined in Table 19.69. Physical problems that may require treatment are listed in Table 19.70.

Table 19.70 Physical stomal problems: treatment options

Obstruction	treat constipation, impaction, bowel obstruction
Recession	treat conservatively unless there are continence problems; surgery
Prolapse	manual reduction; surgery (not if intra-abdominal pressure raised)
Parastomal herniation	treat conservatively unless there are continence problems; surgery
Bleeding	topical sucralfate, 1% alum, silver nitrate; diathermy, laser
Stomal recurrence	diathermy, laser; surgery if causing incontinence
Perforation	use cone irrigation in preference to catheters

Fistulas

Enteric fistulas occur relatively frequently in patients with advanced cancer. Management depends on the type of fistula, the complications caused by the drainage, and the patient's general condition. A mucous fistula, created when the distal colon is brought to the surface after the formation of a permanent colostomy, produces little drainage and can be managed with a simple dry dressing.

Rectal. Rectovaginal and rectovesical fistulas are usually due to advanced pelvic disease and lead to passage of faecal material from the vagina or bladder. Creation of a defunctioning colostomy is the treatment of choice and provides complete relief. Terminally ill patients can be managed conservatively with reassurance, hygiene and skin care.

Enterocutaneous. Enterocutaneous fistulas usually develop as a complication of surgery. A small bowel fistula may produce copious amounts of fluid, leading to fluid and electrolyte depletion, and the presence of digestive enzymes will cause skin damage. Management includes collection of the discharge in a bag or appliance, protection of the skin as set out in the section on stoma care, fluid and electrolyte replacement, and measures to reduce the volume of drainage (Table 19.71). Octreotide is reported to decrease the amount of discharge from enterocutaneous fistulas,[195] but this has not been substantiated in prospective RCTs;[196, 197] there are no controlled studies of octreotide in patients with cancer.[198] A colonic fistula is managed in the same manner as a surgically created colostomy.

Table 19.71 Fistulas: drug treatment to reduce volume

Loperamide	4mg q6h
Hyoscine butylbromide	20mg PO q6h or 60–120mg/24h CSCI
Octreotide	0.1mg SC q8h or 0.25–0.5mg/24h CSCI

Buccal. Buccal fistulas between the mouth or pharynx and the face or neck will lead to leakage of saliva and ingested fluids. Small fistulas can be managed with regularly changed dry dressings. Larger fistulas may be improved with the use of plastic or silicone plugs, shaped or cast to the form of the fistula.

Ascites

Ascites is the accumulation of excess fluid in the peritoneal cavity, and is reported to occur in 15–50% of patients with cancer. Development of ascites in patients with cancer is associated with a life expectancy of a few months only, although some patients with ovarian cancer, lymphoma or other tumours that respond to systemic therapy may fare much better.[199, 200] A number of recent reviews of ascites have been published.[201–204]

Ascites develops if there is raised portal venous pressure (increased hydrostatic pressure), hypoproteinaemia (decreased oncotic pressure), peritoneal disease (fluid production exceeding resorption), or obstruction to the lymphatic channels from the peritoneum (Table 19.72). In patients with cancer, ascites is caused by peritoneal infiltration in about two-thirds of cases.[201] There may be multiple contributing causes as with a patient with extensive liver metastases (causing raised portal venous pressure and hypoalbuminaemia) in addition to peritoneal infiltration. In patients with advanced cancer, hypoproteinaemia is usually due to limited protein intake, the general catabolic state, and poor liver function and this may be compounded by the protein loss associated with repeated paracenteses. Chylous ascites is usually associated with malignant obstruction of the lymphatic system, but can also occur after surgery or radiotherapy.[201, 205]

Table 19.72   Causes of ascites

Raised portal venous pressure	Hypoalbuminaemia
cardiac failure	malnutrition
pericardial effusion, constriction	liver disease: cirrhosis, extensive cancer
IVC obstruction, thrombosis	protein loss (repeated paracenteses)
hepatic vein obstruction, thrombosis	Peritoneal disease
liver disease: cirrhosis, extensive cancer	malignant infiltration
portal vein obstruction, thrombosis	infection
Lymphatic obstruction	
abdominal lymphatics, thoracic duct	

The cancers associated with malignant ascites are usually epithelial carcinomas, particularly cancers of the ovary, colon, stomach, pancreas, breast and lung. Malignant lymphoma is a frequent cause of chylous ascites.

In patients with cancer and ascites, the amount of fluid present is usually considerable and the clinical features obvious. There is uniform abdominal distension with fullness of the flanks and the umbilicus may be flattened or protuberant. Examination shows characteristic shifting dullness and there may be a fluid thrill. Symptoms related to gastric compression and increased intra-abdominal pressure including anorexia, early satiety, nausea, and oesophageal reflux are common. Patients with tense ascites are usually dyspnoeic because of elevation of the diaphragm. Peripheral oedema of the legs and genitalia is common.

Investigations to confirm the presence of ascites are usually unnecessary. Plain x-ray will show a 'ground glass' appearance. Smaller volumes of ascitic fluid, as little as 100–200ml, can be detected on ultrasound or CT scanning.

A diagnostic paracentesis is performed to determine the cause of the ascites. Normal peritoneal fluid is clear. Ascites complicating primary liver disease and cardiac failure is clear and faintly amber. Carcinomatosis produces opaque straw-coloured fluid that may be blood stained. Chylous fluid, indicating lymphatic obstruction, has a milky, yellow or white appearance. Measurement of the serum-ascites albumin gradient (SAAG) (serum albumin concentration minus the ascitic fluid albumin concentration) has been shown to correlate with portal venous pressure and may predict which patients are more likely to respond to diuretic therapy; a SAAG of ≥11g/l is associated with raised portal venous pressure (Table 19.73).[206] Cytological examination will reveal malignant cells in 80–100% of cases where there is peritoneal infiltration, particularly if larger volumes (0.5–1L) are submitted for examination. If chylous ascites is suspected, triglyceride levels should be measured; a level above the serum triglyceride confirms the chylous nature of the fluid.

Table 19.73   Ascitic fluid characteristics

Type response	Colour	Cytology	SAAG	Diuretic
Raised portal venous pressure	clear	–	≥11g/l	yes
Peritoneal infiltration	opaque	+	≤11g/l	no
Lymphatic obstruction	chylous	–	≤11g/l	no

Treatment

The management options for the treatment of ascites are summarized in Table 19.74. The treatment of ascites due to cardiac and liver disease or to venous obstruction is directed at the underlying cause. Ascites unrelated to cancer is treated with appropriate therapy. Systemic or intraperitoneal therapy should be considered for sensitive tumours, as a response will lead to

Table 19.74   Options for the treatment of ascites

Ascites related to cancer
   observation
   systemic or intraperitoneal therapy (sensitive tumours)
   diuretics
       for patients with cirrhosis or extensive liver metastases
       spironolactone 100mg/d PO with frusemide 40mg/d PO
   paracentesis
   peritoneal drain
   peritoneovenous shunt
       for refractory ascites that is not bloody, viscous or loculated
   intraperitoneal therapy
   porto-systemic shunt

Chylous ascites
   corticosteroids, radiotherapy
   systemic therapy (sensitive tumours)
   peritoneovenous shunt

Ascites unrelated to cancer
   appropriate therapy

resolution or control of ascites. Mild ascites, which is neither progressive nor causing symptoms, is managed with reassurance and observation.

Diuretic therapy. Patients with liver disease (due to cirrhosis or extensive hepatic metastases) have portal hypertension and may respond to diuretic therapy in the same way as cirrhotic patients without cancer.[206–208] The recommended therapy is with spironolactone 100 mg/d and frusemide 40 mg/d. The addition of frusemide may augment the action of spironolactone and reduces the risk of significant hyperkalaemia. The response to spironolactone may take up to two weeks and it may be associated with gynaecomastia. The doses may be titrated upward, each few days, to a maximum of spironolactone 400 mg/d and frusemide 160 mg/d. Careful monitoring is required, as some patients may develop intravascular dehydration that can result in renal impairment. Patients may complain of weakness, lethargy and postural hypotension and their clinical condition, electrolytes and renal function should be monitored weekly, at least initially. The diuretic doses are titrated against response and adverse effects, the goal being to control symptoms rather than to render the patient free of ascites. Amiloride is an alternative to spironolactone and has a faster onset of action.[203] Salt and fluid restriction, as might be prescribed for patients with cirrhotic ascites, are usually considered burdensome for patients with advanced cancer.

Paracentesis. Paracentesis is performed using an intravenous or peritoneal dialysis catheter and may be performed as an outpatient procedure or in the patient's home.[209] Ultrasound-guided placement of the catheter is safer, and should be used where it is available. It is usually possible to drain 4–6 litres of ascitic fluid, by gravity, over the first few hours;[210] drainage into vacuum bottles allows the procedure to be completed in half an hour.[209] Drainage for more than six hours is probably unnecessary, as the symptomatic benefit is maximal after the first few litres are removed[211] and drainage is usually minimal after this time. Catheters left in place for longer periods of time increase the risk of infection and fluid loculation. Hypotension or hypovolaemic shock is uncommon in patients with malignant ascites, even though large volumes of fluid may be removed relatively quickly. Care must be taken with patients with hypotension or intravascular dehydration prior to the procedure. The co-administration of intravenous plasma volume expanders or albumin has not been demonstrated to be of benefit in patients with malignant ascites.

Peritoneal drains. Patients with rapidly recurring ascites requiring weekly paracenteses can be considered for the placement of an indwelling catheter. These are tunnelled subcutaneously and the patient or family member can be trained to drain the fluid at home on a daily or weekly basis, as required. These drains provide good symptom relief but are prone to infection.[212–215] There are no studies comparing repeated paracentesis with peritoneal drains.

Peritoneovenous shunt. Peritoneovenous shunting is successful as a palliative measure in some patients with malignant ascites not responding to diuretic therapy or poorly controlled by paracenteses.[200, 202, 216] The lower end is inserted into the peritoneal cavity, the other in the superior vena cava. Shunt insertion is associated with a small but significant operative mortality in patients with malignant ascites.[203] The shunts perform poorly in patients with bloody or viscous ascites and those with loculated fluid. Complications include fever, infection, shunt blockage and coagulopathy. About one-third of shunts require revision or replacement. Laboratory evidence of disseminated intravascular coagulation (DIC) may occur but rarely causes clinical problems. Facilitating haematogenous tumour spread is a theoretical disadvantage, but the incidence of significant dissemination of disease is very low. A comparison of patients with malignant ascites treated by paracentesis and by peritoneovenous shunting showed no difference in survival or quality of life.[217]

Intraperitoneal therapy. Intraperitoneal therapy with various chemotherapy drugs, radioisotopes and biological agents has been employed to inhibit the reaccumulation of fluid.[201, 204] The efficacy of such treatment in patients with advanced disease has not been established in any controlled studies and it has no established place in palliative care. Response seems to depend on the nature of the underlying tumour and is most frequently reported for ovarian cancer. Intraperitoneal triamcinolone may reduce the rate of reaccumulation of malignant ascites.[218]

Chylous ascites. Chylous ascites is due to lymphatic obstruction in the high retroperitoneal region or the mediastinum. Repeated paracenteses will produce only transient improvement. Radiotherapy and corticosteroids can be employed if there is a demonstrable mass obstructing lymphatic flow in the mediastinum or the retroperitoneum. Patients with chylous ascites who have malignant lymphoma may respond well. The use of a peritoneovenous shunt for the management of chylous ascites has been reported.[205]

Portosystemic shunt. Transjugular intrahepatic portosystemic shunt (TIPSS) has been employed for two patients with cancer who had intractable ascites associated with severe portal hypertension. The procedure, which creates an anastomosis between branches of the portal and hepatic veins was well tolerated and provided significant clinical improvement.[219]

Octreotide therapy reduced malignant ascites in two of three patients treated.[220]

Terminal care

Terminally ill patients who are symptomatic of ascites are managed by paracentesis, performed as infrequently as possible.

Liver metastases

The liver is a common site for metastatic disease. More than half of patients with gastrointestinal cancer will develop liver metastases. Other tumours that commonly metastasize to the liver include lung and breast cancer and malignant melanoma.

Most patients with liver metastases are symptomatic (Table 19.75). There is often a general and non-specific decline in the patient's health with anorexia, nausea and weight loss. There may be discomfort or pain in the region of the right costal margin, aggravated by coughing or changes in posture. Marked hepatomegaly may cause abdominal distension and symptoms related to gastric compression. Irritation of the undersurface of the diaphragm will cause pain in the region of the shoulder. Acute severe pain can be caused by small capsular

Table 19.75 Hepatic metastases

General
    anorexia, nausea, weight loss

Pain
    diffuse discomfort or pain in region of liver
    acute severe localized pain due to small capsular tear or perimetastatic haemorrhage
    shoulder pain caused by diaphragmatic irritation

Marked hepatomegaly
    abdominal distension ± jaundice
    gastric compression and gastro-oesophageal reflux
    right lower lobe collapse ± small effusion

tears or perimetastatic haemorrhage. The pain is usually well localized in the right upper quadrant and associated with tenderness and guarding.

Examination usually shows some degree of hepatomegaly, which can be tender and nodular. Jaundice may be present. Patients with marked hepatomegaly may have signs suggestive of collapse of the right lower lobe of the lung, consistent with elevation of the right hemidiaphragm.

The diagnosis of liver metastases is made on the clinical features, abnormal liver function tests and can be confirmed on ultrasound or CT scanning. Biopsy is rarely required to differentiate metastatic disease from other pathology.

Treatment

The treatment options for hepatic metastases are shown in Table 19.76. Systemic therapy should be considered for sensitive tumours.

Table 19.76 Liver metastases in patients with advanced cancer: treatment options

Systemic therapy	chemotherapy, hormonal (sensitive tumours)
Surgery	excision, cryosurgery, injection
Radiotherapy	external, internal (radioisotopes)
Symptomatic	analgesics, antiemetics, dietary manipulation, corticosteroids

Surgery. Surgical resection of liver metastases may be of benefit for a single or small number of lesions but has no role in the treatment of patients with widespread cancer.[221] Intraoperative or percutaneous cryotherapy, in which accessible malignant tissue is destroyed with a cryoprobe, is reported to improve the outlook for small numbers of selected patients.[222] Complications may be severe, including myoglobinuria and acute tubular necrosis, and the role of this technique is not defined. Intralesional injection of absolute alcohol, microwave therapy, and radiofrequency ablation are methods that have been used for primary liver tumours, but their role in the treatment of metastatic disease remains to be defined.[223, 224]

Radiotherapy. Radiotherapy is limited by the tolerance of the normal liver tissue to irradiation. Doses of 24 Gy in 3 Gy fractions will produce significant symptomatic improvement in the majority of patients, with tolerable toxicity.[225] Anorexia, nausea, vomiting and transient abnormalities of the liver function tests occur frequently. Higher doses of irradiation will cause radiation hepatitis associated with portal hypertension and ascites appearing one to three months after treatment. Radioisotopes may allow higher doses of radiation to be selectively delivered to tumour sites.[226]

Symptomatic. The symptomatic treatment of hepatic metastases includes the use of analgesics, antiemetics and dietary modification. Pain is usually well controlled with non-opioid drugs except for episodes of severe acute pain, which are treated with rest and opioid analgesics. Avoidance of fatty foods and the taking of multiple small meals can be helpful.

Corticosteroids will improve symptoms in the majority of patients with hepatic metastases. Prednisolone 25–50 mg/d usually produces a significant reduction in anorexia, nausea and discomfort; it may also improve pruritus, if present. The dose is weaned to the minimum effective dose after a few days. The effect usually lasts for a number of weeks, following which further benefit can sometimes be gained by increasing the dose.

Hepatic failure and encephalopathy

Hepatic failure can occur as a terminal event in patients with extensive hepatic metastases or chronic biliary obstruction. It can also occur in patients with cancer, with or without liver metastases, due to a number of other causes (Table 19.77). Hepatic encephalopathy occurs in patients with impaired liver function, precipitated by a variety of factors (Table 19.78).

Table 19.77   Causes of hepatic failure

Cancer: extensive hepatic replacement, biliary obstruction

Drugs: anticancer, paracetamol, antibiotics, others

Radiation

Alcohol

Viral infection (hepatitis)

Systemic infection

Hepatic vein occlusion, thrombosis (Budd-Chiari syndrome)

Hepatic veno-occlusive disease

Table 19.78   Precipitating factors that may induce hepatic encephalopathy

Increased production and absorption of ammonia and nitrogenous compounds
  excess dietary protein, gastrointestinal bleeding, constipation

Hypovolaemia
  diuretics, haemorrhage, septicaemia, rapid paracentesis

Further liver damage
  drug reactions, alcohol, viral hepatitis, septicaemia

Metabolic disturbance
  uraemia

Drugs causing CNS depression
  sedatives, tranquillizers, opioid analgesics

The clinical features of hepatic failure include jaundice, ascites, peripheral oedema, hepatic encephalopathy and renal failure. The syndrome of hepatic encephalopathy occurs when substances from the intestine reach the brain by porto-systemic shunting, via collateral vessels. Increased blood ammonia levels are responsible for some features of this syndrome but other toxic substances are involved and blood ammonia levels do not always correlate with the clinical state. The clinical features of hepatic encephalopathy vary from a mild disturbance of mental function to coma. In the initial phase there may be apathy, personality alteration and a reversal of the normal sleep pattern.[208] This can progress to an agitated confusional state, leading to somnolence, stupor and coma. There may be a non-rhythmical flapping tremor (asterixis, liver flap) and sweetish musty breath (foetor hepaticus).

Treatment

The treatment of hepatic failure depends on the cause and the stage of the patient's disease and prognosis. In patients who are terminally ill, only measures directed at patient comfort should be considered. In patients not considered terminally ill, the underlying cause is treated as well as measures to treat or prevent the encephalopathy. The treatment involves the withdrawal or treatment of any precipitating cause, dietary protein restriction, and oral lactulose or neomycin to reduce ammonia production. Agitation is treated with diazepam or other benzodiazepine. Hallucinations and psychoses are treated with chlorpromazine or haloperidol. Central nervous system suppressant drugs should be used with caution in patients with hepatic encephalopathy but there is no contraindication to their use for the control of neurological and psychiatric symptoms, especially in the terminally ill.

Biliary tract obstruction

Malignant obstruction of the biliary tract occurs most commonly with carcinoma of the pancreas but can be caused by any tumour infiltrating the region of the porta hepatis.

Biliary tract obstruction is characterized by jaundice, light coloured stools, dark urine and pruritus. Pain occurs less frequently in malignant biliary obstruction than in obstruction due to cholelithiasis. The pathogenesis of the pruritus is complex and multifactorial. Evidence suggests it is partly related to stimulation of dermal itch receptors by bile acids in addition to a central mechanism associated with increased endogenous opioid production by the liver (see Pruritus, Chapter 24).

Liver function tests show elevation of the bilirubin and alkaline phosphatase out of proportion to the elevation in the transaminases. Ultrasonography is the most accurate means of confirming biliary obstruction. It will detect obstruction in up to 90% of cases but is less useful in determining the site and the cause of obstruction; CT scanning is more accurate and MRI cholangiogram is the investigation of choice. Direct cholangiography provides an accurate means of localizing the obstruction. This may be performed either endoscopically (endoscopic retrograde cholangiopancreatography, ERCP) or by the percutaneous cannulation of hepatic ducts (percutaneous transhepatic cholangiography, PTHC). Both constitute invasive procedures and are subject to complications: PTHC may be complicated by sepsis, biliary peritonitis and haemorrhage; and ERCP by pancreatitis, haemorrhage, sepsis and perforation of the biliary tract.

Treatment

The treatment options are listed in Table 19.79. Systemic anticancer therapy should be considered for sensitive tumours. Pruritus will be relieved if the obstruction is overcome or can be palliated with various medications (see Pruritus, Chapter 24).

Relief of obstruction. Relief of obstruction will lead to improvement in liver function and pruritus, and the drainage of bile salts into the bowel will prevent malabsorption and steatorrhoea. The choice of procedure depends on the site of the blockage.[227, 228] A periampullary obstruction may be bypassed surgically or stented endoscopically, whilst obstructions involving the proximal extrahepatic bile ducts usually require catheterization by ERCP or PTHC. Percutaneous transhepatic catheterization may be performed with simple external drainage or with passage of the catheter past the obstruction allowing internal drainage into the intestine. Stents or catheters may be complicated by cholangitis and require regular

Table 19.79 Treatment options for malignant biliary obstruction

Systemic anticancer therapy (sensitive tumours)

Surgical bypass

Endoscopic placement of stent, catheter

Percutaneous transhepatic placement of stent, catheter

Radiotherapy

Symptomatic care
    treatment of pruritus
    corticosteroids

Treatment must be appropriate to the stage of the patient's disease and the prognosis

replacement. External radiotherapy has a limited role in the treatment of biliary obstruction due to the risk of radiation hepatitis. Endoscopic brachytherapy allows radiotherapy to be given to the bile duct with less risk of hepatic toxicity.

Terminal care

The treatment of biliary obstruction in the last days or week of life is symptomatic. If there is doubt about a patient's life expectancy, then non-surgical stenting can be considered, especially if there is severe pruritus.

References

1   Oneschuk, D., Hanson, J. and Bruera, E. (2000). A survey of mouth pain and dryness in patients with advanced cancer. *Supportive Care in Cancer* 8, 372–6.

2   Davies, A.N., Broadley, K. and Beighton, D. (2001). Xerostomia in patients with advanced cancer. *Journal of Pain and Symptom Management* 22, 820–5.

3   Guchelaar, H.J., Vermes, A. and Meerwaldt, J.H. (1997). Radiation-induced xerostomia: pathophysiology, clinical course and supportive treatment. *Supportive Care in Cancer* 5, 281–8.

4   Berger, A.M. and Kilroy, T.J. (2001). Oral Complications. In *Cancer. Principles and Practice of Oncology* (ed. V.T. De Vita, S. Hellman and S.A. Rosenberg). Philadelphia, Lippincott, Williams and Wilkins.

5   Zlotolow, I.M. and Berger, A.M. (2002). Oral manifestations and complications of cancer therapy. In *Principles and Practice of Palliative Care and Supportive Oncology* (ed. A.M. Berger, R.K. Portenoy and D.E. Weissman). Philadelphia, Lippincott, Williams and Wilkins.

6   Sbanotto, A. (2002). Oral complications of cancer. In *Gastrointestinal Symptoms in Patients with Advanced Cancer* (ed. C. Ripamonti and E. Bruera). Oxford, Oxford University Press.

7   Mercadante, S. (2002). Dry mouth and palliative care. *European Journal of Palliative Care* 9, 182–85.

8   Rydholm, M. and Strang, P. (2002). Physical and psychosocial impact of xerostomia in palliative cancer care: a qualitative interview study. *International Journal of Palliative Nursing* 8, 318–23.

9   Radiation Therapy Oncology Group (RTOG)/ European Organisation for Research and Treatment of Cancer (EORTC) (2000). RTOG/EORTC Late Radiation Morbidity Scoring Schema. <www.rtog.org/members/toxicity/late.html>

10 Thomson, W.M. and Williams, S.M. (2000). Further testing of the xerostomia inventory. *Oral Surgery, Oral Medicine, Oral Pathology, Oral Radiology, and Endodontics* 89, 46–50.

11 Chao, K.S. (2002). Protection of salivary function by intensity-modulated radiation therapy in patients with head and neck cancer. *Seminars in Radiation Oncology* 12, 20–5.

12 Buntzel, J., et al. (2002). Amifostine in simultaneous radiochemotherapy of advanced head and neck cancer. *Seminars in Radiation Oncology* 12, 4–13.

13 Anne, P.R. (2002). Phase II trial of subcutaneous amifostine in patients undergoing radiation therapy for head and neck cancer. *Seminars in Oncology* 29, 80–3.

14 Brizel, D.M., et al. (2000). Phase III randomized trial of amifostine as a radioprotector in head and neck cancer. *Journal of Clinical Oncology* 18, 3339–45.

15 Vardy, J., et al. (2002). Life-threatening anaphylactoid reaction to amifostine used with concurrent chemoradiotherapy for nasopharyngeal cancer in a patient with dermatomyositis: a case report with literature review. *Anticancer Drugs* 13, 327–30.

16 Warde, P., et al. (2002). A Phase III placebo-controlled trial of oral pilocarpine in patients undergoing radiotherapy for head-and-neck cancer. *International Journal of Radiation Oncology, Biology and Physics* 54, 9.

17 Buntzel, J., et al. (1998). Radiochemotherapy with amifostine cytoprotection for head and neck cancer. *Supportive Care in Cancer* 6, 155–60.

18 Antonadou, D., et al. (2002). Prophylactic use of amifostine to prevent radiochemotherapy-induced mucositis and xerostomia in head-and-neck cancer. *International Journal of Radiation Oncology, Biology and Physics* 52, 739–47.

19 Davies, A.N. (2000). A comparison of artificial saliva and chewing gum in the management of xerostomia in patients with advanced cancer. *Palliative Medicine* 14, 197–203.

20 Rhodus, N.L. and Bereuter, J. (2000). Clinical evaluation of a commercially available oral moisturizer in relieving signs and symptoms of xerostomia in postirradiation head and neck cancer patients and patients with Sjogren's syndrome. *Journal of Otolaryngology* 29, 28–34.

21 Warde, P., et al. (2000). A phase II study of Biotene in the treatment of postradiation xerostomia in patients with head and neck cancer. *Supportive Care in Cancer* 8, 203–8.

22 Jellema, A.P., et al. (2001). The efficacy of Xialine in patients with xerostomia resulting from radiotherapy for head and neck cancer: a pilot-study. *Radiotherapy and Oncology* 59, 157–60.

23 Horiot, J.C., et al. (2000). Post-radiation severe xerostomia relieved by pilocarpine: a prospective French cooperative study. *Radiotherapy and Oncology* 55, 233–9.

24 Nusair, S. and Rubinow, A. (1999). The use of oral pilocarpine in xerostomia and Sjogren's syndrome. *Seminars in Arthritis and Rheumatism* 28, 360–7.

25 Hawthorne, M. and Sullivan, K. (2000). Pilocarpine for radiation-induced xerostomia in head and neck cancer. *International Journal of Palliative Nursing* 6, 228–32.

26 Jacobs, C.D. and van der Pas, M. (1996). A multicenter maintenance study of oral pilocarpine tablets for radiation-induced xerostomia. *Oncology (Huntington)* 10, 16–20.

27 Niedermeier, W., et al. (1998). Radiation-induced hyposalivation and its treatment with oral pilocarpine. *Oral Surgery, Oral Medicine, Oral Pathology, Oral Radiology, and Endodontics* 86, 541–9.

28 Davies, A.N., et al. (1998). A comparison of artificial saliva and pilocarpine in the management of xerostomia in patients with advanced cancer. *Palliative Medicine* 12, 105–11.

29 Mercadante, S., et al. (2000). The use of pilocarpine in opioid-induced xerostomia. *Palliative Medicine* 14, 529–31.

30 Rydholm, M. and Strang, P. (1999). Acupuncture for patients in hospital-based home care suffering from xerostomia. *Journal of Palliative Care* 15, 20–3.

31 Johnstone, P.A., Niemtzow, R.C. and Riffenburgh, R.H. (2002). Acupuncture for xerostomia: clinical update. *Cancer* 94, 1151–6.

32 Johnson, J.T., et al. (1993). Oral pilocarpine for post-irradiation xerostomia in patients with head and neck cancer. *New England Journal of Medicine* 329, 390–5.

33 LeVeque, F.G., et al. (1993). A multicenter, randomized, double-blind, placebo-controlled, dose-titration study of oral pilocarpine for treatment of radiation-induced xerostomia in head and neck cancer patients. *Journal of Clinical Oncology* 11, 1124–31.

34 Davies, A.N. and Singer, J. (1994). A comparison of artificial saliva and pilocarpine in radiation-induced xerostomia. *Journal of Laryngology and Otology* 108, 663–5.

35   Rieke, J.W., et al. (1995). Oral pilocarpine for radiation-induced xerostomia: integrated efficacy and safety results from two prospective randomized clinical trials. *International Journal of Radiation Oncology, Biology and Physics* 31, 661–9.

36   Hamlar, D.D., et al. (1996). Determination of the efficacy of topical oral pilocarpine for postirradiation xerostomia in patients with head and neck carcinoma. *Laryngoscope* 106, 972–6.

37   Dodd, M.J., et al. (2001). A comparison of the affective state and quality of life of chemotherapy patients who do and do not develop chemotherapy-induced oral mucositis. *Journal of and Pain Symptom Management* 21, 498–505.

38   National Cancer Institute Cancer Therapy Evaluation Program (1998). Common Toxicity Criteria, version 2.0. <http://ctep.cancer.gov/reporting/ctc.html>

39   National Cancer Institute (2002). Oral complications of chemotheraapy and head/neck radiation (PDQ). <http://www.cancer.gov/cancerinfo/pdq/supportivecare/oralcomplications/healthprofessional>

40   Epstein, J.B., et al. (1992). Efficacy of chlorhexidine and nystatin rinses in prevention of oral complications in leukemia and bone marrow transplantation. *Oral Surgery, Oral Medicine, Oral Pathology, Oral Radiology, and Endodontics* 73, 682–9.

41   Foote, R.L., et al. (1994). Randomized trial of a chlorhexidine mouthwash for alleviation of radiation-induced mucositis. *Journal of Clinical Oncology* 12, 2630–3.

42   Adamietz, I.A., et al. (1998). Prophylaxis with povidone-iodine against induction of oral mucositis by radiochemotherapy. *Supportive Care in Cancer* 6, 373–7.

43   Spijkervet, F.K., et al. (1991). Effect of selective elimination of the oral flora on mucositis in irradiated head and neck cancer patients. *Journal of Surgical Oncology* 46, 167–73.

44   Symonds, R.P., et al. (1996). The reduction of radiation mucositis by selective decontamination antibiotic pastilles: a placebo-controlled double-blind trial. *British Journal of Cancer* 74, 312–17.

45   Okuno, S.H., et al. (1997). A randomized trial of a nonabsorbable antibiotic lozenge given to alleviate radiation-induced mucositis. *Cancer* 79, 2193–9.

46   Wijers, O.B., et al. (2001). Mucositis reduction by selective elimination of oral flora in irradiated cancers of the head and neck: a placebo-controlled double-blind randomized study. *International Journal of Radiation Oncology, Biology and Physics* 50, 343–52.

47   El-Sayed, S., et al. (2002). Prophylaxis of radiation-associated mucositis in conventionally treated patients with head and neck cancer: a double-blind, phase III, randomized, controlled trial evaluating the clinical efficacy of an antimicrobial lozenge using a validated mucositis scoring system. *Journal of Clinical Oncology* 20, 3956–63.

48   Osaki, T., et al. (1994). Prophylaxis of oral mucositis associated with chemoradiotherapy for oral carcinoma by Azelastine hydrochloride (Azelastine) with other antioxidants. *Head and Neck* 16, 331–9.

49   Mills, E.E. (1988). The modifying effect of beta-carotene on radiation and chemotherapy induced oral mucositis. *British Journal of Cancer* 57, 416–17.

50   Epstein, J.B. and Wong, F.L. (1994). The efficacy of sucralfate suspension in the prevention of oral mucositis due to radiation therapy. *International Journal of Radiation Oncology, Biology and Physics* 28, 693–8.

51   Carter, D.L., et al. (1999). Double blind randomized trial of sucralfate vs placebo during radical radiotherapy for head and neck cancers. *Head and Neck* 21, 760–6.

52   Cartee, L., et al. (1995). Evaluation of GM-CSF mouthwash for prevention of chemotherapy-induced mucositis: a randomized, double-blind, dose-ranging study. *Cytokine* 7, 471–7.

53   Sprinzl, G.M., et al. (2001). Local application of granulocyte-macrophage colony stimulating factor (GM-CSF) for the treatment of oral mucositis. *European Journal of Cancer* 37, 2003–9.

54   Epstein, J.B., et al. (2001). Benzydamine HCl for prophylaxis of radiation-induced oral mucositis: results from a multicenter, randomized, double-blind, placebo-controlled clinical trial. *Cancer* 92, 875–85.

55   Mahood, D.J., et al. (1991). Inhibition of fluorouracil-induced stomatitis by oral cryotherapy. *Journal of Clinical Oncology* 9, 449–52.

56 Cascinu, S., et al. (1994). Oral cooling (cryotherapy), an effective treatment for the prevention of 5-fluorouracil-induced stomatitis. *European Journal of Cancer. Part B, Oral Oncology.* 30B, 234–6.

57 Barasch, A., et al. (1995). Helium-neon laser effects on conditioning-induced oral mucositis in bone marrow transplantation patients. *Cancer* 76, 2550–6.

58 Bensadoun, R.J., et al. (1999). Low-energy He/Ne laser in the prevention of radiation-induced mucositis. A multicenter phase III randomized study in patients with head and neck cancer. *Supportive Care in Cancer* 7, 244–52.

59 Anderson, P.M., Schroeder, G. and Skubitz, K.M. (1998). Oral glutamine reduces the duration and severity of stomatitis after cytotoxic cancer chemotherapy. *Cancer* 83, 1433–9.

60 Oberbaum, M., et al. (2001). A randomized, controlled clinical trial of the homeopathic medication TRAUMEEL S in the treatment of chemotherapy-induced stomatitis in children undergoing stem cell transplantation. *Cancer* 92, 684–90.

61 Lissoni, P. (2002). Is there a role for melatonin in supportive care? *Supportive Care in Cancer* 10, 110–16.

62 Labar, B., et al. (1993). Prostaglandin E2 for prophylaxis of oral mucositis following BMT. *Bone Marrow Transplantation* 11, 379–82.

63 Loprinzi, C.L., et al. (1990). A controlled evaluation of an allopurinol mouthwash as prophylaxis against 5-fluorouracil-induced stomatitis. *Cancer* 65, 1879–82.

64 Fidler, P., et al. (1996). Prospective evaluation of a chamomile mouthwash for prevention of 5-FU-induced oral mucositis. *Cancer* 77, 522–5.

65 Maciejewski, B., et al. (1991). Acute mucositis in the stimulated oral mucosa of patients during radiotherapy for head and neck cancer. *Radiotherapy and Oncology* 22, 7–11.

66 Dorr, W., et al. (1995). Effects of stimulated repopulation on oral mucositis during conventional radiotherapy. *Radiotherapy and Oncology* 37, 100–7.

67 Pettengell, R., et al. (1992). Granulocyte colony-stimulating factor to prevent dose-limiting neutropenia in non-Hodgkin's lymphoma: a randomized controlled trial. *Blood* 80, 1430–6.

68 Chi, K.H., et al. (1995). Effect of granulocyte-macrophage colony-stimulating factor on oral mucositis in head and neck cancer patients after cisplatin, fluorouracil, and leucovorin chemotherapy. *Journal of Clinical Oncology* 13, 2620–8.

69 Nemunaitis, J., et al. (1995). Phase III randomized, double-blind placebo-controlled trial of rhGM-CSF following allogeneic bone marrow transplantation. *Bone Marrow Transplantation* 15, 949–54.

70 Welte, K., et al. (1996). A randomized phase-III study of the efficacy of granulocyte colony-stimulating factor in children with high-risk acute lymphoblastic leukemia. Berlin-Frankfurt-Munster Study Group. *Blood* 87, 3143–50.

71 Makkonen, T.A., et al. (2000). Granulocyte macrophage-colony stimulating factor (GM-CSF) and sucralfate in prevention of radiation-induced mucositis: a prospective randomized study. *International Journal of Radiation Oncology, Biology and Physics* 46, 525–34.

72 Koukourakis, M.I., et al. (2000). Subcutaneous administration of amifostine during fractionated radiotherapy: a randomized phase II study. *Journal of Clinical Oncology* 18, 2226–33.

73 Hartmann, J.T., et al. (2001). A randomized trial of amifostine in patients with high-dose VIC chemotherapy plus autologous blood stem cell transplantation. *British Journal of Cancer* 84, 313–20.

74 Clarkson, J.E., Worthington, H.V. and Eden, O.B. (2002). Interventions for preventing oral mucositis or oral candidiasis for patients with cancer receiving chemotherapy (excluding head and neck cancer) (Cochrane Review). *Cochrane Database of Systematic Reviews* CD000978.

75 Worthington, H.V., Clarkson, J.E. and Eden, O.B. (2002). Interventions for treating oral mucositis for patients with cancer receiving treatment (Cochrane Review). *Cochrane Database of Systematic Reviews* CD001973.

76 Wadleigh, R.G., et al. (1992). Vitamin E in the treatment of chemotherapy-induced mucositis. *American Journal of Medicine* 92, 481–4.

77 Huang, E.Y., et al. (2000). Oral glutamine to alleviate radiation-induced oral mucositis: a pilot randomized trial. *International Journal of Radiation Oncology, Biology and Physics* 46, 535–9.

78 Loprinzi, C.L., et al. (1997). Phase III controlled evaluation of sucralfate to alleviate stomatitis in patients receiving fluorouracil-based chemotherapy. *Journal of Clinical Oncology* 15, 1235–8.

79 Chiara, S., et al. (2001). Sucralfate in the treatment of chemotherapy-induced stomatitis: a double-blind, placebo-controlled pilot study. *Anticancer Research* 21, 3707–10.

80 Epstein, J.B., et al. (2001). Oral topical doxepin rinse: analgesic effect in patients with oral mucosal pain due to cancer or cancer therapy. *Oral Oncol* 37, 632–7.

81 Cerchietti, L.C., et al. (2002). Effect of topical morphine for mucositis-associated pain following concomitant chemoradiotherapy for head and neck carcinoma. *Cancer* 95, 2230–6.

82 Ehrnrooth, E., et al. (2001). Randomized trial of opioids versus tricyclic antidepressants for radiation-induced mucositis pain in head and neck cancer. *Acta Oncologica* 40, 745–50.

83 Gotzsche, P.C. and Johansen, H.K. (2002). Nystatin prophylaxis and treatment in severely immunodepressed patients (Cochrane Review). *Cochrane Database of Systematic Reviews* CD002033.

84 Worthington, H.V., Clarkson, J.E. and Eden, O.B. (2002). Interventions for preventing oral candidiasis for patients with cancer receiving treatment (Cochrane Review). *Cochrane Database of Systematic Reviews* CD003807.

85 Jacobson, J.M., et al. (1997). Thalidomide for the treatment of oral aphthous ulcers in patients with human immunodeficiency virus infection. National Institute of Allergy and Infectious Diseases AIDS Clinical Trials Group. *New England Journal of Medicine* 336, 1487–93.

86 Comeau, T.B., Epstein, J.B. and Migas, C. (2001). Taste and smell dysfunction in patients receiving chemotherapy: a review of current knowledge. *Support Care Cancer* 9, 575–80.

87 Wickham, R.S., et al. (1999). Taste changes experienced by patients receiving chemotherapy. *Oncology Nursing Forum* 26, 697–706.

88 Silverman, J.E., et al. (1983). Zinc supplementation and taste in head and neck cancer patients undergoing radiation therapy. *Journal of Oral Medicine* 38, 14–16.

89 Ripamonti, C., et al. (1998). A randomized, controlled clinical trial to evaluate the effects of zinc sulfate on cancer patients with taste alterations caused by head and neck irradiation. *Cancer* 82, 1938–45.

90 Twycross, R. and Back, I. (1998). Nausea and vomiting in advanced cancer. *European Journal of Palliative Care* 5, 39–45.

91 Berger, A.M. and Clark-Snow, R.A. (2002). Chemotherapy-related nausea and vomiting. In *Principles and Practice of Palliative Care and Supportive Oncology* (ed. A.M. Berger, R.K. Portenoy and D.E. Weissman). Philadelphia, Lippincott, Williams and Wilkins.

92 Bruera, E. and Sweeney, C. (2002). Chronic nausea and vomiting. In *Principles and Practice of Palliative Care and Supportive Oncology* (ed. A.M. Berger, R.K. Portenoy and D.E. Weissman). Philadelphia, Lippincott, Williams and Wilkins.

93 Mannix, K.A. (2003). Palliation of nausea and vomiting. In *Oxford Textbook of Palliative Medicine, 3rd edition* (ed. D. Doyle, G. Hanks, N. Cherny and K. Calman). Oxford, Oxford University Press.

94 Hesketh, P.J., et al. (1999). Randomized phase II study of the neurokinin 1 receptor antagonist CJ-11, 974 in the control of cisplatin-induced emesis. *Journal of Clinical Oncology* 17, 338–43.

95 Navari, R.M., et al. (1999). Reduction of cisplatin-induced emesis by a selective neurokinin-1-receptor antagonist. L-754,030 Antiemetic Trials Group. *New England Journal of Medicine* 340, 190–5.

96 Van Belle, S., et al. (2002). Prevention of cisplatin-induced acute and delayed emesis by the selective neurokinin-1 antagonists, L-758,298 and MK-869. *Cancer* 94, 3032–41.

97 Rhodes, V.A. and McDaniel, R.W. (1999). The Index of Nausea, Vomiting, and Retching: a new format of the Index of Nausea and Vomiting. *Oncology Nursing Forum* 26, 889–94.

98 Dibble, S.L., et al. (2000). Acupressure for nausea: results of a pilot study. *Oncology Nursing Forum* 27, 41–7.

99 Shen, J., et al. (2000). Electroacupuncture for control of myeloablative chemotherapy-induced emesis: A randomized controlled trial. *Journal of the American Medical Association* 284, 2755–61.

100 Brown, S., et al. (1992). Acupressure wrist bands to relieve nausea and vomiting in hospice patients: do they work? *American Journal of Hospice and Palliative Care* 9, 26–9.

101 Molassiotis, A., et al. (2002). The effectiveness of progressive muscle relaxation training in managing chemotherapy-induced nausea and vomiting in Chinese breast cancer patients: a randomised controlled trial. *Supportive Care in Cancer* 10, 237–46.

102 Twycross, R., Barkby, G. and Hallwood, P. (1997). The use of low dose levomepromazine (methotrimeprazine) in the management of nausea and vomiting. *Progress in Palliative care* 5, 49–53.

103 Critchley, P., et al. (2001). Efficacy of haloperidol in the treatment of nausea and vomiting in the palliative patient: a systematic review. *Journal of Pain and Symptom Management* 22, 631–4.

104 Tramer, M.R., et al. (2001). Cannabinoids for control of chemotherapy induced nausea and vomiting: quantitative systematic review. *British Medical Journal* 323, 16–21.

105 Bagshaw, S.M. and Hagen, N.A. (2002). Medical efficacy of cannabinoids and marijuana: a comprehensive review of the literature. *Journal of Palliative Care* 18, 111–22.

106 Ioannidis, J.P., Hesketh, P.J. and Lau, J. (2000). Contribution of dexamethasone to control of chemotherapy-induced nausea and vomiting: a meta-analysis of randomized evidence. *Journal of Clinical Oncology* 18, 3409–22.

107 Kaiser, R., et al. (2002). Patient-tailored antiemetic treatment with 5-hydroxytryptamine type 3 receptor antagonists according to cytochrome P-450 2D6 genotypes. *Journal of Clinical Oncology* 20, 2805–11.

108 Passik, S.D., et al. (2002). A pilot exploration of the antiemetic activity of olanzapine for the relief of nausea in patients with advanced cancer and pain. *Journal of Pain and Symptom Management* 23, 526–32.

109 Passik, S.D., et al. (2003). A retrospective chart review of the use of olanzapine for the prevention of delayed emesis in cancer patients. *Journal of Pain and Symptom Management* 25, 485–8.

110 Gralla, R.J., et al. (1999). Recommendations for the use of antiemetics: evidence-based, clinical practice guidelines. American Society of Clinical Oncology. *Journal of Clinical Oncology* 17, 2971–94.

111 Italian Group for Antiemetic Research in Radiotherapy (1999). Radiation-induced emesis: a prospective observational multicenter Italian trial. *International Journal of Radiation Oncology, Biology and Physics* 44, 619–25.

112 Tramer, M.R., et al. (1998). Efficacy of 5-HT3 receptor antagonists in radiotherapy-induced nausea and vomiting: a quantitative systematic review. *European Journal of Cancer* 34, 1836–44.

113 Bey, P., et al. (1996). A double-blind, placebo-controlled trial of i.v. dolasetron mesilate in the prevention of radiotherapy-induced nausea and vomiting in cancer patients. *Supportive Care in Cancer* 4, 378–83.

114 Franzen, L., et al. (1996). A randomised placebo controlled study with ondansetron in patients undergoing fractionated radiotherapy. *Annals of Oncology* 7, 587–92.

115 Sykes, A.J., Kiltie, A.E. and Stewart, A.L. (1997). Ondansetron versus a chlorpromazine and dexamethasone combination for the prevention of nausea and vomiting: a prospective, randomised study to assess efficacy, cost effectiveness and quality of life following single-fraction radiotherapy. *Supportive Care in Cancer* 5, 500–3.

116 Kirkbride, P., et al. (2000). Dexamethasone for the prophylaxis of radiation-induced emesis: a National Cancer Institute of Canada Clinical Trials Group phase III study. *Journal of Clinical Oncology* 18, 1960–6.

117 Davis, M.P. and Walsh, D. (2000). Treatment of nausea and vomiting in advanced cancer. *Supportive Care in Cancer* 8, 444–52.

118 Bruera, E., et al. (2000). A double-blind, crossover study of controlled-release metoclopramide and placebo for the chronic nausea and dyspepsia of advanced cancer. *Journal of Pain and Symptom Management* 19, 427–35.

119 Currow, D.C., et al. (1997). Use of ondansetron in palliative medicine. *Journal of Pain and Symptom Management* 13, 302–7.

120 Porcel, J.M., et al. (1998). Antiemetic efficacy of subcutaneous 5-HT3 receptor antagonists in terminal cancer patients. *Journal of Pain and Symptom Management* 15, 265–6.

121 Mystakidou, K., et al. (1998). Comparison of tropisetron and chlorpromazine combinations in the control of nausea and vomiting of patients with advanced cancer. *Journal of Pain and Symptom Management* 15, 176–84.

122 Hardy, J., et al. (2002). A double-blind, randomised, parallel group, multinational, multicentre study comparing a single dose of ondansetron 24 mg p.o. with placebo and metoclopramide 10 mg t.d.s. p.o. in the treatment of opioid-induced nausea and emesis in cancer patients. *Supportive Care in Cancer* 10, 231–6.

123 Lipps, D.C., et al. (1990). Nifedipine for intractable hiccups. *Neurology* 40, 531–2.

124 Ramirez, F.C. and Graham, D.Y. (1992). Treatment of intractable hiccup with baclofen: results of a double-blind randomized, controlled, cross-over study. *American Journal of Gastroenterology* 87, 1789–91.

125 Wilcock, A. and Twycross, R. (1996). Midazolam for intractable hiccup. *Journal of Pain and Symptom Management* 12, 59–61.

126 Walker, P., Watanabe, S. and Bruera, E. (1998). Baclofen, a treatment for chronic hiccup. *Journal of Pain and Symptom Management* 16, 125–32.

127 Eisbruch, A., et al. (2002). Objective assessment of swallowing dysfunction and aspiration after radiation concurrent with chemotherapy for head-and-neck cancer. *International Journal of Radiation Oncology, Biology and Physics* 53, 23–8.

128 Magne, N., et al. (2001). Comparison between nasogastric tube feeding and percutaneous fluoroscopic gastrostomy in advanced head and neck cancer patients. *European Archives of Otorhinolaryngology* 258, 89–92.

129 Keeley, P. (2002). Feeding tubes in palliative care. *European Journal of Palliative Care* 9, 229–31.

130 Heier, S.K., et al. (1995). Photodynamic therapy for obstructing esophageal cancer: light dosimetry and randomized comparison with Nd:YAG laser therapy. *Gastroenterology* 109, 63–72.

131 Lightdale, C.J., et al. (1995). Photodynamic therapy with porfimer sodium versus thermal ablation therapy with Nd:YAG laser for palliation of esophageal cancer: a multicenter randomized trial. *Gastrointestinal Endoscopy* 42, 507–12.

132 Sargeant, I.R., et al. (1997). Radiotherapy enhances laser palliation of malignant dysphagia: a randomised study. *Gut* 40, 362–9.

133 Tan, C.C., et al. (1998). Laser therapy combined with brachytherapy for the palliation of malignant dysphagia. *Singapore Medical Journal* 39, 202–7.

134 Spencer, G.M., et al. (2002). Laser augmented by brachytherapy versus laser alone in the palliation of adenocarcinoma of the oesophagus and cardia: a randomised study. *Gut* 50, 224–7.

135 Sur, R.K., et al. (2002). Prospective randomized trial of HDR brachytherapy as a sole modality in palliation of advanced esophageal carcinoma—an International Atomic Energy Agency study. *International Journal of Radiation Oncology, Biology and Physics* 53, 127–33.

136 Vakil, N., et al. (2001). A prospective, randomized, controlled trial of covered expandable metal stents in the palliation of malignant esophageal obstruction at the gastroesophageal junction. *American Journal of Gastroenterology* 96, 1791–6.

137 Nunes, C.C., et al. (1999). Comparative post operative study of prostheses, with and without an anti-reflux valve system, in the palliative treatment of esophageal carcinoma. *Hepatogastroenterology* 46, 2859–64.

138 Laasch, H.U., et al. (2002). Effectiveness of open versus antireflux stents for palliation of distal esophageal carcinoma and prevention of symptomatic gastroesophageal reflux. *Radiology* 225, 359–65.

139 Costamagna, G., et al. (2003). Prospective evaluation of a new self-expanding plastic stent for inoperable esophageal strictures. *Surgical Endoscopy* 7, 7.

140 Knyrim, K., et al. (1993). A controlled trial of an expansile metal stent for palliation of esophageal obstruction due to inoperable cancer. *New England Journal of Medicine* 329, 1302–7.

141 De Palma, G.D., et al. (1996). Plastic prosthesis versus expandable metal stents for palliation of inoperable esophageal thoracic carcinoma: a controlled prospective study. *Gastrointestinal Endoscopy* 43, 478–82.

142 Siersema, P.D., et al. (1998). Coated self-expanding metal stents versus latex prostheses for esophagogastric cancer with special reference to prior radiation and chemotherapy: a controlled, prospective study. *Gastrointestinal Endoscopy* 47, 113–20.

143 Sanyika, C., Corr, P. and Haffejee, A. (1999). Palliative treatment of oesophageal carcinoma—efficacy of plastic versus self-expandable stents. *South African Medical Journal* 89, 640–3.

144 O'Donnell, C.A., et al. (2002). Randomized clinical trial comparing self-expanding metallic stents with plastic endoprostheses in the palliation of oesophageal cancer. *British Journal of Surgery* 89, 985–92.

145 Mason, R. (1996). Palliation of malignant dysphagia: an alternative to surgery. *Annals of the Royal College of Surgeons of England* 78, 457–62.

146 Adam, A., et al. (1997). Palliation of inoperable esophageal carcinoma: a prospective randomized trial of laser therapy and stent placement. *Radiology* 202, 344–8.

147 Konigsrainer, A., et al. (2000). Expandable metal stents versus laser combined with radiotherapy for palliation of unresectable esophageal cancer: a prospective randomized trial. *Hepatogastroenterology* 47, 724–7.

148 Dallal, H.J., et al. (2001). A randomized trial of thermal ablative therapy versus expandable metal stents in the palliative treatment of patients with esophageal carcinoma. *Gastrointestinal Endoscopy* 54, 549–57.

149 Radiation Therapy Oncology Group (RTOG) (2000). Acute Radiation Morbidity Scoring Criteria. <www.rtog.org/members/toxicity/acute.html>

150 Antonadou, D., et al. (2001). Randomized phase III trial of radiation treatment +/− amifostine in patients with advanced-stage lung cancer. *International Journal of Radiation Oncology, Biology and Physics* 51, 915–22.

151 McGinnis, W.L., et al. (1997). Placebo-controlled trial of sucralfate for inhibiting radiation-induced esophagitis. *Journal of Clinical Oncology* 15, 1239–43.

152 Hawkins, C. and Hanks, G.W. (2000). The gastroduodenal toxicity of nonsteroidal anti-inflammatory drugs: a review of the literature. *Journal of Pain and Symptom Management* 20, 140–51.

153 Huang, J.Q., Sridhar, S. and Hunt, R.H. (2002). Role of Helicobacter pylori infection and non-steroidal anti-inflammatory drugs in peptic-ulcer disease: a meta-analysis. *Lancet* 359, 14–22.

154 Imperiale, T.F. and Birgisson, S. (1997). Somatostatin or octreotide compared with H2 antagonists and placebo in the management of acute nonvariceal upper gastrointestinal hemorrhage: a meta-analysis. *Annals of Internal Medicine* 127, 1062–71.

155 Hawkey, C.J., et al. (1998). Omeprazole compared with misoprostol for ulcers associated with nonsteroidal antiinflammatory drugs. Omeprazole versus Misoprostol for NSAID-induced Ulcer Management (OMNIUM) Study Group. *New England Journal of Medicine* 338, 727–34.

156 Yeomans, N.D., et al. (1998). A comparison of omeprazole with ranitidine for ulcers associated with nonsteroidal antiinflammatory drugs. Acid Suppression Trial: Ranitidine versus Omeprazole for NSAID-associated Ulcer Treatment (ASTRONAUT) Study Group. *New England Journal of Medicine* 338, 719–26.

157 Graham, D.Y., et al. (2002). Ulcer prevention in long-term users of nonsteroidal anti-inflammatory drugs: results of a double-blind, randomized, multicenter, active- and placebo-controlled study of misoprostol vs lansoprazole. *Archives of Internal Medicine* 162, 169–75.

158 Schnoll-Sussman, F. and Kurtz, R.C. (2000). Gastrointestinal emergencies in the critically ill cancer patient. *Seminars in Oncology* 27, 270–83.

159 Loftus, E.V., et al. (1994). Endoscopic treatment of major bleeding from advanced gastroduodenal malignant lesions. *Mayo Clinic Proceedings* 69, 736–40.

160 Savides, T.J., et al. (1996). Severe upper gastrointestinal tumor bleeding: endoscopic findings, treatment, and outcome. *Endoscopy* 28, 244–8.

161 Ripamonti, C., et al. (2001). Clinical-practice recommendations for the management of bowel obstruction in patients with end-stage cancer. *Supportive Care in Cancer* 9, 223–33.

162 Feuer, D.J., et al. (2000). Surgery for the resolution of symptoms in malignant bowel obstruction in advanced gynaecological and gastrointestinal cancer (Cochrane Review). *Cochrane Database of Systematic Reviews* CD002764.

163 Brooksbank, M.A., Game, P.A. and Ashby, M.A. (2002). Palliative venting gastrostomy in malignant intestinal obstruction. *Palliative Medicine* 16, 520–6.

164 Gevers, A.M., et al. (2000). Endoscopic laser therapy for palliation of patients with distal colorectal carcinoma: analysis of factors influencing long-term outcome. *Gastrointestinal Endoscopy* 51, 580–5.

165 Khot, U.P., et al. (2002). Systematic review of the efficacy and safety of colorectal stents. *British Journal of Surgery* 89, 1096–102.

166 Mercadante, S., et al. (2000). Comparison of octreotide and hyoscine butylbromide in controlling gastrointestinal symptoms due to malignant inoperable bowel obstruction. *Supportive Care in Cancer* 8, 188–91.

167 Ripamonti, C., et al. (2000). Role of octreotide, scopolamine butylbromide, and hydration in symptom control of patients with inoperable bowel obstruction and nasogastric tubes: a prospective randomized trial. *Journal of Pain and Symptom Management* 19, 23–34.

168 Mystakidou, K., et al. (2002). Comparison of octreotide administration vs conservative treatment in the management of inoperable bowel obstruction in patients with far advanced cancer: a randomized, double-blind, controlled clinical trial. *Anticancer Research* 22, 1187–92.

169 Hardy, J., et al. (1998). Pitfalls in placebo-controlled trials in palliative care: dexamethasone for the palliation of malignant bowel obstruction. *Palliative Medicine* 12, 437–42.

170 Feuer, D.J. and Broadley, K.E. (2000). Corticosteroids for the resolution of malignant bowel obstruction in advanced gynaecological and gastrointestinal cancer (Cochrane Review). *Cochrane Database of Systematic Reviews* CD001219.

171 Laval, G., et al. (2000). The use of steroids in the management of inoperable intestinal obstruction in terminal cancer patients: do they remove the obstruction? *Palliative Medicine* 14, 3–10.

172 Agra, Y., et al. (1998). Efficacy of senna versus lactulose in terminal cancer patients treated with opioids. *Journal of Pain and Symptom Management* 15, 1–7.

173 Freedman, M.D., et al. (1997). Tolerance and efficacy of polyethylene glycol 3350/electrolyte solution versus lactulose in relieving opiate induced constipation: a double-blinded placebo-controlled trial. *Journal of Clinical Pharmacology* 37, 904–7.

174 Sykes, N.P. (1996). An investigation of the ability of oral naloxone to correct opioid-related constipation in patients with advanced cancer. *Palliative Medicine* 10, 135–44.

175 Meissner, W., et al. (2000). Oral naloxone reverses opioid-associated constipation. *Pain* 84, 105–9.

176 Friedman, J.D. and Dello Buono, F.A. (2001). Opioid antagonists in the treatment of opioid-induced constipation and pruritus. *Annals of Pharmacotherapeutics* 35, 85–91.

177 Liu, M. and Wittbrodt, E. (2002). Low-dose oral naloxone reverses opioid-induced constipation and analgesia. *Journal of Pain and Symptom Management* 23, 48–53.

178 Foss, J.F. (2001). A review of the potential role of methylnaltrexone in opioid bowel dysfunction. *American Journal of Surgery* 182, 19S–26S.

179 Yuan, C.S., et al. (2000). Methylnaltrexone for reversal of constipation due to chronic methadone use: a randomized controlled trial. *Journal of the American Medical Association* 283, 367–72.

180 Yuan, C.S., et al. (2002). Effects of subcutaneous methylnaltrexone on morphine-induced peripherally mediated side effects: a double-blind randomized placebo-controlled trial. *Journal of Pharmacology and Experimental Therapeutics.* 300, 118–23.

181 Davis, M.P. and Walsh, D. (2002). Gastrointestinal motility disorders. In *Gastrointestinal Symptoms in Patients with Advanced Cancer* (ed. C. Ripamonti and E. Bruera). Oxford, Oxford University Press.

182 Martenson, J.A., et al. (2000). Sucralfate in the prevention of treatment-induced diarrhea in patients receiving pelvic radiation therapy: A North Central Cancer Treatment Group phase III double-blind placebo-controlled trial. *Journal of Clinical Oncology* 18, 1239–45.

183 Kneebone, A., et al. (2001). The effect of oral sucralfate on the acute proctitis associated with prostate radiotherapy: a double-blind, randomized trial. *International Journal of Radiation Oncology, Biology and Physics* 51, 628–35.

184 Kouvaris, J., et al. (2003). Amifostine as radioprotective agent for the rectal mucosa during irradiation of pelvic tumors. A phase II randomized study using various toxicity scales and rectosigmoidoscopy. *Strahlentherapie und Onkologie* 179, 167–74.

185 Kilic, D., et al. (2000). Double-blinded, randomized, placebo-controlled study to evaluate the effectiveness of sulphasalazine in preventing acute gastrointestinal complications due to radiotherapy. *Radiotherapy and Oncology* 57, 125–9.

186 Resbeut, M., et al. (1997). A randomized double blind placebo controlled multicenter study of mesalazine for the prevention of acute radiation enteritis. *Radiotherapy and Oncology* 44, 59–63.

187 Martenson, J.A., Jr., et al. (1996). Olsalazine is contraindicated during pelvic radiation therapy: results of a double-blind, randomized clinical trial. *International Journal of Radiation Oncology, Biology and Physics* 35, 299–303.

188 Murphy, J., et al. (2000). Testing control of radiation-induced diarrhea with a psyllium bulking agent: a pilot study. *Canadian Oncology Nursing Journal* 10, 96–100.

189 Lodge, N., et al. (1995). A randomized cross-over study of the efficacy of codeine phosphate versus Ispaghulahusk in patients with gynaecological cancer experiencing diarrhoea during pelvic radiotherapy. *European Journal of Cancer Care* 4, 8–10.

190 Urbancsek, H., et al. (2001). Results of a double-blind, randomized study to evaluate the efficacy and safety of Antibiophilus in patients with radiation-induced diarrhoea. *European Journal of Gastroenterology and Hepatology* 13, 391–6.

191 Yavuz, M.N., et al. (2002). The efficacy of octreotide in the therapy of acute radiation-induced diarrhea: a randomized controlled study. *International Journal of Radiation Oncology, Biology and Physics* 54, 195–202.

192 Denton, A., et al. (2002). Non surgical interventions for late radiation proctitis in patients who have received radical radiotherapy to the pelvis (Cochrane Review). *Cochrane Database Syst Rev* CD003455.

193 Lenfers, B.H., et al. (1999). Substantial activity of budesonide in patients with irinotecan (CPT-11) and 5-fluorouracil induced diarrhea and failure of loperamide treatment. *Annals of Oncology* 10, 1251–3.

194 Zidan, J., et al. (2001). Octreotide in the treatment of severe chemotherapy-induced diarrhea. *Annals of Oncology* 12, 227–9.

195 Alvarez, C., McFadden, D.W. and Reber, H.A. (2000). Complicated enterocutaneous fistulas: failure of octreotide to improve healing. *World Journal of Surgery* 24, 533–7.

196 Scott, N.A., Finnegan, S. and Irving, M.H. (1993). Octreotide and postoperative enterocutaneous fistulae: a controlled prospective study. *Acta Gastroenterologica Belgica* 56, 266–70.

197 Sancho, J.J., et al. (1995). Randomized double-blind placebo-controlled trial of early octreotide in patients with postoperative enterocutaneous fistula. *British Journal of Surgery* 82, 638–41.

198 Gemlo, B. (2002). Enteric fislulae. In *Gastrointestinal Symptoms in Patients with Advanced Cancer* (ed. C. Ripamonti and E. Bruera). Oxford, Oxford University Press.

199 Sadeghi, B., et al. (2000). Peritoneal carcinomatosis from non-gynecologic malignancies: results of the EVOCAPE 1 multicentric prospective study. *Cancer* 88, 358–63.

200 Bieligk, S.C., Calvo, B.F. and Coit, D.G. (2001). Peritoneovenous shunting for nongynecologic malignant ascites. *Cancer* 91, 1247–55.

201 Marincola, F.M. and Schwartzentruber, D.J. (2001). Malignant Ascites. In *Cancer. Principles and Practice of Oncology. 6th edition* (ed. V.T. De Vita, S. Hellman and S.A. Rosenberg). Philadelphia, Lippincott, Williams and Wilkins.

202 Campbell, C. (2001). Controlling malignant ascites. *European Journal of Palliative Care* 8, 187–90.

203 Keen, J. and Fallon, M. (2002). Malignant ascites. In *Gastrointestinal Symptoms in Patients with Advanced Cancer* (ed. C. Ripamonti and E. Bruera). Oxford, Oxford University Press.

204 Thomas, J.R. and von Guten, C.F. (2002). Diagnosis and management of ascites. In *Principles and Practice of Palliative Care and Supportive Oncology* (ed. A.M. Berger, R.K. Portenoy and D.E. Weissman). Philadelphia, Lippincott, Williams and Wilkins.

205 Kaas, R., Rustman, L.D. and Zoetmulder, F.A. (2001). Chylous ascites after oncological abdominal surgery: incidence and treatment. *European Journal of Surgical Oncology* 27, 187–9.

206 Runyon, B.A. (1994). Care of patients with ascites. *New England Journal of Medicine* 330, 337–42.

207 Pockros, P.J., et al. (1992). Mobilization of malignant ascites with diuretics is dependent on ascitic fluid characteristics. *Gastroenterology* 103, 1302–6.

208 Jalan, R. and Hayes, P.C. (1997). Hepatic encephalopathy and ascites. *Lancet* 350, 1309–15.

209 Moorsom, D. (2001). Paracentesis in the home care setting. *Palliative Medicine* 15, 169–70.

210 Stephenson, J. and Gilbert, J. (2002). The development of clinical guidelines on paracentesis for ascites related to malignancy. *Palliative Medicine* 16, 213–18.

211 McNamara, P. (2000). Paracentesis—an effective method of symptom control in the palliative care setting? *Palliative Medicine* 14, 62–4.

212 Lee, A., Lau, T.N. and Yeong, K.Y. (2000). Indwelling catheters for the management of malignant ascites. *Supportive Care in Cancer* 8, 493–9.

213 O'Neill, M.J., et al. (2001). Tunneled peritoneal catheter placement under sonographic and fluoroscopic guidance in the palliative treatment of malignant ascites. *American Journal of Roentgenology* 177, 615–18.

214 Richard, H.M., 3rd, et al. (2001). Pleurx tunneled catheter in the management of malignant ascites. *Journal of Vascular and Interventional Radiology* 12, 373–5.

215 Barnett, T.D. and Rubins, J. (2002). Placement of a permanent tunneled peritoneal drainage catheter for palliation of malignant ascites: a simplified percutaneous approach. *Journal of Vascular and Interventional Radiology* 13, 379–83.

216 Zanon, C., et al. (2002). Palliative treatment of malignant refractory ascites by positioning of Denver peritoneovenous shunt. *Tumori* 88, 123–7.

217 Gough, I.R. and Balderson, G.A. (1993). Malignant ascites. A comparison of peritoneovenous shunting and nonoperative management. *Cancer* 71, 2377–82.

218 Mackey, J.R., et al. (2000). A phase II trial of triamcinolone hexacetanide for symptomatic recurrent malignant ascites. *Journal of Pain and Symptom Management* 19, 193–9.

219 Burger, J.A., et al. (1997). The transjugular stent implantation for the treatment of malignant portal and hepatic vein obstruction in cancer patients. *Annals of Oncology* 8, 200–2.

220 Cairns, W. and Malone, R. (1999). Octreotide as an agent for the relief of malignant ascites in palliative care patients. *Palliative Medicine* 13, 429–30.

221 Sasson, A.R. and Sigurdson, E.R. (2002). Surgical treatment of liver metastases. *Seminars in Oncology* 29, 107–18.

222 Sotsky, T.K. and Ravikumar, T.S. (2002). Cryotherapy in the treatment of liver metastases from colorectal cancer. *Seminars in Oncology* 29, 183–91.

223 Giovannini, M. (2002). Percutaneous alcohol ablation for liver metastasis. *Seminars in Oncology* 29, 192–5.

224 Parikh, A.A., et al. (2002). Radiofrequency ablation of hepatic metastases. *Seminars in Oncology* 29, 168–82.

225 Malik, U. and Mohiuddin, M. (2002). External-beam radiotherapy in the management of liver metastases. *Seminars in Oncology* 29, 196–201.

226 Herba, M.J. and Thirlwell, M.P. (2002). Radioembolization for hepatic metastases. *Seminars in Oncology* 29, 152–9.

227 Roth, L.J. and Pugh, E.J. (1999). The role of endoscopic biliary stents in palliative care. *Palliative Medicine* 13, 63–8.

228 Uthappa, M.C., Ho, S.M. and Boardman, P. (2003). Role of metallic stents in palliative care. *Progress in Palliative care* 11, 3–9.

20

Genitourinary

Haematuria	Urinary infection
Frequency and urgency	Renal failure
Urinary incontinence	Prostatitis, epididymo-orchitis
Hesitancy	Vaginitis, vaginal discharge
Urinary tract obstruction	Uterine bleeding
Urinary catheters	Sexual dysfunction

Haematuria

Haematuria occurs frequently in patients with advanced cancer, although it is often asymptomatic, microscopic, and of limited clinical importance. A number of recent reviews of haematuria have been published.[1, 2]

Table 20.1 Causes of haematuria

Infection	cystitis, prostatitis, urethritis, septicaemia
Malignancy	primary or secondary tumour
Iatrogenic	nephrostomy, ureteric stenting, catheterization, embolization cystitis due to radiation, chemotherapy
Bleeding	diathesis anticoagulants, coagulation disorder, thrombocytopenia primary fibrinolysis
Renal disease	renal vein thrombosis, paraneoplastic glomerular lesions
Urolithiasis	

The common causes of haematuria in patients with cancer are shown in Table 20.1. Macroscopic haematuria occurs in 70% of patients with carcinoma of the bladder and 40% of patients with renal carcinoma. Severe haematuria, sufficient to cause anaemia or produce clots, is usually due to neoplastic infiltration, a coagulation disorder, or cystitis caused by radiation or chemotherapy.

Clinical features

The nature of the haematuria and the associated symptoms often indicate the cause. Haematuria occurring only at the beginning or termination of urination usually indicates a lesion distal to the bladder neck. Haematuria occurring throughout the urinary stream is associated with lesions above the bladder neck. The types of clots may also indicate the source of bleeding: linearly formed clots indicate urethral bleeding, whereas larger, irregular clots usually originate from the bladder. The presence of dysuria, fever and suprapubic tenderness may indicate infection.

Significant haematuria due to a bleeding diathesis is usually accompanied by signs of abnormal bleeding at other sites and coagulation studies will define the cause. However, pathological fibrinolysis, which occurs after local surgery for carcinoma of the prostate, causes severe and persistent haematuria without evidence of systemic bleeding.

Chemotherapy cystitis. Cyclophosphamide and ifosfamide are associated with haemorrhagic cystitis caused by the drug metabolite, acrolein. It usually occurs during or shortly after parenteral treatment, but can occur in patients on chronic oral therapy. Macroscopically the mucosa is oedematous and hyperaemic with multiple bleeding sites and areas of mucosal sloughing and erosion. Microscopically there is mucosal inflammation and ulceration, submucosal granulation tissue and fibrosis. Haemorrhagic cystitis related to the phosphamide drugs can be prevented by giving mesna (sodium mercaptoethane sulfonate), a chelating agent that binds acrolein, and ensuring adequate hydration and urinary output during and after therapy.

Radiation cystitis. Haemorrhagic cystitis is reported to occur in less than 5% of patients following pelvic radiotherapy and the incidence increases with time since irradiation.[3] Radiation leads to bladder wall fibrosis and contraction, as well as the formation of friable, telangiectatic blood vessels (Table 20.2). Macroscopically, the bladder mucosa is pale and bleeds easily on contact. The risk of radiation cystitis can be minimized by ensuring adequate hydration during the period of treatment. Patients requiring urinary drainage during radiotherapy should have a suprapubic rather than urethral catheter.

Table 20.2 RTOG/EORTC grading for late radiation bladder toxicity[4]

0	none
1	slight epithelial atrophy minor telangiectasia (microscopic haematuria)
2	moderate frequency generalized telangiectasia (intermittent macroscopic haematuria)
3	severe frequency and dysuria (bladder capacity <150ml) severe generalized telangiectasia (frequent haematuria)
4	necrosis/contracted bladder (bladder capacity <100ml) severe haemorrhagic cystitis

Assessment

Assessment is aimed at determining the site and cause of the bleeding. Patients with mild or moderate haematuria due to an obvious cause such as infection or catheterization may require no further investigation. Similarly, investigation of patients who are terminally ill should be avoided.

Urine microscopy is performed to confirm the presence of red blood cells (i.e. genuine haematuria), as a number of pigments can produce red or dark brown urine suggesting haematuria (Table 20.3); confirmatory microscopy is not necessary in patients with obvious haemorrhage. Urine microscopy may also show red cell casts (suggestive of glomerular bleeding), leucocytes and bacteria indicative of infection, and malignant cells on cytological examination. Phase contrast microscopy can help identify the site of bleeding: red cells from glomerular bleeding typically have bizarre shapes, whilst those from non-glomerular bleeding are more uniform and appear as target or ghost cells.

Table 20.3   Urinary discolouration not due to haematuria

Pigment	Colour	Condition
Haemoglobin	red/ brown	haemolysis
Methaemoglobin	brown	haemolysis
Urobilinogen	orange	haemolysis
Myoglobin	red	rhabdomyolysis
Bile	brown	obstructive jaundice
Porphyrins	dark red	porphyria
Melanin	brown	melanoma
Carotene	orange	excess carotene containing foods
Anthocyanin	red	excess beetroot, berries
Anthraquinone	red	excess rhubarb
Drugs	red	anthracene laxatives, anthracyclines, flutamide, phenazopyridine, phenindione, phenolphthalein, rifampicin

Further investigation is performed as clinically indicated. Cystoscopy may be required to distinguish between upper and lower urinary tract bleeding. It will allow lateralization of upper tract bleeding as well as direct visualization and treatment of lower tract pathology. Ultrasound, helical CT and MRI scanning may be considered.[5–7] Renal biopsy may be required if a renal lesion is suspected.

Treatment

The treatment is that of the cause although in many cases the bleeding is mild and no specific therapy is needed. Treatment with ethamsylate or tranexamic acid may control mild to moderate bleeding; some advise against the use of tranexamic acid as it may lead to the formation of firm clots that are difficult to remove.[8] Pathological fibrinolysis is treated with aminocaproic acid, which may also be complicated by the formation of tenacious clots.

Severe haematuria. Major haematuria requires intervention or clot retention will develop. A large bore catheter is used to evacuate clots and establish a continuous saline bladder washout; cystoscopy is sometimes required for the initial evacuation of clots. Further treatment measures depend on the cause (Table 20.4).[1, 2, 9] Intravesical alum is frequently effective in stopping bleeding and causes few side effects. Severe and continuing bleeding from haemorrhagic cystitis caused by radiation or chemotherapy can be treated with instillation of silver nitrate or formalin. A cystoscopy and cystogram should be performed before instillation to exclude vesico-ureteric reflux and reduce the risk of ureteric stenosis. Spinal or general anaesthesia is required for formalin instillation. Various treatments can be employed for persistent tumour bleeding (Table 20.4).

Table 20.4 Treatment options for severe haematuria

Catheterization or cystoscopy for clot evacuation
Continuous saline bladder washout to prevent clot formation
Ethamsylate (500mg PO q6h) or tranexamic acid (1g PO q6–8h)
Persistent lower tract bleeding   alum1% solution by continuous washout until urine clear

Persistent tumour bleeding
  cystoscopy for diathermy, laser therapy or endoscopic tumour resection
  external radiotherapy

Persistent bleeding due to radiation or chemotherapy cystitis
  silver nitrate 0.5–1% instilled for 10–20 minutes
  formalin 1–3% instilled for 20–30 minutes (requires anaesthetic)

Fibrinolysis   aminocaproic acid: 5g to start, then 1g/h until bleeding settles, PO or IV infusion
Bleeding from malignant infiltration of kidney   radiotherapy, embolization, surgery

Other reported therapies for haematuria include conjugated oestrogens,[10] intravesical prostaglandins,[1] finasteride for prostatic bleeding,[11] hyperbaric oxygen for radiation cystitis,[12] and radiofrequency ablation for bleeding renal lesions.[13] A Cochrane review of treatments for late radiation cystitis yielded no RCTs and little evidence on which to base conclusions or recommendations.[14]

Terminal care

A conservative approach is adopted whenever possible. Bleeding causing ureteric colic or clot retention is managed by the simplest and least invasive procedures that effectively control the symptoms.

Frequency and urgency

Normal micturition depends on intact sympathetic and parasympathetic innervation of the bladder (Table 20.5). The urethral sphincter is under voluntary control, innervated from sacral roots S2–4 via the pudendal nerve.

Table 20.5 Normal voiding

Innervation	Parasympathetic	Sympathetic
from segments	S2–4	T10–12, L1
via	hypogastric nerves	pelvic nerves
mediated by	acetylcholine	noradrenaline
effect on detrusor	contracts	relaxes
effect on sphincter	relaxes	contracts
inhibited by	anticholinergic drugs	sympathetic nerve damage

The causes of frequency are shown in Table 20.6. Frequency in combination with large urine volumes or bladder abnormalities will cause urgency. Clinical assessment, urine examination (chemical, microscopy, culture and cytology), and monitoring the urinary volume will usually define the cause.

Table 20.6   Causes of frequency

Polyuria
    high fluid intake, diuretic therapy
    diabetes mellitus, diabetes insipidus
    hypercalcaemia

Inflammation
    infection: cystitis, prostatitis, urethritis
    chemotherapy, radiotherapy
    foreign bodies: stents, calculi

Diminished bladder capacity
    tumour, including extrinsic compression
    surgery
    post radiation, chemotherapy

Detrusor instability/hyperactivity
    neurological: CNS, spinal, pelvic nerve lesions
    infection
    anxiety

Lower urinary tract obstruction
    tumour, strictures, prostatomegaly, faecal impaction

Treatment

The treatment is that of the cause. Polyuria is corrected, and infection and outflow obstruction are treated appropriately.

Drug therapy. A small proportion of patients, including those with chronic bladder damage and those with neurological lesions, suffer persistent and troublesome frequency. Treatment with one of the anticholinergic agents that also have smooth muscle relaxant activity (Table 20.7) can be helpful, although anticholinergic side effects may be troublesome if there is urinary outlet or gastrointestinal obstruction. In the terminal care setting, hyoscine butylbromide can be given by subcutaneous infusion. Antidepressants may also be useful,

Table 20.7   Examples of bladder relaxant medications

Anticholinergic	oxybutynin	2.5–5mg PO q6–8h
	tolterodine	2mg q12h
	flavoxate	100–200mg PO q6–8h
	hyoscine butylbromide	30–180mg/24h CSCI
Antidepressant	amitriptyline	25–50mg PO nocte
	imipramine	25–50mg PO nocte
Local anaesthetic	phenazopyridine	100–200mg PO q8h

probably because of their anticholinergic action. Phenazopyridine has a local anaesthetic or topical analgesic action in the urinary tract and is effective in relieving frequency or urgency associated with dysuria.

Urinary incontinence

Urinary incontinence, or the involuntary passage of urine, is common in patients with advanced cancer and the elderly.[15] It can be the cause of severe embarrassment for the patient and cause serious irritation of the skin and perineum. The causes of incontinence, classified by the different pathological mechanisms, are listed in Table 20.8.

Table 20.8 Causes of urinary incontinence

Overflow incontinence	
bladder outlet obstruction	malignant infiltration, prostatic hypertrophy
	faecal impaction, strictures, calculi
detrusor failure	anticholinergic drugs, anticholinergic side effects
	CNS, spinal cord or sacral nerve root lesions
	somnolence, confusion, dementia
	general weakness and debility
Stress incontinence	
sphincter insufficiency	spinal cord or sacral nerve root lesions
	pelvic, urological surgery
	malignant infiltration
	multiparity (prolapse), postmenopausal
Urge incontinence	
detrusor hyperactivity	polyuria, infection, inflammation
or instability	malignant infiltration
	post radiation, chemotherapy
	CNS, spinal cord or sacral nerve root lesions
	anxiety
Continuous incontinence	
fistulas	malignant infiltration, radiotherapy, surgery

Patients with overflow incontinence complain of suprapubic pain, urgency and the frequent passage of small amounts of urine; the post-voiding residual urine volume is high. Stress incontinence leads to voiding when the patient coughs or laughs, lifts or strains; the amount of urine voided is normal or low and the post-voiding residual urine volume is low. Urge incontinence occurs when there is detrusor instability or damage to the sacral nerve roots which innervate the bladder; the post-voiding residual volume is low. Continuous incontinence or the persistent dribbling of urine occurs when a ureterovaginal or vesicovaginal fistula develops as a result of malignant infiltration, surgery or radiotherapy.

The cause of urinary incontinence is usually evident from the history and examination, including pelvic examination and urinalysis. A record of the patient's voiding habits on a voiding chart is useful for treatment planning. The post-voiding residual volume can be measured by portable ultrasound at the bedside. Instillation of methylene blue into the bladder will demonstrate a fistula.

Treatment

Treatment depends on the type of incontinence and the cause (Table 20.9).[15, 16]

Table 20.9   Incontinence: treatment options

Bladder outlet obstruction
    relief of obstruction: surgery, radiotherapy
    treatment of faecal impaction
    stop drugs causing sedation or anticholinergic effects
    regular voiding, management of fluids
    α-blocker: prazosin 0.5–1mg PO q12h

Detrusor failure
    stop drugs causing sedation or anticholinergic effects
    α-blocker: prazosin 0.5–1mg PO q12h
    cholinergic: bethanechol 5–30mg PO q6h

Stress incontinence
    regular voiding, management of fluids
    pelvic muscle exercises, oestrogens, condom drainage
    adrenergic: ephedrine 25–50mg PO q8h
    antidepressant: doxepin or imipramine 25–50mg PO nocte
    surgery, collagen implant

Urge incontinence
    regular voiding, management of fluids
    pelvic floor exercises
    anticholinergic drugs (see Table 20.7)

General measures. Correctable causes should be sought and treated appropriately, where possible (Table 20.10). Access to toilet facilities is important, as well as the ability to use them or the availability of someone to provide assistance. A variety of non-surgical interventions including pelvic floor muscle training and prompted voiding are of benefit to some patients although there are few controlled studies.[17–20] Regular voiding is encouraged and may reduce the degree of incontinence. Patients incapable of independent toileting should be toileted regularly according to a consistent schedule; others may benefit from habit training or prompted voiding. Fluid loads and foods with diuretic action such as coffee and alcohol are avoided, especially in the evening. Drugs that cause significant sedation should also be avoided. Attention to perineal skin care is important.

Overflow incontinence. Treatment of incontinence related to bladder outlet obstruction may involve surgery, radiotherapy, or correction of faecal impaction. Drugs causing sedation

Table 20.10   Urinary incontinence: potentially correctable causes

Restricted mobility	Delirium
Urinary infection	Depression
Faecal impaction	Anxiety
Oestrogen deficiency	Excess fluids
Other medications	Diuretics

or anticholinergic effects are stopped, if feasible. Some patients can be managed by regular voiding every 2 to 4 hours to prevent overdistension of the bladder. Treatment with an α-blocker such as prazosin will improve urinary flow and bladder emptying; the main adverse effect is postural hypotension. Bladder catheterization may be necessary in the short term and is the only treatment required for terminally ill patients.

Detrusor failure. Detrusor failure due to drugs that cause sedation or anticholinergic effects may respond to dose reduction or withdrawal. Treatment with an α-blocker is frequently helpful. Cholinergic drugs like bethanechol will stimulate detrusor function but are rarely useful unless the bladder weakness is due to an anticholinergic drug that cannot be stopped. Bethanechol cannot be used if there is outlet obstruction; other adverse effects include gastrointestinal colic and sweating. Patients with detrusor failure due to spinal cord disease, but with intact sacral reflexes, can be taught to void by reflex stimulation of the lower abdomen or perineum.

Stress incontinence. Stress incontinence may be improved by a programme of regular voiding and exercises to strengthen pelvic musculature. Topical or systemic oestrogens are frequently prescribed for incontinence in postmenopausal women, although a 1996 review[16] showed only limited evidence of efficacy, and more recent studies have not shown benefit.[21, 22] Women with pelvic prolapse may be helped by the insertion of a pessary. Some recommend the intermittent use of a penile clamp or condom drainage for men with incontinence. Adrenergic drugs such as ephedrine will increase sphincter tone although troublesome adverse effects including tremor, palpitations and hypertension limit the usefulness of these drugs. Therapy with an antidepressant will help some patients with detrusor weakness. Endoscopic injection of collagen implant into the tissues around the bladder neck, to create increased tissue bulk, helps some patients.[23]

Urge incontinence. The treatment of urge incontinence is described in the section on Frequency and Urgency. A Cochrane review reported significant improvement in symptoms with the use of anticholinergic drugs.[24] Incontinence occurring at night can be treated with desmopressin (DDAVP), 20–40μg by intranasal spray, at bedtime.

Fistulas. Regular voiding may be of assistance as the amount of drainage from a fistula is less if the bladder is empty. For patients with a longer life expectancy, urinary surgical diversion can be considered. For patients with a shorter life expectancy, management is by catheterization that will reduce urine leakage through the fistula although incontinence pads and special attention to perineal skin care are still necessary.

Terminal care

The treatment of urinary incontinence is by catheterization.

Hesitancy

Urinary hesitancy, an abnormal delay between attempting to void and the start of micturition, may be caused by bladder outflow obstruction or detrusor weakness (Table 20.11). The cause of urinary hesitancy is usually clinically evident.

Treatment. Where possible and appropriate, the specific cause is treated. If hesitancy is due to the side effects of drugs, the doses are modified where possible. The α-adrenoreceptor antagonist drugs (Table 20.12) are of benefit to some patients, but all may cause severe postural hypotension with the first dose, particularly in patients taking diuretics or antihypertensive medications. Treatment should be initiated at a low dose and gradually titrated upward. The

Table 20.11 Causes of urinary hesitancy

Bladder outflow obstruction
    malignant infiltration
    prostatic enlargement, carcinoma
    faecal impaction
    stricture

Detrusor weakness
    anticholinergic drugs: scopolamine, atropine
    anticholinergic side effects: antidepressants, phenothiazines, haloperidol, antihistamines
    CNS, spinal cord or sacral nerve root lesions
    spinal analgesia
    sedation
    general weakness and debility

Table 20.12 Drug treatment of urinary hesitancy

α-adrenoreceptor antagonists
    prazosin 0.5–1mg PO q12h, and titrate
    tamsulosin 400µg/d
    terazosin 1mg nocte, and titrate
    indoramin 20mg nocte, and titrate

Anticholinergic
    bethanechol 10–30mg PO q8h

'start low and go slow'

anticholinergic agent, bethanechol, helps some patients but adverse effects of abdominal colic, salivation, flushing and sweating may be troublesome. For patients too weak to sit or stand, nursing assistance to a more suitable position may help, but catheterization is often necessary.

Urinary tract obstruction

Urinary tract obstruction occurs not infrequently in patients with advanced cancer and may lead to renal failure if not treated. Many reviews of urinary tract obstruction have been published.[1,2,9]

The causes of urinary tract obstruction are listed in Table 20.13. Cancers of the kidney, renal pelvis and ureter will cause unilateral obstruction. Cancers of the bladder, prostate, cervix, endometrium and rectum may cause unilateral or bilateral ureteric obstruction in the pelvis. Marked retroperitoneal lymphadenopathy as occurs with lymphoma can cause bilateral ureteric obstruction.

Lower urinary tract obstruction usually presents as retention and the finding of a large urine volume on catheterization is diagnostic. Upper urinary tract obstruction may be insidious and asymptomatic, and diagnosis requires some form of imaging. Ultrasound or CT scanning is usually diagnostic; if doubt remains, cystoscopy and retrograde pyelography should be performed.

Treatment

Treatment decisions for urinary tract obstruction must take into account the stage of the patient's disease, the anticipated life expectancy, and whether or not further anticancer therapy is available.

Lower tract obstruction. Lower urinary tract obstruction usually requires catheterization, at least temporarily. If urethral catheterization is not possible, a suprapubic catheter is inserted.

Table 20.13 Causes of urinary tract obstruction

Upper tract (renal pelvis, ureter)	Lower tract (bladder, urethra)
infiltration, compression by tumour	infiltration, compression by tumour
stricture: surgery, radiotherapy	benign enlargement of prostate
calculi	blood clots
blood clots	calculi
retroperitoneal fibrosis	infection
	urethral stricture
	faecal impaction
	detrusor failure
	anticholinergic drugs
	anticholinergic side effects of drugs
	neurogenic

Treatment of obstructing tumour may involve surgery, radiotherapy, endoscopic resection or laser therapy. Haematuria, calculi, infection and faecal impaction are treated appropriately. Urethral strictures are treated by dilatation. Resection of benign prostatic disease can be considered if it is a major factor causing obstruction. Urethral stents can be used for patients who would otherwise require permanent catheterization but wish to remain catheter-free.[2]

Upper tract obstruction. Treatment is by cystoscopy and retrograde ureteric stenting or by a percutaneous nephrostomy inserted under radiological control. Antegrade ureteric stenting via the nephrostomy can be attempted several days later when local bleeding and swelling have settled. If successful, this will allow closure of the percutaneous nephrostomy. If ureteric stenting cannot be achieved, usually due to destruction of the ureteric orifices by carcinoma of the bladder, the nephrostomy is left in place permanently or some form of surgical urinary diversion considered. Ureteric stents may occlude, in which situation a cystogram will fail to show reflux of dye up the stent. Ureteric stents are routinely changed each 3 to 6 months.

Bilateral ureteric obstruction (or unilateral obstruction in a patient with a single functioning kidney) requires urgent intervention if renal function is to be preserved. However, careful consideration of the stage of the patient's disease and prognosis is required before embarking on therapy. For patients with advanced disseminated disease and no effective anticancer treatment available, allowing them to die with progressive uraemia, without submitting them to invasive procedures, may be the less distressing course.

Post-obstruction diuresis. Relief of urinary obstruction frequently causes a post-obstruction diuresis. The urine volume may be very large, causing significant electrolyte imbalance and requiring careful replacement therapy.

Terminal care

Lower urinary tract obstruction is relieved by catheterization; other investigations or therapy are inappropriate. Upper urinary tract obstruction with renal impairment developing in the last week or days of life should be managed conservatively and symptomatically.

Urinary catheters

Urinary catheters are commonly used for the management of acute retention, but long-term catheterization may be required for some patients with advanced cancer. An alternative for some patients is intermittent self-catheterization.[25] The indications for long-term catheterization are listed in Table 20.14.

Table 20.14 Indications for long-term urinary catheterization

Atonic bladder
Persistent obstruction
Persistent incontinence
Management of pressure sore complicated by incontinence
Perineal ulceration or infection complicated by incontinence
Avoidance of painful movement required to change clothes and bed linen
Patient comfort (terminally ill patients)

Infection. Regular irrigation delays the development of obstruction but increases the risk of infection. Prophylactic antibiotics do not prevent bacteriuria or reduce the incidence of urinary infections. Antibiotics should be considered if there are clinical signs of infection or repeated catheter blockages. Asymptomatic bacteriuria does not warrant treatment except for urease-producing organisms (most commonly *Proteus mirabilis*), which greatly increase the risk of calculus formation. A urinary antiseptic, methenamine hippurate, should be considered for patients with long term indwelling catheters; it requires urinary acidification to be effective.[26, 27]

Bypassing. Bypassing may be due to catheter obstruction or irritation of the bladder by the catheter. Obstruction is treated by flushing the catheter clear or by replacing it. For patients with a small or contracted bladder, the catheter balloon is inflated to only 5–10 ml (rather than the maximum volume written on the catheter) to avoid detrusor stimulation. Catheter bypassing is not treated by inserting a larger catheter, which may cause more irritation. Some patients will benefit from the use of antispasmodic and bladder relaxant drugs (see Table 20.7).

Suprapubic catheters. A suprapubic urinary catheter is used if urethral catheterization is not possible and if catheterization is necessary during the course of pelvic radiotherapy. The principles of catheter care are the same. The advantages of a suprapubic catheter include greater patient comfort, fewer infections (prostatitis, epididymitis), avoidance of urethral strictures, and ease with which the patient can be given a trial of voiding by clamping the tube intermittently.

Urinary infection

Patients with advanced cancer are prone to urinary infection (Table 20.15). The diagnosis is established by the appropriate microbiological tests. The differential diagnosis includes non-infective causes of dysuria, as may result from the passage of urine over any inflamed mucosa.

Treatment

Treatment of urinary infection includes appropriate antibiotics, correction of predisposing factors (where feasible), analgesia, urinary alkalinization, and encouragement regarding

Table 20.15 Predisposition to urinary infection in patients with cancer

General	immunosuppression: cancer, therapy general debility
Obstruction, stasis	malignant infiltration, compression neurogenic bladder
Tissue damage	cystitis: radiotherapy, chemotherapy surgery
Iatrogenic	catheters, ureteric stents, nephrostomy tubes
Fistulas	

fluid intake. Treatment of obstruction should be considered, if feasible, as urinary infection is difficult to eradicate in the presence of persistent obstruction. A Cochrane review of the use of cranberry products to treat urinary infection found no RCTs on which to base recommendations.[28] Patients with chronic urinary infection may benefit from a topical urinary analgesic (phenazopyridine) or drugs that reduce the detrusor sensitivity such as oxybutynin or flavoxate.

Preventive. For patients without indwelling devices, maintenance antibiotic therapy with nitrofurantoin, ciprofloxacin or trimethoprim may reduce the incidence of recurrent urinary infection.[29, 30] Cochrane reviews of methenamine[27] and cranberry products[31] reported the size and quality of available trials were insufficient to provide conclusive evidence for their use; a more recently published trial showed cranberry lingonberry juice to be effective in preventing recurrent urinary infection.[32] For patients with indwelling catheters or stents, antibiotics do not reduce the incidence of bacteriuria or lower urinary tract infections. Asymptomatic bacteriuria usually warrants no therapy except for urease-producing organisms such as *Proteus mirabilis* (which predispose to calculus formation) or if repeated catheter blockage is a problem; antibiotic therapy will not eradicate the infection and may encourage the development of drug resistance. Treatment with methenamine hippurate has been reported to reduce the frequency of infection and infection-related catheter blockage, but a Cochrane review concluded that the evidence that methenamine reduced the incidence of urinary infection was inconclusive.[27]

Renal failure

Renal failure may be due to pre-renal factors, intrinsic renal disease, or post-renal factors (Table 20.16). In practice, renal failure is frequently multifactorial.[2]

Pre-renal factors. Reduction in the plasma volume or the effective circulating blood volume due to any cause will reduce renal perfusion and can predispose to renal failure. Renal failure can occur in association with advanced liver disease (of whatever cause) in the absence of any primary renal disorder. This hepatorenal syndrome is due to a functional decline in renal perfusion caused by multiple factors including hypoalbuminaemia and peripheral vasodilatation.

Intrinsic renal disease. Various types of immunologically mediated glomerular disease occur in association with malignant disease, which may manifest as either renal failure or the nephrotic syndrome. The injection of radiological contrast media may cause renal impairment due to ischaemic tubular cell damage; this is more likely to occur in patients who are

Table 20.16 Causes of renal impairment in patients with cancer

Pre-renal
    inadequate fluid intake
    vomiting, diarrhoea, gastrointestinal fistulas
    polyuria: hypercalcaemia, diabetes insipidus and mellitus, diuretics
    haemorrhage
    sepsis and shock
    liver disease (hepatorenal syndrome)
    third space fluid accumulation: ascites, bowel obstruction, vena caval obstruction
    pericardial tamponade, cardiac failure

Renal
    tumour infiltration
    tumour-associated glomerular disease
    metabolic: hypercalcaemia, hyperuricaemia, tumour lysis syndrome
    hyperviscosity: paraproteinaemia, polycythaemia, hyperleucocytosis
    amyloidosis
    disseminated intravascular coagulation (DIC)
    renal vein thrombosis
    radiation
    radiological contrast media
    drugs
        antitumour: cisplatin, methotrexate, nitrosoureas, ifosfamide
        antibiotics: aminoglycosides, amphotericin, penicillins, sulfonamides
        other: allopurinol, NSAIDs, cyclosporin
    pyelonephritis

Post-renal (see Urinary Tract Obstruction)

dehydrated and those with pre-existing renal impairment, diabetes mellitus or myeloma. Renal damage by drugs is more likely to occur in patients with pre-existing renal impairment and in those who are dehydrated, elderly or debilitated; potentially nephrotoxic agents should be withheld or the doses modified in these situations.

Post-renal factors. The causes of renal failure due to post-renal factors are discussed in the section on Urinary Tract Obstruction.

Treatment

The treatment of renal failure is directed at the cause, where possible and appropriate. If impairment is mild, no further treatment may be necessary although other nephrotoxic influences need to be avoided. If renal failure is severe, treatment decisions will depend on the stage of the patient's disease and life expectancy. Patients for whom other anticancer therapy is available and those whose life expectancy is longer (except for renal failure) may appropriately be managed by dialysis, either temporarily until renal function recovers, or indefinitely. Other patients with advanced cancer, for whom further anticancer therapy is not available and whose life expectancy (before the onset of renal failure) was short, may best be treated without dialysis.

Patients with progressively deteriorating renal function require palliation of symptoms associated with uraemia including nausea and vomiting, tiredness and weakness, pruritus and dyspnoea.[33] Renal failure alters the pharmacokinetics of many drugs and careful observation for signs of toxicity is required. Some of the medications used in palliative care need to be given in reduced doses to avoid toxicity (Table 20.17).[33]

Table 20.17 Medication guidelines for patients with renal impairment

	Reduced dose	No change
Analgesics	opioids paracetamol (acetaminophen)	NSAIDs
Adjuvants	gabapentin	carbamazepine corticosteroids tricyclic antidepressants mexiletine
Anxiolytics		benzodiazepines
Antidepressants		tricyclic antidepressants fluoxetine sertraline
Antipsychotics		chlorpromazine levomepromazine haloperidol
Anticonvulsants	gabapentin	carbamazepine phenytoin
Antiemetics	metoclopramide	prochlorperazine
Antidyspeptics	H_2-receptor antagonists	proton pump inhibitors

Terminal care

The development of oliguria or anuria during the last days of life requires no investigation or therapy unless it is associated with pain or increased dyspnoea.

Prostatitis, epididymo-orchitis

Inflammation and infection of the prostate gland can occur after catheterization and endoscopy or following pelvic irradiation. The patient complains of dysuria, pain in the lower back and perineum, and is febrile. The prostate gland is swollen and exquisitely tender. The responsible organism can usually be identified from urine examination, the most frequent being *E. coli*. Treatment is with appropriate antibiotics.

Epididymitis and epididymo-orchitis occur secondary to obstruction of the lower urinary tract, in association with prostatitis, or following genitourinary tract manipulation. Initially there can be tender swelling of the epididymis alone, which usually progresses rapidly to orchitis and painful swelling of the scrotum. There may be a urethral discharge or dysuria and the responsible organism can usually be identified on examination of the urine; *E. coli* and other gram-negative bacteria are the most frequent cause. Treatment is with appropriate antibiotics in conjunction with bed rest, analgesia and the use of a scrotal sling.

Vaginitis, vaginal discharge

Patients with cancer are prone to the development of vaginitis because of general immunosuppression and the frequent use of antibiotics and corticosteroids. Chemotherapy or radiotherapy may cause vaginal inflammation that is frequently complicated by secondary infection. More serious and troublesome vaginitis occurs with local tumour recurrence, radionecrosis, and faecal or urinary fistulas.

Vaginitis will cause pain and discharge usually associated with perineal discomfort. If associated with tumour, radionecrosis or a faecal fistula, there may be considerable odour.

Treatment The management options are outlined in Table 20.18. Whatever the cause, secondary infection is common and is treated with appropriate antimicrobial therapy and attention to local hygiene. Metronidazole suppositories may reduce odour associated with tumour infiltration, fistulas or radionecrosis. Persistent vaginitis following radiotherapy is treated with topical oestrogen cream. Radionecrosis may require surgical debridement. The use of polymer gels such as Intrasite to cover vaginal wounds may not aid healing, but can greatly reduce discharge and odour. Faecal and urinary fistulas usually require surgical diversion, except in the terminally ill.

Table 20.18 Vaginitis: treatment options

Infection	appropriate antimicrobial therapy attention to local hygiene
Chemotherapy	treat secondary infection
Radiation	acute: treat secondary infection chronic: topical oestrogens
Tumour	diathermy, laser, radiotherapy, surgery treat secondary infection metronidazole suppositories (for odour)
Fistulas	rectovaginal: colostomy vesicovaginal: urinary diversion

Abnormal uterine bleeding

The various abnormalities of uterine bleeding and their common causes are shown in Table 20.19.

Table 20.19 Abnormalities of uterine bleeding

Menorrhagia (heavy periods occurring regularly)
    idiopathic, dysfunctional
    uterine fibroid, IUD
    bleeding diathesis	

Irregular heavy bleeding anovulatory cycles	

Non-menstrual bleeding
    postcoital
    intermenstrual
    postmenopausal
	
	infection, polyp, tumour, bleeding diathesis
	progesterone-only pill, dysfunctional
	cancer, radiation, infection, hormonal therapy, bleeding diathesis

Amenorrhoea
    hysterectomy
    oestrogen deficiency
    hormonal therapy
	
	oophorectomy, chemotherapy, radiotherapy
	tamoxifen, progestogens

Treatment. Postmenopausal bleeding in patients with cancer is most frequently due to progestogen or tamoxifen therapy given for breast cancer, but an assessment needs to be made to exclude cervical and uterine pathology. Bleeding due to hormonal therapy simply requires reassurance. The treatment of bleeding due to recurrent tumour may include surgery, irradiation or local treatment with diathermy or laser. There will be signs of abnormal bleeding at other sites if uterine bleeding is caused by a systemic bleeding diathesis.

Amenorrhoea occurs with ovarian removal or failure and after hysterectomy. Treatment with tamoxifen or a progestogen for breast cancer can also cause amenorrhoea. Hormone replacement therapy is appropriate for women who do not have hormone sensitive tumours.

Sexual dysfunction

Cancer and its treatment are major causes of sexual dysfunction, both physical and psychological, although it is frequently not discussed or treated.[34, 35] This may be due to embarrassment about discussing sexual issues on the part of the patient or the doctor, or the belief that older or sick patients have no sexual interest. Health care professionals need to be prepared to provide reassurance, explanation and advice on sexual matters.

Normal sexual response. The normal sexual response may be divided into three phases—desire, arousal and orgasm (Table 20.20). Each phase has defined physiological requirements, abnormalities or inhibition of which lead to sexual dysfunction. Dyspareunia, or the development of pain during or immediately after sexual intercourse, is a powerful inhibitor of all phases of sexual activity.

Table 20.20 The normal sexual response

Desire - the initiation phase
sexual interest or motivation
physiological requirements: CNS, hormones
Arousal - the stimulatory phase
sexual excitement: penile erection, vaginal expansion and lubrication
physiological requirements: CNS, hormones, intact sacral nerves
Orgasm
sensation of orgasmic pleasure
rhythmic contractions of genital muscles, emission in the male
physiological requirements: CNS, sensory and autonomic sacral nerves

Psychological factors. Sexual dysfunction due to psychological factors, difficulties with communication, and marital discord can precede the diagnosis of cancer or may be precipitated or aggravated by it (Table 20.21). The emotional consequences of cancer, including depression and anxiety, often have profound effects on both the patient's sexuality and sexual function. Patients with cancer may feel that their bodies are contaminated or unclean and problems related to an altered body image (such as caused by mastectomy, limb amputation or colostomy) can inhibit sexual desire or activity. Patients or their partners may fear that sexual activity may be too vigorous or lead to further spread of the disease. It is not uncommon to be asked whether the partner is at risk of contracting cancer as a result of sexual activity.

Physical factors. Physical factors play a major role in sexual dysfunction in patients with cancer. General ill health, physical weakness and pain all contribute to lessened desire.

Table 20.21 Causes of sexual dysfunction

Psychological
    depression, anxiety
    altered body image, poor self esteem
    fears regarding the patient's physical condition
    fears about cancer being contagious
    pre-existing sexual and marital problems

Physical
    general ill health, physical weakness, pain
    medications: CNS depressants, anticholinergics
    physical abnormalities due to the presence of cancer
    adverse effects of therapy: surgery, radiation, chemotherapy, hormone therapy

Medications, particularly those causing CNS depression or anti-cholinergic effects, impair sexual desire and function. Abnormalities or deformities due to the presence of cancer can make sexual activity difficult and sexual function can be greatly affected by surgery, radiotherapy, chemotherapy and hormone treatment.

Sexual dysfunction in females

In women treated for cancer there is evidence for a reduction in all phases of the sexual response—desire, arousal and orgasm—and an increased incidence of dyspareunia. Causes of sexual dysfunction are listed in Table 20.22.

Table 20.22 Female sexual dysfunction

Diminished desire
    general physical and psychological factors (Table 20.21)
    any cause of dyspareunia

Decreased arousal
    any factor causing decreased desire
    any cause of dyspareunia
    oestrogen deficiency: surgery, radiotherapy, chemotherapy, postmenopausal
    pelvic autonomic nerve damage: surgery, tumour
    vaginal mucosal atrophy: oestrogen deficiency, postmenopausal, radiotherapy

Difficulty achieving orgasm
    any factor causing decreased desire, arousal
    any cause of dyspareunia

Dyspareunia
    vaginal mucositis, ulceration: radiotherapy, chemotherapy, infection
    atrophic vaginal mucosa: oestrogen deficiency, radiotherapy
    vaginal fibrosis, stenosis: radiotherapy, surgery
    vaginal surgery
    pelvic adhesions: surgery, radiotherapy
    pelvic mass
    psychological factors

Treatment. The treatment of sexual dysfunction related to cancer treatment is, where possible, that of the cause. A Cochrane review of female sexual dysfunction following pelvic radiotherapy found a paucity of quality evidence on which to base recommendations.[36] Systemic hormonal replacement therapy should be considered for women with ovarian failure who do not have hormone sensitive tumours. For women with hormone sensitive tumours, problems related to vaginal mucosal atrophy can be treated with small doses of topical oestrogens or adequate lubrication used before intercourse. Vaginitis due to chemotherapy or radiotherapy requires intensive local hygiene and douching, and the use of metronidazole vaginal suppositories is helpful. Infection should be treated with appropriate antimicrobial therapy. When requested, simple explanation and reassurance regarding sexual matters, as well as advice on how to overcome physical problems and handicaps, can be of great benefit to the patient.

Sexual dysfunction in males

Men treated for cancer are susceptible to various disorders of sexual function, the most frequent being impotence or inability to achieve and maintain an erection (Table 20.23). Lack of sexual desire can relate to androgen deficiency but is more likely to be associated with the general physical and psychological factors listed in Table 20.21. Impotence can occur as a result of testosterone deficiency or other physical disease but is often due to psychological factors. Damage to the pelvic sympathetic nerves by surgery or tumour leads to retrograde ejaculation into the bladder. However, it is rare for the sensation of orgasm to be lost, and where orgasm cannot be achieved, lack of desire or psychological problems should be suspected. Dyspareunia is uncommon in men but can occur secondary to urethritis caused by radiotherapy or infection.

Table 20.23 Male sexual dysfunction

Lack of desire
    general physical and psychological problems (Table 20.21)
    androgen deficiency

Failure of erection
    any factor causing decreased desire
    androgen deficiency: orchidectomy, radiation, chemotherapy, hormone therapy
    pelvic radiotherapy
    pelvic autonomic nerve damage: surgery, tumour
    spinal cord, cauda equina lesion: tumour
    psychogenic
    chronic or pre-existing erectile dysfunction
    medication: alcohol, antihypertensives, antidepressants, tranquillizers

Absence of ejaculation
    androgen deficiency
    absence of semen: prostatectomy, cystectomy
    retrograde ejaculation: sympathetic nerve damage

Absence of orgasm
    any factor causing decreased desire, arousal
    psychogenic

Dyspareunia
    urethritis: radiotherapy, infection

Treatment

The management of male sexual dysfunction is directed at the cause, where possible. Psychological and psychosocial factors that lead to complaints of sexual dysfunction need to be assessed and managed appropriately. Testosterone deficiency may be treated with systemic replacement therapy except in men with prostate cancer. A significant proportion of men with pelvic disease or androgen deficiency are capable of a reasonable degree of sexual activity given the desire and an understanding partner.

Selective phosphodiesterase-5 inhibitors. The treatment of erectile dysfunction was revolutionized by the introduction of the selective phosphodiesterase-5 inhibitor, sildenafil. In a meta-analysis of RCTs involving more than 6000 men, treatment with sildenafil was significantly more likely than placebo to lead to successful sexual intercourse (Table 20.24).[37] Sildenafil is effective in a similar proportion of men who have undergone proctectomy or prostatectomy. The usual starting dose is 50mg, taken about one hour before sexual activity. This can be increased to 100mg, depending on efficacy and tolerance. The starting dose for older patients and those with hepatic or renal impairment is 25mg. Side effects include flushing, headache, dyspepsia and visual disturbance, which are usually mild and transient. There is no significant association with severe cardiovascular events or death, although sildenafil is contraindicated in patients taking nitrate or nitrite medications in any form. Men with chemotherapy-related hypogonadism may benefit from combined therapy with testosterone and sildenafil.[38] A second selective phosphodiesterase-5 inhibitor, vardenafil, showed similar efficacy in initial clinical trials.[39]

Table 20.24 Meta-analysis of sildenafil RCTs

Author	n	Intervention	Outcome
Fink[37]	6659	sildenafil	sildenafil: no. with ≥1 successful intercourse: 83 vs 45%;
	27 RCTs	vs placebo	proportion intercourse attempts successful: 57 vs 21%

References

1 Russo, P. (2000). Urologic emergencies in the cancer patient. *Seminars in Oncology* 27, 284–98.

2 Arrison, D.P., Hirshberg, S.J. and Greenberg, R.E. (2002). Urologic issues of palliative care. In *Principles and Practice of Palliative Care and Supportive Oncology* (ed. A.M. Berger, R.K. Portenoy and D.E. Weissman). Philadelphia, Lippincott, Williams and Wilkins.

3 Crew, J.P., Jephcott, C.R. and Reynard, J.M. (2001). Radiation-induced haemorrhagic cystitis. *European Urology* 40, 111–23.

4 Radiation Therapy Oncology Group (RTOG)/ European Organisation for Research and Treatment of Cancer (EORTC) (2000). RTOG/EORTC Late Radiation Morbidity Scoring Schema. <www.rtog.org/members/toxicity/late.html>

5 Datta, S.N., et al. (2002). Urinary tract ultrasonography in the evaluation of haematuria—a report of over 1,000 cases. *Annals of the Royal College of Surgeons of England* 84, 203–5.

6 Lammle, M., et al. (2002). Reliability of MR imaging-based virtual cystoscopy in the diagnosis of cancer of the urinary bladder. *American Journal of Roentgenology* 178, 1483–8.

7 Lang, E.K., et al. (2002). Computerized tomography tailored for the assessment of microscopic hematuria. *Journal of Urology* 167, 547–54.

8 Schultz, M. and van der Lelie, H. (1995). Microscopic haematuria as a relative contraindication for tranexamic acid. *British Journal of Haematology* 89, 663–4.

9 Walther, M.M. (2001). Urologic emergencies. In *Cancer. Principles and Practice of Oncology.6th edition* (ed. V.T. De Vita, S. Hellman and S.A. Rosenberg). Philadelphia, Lippincott, Williams and Wilkins.

10 Ordemann, R., et al. (2000). Encouraging results in the treatment of haemorrhagic cystitis with estrogen—report of 10 cases and review of the literature. *Bone Marrow Transplantation* 25, 981–5.

11 Foley, S.J., et al. (2000). A prospective study of the natural history of hematuria associated with benign prostatic hyperplasia and the effect of finasteride. *Journal of Urology* 163, 496–8.

12 Mayer, R., et al. (2001). Hyperbaric oxygen—an effective tool to treat radiation morbidity in prostate cancer. *Radiotherapy and Oncology* 61, 151–6.

13 de Baere, T., et al. (2002). Radio frequency ablation of renal cell carcinoma: preliminary clinical experience. *Journal of Urology* 167, 1961–4.

14 Denton, A.S., Clarke, N.W. and Maher, E.J. (2002). Non-surgical interventions for late radiation cystitis in patients who have received radical radiotherapy to the pelvis (Cochrane Review). *Cochrane Database of Systematic Reviews* CD001773.

15 Scientific Committee of the First International Consultation on Incontinence (2000). Assessment and treatment of urinary incontinence. *Lancet* 355, 2153–8.

16 Fantl, J.A., Newman, D.K. and Colling, J. (1996). *Urinary incontinence in adults: acute and chronic management. Clinical Practice Guideline.* Rockville, MD: Agency for Health Care Policy and Research (AHCPR).

17 Moore, K.N. and Dorey, G.F. (1999). Conservative treatment of urinary incontinence in men: a review of the literature. *Physiotherapy* 85, 77–87.

18 Berghmans, L.C., et al. (2000). Conservative treatment of urge urinary incontinence in women: a systematic review of randomized clinical trials. *British Journal of Urology* 85, 254–63.

19 Eustice, S., Roe, B. and Paterson, J. (2000). Prompted voiding for the management of urinary incontinence in adults (Cochrane Review). *Cochrane Database of Systematic Reviews* CD002113.

20 Hay-Smith, E.J., et al. (2001). Pelvic floor muscle training for urinary incontinence in women (Cochrane Review). *Cochrane Database of Systematic Reviews* CD001407.

21 Grady, D., et al. (2001). Postmenopausal hormones and incontinence: the Heart and Estrogen/Progestin Replacement Study. *Obstetrics and Gynecology* 97, 116–20.

22 Ouslander, J.G., et al. (2001). Effects of oral estrogen and progestin on the lower urinary tract among female nursing home residents. *Journal of the American Geriatric Society* 49, 803–7.

23 Glazener, C.M. and Cooper, K. (2002). Bladder neck needle suspension for urinary incontinence in women (Cochrane Review). *Cochrane Database of Systematic Reviews* CD003636.

24 Hay Smith, J., et al. (2002). Anticholinergic drugs versus placebo for overactive bladder syndrome in adults (Cochrane Review). *Cochrane Database of Systematic Reviews* CD003781.

25 Hunt, G.M., Oakeshott, P. and Whitaker, R.H. (1996). Intermittent catheterisation: simple, safe, and effective but underused. *British Medical Journal* 312, 103–7.

26 Norberg, A., et al. (1980). Randomized double-blind study of prophylactic methenamine hippurate treatment of patients with indwelling catheters. *European Journal of Clinical Pharmacology* 18, 497–500.

27 Lee, B., et al. (2002). Methenamine hippurate for preventing urinary tract infections (Cochrane Review). *Cochrane Database of Systematic Reviews* CD003625.

28 Jepson, R.G., Mihaljevic, L. and Craig, J. (2000). Cranberries for treating urinary tract infections (Cochrane Review). *Cochrane Database of Systematic Reviews* CD001322.

29 Raz, R. and Boger, S. (1991). Long-term prophylaxis with norfloxacin versus nitrofurantoin in women with recurrent urinary tract infection. *Antimicrobial Agents and Chemotherapy* 35, 1241–2.

30 Biering-Sorensen, F., et al. (1994). Ciprofloxacin as prophylaxis for urinary tract infection: prospective, randomized, cross-over, placebo controlled study in patients with spinal cord lesion. *Journal of Urology* 151, 105–8.

31 Jepson, R.G., Mihaljevic, L. and Craig, J. (2001). Cranberries for preventing urinary tract infections (Cochrane Review). *Cochrane Database of Systematic Reviews* CD001321.

32 Kontiokari, T., et al. (2001). Randomised trial of cranberry-lingonberry juice and Lactobacillus GG drink for the prevention of urinary tract infections in women. *British Medical Journal* 322, 1571.

33 Cohen, L.M., et al. (2001). Renal palliative care. In *Palliative care for non-cancer patients* (ed. J.M. Addington-Hall and I.J. Higginson). Oxford, Oxford University Press.

34 Ganz, P.A., Litwin, M.S. and Myerowitz, B.E. (2001). Sexual problems. In *Cancer. Principles and Practice of Oncology. 6th edition* (ed. V.T. De Vita, S. Hellman and S.A. Rosenberg). Philadelphia, Lippincott, Williams and Wilkins.

35 Ofman, U.S. (2002). Disorders of sexuality and reproduction. In *Principles and Practice of Palliative Care and Supportive Oncology* (ed. A.M. Berger, R.K. Portenoy and D.E. Weissman). Philadelphia, Lippincott, Williams and Wilkins.

36 Denton, A.S. and Maher, E.J. (2003). Interventions for the physical aspects of sexual dysfunction in women following pelvic radiotherapy (Cochrane Review). *Cochrane Database of Systematic Reviews* CD003750.

37 Fink, H.A., et al. (2002). Sildenafil for male erectile dysfunction: a systematic review and meta-analysis. *Archives of Internal Medicine* 162, 1349–60.

38 Chatterjee, R., et al. (2002). Management of erectile dysfunction by combination therapy with testosterone and sildenafil in recipients of high-dose therapy for haematological malignancies. *Bone Marrow Transplantion* 29, 607–10.

39 Porst, H., et al. (2001). The efficacy and tolerability of vardenafil, a new, oral, selective phospho-diesterase type 5 inhibitor, in patients with erectile dysfunction: the first at-home clinical trial. *International Journal of Impotence Research* 13, 192–9.

21

Cardiovascular

Cardiac complications	Oedema
Acute pericarditis	SVC obstruction
Pericardial effusion	IVC obstruction
Constrictive pericarditis	Lymphoedema

Cardiac complications of cancer and cancer treatment

Cardiac disease occurring in patients with cancer is more frequently due to pre-existing ischaemic heart disease, but cancer and its treatment may cause and aggravate a number of conditions (Table 21.1).[1,2]

Table 21.1 Cardiac complications of cancer and cancer treatment

Myocardial ischaemia	radiotherapy, chemotherapy
Arrhythmias	malignant infiltration, chemotherapy, radiotherapy
Cardiomyopathy	chemotherapy, radiotherapy
Acute pericardial disease	malignant infiltration, radiation, chemotherapy, infection
Chronic pericardial disease	radiotherapy: effusion, constriction malignant encasement

Myocardial ischaemia. Acute myocardial ischaemia and infarction have been reported after the administration of some chemotherapy drugs, including fluorouracil, vinca alkaloids, interferon and interleukin-2. Cardiac irradiation is associated with accelerated coronary artery disease that becomes clinically manifest a few to many years after treatment; the incidence is less with modern radiotherapy techniques that limit the radiation dose to the heart. Provided it is justified by the prognosis due to cancer, investigation and treatment of myocardial ischaemia are the same as for patients without cancer.

Cardiomyopathy. Cardiomyopathy causing cardiac failure may occur after chemotherapy. This is classically associated with anthracycline therapy and the effect may be potentiated by other drugs (e.g. paclitaxel) or mediastinal irradiation. Cardiac failure is also reported with other agents including interferon, interleukin-2 and trastuzumab (Herceptin). Treatment with an angiotensin converting enzyme (ACE)-inhibitor leads to improvement for most patients; traditional therapy with digoxin, diuretics and vasodilators is often ineffective. Many asymptomatic patients previously treated with anthracyclines have compromised cardiac function, which may predispose to the subsequent development of cardiac failure. Radiation may cause myocardial fibrosis, which is usually mild in degree and asymptomatic.

Arrhythmias. Acute arrhythmias have been associated with the administration of a variety of chemotherapy drugs including anthracyclines, taxanes, vinca alkaloids, fluorouracil, interferon and interleukin-2. Mediastinal irradiation is associated with an increased incidence of arrhythmias, the most common clinically significant abnormality being complete atrioventricular block. This occurs after a mean of 12 years following therapy and is attributed to radiation-induced fibrosis of the conduction system. Malignant disease involving the pericardium or mediastinum is associated with cardiac arrhythmias, presumably due to infiltration of the cardiac conduction system.

Acute pericarditis

Acute pericarditis is reported following the administration of all-trans retinoic acid (ATRA), anthracycline drugs and high dose cyclophosphamide. Acute pericarditis due to irradiation occurs during or up to a few months after treatment. The patient complains of anterior chest pain and a pericardial rub is heard on examination. Clinically mild pericarditis can be managed by careful observation and treatment with a corticosteroid or NSAID. If symptoms are more severe or there is evidence of significant effusion on echocardiography, pericardiocentesis is performed for diagnostic and therapeutic purposes (see below). Acute pericarditis can also be caused by infection.

Pericardial effusion

Malignant pericardial effusions occur in less than 5% of patients with cancer, but the incidence may be nearer 20% in patients with lung cancer.[3, 4] Effusions usually develop in patients with advanced metastatic disease and the overall median survival is less than 6 months, although patients with tumours sensitive to radiotherapy or systemic therapy may survive considerably longer. A number of recent reviews of the management of pericardial effusion have been published.[5, 6]

Pericardial effusions in patients with cancer are most commonly due to malignant infiltration; other causes include radiotherapy, uraemia and infection (Table 21.2). Cancer can involve the pericardium by direct extension, retrograde lymphatic infiltration or haematogenous spread. Lymphatic obstruction in the mediastinum can also lead to the development of a pericardial effusion. Lung and breast cancers and the haematological malignancies account for three-quarters of malignant pericardial effusions. Radiotherapy may cause pericardial effusion either as an acute (weeks/months) or late (years) adverse effect; the latter is often accompanied by signs of pericardial constriction.

The clinical features depend on the volume of pericardial fluid, the rate of accumulation, and the underlying cardiac function. The pericardium normally contains less than 50 ml of fluid, but may accommodate several hundred millilitres if the accumulation is slow. If the increase is rapid, serious symptoms and signs can develop with small changes in the pericardial fluid volume. Pericardial tamponade exists when the amount of fluid present is sufficient to cause significant impairment of cardiac function.

Table 21.2 Pericardial disease

Effusion
    malignant infiltration
    mediastinal lymphatic obstruction
    radiation
        acute pericarditis
        late pericardial effusion ± constriction
    uraemia
    infection

Constriction
    malignant encasement
    radiation

Patients present with dyspnoea and may also have orthopnoea and cough. Compromised cardiac function causes weakness, fatigue, dizziness, peripheral oedema and abdominal swelling. Typical pericardial chest pain is frequently absent. On examination, the patient is anxious, sitting upright and leaning forward. There is a tachycardia, reduced systolic blood pressure and raised venous pressure. Pulsus paradoxus, the reduction of the pulse volume or a fall in the systolic blood pressure of more than 10mm Hg occurring during inspiration, is present. The heart sounds are typically distant or soft and there may be a pericardial rub. Pleural effusions, hepatomegaly and peripheral oedema are common.

A chest x-ray may show enlargement of the cardiac shadow, which classically takes on a globular or boot-shaped appearance. A normal cardiac shadow does not exclude tamponade, especially in patients who have had previous radiotherapy. The x-ray may also show pleural effusions. An ECG may show diminished voltages compared to an earlier trace but is frequently unhelpful and shows non-specific changes ST and T-wave changes. Echocardiography will confirm the presence of an effusion, define its position and distribution, and provide an assessment of cardiac function. A CT scan will document the presence and distribution of an effusion but does not assess the effect on cardiac function.

Treatment

Patients presenting with haemodynamic instability or significant symptoms are treated by echocardiographically guided pericardiocentesis, which is reported to be successful in more than 95% of cases with minimal morbidity and no mortality.[6] A drain tube can be inserted to allow further drainage or for subsequent instillation therapy. Failure of pericardiocentesis to relieve the signs of cardiac compression indicates that coexistent constriction is present, due either to radiation fibrosis or neoplastic encasement.

Cytological examination of the pericardial fluid is reported to be positive in 65–90% of patients with malignant pericardial effusions.[6]

Recurrent effusions will develop in about half of patients with a malignant pericardial effusion treated by pericardiocentesis alone. A variety of further treatment procedures have been advocated (Table 21.3) and treatment decisions need to be individualized and take into account the patient's anticipated life expectancy. Systemic therapy should be given for sensitive tumours.

Extended catheter drainage. The pericardial catheter is left in place for a number of days until the daily drainage is less than 25–50 ml and a check echocardiograph shows satisfactory drainage. Inflammation related to the catheter is presumed to lead to some pericardial sclerosis. This is associated with no significant side effects and the recurrence rate is 12%.[7]

Table 21.3 Pericardial effusion: treatment options

Pericardiocentesis
    to correct haemodynamic abnormalities
    to obtain fluid for diagnostic examination

Malignant infiltration
    extended catheter drainage
    instillation of sclerosants, cytotoxic agents
    surgical pericardial window
    radiotherapy
    systemic therapy (sensitive tumours)

Radiation-induced
    early: observe, NSAID
    late: no treatment unless constriction also present

Other causes (e.g. uraemia, infection)
    appropriate therapy

Intrapericardial instillation therapy. Intrapericardial instillation of sclerosing agents has been used to control malignant pericardial effusions. The most frequently used sclerosant in the past was tetracycline, and more recent studies have used doxycycline or bleomycin. Repeated treatments on a daily or second daily basis (an average of 3) are required and adverse effects include fever, chest pain and arrhythmias. A comparison of doxycycline and bleomycin showed them to be equally effective, but bleomycin was associated with significantly less adverse effects.[8] Compared to surgical interventions, sclerosant therapy is associated with less patient morbidity and cost.[9] There are no RCTs to determine which sclerosant is better or whether sclerosant therapy is superior to extended catheter drainage alone. Other agents that have been recommended for intrapericardial instillation include cytotoxic drugs, radiopharmaceuticals, and interleukin-2.[5, 6, 10–14]

Surgery. The most popular surgical approach is the subxiphoid pericardiectomy.[5, 6] This involves the surgical creation of a pericardial window or opening in the parietal pericardium that allows fluid to drain into the pericardiac tissues; postoperatively, an intrapericardial drain is left in place until the drainage is minimal. Follow-up studies indicate the effectiveness of this technique does not depend on an aperture through which fluid continues to drain but on the development of pericardial sclerosis, which is possibly caused by the extended catheter drainage.[15] Another surgical approach is to create a pericardial window at thoracoscopy that allows drainage of pericardial fluid into the left pleural space.

Radiotherapy. Radiotherapy is reported to control malignant pericardial effusions in two-thirds of cases.[10] The response rate is highest with lymphoma and breast cancer, but it is also effective for some patients with less radiosensitive tumours.

Constrictive pericarditis

Constrictive pericardial disease in patients with cancer is due to either radiation fibrosis or neoplastic encasement. It is most frequently diagnosed when the removal of pericardial fluid fails to improve cardiac function.

Patients with constrictive pericarditis complain of dyspnoea and cough. Examination shows elevated venous pressure, a small pulse volume and lowering of the systolic blood pressure. Pulsus paradoxus is usually absent. Pleural effusions, hepatomegaly, ascites and dependent oedema are common.

The diagnosis is usually established by echocardiography but sometimes requires cardiac catheterization. If there is a significant effusion present, the diagnosis may be missed until the effusion has been drained. A chest x-ray frequently shows a normal cardiac shadow.

Treatment

The treatment of pericardial constriction depends on the cause (Table 21.4), as well as the stage of the patient's disease and prognosis. Patients with constrictive pericarditis due to radiotherapy can be considered for pericardiectomy. For patients with malignant encasement, pericardiectomy is frequently not feasible and pericardial irradiation should be considered.

Table 21.4 Pericardial constriction: treatment options

Radiotherapy fibrosis	pericardiectomy
Tumour encasement	systemic therapy (sensitive tumours) radiotherapy pericardiectomy

Oedema

Oedema is a frequent complaint in patients with advanced cancer. Localized oedema is due to local venous or lymphatic obstruction, local inflammation or infection, or reduced mobility. Generalized oedema is due to increased capillary venous pressure or reduced oncotic pressure.[16] In patients with advanced cancer, oedema is likely to be multifactorial (Table 21.5).

Table 21.5 Oedema

Localized
    venous or lymphatic obstruction
    inflammation, infection
    reduced mobility, immobilization

Generalized
    raised capillary venous pressure
        cardiac failure
        salt and water retention
            drugs: corticosteroids, NSAIDs, progestogens
            cardiac, renal or hepatic impairment
        vena caval obstruction
        raised intra-abdominal pressure
        fluid overload (iatrogenic)
        peripheral venous insufficiency
        decreased physical activity
    decreased oncotic pressure (hypoproteinaemia)
        poor dietary intake, malabsorption
        hepatic impairment
        catabolic state associated with cancer
        repeated aspiration of (protein-rich) effusions
        nephrotic syndrome

Oedema associated with raised capillary venous pressure is peripheral and dependent and is more marked in the evening. In cardiac failure and other fluid overload states, examination shows raised jugular venous pressure without postural hypotension. Oedema associated with reduced capillary oncotic pressure is generalized with swelling of the face and hands and is more noticeable in the morning. Examination often shows postural hypotension without elevation of the venous pressure.

Treatment. The treatment is that of the cause, where possible. Infusions of protein or albumin are of little or no benefit. Strict fluid and salt restriction usually have no effect and may compromise the quality of life. Diuretic therapy, employing a combination of frusemide with spironolactone or amiloride, is of benefit to some patients. Patients with cardiac failure can be treated with digoxin, vasodilators and angiotensin converting enzyme (ACE)-inhibitors. Drugs predisposing to fluid retention should be stopped, if possible. Patients with dependent oedema should be encouraged to exercise and the increased swelling that occurs through the day can be minimized by using full-length compression stockings. When resting, these patients should be lying flat with their legs elevated on several pillows.

Superior vena caval obstruction

Superior vena caval (SVC) obstruction is reported to occur less often in patients with advanced disease than at the time of initial diagnosis. It can cause distressing symptoms but is very amenable to palliation. A number of recent reviews of this topic have been published. [17, 18]

Superior vena caval (SVC) obstruction is usually due to compression or invasion by tumour, with or without secondary thrombus formation. Primary lung cancer accounts for two thirds of cases but it can occur with any tumour involving the mediastinum. Less commonly, thrombosis occurs secondary to a centrally placed catheter. Occasionally, there is a benign cause such as fibrosis caused by previous mediastinal irradiation.

The common presenting symptoms are dyspnoea, facial swelling and a feeling of fullness in the head. There may be other symptoms related to mediastinal disease including cough, dysphagia, chest pain or hoarseness. Neurological symptoms include headache, dizziness, blurred vision and syncope, all of which are aggravated or precipitated by leaning forward or stooping. Examination shows venous distention in the neck and on the chest wall; there are dilated veins on the backs of the hands that do not collapse when the arm is elevated. There is oedema of the face, neck and upper limbs as well as conjunctival oedema and retinal vein dilatation.

The diagnosis can usually be made on clinical grounds. A chest x-ray or CT scan should be performed to confirm that the obstruction is due to tumour. Helical (spiral) CT venography is currently the most accurate investigation to determine the cause and location of the obstruction.

Treatment

Traditionally regarded as an oncological emergency, SVC obstruction is not immediately life threatening unless adjacent structures such as the trachea or pericardium are involved.

General measures. General symptomatic measures include bed rest with the head elevated and oxygen therapy, which will reduce cardiac output and venous pressure. Diuretic therapy with fluid and salt restriction has been used in the past but dehydration may increase the risk of thrombosis. Corticosteroid therapy (dexamethasone16–24 mg/d) is of benefit to some patients, although its value has never been proven; it will be effective in patients with steroid-sensitive tumours such as lymphoma and may reduce tumour-associated oedema in other cases.

Endovascular therapy. Endovascular therapy is now the initial treatment of choice for SVC obstruction. The endovascular placement of expandable metal stents, with or without balloon angioplasty, provides rapid and durable relief of obstruction with few side effects in experienced hands. [19–23] A Cochrane review reported relief of obstruction by stent insertion in 95% of cases; re-stenting was required in 11% and the overall long-term patency rate was 92%.[17] Patients with thrombosis can also be treated with catheter-directed thrombolysis, although this may increase the complication rate.[17, 24] Compared to radiotherapy, stenting provides much more rapid relief and is effective whether the obstruction is primarily due to tumour, thrombosis or fibrosis.

Anticancer treatment. SVC obstruction caused by tumour is traditionally treated with radiotherapy. Chemotherapy can be considered for small cell lung cancer or lymphoma, depending on what previous treatment has been given.

Catheter-associated thrombosis. Patients with catheter-associated thrombosis are traditionally managed by removal of the catheter and anticoagulation. More recent reports describe the use of thrombolytic therapy, transluminal angioplasty and stent insertion for the treatment of catheter-induced SVC thrombosis.[18, 25]

Inferior vena caval obstruction

The inferior vena cava (IVC) may be obstructed by compression, direct infiltration or thrombosis. Lesser degrees of IVC obstruction often pass unnoticed except for some peripheral oedema, due to the availability of collateral venous circulation. Complete IVC obstruction causes marked swelling of the lower limbs and there is pitting oedema extending up to at least the level of the iliac crests, including the perineum and external genitalia. There is venous dilatation on the anterior abdominal wall and there may be ascites.[26]

Treatment

IVC obstruction occurs most commonly in the terminal phase and treatment is symptomatic. For patients who are not terminal, consideration can be given to stenting and thrombolytic therapy as used for SVC obstruction, although experience is limited.[27, 28]

Lymphoedema

Lymphoedema is oedema or tissue swelling caused by failure of regional lymphatic drainage. It occurs in about 30% of women who had axillary dissection performed in the course of treatment for breast cancer, and the incidence is higher in those who also received radiation to the axilla.[29] It results in disfigurement and impaired function, as well as pain and psychological distress. A number of recent reviews of the management of lymphoedema have been published.[30, 31]

Lymphoedema in patients with cancer is caused by obstruction or interruption of the lymphatic system by surgery, radiotherapy or tumour. It develops most frequently after surgical lymphadenectomy or radiotherapy to the inguinal region or axilla and the incidence is further increased if both modalities of treatment are used. Limbs affected by lymphoedema are particularly prone to cellulitis and each episode of infection can aggravate the degree of oedema.

Lymphoedema is unsightly, uncomfortable and compromises function. Patients complain of swelling and about half report pain.[32] Examination shows non-pitting oedema that does not resolve with rest or elevation. In chronic lymphoedema the skin is thickened due to interstitial fibrosis in the subcutaneous tissues and there may be lymphangiomas (dilated skin lymphatics that look like blisters) or cutaneous hyperkeratosis (warty, scaly skin).[33] The development of malignant lymphangiosarcoma (Stewart-Treves syndrome) is a rare (<0.5%) but documented complication of chronic lymphoedema.[34] In addition to its physical effects, lymphoedema has been demonstrated to have adverse effects on patients' mental health and quality of life.[35–37]

Treatment

In patients with advanced cancer, treatment is often directed at comfort and preventing deterioration, but patients with a better life expectancy may achieve significant physical and psychological improvement with some of the more active therapies.

General measures. There needs to be scrupulous care of the skin and nails as well as the avoidance of any injuries, however minor, which might lead to infection (Table 21.6). If infection occurs it is treated promptly with antibiotics, which often need to be continued for several weeks.

Table 21.6   Treatment of lymphoedema

General skin and nail care
    avoid trauma
        protective garments, gloves
        no injections, venepunctures
        electric razor, nail clippers not scissors
        insect repellents, sun blockout creams
    moisturizing creams
    prompt cleansing and topical antiseptic for any cuts, injuries
    prompt and adequate treatment of cellulitis

Support garments

Exercise

Massage

Compression pumps

Drug therapy

Surgery

Support garments. Patients are fitted with a well-fitting compression sleeve or stocking. A support garment should feel comfortable and not tight—the aim is not to reduce limb volume but to prevent further fluid accumulation.

Exercise. Patients are encouraged to use the limb as normally as possible, as active movement may improve lymph drainage. The affected limb can be elevated when resting. Patients with leg oedema should avoid prolonged periods of standing.

Massage. A variety of different massage techniques or methods of manual lymphatic drainage, collectively known as decongestive lymphoedema therapy (DLT), have been advocated for the initial intensive treatment of lymphoedema.[38, 39] The aim is to stimulate lymph flow in more proximal normal lymphatics, which in turn allows better drainage from the lymphoedematous area. These techniques are widely used although long-term benefit has not been demonstrated in some RCTs (Table 21.7). An RCT of multilayer bandaging was beneficial when used as initial therapy.[40] Following the initial intensive treatment, patients can be instructed to perform self-massage that, performed once or twice a day, is of benefit to many patients. Massage is started on the trunk adjacent to the swollen limb, stroking the skin away from the limb; the process is continued progressively down the limb. The massage strokes should be firm enough to move the skin but not redden it. Support garments are worn between treatments.

Table 21.7 Physical therapy for lymphoedema: RCTs

Author	n	Intervention	Outcome
Bertelli[41]	74	compression sleeve ± electrically stimulated lymphatic drainage	no differences at 6 mo
Hornsby[42]	25	± graduated compression sleeve	compression sleeve: ↓ oedema
Johansson[43]	38	compression bandaging ± initial MLD	MLD: ↓ oedema (pNS)
Andersen[44]	42	standard therapy ± initial MLD	no differences at 12 mo
Badger[40]	90	compression garment ± initial MLB	MLB: doubled the ↓ in oedema at 24 w (pS)
Williams[45]	31	± MLD	MLD: ↓ excess limb volume, ↓ dermal thickness (pS)

MLB: multilayer bandaging; MLD: manual lymphatic drainage

Compression pumps. Compression pumps provide intermittent sequential pneumatic compression of the limb, repetitively massaging the limb in a central direction. Pumps need to be used daily or at least several times a week, indefinitely, with support garments worn between treatments. Pumps cannot be used if there is evidence of infection or thrombosis of the affected limb. Clinical experience is that compression pumps are of benefit if used regularly over longer periods; the negative results of the RCTs in which compression pumps were used for only a few weeks are of questionable clinical relevance.[46, 47] Pumps will prevent progression or produce gradual improvement for some patients.

Drug therapy. Benzopyrones are a group of naturally occurring substances, some of which are beneficial in the treatment of high-protein oedemas. They act by reducing capillary permeability, lessening the accumulation of fluid, and by stimulating macrophage activity in the oedematous tissues, which may promote the breakdown and removal of fibrous tissue. The initial studies of coumarin were positive, but the largest and most recent study showed no benefit (Table 21.8). In addition, hepatotoxicity was reported in 6% of the patients in this study, which is in keeping with anecdotal case reports of severe liver dysfunction, including two deaths, which have lead to the prohibition of coumarin in several countries. RCTs of oxerutin and other flavenoids are uniformly positive (Table 21.8), although the clinical improvement in some studies is quite modest. A review of benzopyrone therapy showed that the reduction in oedema obtained with decongestive lymphoedema therapy (DLT) was significantly greater in patients pre-treated with benzopyrones, and that the effect of DLT is more durable in those who continue to take benzopyrones.[48] These observations would be consistent with benzopyrone-induced breakdown of fibrous tissue by macrophages.

Table 21.8 Drug therapy of lymphoedema: RCTs

Author	n	Intervention	Outcome
Desprez-Curely[49]	92	coumarin 135mg/d + troxerutin 810mg/d vs placebo	↓ oedema at 6 mo
Piller[50]	40	oxerutin 3g/d vs placebo	↓ oedema at 6 mo (pS)
Casley-Smith[51]	52	coumarin 400mg/d vs placebo	↓ oedema at 6 mo (pS)
Taylor[52]	31	oxerutin 3g/d vs placebo	↓ oedema at 24 w
Mortimer[53]	46	oxerutin 3g/d vs placebo	↓ oedema at 6 mo
Cluzan[54]	57	flavenoid (ruscus + hesperidin) vs placebo	↓ oedema at 3 mo (pS)
Pecking[55]	104	micronized purified flavenoid fraction vs placebo	↓ oedema at 6 mo (pNS)
Loprinzi[56]	140	coumarin 400mg/d vs placebo	no difference at 6 mo 6% hepatotoxicity

Diuretic therapy is of no benefit in lymphoedema, and improvement suggests significant co-existing venous obstruction or cardiac failure. Patients with lymphoedema secondary to metastatic involvement of the regional lymph nodes may respond to corticosteroids.

Surgery. A variety of surgical procedures have been advocated for the treatment of lymphoedema, including excision of excessive tissue and bypass surgery for the lymphatic obstruction, but the role of these procedures is not established.[57,58] In patients with concomitant venous obstruction, endovascular venoplasty and stent placement leads to clinical improvement.[59]

References

1   Steinherz, L.J. and Yahalom, J. (2001). Cardiac toxicity. In *Cancer. Principles and Practice of Oncology. 6th edition* (ed. V.T. De Vita, S. Hellman and S.A. Rosenberg). Philadelphia, Lippincott, Williams and Wilkins.

2   Davies, M.J., Schultz, M.Z. and Murren, J.R. (2002). Cardiopulmonary toxicity of cancer therapy. In *Principles and Practice of Palliative Care and Supportive Oncology* (ed. A.M. Berger, R.K. Portenoy and D.E. Weissman). Philadelphia, Lippincott, Williams and Wilkins.

3   Klatt, E.C. and Heitz, D.R. (1990). Cardiac metastases. *Cancer* 65, 1456–9.

4   Tamura, A., et al. (1992). Cardiac metastasis of lung cancer. A study of metastatic pathways and clinical manifestations. *Cancer* 70, 437–42.

5   Schrump, D.S. and Nguyen, D.M. (2001). Malignant pleural and pericardial effusions. In *Cancer. Principles and Practice of Oncology. 6th edition* (ed. V.T. De Vita, S. Hellman and S.A. Rosenberg). Philadelphia, Lippincott, Williams and Wilkins.

6   Ruckdeschel, J.C. and Robinson, L.A. (2002). Management of pleural and pericardial effusions. In *Principles and Practice of Palliative Care and Supportive Oncology* (ed. A.M. Berger, R.K. Portenoy and D.E. Weissman). Philadelphia, Lippincott, Williams and Wilkins.

7   Tsang, T.S., et al. (2000). Outcomes of primary and secondary treatment of pericardial effusion in patients with malignancy. *Mayo Clinic Proceedings* 75, 248–53.

8   Liu, G., et al. (1996). Prospective comparison of the sclerosing agents doxycycline and bleomycin for the primary management of malignant pericardial effusion and cardiac tamponade. *Journal of Clinical Oncology* 14, 3141–7.

9   Anderson, T.M., et al. (2001). Pericardial catheter sclerosis versus surgical procedures for pericardial effusions in cancer patients. *Journal of Cardiovascular Surgery (Torino)* 42, 415–19.

10   Vaitkus, P.T., Herrmann, H.C. and LeWinter, M.M. (1994). Treatment of malignant pericardial effusion. *Journal of the American Medical Association* 272, 59–64.

11   Colleoni, M., et al. (1998). Intracavitary chemotherapy with thiotepa in malignant pericardial effusions: an active and well-tolerated regimen. *Journal of Clinical Oncology* 16, 2371–6.

12   Dempke, W. and Firusian, N. (1999). Treatment of malignant pericardial effusion with 32P-colloid. *British Journal of Cancer* 80, 1955–7.

13   Moriya, T., et al. (2000). Controlling malignant pericardial effusion by intrapericardial carboplatin administration in patients with primary non-small-cell lung cancer. *British Journal of Cancer* 83, 858–62.

14   Lissoni, P., et al. (2001). Progress report on the palliative therapy of 100 patients with neoplastic effusions by intracavitary low-dose interleukin-2. *Oncology* 60, 308–12.

15   Sugimoto, J.T., et al. (1990). Pericardial window: mechanisms of efficacy. *Annals of Thoracic Surgery* 50, 442–5.

16   Diskin, C.J., et al. (1999). Towards an understanding of oedema. *British Medical Journal* 318, 1610–13.

17   Rowell, N.P. and Gleeson, F.V. (2001). Steroids, radiotherapy, chemotherapy and stents for superior vena caval obstruction in carcinoma of the bronchus (Cochrane Review). *Cochrane Database of Systematic Reviews* CD001316.

18   Yahalom, J. (2001). Superior vena cava syndrome. In *Cancer. Principles and Practice of Oncology. 6th edition* (ed. V.T. De Vita, S. Hellman and S.A. Rosenberg). Philadelphia, Lippincott, Williams and Wilkins.

19   Nicholson, A.A., et al. (1997). Treatment of malignant superior vena cava obstruction: metal stents or radiation therapy. *Journal of Vascular and Interventional Radiology* 8, 781–8.

20   Schindler, N. and Vogelzang, R.L. (1999). Superior vena cava syndrome. Experience with endovascular stents and surgical therapy. *Surgical Clinics of North America* 79, 683–94.

21   Lanciego, C., et al. (2001). Stenting as first option for endovascular treatment of malignant superior vena cava syndrome. *American Journal of Roentgenology* 177, 585–93.

22   Marcy, P.Y., et al. (2001). Superior vena cava obstruction: is stenting necessary? *Supportive Care in Cancer* 9, 103–7.

23   Wilson, E., et al. (2002). Radiological stenting provides effective palliation in malignant central venous obstruction. *Clinical Oncology* 14, 228–32.

24   Kee, S.T., et al. (1998). Superior vena cava syndrome: treatment with catheter-directed thrombolysis and endovascular stent placement. *Radiology* 206, 187–93.

25   Morales, M., et al. (2000). Treatment of catheter-induced thrombotic superior vena cava syndrome: a single institution's experience. *Supportive Care in Cancer* 8, 334–8.

26   Hassan, B., et al. (1999). The management of inferior vena cava obstruction complicating metastatic germ cell tumors. *Cancer* 85, 912–18.

27   Fletcher, W.S., et al. (1998). Results of treatment of inferior vena cava syndrome with expandable metallic stents. *Archives of Surgery* 133, 935–8.

28   Sato, T., et al. (2001). Successful treatment for the IVC syndrome due to recurrence of colon cancer—chemotherapy in combination with the use of the expandable metallic stent placement. *Hepatogastroenterology* 48, 1048–9.

29   Ganz, P.A. (1999). The quality of life after breast cancer—solving the problem of lymphedema. *New England Journal of Medicine* 340, 383–5.

30   Twycross, R., Jenns, K. and Todd, J. (ed.) (2000). *Lymphoedema*. Oxford, Radcliffe Medical Press.

31   Farncombe, M.L. and Robertson, E.D. (2002). Lymphedema. In *Principles and Practice of Palliative Care and Supportive Oncology* (ed. A.M. Berger, R.K. Portenoy and D.E. Weissman). Philadelphia, Lippincott, Williams and Wilkins.

32   Twycross, R. (2000). Pain in lymphoedema. In *Lymphoedema* (ed. R. Twycross, K. Jenns and J. Todd). Oxford, Radcliffe Medical Press.

33 Mortimer, P.S. (1998). The pathophysiology of lymphedema. *Cancer* 83, 2798–802.

34 Keeley, V. (2000). Clinical features of lymphoedema. In *Lymphoedema* (ed. R. Twycross, K. Jenns and J. Todd). Oxford, Radcliffe Medical Press.

35 Velanovich, V. and Szymanski, W. (1999). Quality of life of breast cancer patients with lymphedema. *American Journal of Surgery* 177, 184–7.

36 Woods, M. (2000). Psychosocial aspects of lymphoedema. In *Lymphoedema* (ed. R. Twycross, K. Jenns and J. Todd). Oxford, Radcliffe Medical Press.

37 Coster, S., Poole, K. and Fallowfield, L.J. (2001). The validation of a quality of life scale to assess the impact of arm morbidity in breast cancer patients post-operatively. *Breast Cancer Research and Treatment* 68, 273–82.

38 Jenns, K. (2000). Management strategies. In *Lymphoedema* (ed. R. Twycross, K. Jenns and J. Todd). Oxford, Radcliffe Medical Press.

39 Cohen, S.R., Payne, D.K. and Tunkel, R.S. (2001). Lymphedema: strategies for management. *Cancer* 92, 980–7.

40 Badger, C.M., Peacock, J.L. and Mortimer, P.S. (2000). A randomized, controlled, parallel-group clinical trial comparing multilayer bandaging followed by hosiery versus hosiery alone in the treatment of patients with lymphedema of the limb. *Cancer* 88, 2832–7.

41 Bertelli, G., et al. (1991). Conservative treatment of postmastectomy lymphedema: a controlled, randomized trial. *Annals of Oncology* 2, 575–8.

42 Hornsby, R. (1995). The use of compression to treat lymphoedema. *Professional Nurse* 11, 127–8.

43 Johansson, K., et al. (1999). Effects of compression bandaging with or without manual lymph drainage treatment in patients with postoperative arm lymphedema. *Lymphology* 32, 103–10.

44 Andersen, L., et al. (2000). Treatment of breast-cancer-related lymphedema with or without manual lymphatic drainage—a randomized study. *Acta Oncologica* 39, 399–405.

45 Williams, A.F., et al. (2002). A randomized controlled crossover study of manual lymphatic drainage therapy in women with breast cancer-related lymphoedema. *European Journal of Cancer Care* 11, 254–61.

46 Dini, D., et al. (1998). The role of pneumatic compression in the treatment of postmastectomy lymphedema. A randomized phase III study. *Annals of Oncology* 9, 187–90.

47 Johansson, K., et al. (1998). A randomized study comparing manual lymph drainage with sequential pneumatic compression for treatment of postoperative arm lymphedema. *Lymphology* 31, 56–64.

48 Casley-Smith, J.R. (1996). Treatment of lymphedema by complex physical therapy, with and without oral and topical benzopyrones: what should therapists and patients expect. *Lymphology* 29, 76–82.

49 Desprez-curely, J.P., et al. (1985). Benzopyrones and post-mastectomy lymphedemas. Double-blind trial of placebo versus sustained release coumarin with trioxyethylrutin (TER). *Progress in Lymphology* 10, 203–5.

50 Piller, N.B., Morgan, R.G. and Casley-Smith, J.R. (1988). A double-blind, cross-over trial of O-(beta-hydroxyethyl)-rutosides (benzo-pyrones) in the treatment of lymphoedema of the arms and legs. *British Journal of Plastic Surgery* 41, 20–7.

51 Casley-Smith, J.R., Morgan, R.G. and Piller, N.B. (1993). Treatment of lymphedema of the arms and legs with 5,6-benzo-[alpha]-pyrone. *New England Journal of Medicine* 329, 1158–63.

52 Taylor, H.M. and al, e. (1993). A double-blind clinical trial of hydroxyethylrutosides in obstructive arm lymphoedema. *Phlebology* 8, 22–8.

53 Mortimer, P.S. and al, e. (1995). A double-blind, randomized, parallel-group, placebo-controlled trial of O-(ß-hydroxyethyl)-rutosides in chronic arm oedema resulting from breast cancer treatment. *Phlebology* 10, 51–5.

54 Cluzan, R.V., et al. (1996). Treatment of secondary lymphedema of the upper limb with CYCLO 3 FORT. *Lymphology* 29, 29–35.

55 Pecking, A.P., et al. (1997). Efficacy of Daflon 500 mg in the treatment of lymphedema (secondary to conventional therapy of breast cancer). *Angiology* 48, 93–8.

56 Loprinzi, C.L., et al. (1999). Lack of effect of coumarin in women with lymphedema after treatment for breast cancer. *New England Journal of Medicine* 340, 346–50.

57 Brorson, H. (2000). Liposuction gives complete reduction of chronic large arm lymphedema after breast cancer. *Acta Oncologica* 39, 407–20.

58 Koshima, I., et al. (2000). Supermicrosurgical lymphaticovenular anastomosis for the treatment of lymphedema in the upper extremities. *Journal of Reconstructive Microsurgery* 16, 437–42.

59 Szuba, A., Razavi, M. and Rockson, S.G. (2002). Diagnosis and treatment of concomitant venous obstruction in patients with secondary lymphedema. *Journal of Vascular and Interventional Radiology* 13, 799 803.

22

Haematological

Anaemia	Thrombosis
Polycythaemia	Bleeding
Leucocyte disorders	Hyperviscosity
Platelet disorders	Splenomegaly, hypersplenism
Coagulation disorders	

Anaemia

Cause

Anaemia occurs at some stage in most patients with cancer. It may be due to a variety of causes (Table 22.1) and is frequently multifactorial. Some distinguishing laboratory features are listed in Table 22.2. A number of recent reviews of anaemia in patients with cancer have been published.[1-3]

Table 22.1 Classification of anaemia

Decreased red cell production	Increased red cell production
anaemia of chronic disease	autoimmune haemolytic anaemia
chemotherapy, radiotherapy	microangiopathic haemolytic anaemia
marrow infiltration	infection
iron deficiency	hypersplenism
megaloblastic anaemia	Increased plasma volume (spurious anaemia)
myelodysplasia	paraproteinaemia
pure red cell aplasia	inappropriate ADH
Red blood cell loss	
bleeding	

Anaemia of chronic disease. This is the most common type of anaemia seen in patients with cancer. It is usually a diagnosis of exclusion, no other cause for anaemia being found. It is due to a combination of low erythropoietin levels, inefficient erythropoiesis and iron utilization, as well as some reduction in red cell survival. Investigations show a normochromic normocytic anaemia; there may be some microcytosis suggesting iron deficiency. The serum iron and iron binding capacity are reduced and the serum ferritin level is normal or increased.

Chemotherapy, radiotherapy. Chemotherapy and radiotherapy suppress the proliferative capacity of the bone marrow, causing pancytopenia with leucopenia and thrombocytopenia as well as anaemia. The severity depends upon the intensity of the chemotherapy or the volume of bone marrow irradiated. Given together or sequentially, the effects may be additive.

Bone marrow infiltration. Bone marrow infiltration occurs frequently in the lymphoproliferative disorders and with solid tumours, particularly those from the breast, lung and prostate. The equivalent of marrow infiltration occurs in all the myeloproliferative disorders. Marrow infiltration produces a leucoerythroblastic blood film with immature white cells, some immature erythrocytes (nucleated red cells, normoblasts) and red cell changes similar to those seen in myelofibrosis: there is marked variation in the size and shape of the red cells (anisopoikilocytosis) with the presence of 'tear-drop' poikilocytes. If infiltration is severe or diffuse, there will be pancytopenia in addition to leucoerythroblastic changes.

Iron deficiency and bleeding. Iron deficiency anaemia occurs most frequently as a result of bleeding. It produces a hypochromic microcytic anaemia. The serum iron is reduced, the iron binding capacity elevated and the serum ferritin level reduced.

Megaloblastic anaemia. Vitamin B_{12} deficiency occurs following gastrectomy, removal of the terminal ileum, or as a result of coincidental pernicious anaemia. Folate deficiency occurs as a result of malabsorption or poor dietary intake. The body has limited stores of folic acid and deficiency may develop within days in seriously ill patients. Vitamin B_{12} or folate deficiency produces a macrocytic anaemia with hypersegmented neutrophils and some degree of neutropenia and thrombocytopenia. Measurement of the serum vitamin B_{12} and folate levels will document deficiency. The bone marrow examination will show megaloblastic change. Similar macrocytic anaemia with megaloblastic change in the bone marrow, but without vitamin B_{12} or folate deficiency, occurs with certain antimetabolite drugs including cytosine arabinoside, methotrexate, fluorouracil and thioguanine. Macrocytic anaemia without vitamin B_{12} or folate deficiency and without megaloblastic change in the marrow can occur with liver disease, myelodysplasia, sideroblastosis and hypothyroidism.

Myelodysplasia. The myelodysplastic syndromes are characterized by ineffective production of one or more cell lines in the bone marrow and may show megaloblastic or sideroblastic change. Myelodysplasia may occur secondary to previous cytotoxic therapy; it may precede the development of acute leukaemia or follow a chronic course.

Pure red cell aplasia. This rare condition is often associated with cancer, particularly thymomas. Investigations show anaemia, a reduced reticulocyte count and a bone marrow with reduced or absent erythropoiesis.

Autoimmune haemolytic anaemia. Autoimmune haemolytic anaemia, in which antibodies reactive against red cells lead to haemolysis, occurs commonly with chronic lymphocytic leukaemia and other lymphoproliferative disorders; it occurs infrequently with solid tumours. Investigation shows anaemia, reticulocytosis, reduced haptoglobin and increased bilirubin levels. The antiglobulin test is positive. With 'warm' antibodies (reactive at 37°C) the blood film shows spherocytes; with 'cold' antibodies (reactive at lower temperatures) the blood film shows red cell agglutination.

Microangiopathic haemolytic anaemia. Microangiopathic haemolytic anaemia is often associated with disseminated mucin-secreting adenocarcinomas. Investigation shows haemolytic anaemia with microangiopathic red cell changes (fragmentation, schistocytes), due to mechanical damage caused by tumour-induced fibrin deposition and thrombi in the microvasculature. There may be evidence of disseminated intravascular coagulation and thrombocytopenia.

Hypersplenism. Some degree of increased red cell destruction or haemolytic anaemia occurs with splenomegaly of any cause, including liver disease and the haematological malignancies. Marrow examination shows erythroid hyperplasia.

Relative or spurious anaemia. This occurs when the plasma volume is expanded by the presence of a paraprotein or due to salt and water retention caused by inappropriate secretion of antidiuretic hormone.

Clinical features

The clinical features depend on the severity of the anaemia, the speed of onset, and the patient's age and cardiopulmonary reserve. Acute haemorrhage is associated with tachycardia, dyspnoea and hypotension. More frequently, anaemia develops slowly and is only mild to moderate in degree. Patients complain of tiredness, weakness and fatigue. There is often shortness of breath on exertion and angina may be exacerbated. There can be dizziness due to postural hypotension and cognitive function may be impaired. Examination shows pallor of the mucous membranes and there may be signs of cardiac failure. Splenomegaly may be present due to the underlying condition or to haemolytic anaemia. Patients with haemolysis may be jaundiced.

The effects of anaemia on functional ability and quality of life have been measured using the FACT-An, a subscale of the Functional Assessment of Cancer Therapy (FACT)

Table 22.2   Laboratory evaluation of anaemia

Microcytic anaemia: MCV <80 fl	
se Fe ↓, IBC ↑, ferritin ↓	iron deficiency, bleeding
se Fe ↓, IBC ↓, ferritin N or ↓	anaemia of chronic disease
se Fe N, IBC N, ferritin N or ↓	haemoglobinopathy
Macrocytic anaemia: MCV >95 fl	
B_{12} or folate ↓	B_{12} or folate deficiency
B_{12} and folate N	
marrow megaloblastic	cytotoxic therapy
marrow not megaloblastic	liver disease, myelodysplasia, sideroblastosis, hypothyroidism
Reticulocytes ↑	haemolysis
Normocytic anaemia: MCV 80-95 fl	
Reticulocytes ↑	
DAT positive	autoimmune haemolytic anaemia
DAT negative	non-autoimmune haemolytic anaemia
	acute blood loss
	marrow infiltration (leucoerythroblastic)
	microangiopathic haemolytic anaemia
Reticulocytes N or ↓	
anaemia only	anaemia of chronic disease
	pure red cell aplasia
pancytopenia	chemotherapy, radiotherapy

se Fe: serum iron; IBC : serum iron binding capacity; B_{12} and folate: serum vitamin B_{12} and folate measurements; MCV: mean corpuscular volume of red blood cells; DAT: direct antiglobulin test; ↑, ↓, N: increased, reduced, normal questionnaire.[4] FACT-An scores clearly differentiate between patients with low and high haemoglobin levels, and can be used to assess the effect of treatments [5] and to compare different groups of patients.

If the anaemia is mild or the cause obvious, further investigation is often unnecessary. If it is severe, an attempt should be made to define the cause (Table 22.2), as many anaemias are amenable to therapy. The mild anaemia that occurs with terminal cancer should not be investigated.

Treatment

The treatment of anaemia depends on the cause, the speed of onset, the severity of the symptoms, and the stage of the patient's disease and the prognosis.

Anaemia of chronic disease. The anaemia of chronic disease is rarely severe and the treatment is that of the underlying disease. Haematinic therapy with iron, vitamin B_{12} or folate is ineffective. Transfusion may provide temporary symptomatic improvement.

Chemotherapy, radiotherapy. Anaemias due to chemotherapy and radiotherapy usually resolve spontaneously and transfusion can be given in the interim if required for symptoms.

Bone marrow infiltration. Anaemia due to marrow infiltration responds to treatment of the underlying condition, where possible.

Iron deficiency. Iron deficiency anaemia is treated with replacement therapy and by treatment of the cause of bleeding. Oral or parenteral iron or transfusion can be used, depending on the severity and speed of onset of the anaemia.

Megaloblastic anaemia. Megaloblastic anaemia due to vitamin B_{12} or folate deficiency can be corrected by appropriate replacement therapy. The megaloblastic changes that occur secondary to cytotoxic therapy are self-limiting.

Autoimmune haemolytic anaemia. Anaemia due to cold agglutinins is usually mild and chronic although there can be haemolytic crises precipitated by cold exposure. Treatment is directed at the underlying lymphoproliferative disease; corticosteroids and splenectomy are often ineffective. Anaemia due to 'warm' antibodies may respond to corticosteroids and, if necessary, splenectomy. Patients with solid tumours respond less often to corticosteroids and treatment is directed at the underlying tumour.

Microangiopathic haemolytic anaemia. Treatment of microangiopathic haemolytic anaemia is usually unsuccessful except where there is effective treatment for the underlying malignancy, as with hormonal therapy for breast or prostate cancer.

Transfusion Decisions regarding blood transfusions for patients with advanced cancer depend on the stage of the disease and life expectancy, as well as the speed of onset and severity of the symptoms of anaemia. Acute anaemia due to blood loss or serious infection usually requires transfusion. Recommendations regarding the level at which patients with chronic anaemia should be transfused are listed in Table 22.3.

The complications of transfusion are summarized in Table 22.4.[6] Allergic reactions after transfusion of ABO-compatible blood are mostly non-specific reactions against constituents of the donor plasma. Fevers, chills, urticaria or hives that occur are treated with antihistamines or corticosteroids. With repeated transfusion, the recipient may develop antibodies to HLA and granulocyte-specific antigens on donor platelets and leucocytes, causing febrile and allergic reactions. Treatment is with leucocyte-poor red cells or by transfusion through a special filter. Transmission of hepatitis and other viruses remains a major concern.

In palliative care, transfusion is reported to benefit a significant proportion of patients, both in terms of physical symptoms and the overall sense of well being.[7]

Table 22.3   Indications for blood transfusion

Acute anaemia

Chronic anaemia
    Hb <8–9 g/dl and symptomatic
    Hb 8–9 g/dl and   continued or likely haemorrhage
                           planned surgery
                           planned radiotherapy
                           planned chemotherapy
                           serious infection
                           doubt whether transfusion would be of symptomatic benefit
                           unexplained weakness, fatigue or dyspnoea
    Hb >9–10 g/dl and symptomatic (as a result of cardiac or respiratory insufficiency)

Table 22.4   Complications of transfusion

Major haemolytic transfusion reaction (ABO incompatibility)

Delayed haemolytic transfusion reaction (Kidd incompatibility)

Infected blood

Allergic reactions
    antibodies to donor plasma constituents
    antibodies to donor platelet HLA and leucocyte antigens
    anti-IgA antibodies in IgA deficient patients

Transmission of infection

Volume overload

Aggravation of hyperviscosity

Hypocalcaemia (massive transfusion)

Erythropoietin. Patients with the anaemia of chronic disease, including cancer patients, have low endogenous erythropoietin levels and reduced bone marrow response to it.[3, 8] Treatment with epoetin (recombinant human erythropoietin) leads to a significant increase in haemoglobin, reduction in transfusion requirement, and improvement in fatigue and quality of life for some patients receiving chemotherapy or radiation.[3, 5, 8–12] It is usually given three times weekly (150U/kg SC); the dose may be doubled if there is no haematological response after four weeks, but should be stopped if there is no improvement after a further four weeks. Iron deficiency should be excluded as a reason for non-response. Once-weekly treatment (epoetin 40,000U SC) is reported to produce equivalent benefits to thrice-weekly therapy.[13] Epoetin is generally well tolerated, although there are reports of rare cases of pure red cell aplasia in patients with renal failure.[14] Epoetin therapy is expensive.

The role of epoetin in the palliative care setting remains to be defined.[15] Epoetin treatment for patients not receiving chemotherapy showed an increase in haemoglobin and a reduction in transfusion requirement, as well as improvement in the quality of life for those showing haematological response.[16] RCTs indicate benefit for some patients with advanced solid tumours and for patients with haematological malignancies and anaemia requiring transfusion (Table 22.5).

Table 22.5 Epoetin (EPO) therapy for patients with advanced cancer: RCTs

Author	n	Patients/Intervention	Outcome
Henry[19]	112	anaemia, no chemotherapy epoetin vs placebo	EPO: 40% responded, with ↑ Hb and ↑ QOL (both pS)
Daneryd[20]	108	cachexia, no chemotherapy epoetin vs placebo	EPO: prevented anaemia, preserved exercise tolerance (both pS)
Johansson[21]	180	refractory prostate cancer, anaemia epoetin low dose vs high dose	higher dose: ↑ Hb in 47 vs 25%, ↓ transfusions and ↑ QOL (all pS)
Osterborg[22]	349	Haem. malignancies requiring transfusion: epoetin vs placebo	EPO: 67 vs 27% response: ↑ Hb, ↓ transfusion, ↑ QOL (all pS)

Darbepoetin is a new analogue of erythropoietin that has a longer serum half-life and requires administration less often (each 1 to 3 weeks). It produces similar benefits to epoetin for patients with cancer and anaemia.[17, 18]

Polycythaemia (erythrocytosis)

Polycythaemia is defined as an elevation of the haemoglobin or haematocrit (packed cell volume, PCV) above the upper limit of the normal range.

The causes of polycythaemia are listed in Table 22.6. In spurious or relative polycythaemia the elevated haematocrit is due to contraction of the plasma volume. Polycythaemia vera is a malignant myeloproliferative disorder. Secondary polycythaemia occurs with hypoxia and a number of uncommon conditions associated with increased erythropoietin levels.

Table 22.6 Causes of polycythaemia

Relative or spurious polycythaemia
    dehydration, diuretic therapy

True or absolute polycythaemia
    primary
        polycythaemia vera
    secondary
        hypoxia
            lung disease, cyanotic congenital heart disease, high altitude
    increased erythropoietin
        renal disease
        androgen therapy
        renal adenocarcinoma, hepatoma, cerebellar haemangioblastoma, adrenal and ovarian tumours, uterine myomata

Patients with polycythaemia vera have an increased incidence of both thrombosis and haemorrhage; most have splenomegaly and many complain of pruritus. Severe polycythaemia causes a hyperviscosity syndrome, which leads to headaches and dizziness, visual disturbance, angina and heart failure, abdominal pain, and claudication. Haematological investigation shows a panmyelosis, with elevation of the neutrophil and platelet counts in addition to the haemoglobin, and hyperplasia of all cell lines in the bone marrow.

Patients with polycythaemia secondary to hypoxia may be cyanosed and will have reduced arterial oxygen tension and signs of underlying cardiac or lung disease. Significant hyperviscosity is uncommon. With tumour-associated polycythaemia, the haematocrit is only mildly elevated and the patient asymptomatic.

Treatment

Polycythaemia vera requires treatment to prevent the complications of thrombosis and haemorrhage. Venesection or phlebotomy will reduce the blood volume and haematocrit and control the symptoms of hyperviscosity. Venesection alone may be adequate if the abnormalities are mild, but myelosuppressive treatment with cytotoxic therapy or radioactive phosphorus (^{32}P) is often required. The aim is to keep the haematocrit at or near the upper limit of normal, especially if surgery is planned.

Patients with polycythaemia secondary to hypoxia rarely require haematological therapy. Despite marked elevation of the haematocrit, the patient is asymptomatic and there is no major risk of bleeding or thrombosis. Patients with symptoms of hyperviscosity or right heart failure may benefit from cautious venesection. The treatment of other secondary polycythaemias is directed at the cause. Relative polycythaemia is treated by correction of dehydration or modification of diuretic therapy.

Leucocyte disorders

Leucocytosis

Leucocytosis is a frequent finding in patients with advanced cancer. The common causes, classified according to the cell line involved, are shown in Table 22.7. In the setting of advanced cancer, recognition of the numerous causes of leucocytosis can avoid unnecessary investigation or treatment for suspected infection.

Neutrophilia associated with solid tumours is caused by tumour necrosis or tumour production of ACTH-like proteins and colony stimulating factors. Eosinophilia occurs with various types of cancer or can be due to other relatively common but unrelated conditions including allergy, dermatitis and parasitic infection. Basophilia occurs with the chronic myeloproliferative disorders and indicates a poor prognosis. Monocytosis occurs frequently with both solid tumours and haematological malignancies. Lymphocytosis may occur with lymphocytic leukaemia, lymphoma, solid tumours and viral infection. Lymphocyte surface marker analysis shows the lymphocytosis associated with solid tumours or infections to be polyclonal in nature, whilst that associated with lymphoproliferative disorders is monoclonal. If required, the treatment of leucocytosis is that of the underlying cause.

Hyperleucocytosis. Hyperleucocytosis, defined as a white cell count of $>100 \times 10^9$/l, may cause hyperviscosity with intravascular stasis in the capillary circulation leading to local tissue hypoxia. Hyperviscosity depends on the cell size and deformability as well as the count: it occurs commonly in myeloid leukaemia but rarely in chronic lymphocytic leukaemia. Treatment needs to be initiated before irreversible cerebral or pulmonary damage occurs. Treatment consists of reducing the count as quickly as possible, employing cytotoxic drugs or leucopheresis. Blood transfusion is contraindicated during the initial phase because it exacerbates hyperviscosity.

Table 22.7 Causes of leucocytosis

Myeloid leucocytosis	
Predominantly mature neutrophils	
solid tumours	corticosteroids
myeloproliferative disorders	post splenectomy
chemotherapy-recovery phase	inflammation and tissue necrosis
colony stimulating factor therapy	infection
Leukaemoid (with circulating immature leucocytes)	
myeloid leukaemia	chemotherapy-recovery phase
myeloproliferative	disorders infection
marrow infiltration	inflammation
Eosinophilia	
allergic disorders	Hodgkin's disease
parasitic infection	myeloproliferative disorders
dermatitis	
Basophilia	
myeloproliferative disorders	
Monocytosis	
monocytic leukaemia	inflammation
solid tumours	infection
Lymphocytosis	
lymphoid leukaemia	infection
lymphoma	drugs

Sweet's syndrome. This is the association of neutrophilia, pyrexia, painful cutaneous plaques and arthralgia occurring in patients with cancer. The treatment is that of the underlying disease; there may be symptomatic improvement with corticosteroids.

Leucopenia

Lymphopenia. Lymphopenia occurs frequently as a result of chemotherapy, radiotherapy or treatment with corticosteroids. It requires no investigation or treatment.

Neutropenia. Causes of neutropenia are listed in Table 22.8. Neutropenia predisposes to infection, the risk being proportional to the severity and duration. Neutropenia also leads to mucositis, especially of the gastrointestinal tract. Treatment-related neutropenia usually

Table 22.8 Causes of neutropenia

Cancer treatment	chemotherapy, radiotherapy
Marrow infiltration	
Megaloblastosis	vitamin B_{12}, folic acid deficiency
Infection	
Hypersplenism	
Drug-induced	antibiotics, NSAIDs, carbamazepine, diuretics, oral hypoglycaemics, antidepressants, phenothiazines

resolves spontaneously. The haematopoietic growth factors, G-CSF and GM-CSF, reduce the severity and duration of the neutropenia caused by chemotherapy, as well as the incidence and severity of infections related to it.[8] In other situations, treatment should be directed at the underlying cause.

Platelet disorders

Thrombocytosis

Thrombocytosis, or elevation of the platelet count above $400 \times 10^9/l$, occurs in about one third of patients with cancer. The causes are listed in Table 22.9.

Table 22.9 Causes of thrombocytosis

Chronic myeloproliferative disorders: ET, PRV, CML
Other cancers: solid tumours, lymphomas
Haemorrhage
Postoperative
Splenectomy
Chemotherapy: recovery phase
Other: infection, inflammation, haemolysis, vincristine therapy

Marked elevation of the platelet count (over $800–1000 \times 10^9/l$) occurs in the chronic myeloproliferative disorders—essential thrombocythaemia (ET), polycythaemia vera (PRV) and chronic myeloid leukaemia (CML). It predisposes to both thrombosis and haemorrhage and may also be associated with a syndrome of burning pain in the hands and feet. The risk of thrombosis is proportional to the degree of thrombocytosis but also depends on other factors including the patient's age and mobility, the degree of atherosclerosis, and the presence of any other factors predisposing to thrombosis. Treatment is by myelosuppressive therapy with either cytotoxic drugs or radioactive phosphorus (^{32}P). Normalization of the count reduces the risk of thrombosis and haemorrhage to near normal. If surgery is planned, the count should be reduced to as near normal as possible preoperatively and care should be taken that postoperative anticoagulation is adequate. Treatment with aspirin or NSAID does not reduce the incidence of thrombosis and can predispose to bleeding; they are useful in treating the syndrome of painful fingers and toes.

The thrombocytosis that occurs with other tumours and due to the other causes listed in Table 22.9 is usually mild in degree (platelet count $400–800 \times 10^9/l$) and does not require specific treatment. Other factors predisposing to thrombosis need to be avoided or treated and care taken that postoperative anticoagulation is adequate.

Thrombocytopenia

Thrombocytopenia, or a platelet count of less than $150 \times 10^9/l$, may occur in patients with cancer for a variety of reasons (Table 22.10). Bone marrow examination should be considered for patients with platelet counts $<70 \times 10^9/l$ for which the cause is not apparent. This

Table 22.10   Causes of thrombocytopenia

Diminished platelet production
    marrow infiltration: solid tumours, haematological malignancies
    cancer treatment: chemotherapy, radiotherapy
    drugs: thiazides, alcohol, oestrogens, interferon
    vitamin B_{12} or folate deficiency
    viral infection

Increased platelet destruction
    non-immune
        infection
        disseminated intravascular coagulation (DIC)
        thrombotic thrombocytopenic purpura (TTP)
        haemolytic uraemic syndrome
        microangiopathic haemolytic anaemia
    immune
        drugs: NSAIDs, antibiotics, anticonvulsants, quinine, diuretics, heparin, hypnotics
        lymphoproliferative disorders
        solid tumours
        idiopathic (ITP)

Platelet sequestration: hypersplenism

Platelet loss: haemorrhage, extracorporeal circulation (pheresis, dialysis)

will distinguish impaired production from increased peripheral destruction and will demonstrate marrow infiltration if present.

The risk of bleeding depends on the degree of thrombocytopenia (Table 22.11) and will be greater if there is also abnormal platelet function (see below).

Table 22.11   Thrombocytopenia and bleeding

Platelet count	
>50x10^9/l	easy bruising, spontaneous bleeding rare
20–50x10^9/l	excessive bruising, increased bleeding with trauma, procedures
<20x10^9/l	significant risk of spontaneous bleeding

Treatment. The treatment of thrombocytopenia depends on the cause and severity. Any drugs that might cause thrombocytopenia or diminished platelet function should be stopped if possible. For thrombocytopenia due to diminished production, the treatment is that of the cause. If severe, platelet transfusions may be required. Thrombocytopenia due to increased platelet destruction may improve with treatment of the underlying cause. Treatment of immune thrombocytopenia with corticosteroids is usually successful but frequently transient, and other therapies need to be considered including intravenous immunoglobulin, danazol, splenectomy and immunosuppression. Treatment of thrombocytopenia due to hypersplenism is that of the underlying cause; patients with massive splenomegaly causing severe physical symptoms or thrombocytopenia may be considered for splenectomy or splenic irradiation.

Abnormal platelet function

Abnormalities of platelet aggregation or release reactions and diminished platelet adhesiveness can cause a bleeding tendency. Bleeding may occur when the platelet count is normal or be more severe than expected from the degree of thrombocytopenia.

Abnormal platelet function may be due to intrinsic abnormalities in the platelets or to the secondary effects of uraemia, paraproteinaemia or drugs (Table 22.12). In addition, the elevated levels of fibrin degradation products in patients with cancer and chronic disseminated intravascular coagulation (DIC), may lead to coating of the platelet surface and abnormal platelet function. Drug-induced platelet dysfunction will resolve if the drug is stopped. The intrinsic abnormalities that occur in dyshaemopoietic conditions are not correctable and platelet transfusions are required for significant bleeding. Abnormal platelet function due to uraemia or paraproteinaemia will improve with treatment of the underlying cause.

Table 22.12 Abnormal platelet function

Dyshaemopoiesis	myeloid leukaemia, myelodysplasia chronic myeloproliferative disorders
Drugs	aspirin, NSAIDs, penicillins
Other	uraemia, paraproteinaemia, DIC

Platelet transfusions

Platelet transfusions are indicated for patients with severe thrombocytopenia or marked platelet dysfunction who have active bleeding. Prophylactic platelet transfusion is considered if there are lesions with significant risk of haemorrhage, if surgery is planned, or if a further fall in the platelet count is anticipated.[23]

Platelet transfusions are usually given from random donors and a significant proportion of patients receiving repeated platelet transfusions will develop antibodies to HLA antigens on the donor platelets, resulting in febrile reactions and poor incremental responses to transfusion. Such alloimmunization is documented by the demonstration of HLA antibodies in the recipient's blood and future platelet transfusions are best obtained from HLA-matched single donors.

The efficacy of platelet transfusion is related to the post-transfusion increment in the platelet count. The count should be checked after 1 and 24 hours. A poor 1-hour increment suggests alloimmunization. A poor increment at 24 hours may occur with alloimmunization and also with bleeding, fever, infection, hypersplenism and DIC.

Coagulation disorders

Normal coagulation

Normal coagulation involves complex interrelationships between the blood vessel wall, the platelets and the coagulation factors (Figure 22.1). Endothelial injury releases tissue factors that activate both the platelet system and the coagulation factors. These two systems are interdependent and each facilitates the other. Activation of platelets causes adhesion, release reactions and aggregation and results in a mass of aggregated platelets. Activation of the coagulation system results in the formation of thrombin, which converts fibrinogen to fibrin. Fibrin and aggregated platelets make up the primary haemostatic plug or blood clot. Another system, the fibrinolytic system, produces plasmin, which is capable of lysing thrombus. Under normal circumstances, there is a balance between these two systems, the fibrinolytic system clearing any thrombus formed.

Figure 22.1   Normal coagulation

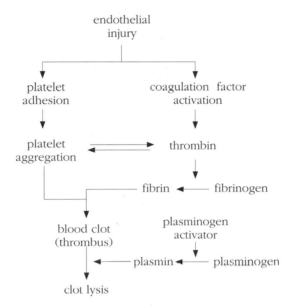

Disorders of coagulation

Haemorrhage. Bleeding can occur with a low platelet count (thrombocytopenia), abnormal platelet function (thrombocytopathy), or coagulation factor deficiencies. Fibrinogen depletion by consumption (in disseminated intravascular coagulation) or degradation (in primary fibrinolysis) will also lead to haemorrhage.

Thrombosis. Thrombosis will occur if there is stimulation of the coagulation pathways without a compensatory increase in fibrinolysis.

Disseminated intravascular coagulation (DIC). Activation of the platelet and coagulation factor pathways leads DIC. The acute fulminant form of DIC occurs with sepsis or promyelocytic leukaemia and is uncommon. It causes thromboses in the microvasculature as well as consumption and depletion of both platelets and coagulation factors, causing serious haemorrhage.

Chronic DIC can be demonstrated in as many as 75% of patients with malignant disease.[24] Sophisticated laboratory tests show increased turnover or consumption of clotting factors, platelets and fibrinogen in association with elevated levels of fibrin degradation products. Routine laboratory tests may be essentially normal or may show signs of compensated intravascular coagulation including thrombocytosis and elevated levels of fibrinogen and D-dimer. The majority of these patients are completely asymptomatic, but there is evidence that many of the thrombotic events in patients with cancer are part of a hypercoagulable state related to chronic DIC, initiated by tumour-related procoagulants.

Primary fibrinolysis. Plasminogen activators released by tumour cells (usually prostate cancer) lead to increased levels of plasmin which act on fibrinogen and cause hypofibrinogenaemia and clinical bleeding.

Thrombosis

About 15% of patients with malignant disease suffer clinically evident thrombosis although the incidence at postmortem examination is higher. Many of the accepted risk factors for the development of thrombosis are particularly relevant to patients with cancer (Table 22.13).

Table 22.13 Clinical risk factors for thrombosis

Surgical or non-surgical trauma
Older age
Immobilization: prolonged, paralysis
Malignant disease
Previous thromboembolism
Cardiac failure
Obesity
Oestrogens: exogenous oestrogens, contraceptive pill, pregnancy
Corticosteroids

Table 22.14 Predisposition to thrombosis in malignant disease

Vessel wall abnormalities
malignant invasion
ischaemic damage, hypoxia
corticosteroid therapy
new vessel formation within tumours
Reduced flow
immobilization, bed rest
malignant invasion, compression
congestive heart failure, oedematous states
hyperviscosity syndromes
intravascular catheters
Platelet abnormalities
thrombocytosis
platelet activation by tumour cell products
Coagulation factor abnormalities
increased factor levels: oestrogens
increased levels of activated factors: tumour-associated procoagulants
decreased hepatic clearance of activated factors: liver disease

Thrombosis may result from abnormalities of the vessel wall, changes in blood flow, or abnormalities of the blood itself (Table 22.14).[25] Blood vessel walls may be damaged by malignant invasion or hypoxia and corticosteroid therapy is thought to reduce the levels of natural anticoagulant in the endothelial wall. Normal blood flow serves to keep platelets away from the endothelium and to disperse any activated coagulation factors; reduced flow or stasis, for whatever reason, will predispose to thrombosis. Secretion of procoagulant or platelet activating substances, by either the tumour cells or the monocytes that form part of the immune response to the tumour, will predispose to thrombosis. If liver disease is present, there will be diminished hepatic clearance of activated factors, also predisposing to thrombosis. As discussed above, there is evidence that many of the thrombotic events in patients with cancer (Table 22.15) are part of a hypercoagulable state related to disseminated intravascular coagulation (DIC).[24]

Table 22.15 Thrombotic syndromes in cancer

Venous thrombosis	Iatrogenic
Disseminated intravascular coagulation	vascular catheters
acute, fulminant	peritoneovenous shunts
chronic	chemotherapy
venous thrombosis	venous thrombosis
Trousseau's syndrome	hepatic veno-occlusive disease
non-bacterial thrombotic endocarditis	microangiopathic haemolytic anaemia
microangiopathic haemolytic anaemia	hormones: oestrogens, corticosteroids
microvascular arterial thrombosis	

Venous thrombosis

The signs and symptoms of venous thrombosis are no different to those in patients without malignancy and the diagnosis is made in the same manner with venography, ultrasonography or venous pool scanning. A negative test for D-dimer is useful in excluding a diagnosis of thrombosis.[26]

Standard therapy. Standard treatment for venous thrombosis is anticoagulation with intravenous unfractionated heparin (UH), followed by oral warfarin.[27, 28] These may be contraindicated in certain circumstances (Table 22.16) and careful consideration is necessary before starting anticoagulation for the palliative care patients. Surgical placement of vena caval filters may be of value in certain situations, and thrombolytic therapy may be considered in exceptional circumstances.

Intravenous heparin, monitored by the activated partial thromboplastin time (APTT), will prevent further thrombus formation and aid the resolution of acute symptoms. Oral warfarin therapy is commenced a day or two later. Heparin is continued for a few days until warfarin levels are stable, as measured by the International Normalized Ratio (INR) (Table 22.17). It is customary to give warfarin for a period of 3 to 6 months, although the optimal duration of therapy remains uncertain.[29, 30]

Heparin can be given by subcutaneous injection each 8–12 hours. This may cause local bruising but is valuable for patients requiring continued heparin therapy and those being treated at home. Subcutaneous heparin therapy is monitored in the same way as intravenous therapy.

Table 22.16 Contraindications to anticoagulant therapy

Absolute	Relative
significant active bleeding	recent bleeding
severe bleeding tendency	bleeding tendency
recent brain or spinal cord surgery	active peptic ulceration
	recent major surgery
	cerebral metastases
	uncontrolled hypertension
	severe renal failure
	severe hepatic failure
	terminally ill

Complications of standard anticoagulation with unfractionated heparin and warfarin include haemorrhage and the development of recurrent thrombosis, and there is good evidence that these are more likely to occur in patients with cancer.[31–34] Significant bleeding occurs in 5–10% of patients, which may be life threatening, due either to over-anticoagulation or to the presence of other lesions prone to haemorrhage such as a peptic ulcer. Recurrent thrombosis whilst on warfarin may be due to inadequate anticoagulation or to 'warfarin resistance' that occurs with cancer.[31] Recurrence despite adequate anticoagulation can be treated with heparin, followed by more intensive warfarin therapy (target INR 3–4), or by continued heparin therapy.

Table 22.17 Management of venous thrombosis

Initial therapy	
heparin	5–10d IV; APTT 1.5–2.5 x normal
alternatives	vena caval filter (heparin contraindicated)
	SC heparin (home care)
	no anticoagulation (terminal care)
Continuation therapy	
warfarin	3–6 mo PO; INR 2–3
alternatives	no treatment (advanced disease)
	continued heparin (evidence of DIC)
Recurrent thrombosis on warfarin	
heparin	then warfarin to INR of 2–3 (or higher)
alternatives	continued heparin (evidence of DIC or INR was therapeutic)
	vena caval filter
	no treatment (advanced disease)
Recurrent thrombosis after completing warfarin therapy	
heparin	then warfarin to INR of 2–3
alternatives	continued heparin (evidence of DIC)
	no treatment (advanced disease)
	vena caval filter

Continued treatment with heparin should be considered for patients who have either definite or presumptive evidence of underlying DIC, including patients with recurrent thrombosis on warfarin therapy and those with multiple or arterial thromboses (Table 22.17). Warfarin is ineffective in preventing recurrent thromboses in patients with cancer-related DIC and heparin therapy may need to be continued indefinitely.

Patients with cancer receiving warfarin require more frequent laboratory monitoring than patients without malignant disease. Features commonly associated with advancing cancer, including poor nutritional intake and progressive liver dysfunction, will predispose to over-anticoagulation.

Another major problem with warfarin therapy is the frequent interaction with other drugs, which may either enhance or reduce activity. This problem is usually managed by instructing the patient to take other medications in the same dose every day, but this may not be feasible for the palliative care patient requiring repeated changes of drugs or doses, and makes frequent laboratory testing necessary.

Low molecular weight heparins (LMWHs). A number of LMWH preparations are now available that are effective in the prevention and treatment of venous thrombosis, and which may be particularly useful for the management of patients with cancer and thrombosis. They are administered subcutaneously, are associated with less haemorrhage, do not require laboratory monitoring, and are suitable for home treatment.[27, 35–37]

Cochrane reviews indicate that fixed-dose subcutaneous LMWH is as effective as titrated intravenous unfractionated heparin in the initial treatment of venous thromboembolism, is associated with less haemorrhage, and may be able to be given as a single daily injection.[38–40] Continued therapy with LMWH is at least as effective as warfarin in preventing recurrent thrombosis and is associated with significantly less haemorrhage.[36] In patients with cancer, continued therapy with LMWH avoids the difficulties and inadequacies of warfarin therapy (see above). The results of a single RCT comparing enoxaprin and warfarin therapy for 3 months reported less haemorrhage and recurrent thrombosis in the LMWH group (21 vs 10.5%), although this did not reach statistical significance.[41] LMWHs may be more expensive and less convenient to administer, but are significantly safer and may be more effective in the palliative care population.

Vena caval filters. Vena caval filters reduce the incidence of pulmonary embolism in patients for whom anticoagulant therapy is contraindicated or associated with serious complications.[42–44] Vena cava filters are not of use if the thrombosis involves the vena cava itself or in patients with chronic DIC who develop thromboses at multiple sites. Clear guidelines for the use of vena caval filters in the management of patients with cancer are still to be established.

Thrombolytic therapy. The thrombolytic agent, recombinant tissue plasminogen activator (TPA), can be used in the treatment of thrombosis and pulmonary embolism.[45] TPA is not associated with the immunological reactions seen with the thrombolytic agents used in the past, streptokinase and urokinase [27]. The thrombolytic agents convert plasminogen to plasmin, leading to rapid clot lysis with relief of oedema and cardiopulmonary complications, but there are substantial risks of serious haemorrhage. The contraindications and indications for thrombolytic therapy for patients with cancer are shown in Table 22.18; in most instances the risks outweigh the potential benefits. The presence of intracranial disease is an absolute contraindication and it is usually advised that patients be scanned for occult cerebral metastases before commencing thrombolytic therapy.

The other indication for thrombolytic therapy is to treat central venous catheter dysfunction caused by a thrombus at the tip of the catheter. A small dose of TPA is injected, the

Table 22.18   Thrombolytic therapy in cancer patients

Contraindications
  intracranial pathology
  recent (less than 10 days) surgery
  active or recent bleeding
  bleeding diathesis
  presence of lesions prone to haemorrhage

Indications
  pulmonary embolism: massive embolism with cardiac decompensation
  no contraindications and a reasonable life expectancy
  venous catheter dysfunction

volume adjusted so that it will just fill the occluded catheter, and left in place for between 30 minutes and 2 hours.[46, 47] This treatment has a high success rate and can be repeated as often as necessary without risk of systemic bleeding.

Thrombosis associated with disseminated intravascular coagulation (DIC)

As already noted, specialized investigations show that many patients with cancer have evidence of DIC and this is thought to be the basis of the various thrombotic syndromes seen in these patients.

Venous thromboses occurring in patients with chronic DIC are more likely to be recurrent and multiple. Continued therapy with heparin, rather than warfarin, is necessary to prevent recurrence. This is continued indefinitely or until there is tumour control.

Trousseau's syndrome is recurrent superficial thrombophlebitis, which is characteristically associated with intra-abdominal cancer. The thromboses involve veins on either the limbs or the trunk and may resolve spontaneously within a few days. If the symptoms are mild, no treatment other than reassurance is required. Treatment with heparin is indicated if symptoms are troublesome or if there is frequent recurrence.

Non-bacterial thrombotic endocarditis, also known as marantic endocarditis, involves thrombus formation on the cardiac valves. It is reported to occur in 7% of patients with lung cancer and less commonly with other tumours. The diagnosis is made by detection of a new cardiac murmur with signs of peripheral arterial embolization and is confirmed on echocardiography.

Microangiopathic haemolytic anaemia occurs with mucin-secreting adenocarcinomas and is usually associated with DIC.

Hepatic vein thrombosis (Budd-Chiari syndrome) is associated with myeloproliferative syndromes. The clinical features include abdominal pain, hepatosplenomegaly, ascites, and distention of the abdominal wall veins.

Microvascular arterial thrombosis occurs in patients with chronic DIC, especially those with polycythaemia vera or essential thrombocythaemia. Involvement of the vessels in the limbs can produce excruciating pain in the hands or feet with few physical signs; if severe, ischaemic changes may develop. Involvement of cerebral vessels may produce a variety of neurological and visual symptoms. Therapy is with aspirin and treatment of the underlying condition, including the control of any thrombocytosis.

Acute fulminant DIC has clinical features related to microvascular thromboses and to a severe coagulopathy. The former may produce ischaemia, cyanosis and even gangrene of the fingers or toes and abnormalities of lung, kidney and cerebral function. The coagulopathy is characterized by severe generalized bleeding. Treatment is that of the underlying cause and by the energetic replacement of clotting factors and platelets; the use of heparin is controversial.

Terminal care

Decisions regarding the treatment of venous thrombosis in patients who are terminally ill can be difficult. Heparin therapy will reduce the pain and swelling in the leg and can hasten resolution of chest pain and dyspnoea from pulmonary embolism. Whether heparin is employed depends on the severity of the symptoms and the patient's estimated life expectancy. Heparin therapy does not necessarily require hospitalization as heparin (or a LMWH preparation) can be given by subcutaneous injection at home. Warfarin therapy is not indicated.

Iatrogenic thrombosis

Vascular catheters. Intravenous catheters, particularly if used for the delivery of chemotherapy, will cause local phlebitis due to physical and chemical irritation or sepsis. Indwelling intravenous and intra-arterial catheters are associated with an increased incidence of local thrombosis.

Peritoneovenous shunts. The use of peritoneovenous shunting for the treatment of ascites may cause DIC and predispose to thrombosis.

Chemotherapy. Hepatic veno-occlusive disease may occur after treatment with dacarbazine or following chemotherapy given before bone marrow transplantation. It presents with the acute onset of painful hepatomegaly without jaundice and the diagnosis is made on liver biopsy. Microangiopathic haemolytic anaemia with DIC can occur after mitomycin therapy.

Hormonal therapy. The treatment of prostatic carcinoma with oestrogens in the past was associated with a significantly increased morbidity and mortality from thrombosis. Corticosteroids and tamoxifen are associated with an increased incidence of thrombosis.

Bleeding disorders

Many patients with cancer develop abnormal bruising or bleeding.[25, 48] The responsible conditions are arbitrarily divided into those in which the signs are frequently confined to the skin (purpura) and those causing generalized bleeding.

Purpura

Purpura is defined as bleeding into the skin or mucous membranes. The smallest purpuric spots (<3 mm) are called petechiae; larger lesions are called ecchymoses. The common causes are listed in Table 22.19.

Mechanical purpura occurs at pressure areas or under adhesive bandages; paroxysmal coughing or violent retching can produce purpura over the head and neck as well as conjunctival haemorrhage. Orthostatic purpura is seen on the lower legs in oedematous states. Purpura simplex or easy bruising consists of purpura or ecchymoses that develop in response to otherwise trivial trauma; it is common in women of reproductive age and requires no specific therapy. Senile purpura is the same as purpura simplex except that it occurs in older people and requires only reassurance. Patients with Cushing's syndrome or receiving corticosteroids develop a similar syndrome, which is reversible once the drug is withdrawn. Vitamin C deficiency causes perifollicular haemorrhages in the skin in association with swollen bleeding

Table 22.19   Causes of purpura

Mechanical purpura	Allergic purpura (Henoch-Schönlein)
Orthostatic purpura	Infection
Purpura simplex ('easy bruising')	Paraproteinaemia
Senile purpura	Thrombocytopenia (see Table 22.10)
Cushing's syndrome, corticosteroids	Abnormal platelet function (see Table 22.12)
Vitamin C deficiency	Coagulation abnormalities (see Table 22.20)
Amyloidosis	

gums; treatment is with vitamin C. Amyloidosis can involve the cutaneous vessels and produce purpura that often affects the eyelids. Paraproteinaemia may cause purpura if the abnormal protein has cryoglobulin properties or by interference with platelet function. In addition, any of the conditions that cause a generalized bleeding diathesis can cause purpura.

Generalized bleeding

Generalized bleeding may occur as a result of thrombocytopenia, abnormal platelet function or a disorder of coagulation (Table 22.20). The diagnosis of the cause of clinical bleeding is based on laboratory investigations.

Table 22.20   Causes of generalized bleeding

Thrombocytopenia (see Table 22.10)
Abnormal platelet function (see Table 22.12)
Coagulation abnormalities
vitamin K deficiency (see Table 22.21)
liver disease
anticoagulation: heparin, warfarin
coagulation factor inhibitors
disseminated intravascular coagulation (DIC)
fibrinolysis: pathological, therapeutic

Vitamin K. Vitamin K is necessary for the hepatic production of a number of clotting factors, including factors II, VII, IX and X. Vitamin K is contained in leafy green vegetables but the prime source is bacterial synthesis in the intestine. It is a fat-soluble vitamin and requires a functional biliary system for absorption. The causes of vitamin K deficiency are shown in Table 22.21. The liver is responsible for the synthesis of most coagulation factors and hepatic disease can lead to deficiencies in some or all of these factors.

The treatment of vitamin K deficiency is that of the cause. Providing there is adequate liver function and no malabsorption, oral supplements can be given. Parenteral therapy (vitamin K 5–10mg IM or SC) will correct or shorten the prothrombin time within 12 to 24 hours. For patients with active bleeding or severe hepatic dysfunction, transfusion of plasma is required.

Coagulation factor inhibitors. Circulating coagulation factor inhibitors associated with a clinical bleeding diathesis are rare but have been reported with a variety of cancers. These may

Table 22.21 Vitamin K deficiency

Decreased intake

Decreased production in small bowel
    small bowel disease
    antibiotics

Decreased absorption
    small bowel resection, bypass
    small bowel disease (malabsorption)
    biliary obstruction (intrahepatic or extrahepatic)
    cholestyramine

Decreased utilization
    liver disease
    coumarin anticoagulants

be antibodies directed against specific clotting factors or a paraprotein that non-specifically interferes with coagulation and fibrin formation.

DIC. Acute disseminated intravascular coagulation, which occurs as a result of sepsis or shock and in association with mucin secreting adenocarcinomas or acute leukaemia, causes depletion of clotting factors, fibrinogen and platelets. Treatment is with replacement of clotting factors and platelets and treatment of the underlying cause; whether or not heparin should be used is controversial.

Fibrinolysis. Primary fibrinolysis occurs with the use of the thrombolytic agent, tissue plasminogen activator (TPA), and in patients with carcinoma of the prostate. The latter usually manifests as severe postoperative bleeding following urological surgery. Treatment is with clotting factor replacement. The fibrinolytic inhibitor aminocaproic acid can be used but may increase the risk of thrombosis.

Local tumour bleeding

Patients with advanced cancer may suffer troublesome local bleeding, usually related to recurrent tumour, for which a variety of treatments can be considered (Table 22.22).[48]

Table 22.22 Treatment options for local bleeding

Local therapy	Topical therapy
radiotherapy	epinephrine (adrenaline) 1:1000
diathermy, laser, cryotherapy	thrombin
embolization	tranexamic acid: 500mg tab dissolved in 5 ml
Systemic therapy	aluminum astringents: 1% alum solution
correction of bleeding diathesis	sucralfate paste
tranexamic acid 1g PO q8h	haemostatic dressings e.g. calcium alginate
aminocaproic acid 1g PO q6h	silver nitrate sticks

Topical therapy. A variety of agents can be applied topically to control local bleeding, including adrenaline (epinephrine), thrombin and tranexamic acid. Aluminium astringents such as 1% alum solution or sucralfate may be useful; sucralfate paste is prepared by dispersing one 1g tablet in 5 ml of water soluble gel (e.g. KY jelly). Sclerosing agents such as phenol and silver nitrate are best avoided as they cause tissue damage. A number of haemostatic dressings containing compounds such as calcium alginate are available which will promote local haemostasis.

Local therapy. Local radiotherapy is the standard treatment for local tumour-related bleeding which is not responding to topical therapy. In some situations, local tumour bleeding is amenable to diathermy, laser treatment or cryotherapy. Persistent local bleeding, such as that due to a carcinoma of the kidney, may be treated by embolization.

Systemic therapy. Any systemic bleeding diathesis is corrected. Administration of a fibrinolytic inhibitor, tranexamic acid or aminocaproic acid, is reported to be effective in controlling troublesome tumour-related bleeding.[49] Fibrinolytic inhibitor therapy may predispose to thrombosis but the frequency with which this occurs is not documented.

Hyperviscosity syndrome

The hyperviscosity syndrome occurs when the whole blood viscosity is increased sufficiently to cause interference with the microcirculation.

Hyperviscosity may be caused by excessive amounts of protein in paraproteinaemia (multiple myeloma, Waldenstrom's macroglobulinaemia), hyperleucocytosis in myeloid leukaemia, or erythrocytosis in polycythaemia vera.

The clinical features are outlined in Table 22.23. The bleeding tendency is variously related to abnormal platelet function, interference with coagulation factor function and fibrin deposition, and inability of the microcirculation to vasoconstrict due to the increased total blood volume. The hyperviscosity syndrome, untreated, can cause irreversible damage to the brain, eyes, kidney and lung and can be fatal.

Table 22.23   Clinical features of the hyperviscosity syndrome

Bleeding	purpura and mucosal haemorrhage
Neurological	headache, nausea, dizziness ataxia, dysarthria confusion, somnolence, coma, seizures
Visual	blurred vision, diplopia, blindness distended retinal veins, haemorrhages, papilloedema
Cardiac	dyspnoea, angina, congestive heart failure
Renal	renal impairment
Pulmonary	cough, dyspnoea, respiratory impairment

Treatment. Treatment comprises physical removal of the cause of the hyperviscosity as well as therapy for the underlying disorder: leucopheresis and chemotherapy for myeloid leukaemia, venesection and myelosuppressive therapy for polycythaemia vera, and plasmapheresis and chemotherapy for paraproteinaemia. Blood transfusion should not be given until hyperviscosity is controlled.

Splenomegaly and hypersplenism

The causes of splenomegaly in patients with cancer are listed in Table 22.24. Splenomegaly may cause left upper quadrant pain and tenderness, with or without pain referred to the region of the left shoulder. Acute pleuritic-type pain with marked local tenderness may occur with capsular haemorrhage or infarction. Massive splenomegaly can cause considerable abdominal discomfort and swelling associated with anorexia, postprandial fullness, nausea, irritable bowel, and urinary frequency.

Table 22.24   Causes of splenomegaly

Infection	viral, bacterial, fungal, parasitic
Infiltration	myeloid leukaemia (acute and chronic) chronic myeloproliferative disorders lymphocytic leukaemia (acute and chronic) malignant lymphoma solid tumour metastases
Vascular	cardiac: congestive failure, pericardial constriction hepatic vein obstruction: thrombosis, tumour, veno-occlusive disease liver disease with portal hypertension portal vein obstruction or thrombosis splenic vein obstruction or thrombosis
Haemolysis	

The treatment of the physical symptoms related to splenomegaly is symptomatic and directed at the underlying cause. Patients with massive splenomegaly can be considered for palliative splenectomy if their symptoms are sufficiently debilitating and their life expectancy is otherwise reasonable. Care must be taken to ensure there is adequate bone marrow reserve, particularly in myelofibrosis where the spleen may be responsible for a significant portion of haemopoiesis. Patients with myeloproliferative disorders can develop extreme thrombocytosis postsplenectomy with platelet counts of 1,000–5,000 x 10^9/l and preoperative myelosuppressive therapy should be considered. Patients with massive splenomegaly and significant symptoms who are not suitable for surgery can often be well palliated with low doses of irradiation given to the spleen.[50]

Hypersplenism. Hypersplenism is the reduction in the peripheral blood cell counts due to an increase in the filtering and phagocytic functions associated with splenomegaly. Treatment depends on the severity of the cytopenias and, where possible, the cause is treated. Splenectomy occasionally has to be considered.

References

1   Frenkel, E.P., Bick, R.L. and Rutherford, C.J. (1996). Anemia of malignancy. *Hematology/Oncology Clinics of North America* 10, 861–73.

2   Arnold, S.M., et al. (2001). Paraneoplastic syndromes. In *Cancer. Principles and Practice of Oncology. 6th edition* (ed. V.T. De Vita, S. Hellman and S.A. Rosenberg). Philadelphia, Lippincott, Williams and Wilkins.

3   Daniel, D.B., Johnston, E.M. and Crawford, J. (2002). Hematologic support of the cancer patient. In *Principles and Practice of Palliative Care and Supportive Oncology* (ed. A.M. Berger, R.K. Portenoy and D.E. Weissman). Philadelphia, Lippincott, Williams and Wilkins.

4   Cella, D. (1998). Factors influencing quality of life in cancer patients: anemia and fatigue. *Seminars in Oncology* 25, 43–6.

5 * Cella, D., et al. (2003). Epoetin alfa treatment results in clinically significant improvements in quality of life in anemic cancer patients when referenced to the general population. *Journal of Clinical Oncology* 21, 366–73.

6 Goodnough, L.T., et al. (1999). Transfusion medicine. First of two parts—blood transfusion. *New England Journal of Medicine* 340, 438–47.

7 Gleeson, C. and Spencer, D. (1995). Blood transfusion and its benefits in palliative care. *Palliative Medicine* 9, 307–13.

8 Griffin, J.D. (2001). Hematopoietic growth factors. In *Cancer. Principles and Practice of Oncology* (ed. V.T. De Vita, S. Hellman and S.A. Rosenberg). Philadelphia, Lippincott, Williams and Wilkins.

9 Sweeney, P.J., et al. (1998). Effect of subcutaneous recombinant human erythropoietin in cancer patients receiving radiotherapy: final report of a randomized, open-labelled, phase II trial. *British Journal of Cancer* 77, 1996–2002.

10 Seidenfeld, J., et al. (2001). Epoetin treatment of anemia associated with cancer therapy: a systematic review and meta-analysis of controlled clinical trials. *Journal of the National Cancer Institute* 93, 1204–14.

11 Turner, R., et al. (2001). Epoetin alfa in cancer patients: evidence-based guidelines. *Journal of Pain and Symptom Management* 22, 954–65.

12 Rizzo, J.D., et al. (2002). Use of epoetin in patients with cancer: evidence-based clinical practice guidelines of the American Society of Clinical Oncology and the American Society of Hematology. *Journal of Clinical Oncology* 20, 4083–107.

13 Gabrilove, J.L., et al. (2001). Clinical evaluation of once-weekly dosing of epoetin alfa in chemotherapy patients: improvements in hemoglobin and quality of life are similar to three-times-weekly dosing. *Journal of Clinical Oncology* 19, 2875–82.

14 Casadevall, N., et al. (2002). Pure red-cell aplasia and antierythropoietin antibodies in patients treated with recombinant erythropoietin. *New England Journal of Medicine* 346, 469–75.

15 Bottomley, A., et al. (2002). Human recombinant erythropoietin and quality of life: a wonder drug or something to wonder about? *Lancet Oncology* 3, 145–53.

16 Quirt, I., et al. (2002). Epoetin alfa in patients not on chemotherapy—Canadian data. *Seminars in Oncology* 29, 75–80.

17 Glaspy, J.A., et al. (2002). Darbepoetin alfa given every 1 or 2 weeks alleviates anaemia associated with cancer chemotherapy. *British Journal of Cancer* 87, 268–76.

18 Hedenus, M., et al. (2002). Randomized, dose-finding study of darbepoetin alfa in anaemic patients with lymphoproliferative malignancies. *British Journal of Haematology* 119, 79–86.

19 Henry, D.H. and Abels, R.I. (1994). Recombinant human erythropoietin in the treatment of cancer and chemotherapy-induced anemia: results of double-blind and open-label follow-up studies. *Seminars in Oncology* 21, 21–8.

20 Daneryd, P., et al. (1998). Protection of metabolic and exercise capacity in unselected weight-losing cancer patients following treatment with recombinant erythropoietin: a randomized prospective study. *Cancer Research* 58, 5374–9.

21 Johansson, J.E., et al. (2001). Efficacy of epoetin beta on hemoglobin, quality of life, and transfusion needs in patients with anemia due to hormone-refractory prostate cancer—a randomized study. *Scandinavian Journal of Urology and Nephrology* 35, 288–94.

22 Osterborg, A., et al. (2002). Randomized, double-blind, placebo-controlled trial of recombinant human erythropoietin, epoetin Beta, in hematologic malignancies. *Journal of Clinical Oncology* 20, 2486–94.

23 Schiffer, C.A., et al. (2001). Platelet transfusion for patients with cancer: clinical practice guidelines of the American Society of Clinical Oncology. *Journal of Clinical Oncology* 19, 1519–38.

24 Bick, R.L. (2003). Disseminated intravascular coagulation current concepts of etiology, pathophysiology, diagnosis, and treatment. *Hematology/Oncology Clinics of North America* 17, 149–76.

25 Bick, R.L., Strauss, J.F. and Frenkel, E.P. (1996). Thrombosis and hemorrhage in oncology patients. *Hematology/Oncology Clinics of North America* 10, 875–907.

26 ten Wolde, M., et al. (2002). The clinical usefulness of D-dimer testing in cancer patients with suspected deep venous thrombosis. *Archives of Internal Medicine* 162, 1880–4.

27 Blann, A.D., Landray, M.J. and Lip, G.Y. (2002). ABC of antithrombotic therapy: An overview of antithrombotic therapy. *British Medical Journal* 325, 762–5.

28 Turpie, A.G., Chin, B.S. and Lip, G.Y. (2002). ABC of antithrombotic therapy: Venous thromboembolism: treatment strategies. *British Medical Journal* 325, 948–50.

29 Pinede, L., et al. (2000). Comparison of long versus short duration of anticoagulant therapy after a first episode of venous thromboembolism: a meta-analysis of randomized, controlled trials. *Journal of Internal Medicine* 247, 553–62.

30 Hutten, B.A. and Prins, M.H. (2000). Duration of treatment with vitamin K antagonists in symptomatic venous thromboembolism (Cochrane Review). *Cochrane Database of Systematic Reviews* CD001367.

31 Bauer, K.A. (2000). Venous thromboembolism in malignancy. *Journal of Clinical Oncology* 18, 3065–7.

32 Hutten, B.A., et al. (2000). Incidence of recurrent thromboembolic and bleeding complications among patients with venous thromboembolism in relation to both malignancy and achieved international normalized ratio: a retrospective analysis. *Journal of Clinical Oncology* 18, 3078–83.

33 Luk, C., et al. (2001). Extended outpatient therapy with low molecular weight heparin for the treatment of recurrent venous thromboembolism despite warfarin therapy. *American Journal of Medicine* 111, 270–3.

34 Prandoni, P., et al. (2002). Recurrent venous thromboembolism and bleeding complications during anticoagulant treatment in patients with cancer and venous thrombosis. *Blood* 100, 3484–8.

35 Schafer, A.I. (1996). Low-molecular-weight heparin—an opportunity for home treatment of venous thrombosis. *New England Journal of Medicine* 334, 724–5.

36 van der Heijden, J.F., Prins, M.H. and Buller, H.R. (2000). For the initial treatment of venous thromboembolism: are all low molecular-weight heparin compounds the same? *Thrombosis Research* 100, V121–30.

37 Breddin, H.K., et al. (2001). Effects of a low-molecular-weight heparin on thrombus regression and recurrent thromboembolism in patients with deep-vein thrombosis. *New England Journal of Medicine* 344, 626–31.

38 Siragusa, S., et al. (1996). Low-molecular-weight heparins and unfractionated heparin in the treatment of patients with acute venous thromboembolism: results of a meta-analysis. *American Journal of Medicine* 100, 269–77.

39 van Den Belt, A.G., et al. (2000). Fixed dose subcutaneous low molecular weight heparins versus adjusted dose unfractionated heparin for venous thromboembolism (Cochrane Review). *Cochrane Database of Systematic Reviews* CD001100.

40 van Dongen, C.J., Mac Gillavry, M.R. and Prins, M.H. (2003). Once versus twice daily LMWH for the initial treatment of venous thromboembolism (Cochrane Review). *Cochrane Database of Systematic Reviews* CD003074.

41 Meyer, G., et al. (2002). Comparison of low-molecular-weight heparin and warfarin for the secondary prevention of venous thromboembolism in patients with cancer: a randomized controlled study. *Archives of Internal Medicine* 162, 1729–35.

42 Schwarz, R.E., et al. (1996). Inferior vena cava filters in cancer patients: indications and outcome. *Journal of Clinical Oncology* 14, 652–7.

43 Jarrett, B.P., Dougherty, M.J. and Calligaro, K.D. (2002). Inferior vena cava filters in malignant disease. *Journal of Vascular Surgery* 36, 704–7.

44 Marcy, P.Y., et al. (2002). Cost-benefit assessment of inferior vena cava filter placement in advanced cancer patients. *Supportive Care in Cancer* 10, 76–80.

45 Agnelli, G., Becattini, C. and Kirschstein, T. (2002). Thrombolysis vs Heparin in the Treatment of Pulmonary Embolism. A Clinical Outcome–Based Meta-analysis. *Archives of Internal Medicine* 162, 2537–41.

46 Deitcher, S.R., et al. (2002). Safety and efficacy of alteplase for restoring function in occluded central venous catheters: results of the cardiovascular thrombolytic to open occluded lines trial. *Journal of Clinical Oncology* 20, 317–24.

47 Timoney, J.P., et al. (2002). Safe and cost effective use of alteplase for the clearance of occluded central venous access devices. *Journal of Clinical Oncology* 20, 1918–22.

48 Pereira, J., Mancini, I. and Bruera, E. (2000). The management of bleeding in advanced cancer patients. In *Topics in Palliative Care* (ed. R. Portenoy and E. Bruera). New York, Oxford University Press.

49 Dean, A. and Tuffin, P. (1997). Fibrinolytic inhibitors for cancer-associated bleeding problems. *Journal of Pain and Symptom Management* 13, 20–4.

50 Bouabdallah, R., et al. (2000). Safety and efficacy of splenic irradiation in the treatment of patients with idiopathic myelofibrosis: a report on 15 patients. *Leukemia Research* 24, 491–5.

23

Musculoskeletal

Muscle weakness	Myoclonus
Muscle cramps	Hypertrophic osteoarthropathy
Muscle spasm	Bone metastases

Muscle weakness

Generalized weakness is an almost universal symptom of advanced cancer. In the majority it is a sign of advancing disease, due to a combination of cachexia, anorexia and poor nutrition, and immobility. Damage or disease affecting any part of the central or peripheral nervous system can produce muscle weakness, which may be focal or localized. Other causes include metabolic and myopathic disorders (Table 23.1), some of which may respond to treatment. Where possible, the treatment is that of the underlying cause.

Polymyositis and dermatomyositis. These syndromes have an association with both cancer and connective tissue diseases.[1, 2] The myositis may develop before or after the diagnosis

Table 23.1 Muscle weakness

Muscle wasting secondary to progression of cancer
    cachexia
    anorexia and poor nutrition
    immobility

Central or peripheral nervous system disease, damage

Metabolic
    hypercalcaemia, hypokalaemia, hypomagnesaemia
    hyperthyroidism, hypoadrenalism
    dehydration

Anaemia

Myopathic syndromes
    polymyositis, dermatomyositis
    myaesthenic syndrome (Lambert-Eaton)
    corticosteroid myopathy: iatrogenic, ectopic ACTH

of cancer. Muscle pain and tenderness are common and a proximal muscular weakness develops over weeks or months. Dermatomyositis is distinguished by the presence of a violaceous or erythematous rash symmetrically involving the periorbital skin, with blotch patches on the cheeks and nose and over the knuckles and elbows. Investigations show elevation of the ESR and creatine phosphokinase, a myopathic pattern on EMG examination, and inflammation and muscle fibre necrosis on biopsy. The myositis syndromes are often associated with cancer of the lung, breast and ovary, less commonly with leukaemia and lymphoma. Control of the underlying tumour may lead to improvement in the myopathy in some cases.[1] Treatment with corticosteroids and immunosuppressive agents benefits some patients. Intravenous immunoglobulin has been used for severe cases, but may only be of benefit in patients without an associated malignancy.[3, 4]

Myasthenic (Lambert-Eaton) syndrome. This uncommon syndrome usually occurs in association with small cell carcinoma of the lung. It is caused by an antibody directed against the calcium channels in the presynaptic membrane of the neuromuscular junction, resulting in impaired release of acetylcholine. It is characterized by proximal muscle weakness, which initially involves the legs. It may progress to involve the arms and the extraorbital and bulbar muscles in some patients.[5] There may be transient improvement in strength following exercise, distinguishing it from true myasthenia. EMG examination shows characteristic abnormalities. The neurological symptoms may improve with successful control of the underlying malignancy, corticosteroids, immunosuppression, or intravenous immunoglobulin. The anticholinesterase agent, pyridostigmine (60–180mg q6h), and drugs that enhance acetylcholine release, diaminopyridine (10–20mg q6h) and guanidine, are also reported to be effective.[6]

Corticosteroid myopathy. Patients treated with corticosteroids for more than a few weeks are at risk of developing proximal muscle weakness, which if severe can be debilitating. The onset is usually insidious, but can be accelerated by immobility. Patients have difficulty standing from a chair and climbing stairs. Treatment includes explanation to the patient, exercise and physiotherapy, and an attempt can be made to wean the dose. Myopathy occurs more frequently with fluorinated steroids, and substitution of prednisolone for dexamethasone should be considered.[7] The myopathy will improve within a few weeks of stopping corticosteroid therapy although this is frequently not possible in patients with advanced cancer.

Patients with tumours secreting ectopic ACTH may also develop proximal myopathy. This may improve with successful control of the underlying tumour. If this cannot be achieved, drugs that inhibit adrenal corticosteroid production, such as aminoglutethimide or metyrapone, can be used. Treatment with these drugs produces adrenal suppression and patients require corticosteroid replacement at physiological dosage. There may be improvement in the myopathy as the levels of circulating corticosteroids return to normal.

Muscle cramps

Muscle cramps are acute painful muscular contractions. They can occur spontaneously, after minor muscle movement, or after forceful contraction. The rate of resolution is variable and there may be persisting muscle twitching and residual tenderness. A muscle cramp usually resolves with passive stretching of the muscle. Muscle cramps are thought to be due to hyperexcitability of the intramuscular portion of the motor nerve.

Cramps can occur in well people during or after strenuous exercise (Table 23.2). A small proportion of healthy young adults will experience nocturnal cramps, the incidence increasing with age. Cramps may occur in patients with cancer for a variety of other reasons including abnormalities of the motor neurone, metabolic disturbances or treatment with certain drugs, particularly diuretics.[8]

Table 23.2 Causes of muscle cramps

Idiopathic
    resting: post-exercise, nocturnal
    during exercise

Pathological
    neuromuscular
        nerve root damage by tumour, radiotherapy
        paraneoplastic neuromyopathy
        peripheral neuropathy due to chemotherapy
        polymyositis, dermatomyositis
    metabolic
        dehydration, hypocalcaemia, hypomagnesaemia, uraemia
        anxiety with hyperventilation
    drugs
        diuretics, platinum, prednisolone, progestogens

Tetany. Tetany is a cramp-like involuntary spasm usually involving distal muscles, as in carpopedal spasm. It occurs with hypocalcaemia and hypomagnesaemia, but is most frequently seen with hyperventilation in patients with anxiety. In this situation, the respiratory alkalosis increases the binding of calcium to albumin, reducing the level of ionized calcium in the serum. Treatment is by correction of the metabolic abnormality or, in the case of hyperventilation, teaching breathing control and relaxation exercises.

Treatment

Acute cramp is treated by passive stretching of the involved muscles. Regular active or passive stretching may reduce the incidence of recurrent cramps. Treatment of muscle cramps includes the correction of metabolic abnormalities, withholding drugs that may be responsible, and the treatment of nerve infiltration or compression.[8] Where there is no reversible cause one of the membrane-stabilizing agents can be used. Quinine sulfate (300mg at night) usually controls nocturnal cramps.[9] Anticonvulsants may be useful in controlling daytime cramps.[10] Corticosteroids can be of benefit in the neuropathic syndromes. Diazepam can be useful, particularly for anxious patients.

Muscle spasm

Spasm secondary to bone disease. Painful bone metastases or pathological fractures are often associated with muscle spasm, which serves to protect and splint the painful area. Treatment is directed at the underlying bone disease. The use of diazepam can be considered if the muscle spasm itself is causing significant pain.

Neuropathic spasm. Disease or damage to the brain or spinal cord can cause spasticity of the limbs and trunk, which may be associated with painful muscle spasms. Treatment is of the causative pathology, if possible, and by physiotherapy. Spasticity and troublesome muscle spasm can be treated with a skeletal muscle relaxant (Table 23.3),[11] although this may result in diminished mobility for the patient if there is significant reduction in general muscle tone. Doses should be increased gradually and titrated against effect. Diazepam is given in anxiolytic doses, the main adverse effect being sedation. Baclofen acts at a spinal level but can also cause significant drowsiness; sudden withdrawal may cause seizures. Dantrolene acts peripherally and may cause less sedation. Local intramuscular injection of botulinum toxin A prevents the release of acetylcholine and has been used for the treatment of spasticity following stroke.[12] It has the advantage of having no central adverse effects but presently has no defined role in palliative care.

Table 23.3 Treatment of muscle spasm

Drug	Dose	Adverse effects
Diazepam	2mg q8h & titrate	sedation
Baclofen	5mg q8h & titrate	weakness, sedation, nausea, hypotension
Tizanidine	2–4mg/d & titrate	sedation, weakness, xerostomia, hypotension
Dantrolene	25mg/d & titrate	weakness, sedation, diarrhoea

Myoclonus

Myoclonus is random involuntary jerking involving single muscles or muscle groups. Myoclonus is not necessarily pathological and includes the muscle jerk or start sometimes experienced whilst falling asleep.

Multifocal myoclonus is associated with brain damage, neurological degenerative disease, and viral infections involving the central nervous system. Children with neuroblastoma may develop the opsoclonus-myoclonus syndrome. In the palliative care setting, myoclonus may be associated with hepatic or renal failure, severe hyponatraemia, and is seen as part of the terminal restlessness syndrome. Multifocal myoclonus may occur with any opioid analgesic and is most frequently seen with pethidine (meperidine).

Treatment

Treatment is directed at the cause, where possible. Opioid-related myoclonus is treated by dose reduction, if feasible, or by switching to an alternative opioid. Clonazepam, midazolam[13] and gabapentin[14] usually control myoclonus. In the terminal care setting, midazolam (2.5–10 mg SC hourly until controlled, followed by 10–60 mg/24h CSCI) is usually effective.

Hypertrophic osteoarthropathy

Hypertrophic osteoarthropathy (HOA) is a paraneoplastic syndrome comprising clubbing of the fingers and toes, polyarthritis, and periostitis.[15, 16] The joints most frequently involved are the wrists, ankles, knees and elbows; symptoms range from mild arthralgia to severe inflammatory arthritis. Periostitis occurs most commonly at the distal ends of the radius and ulna or the tibia and fibula and can cause severe burning pain, which is relieved by elevation. HOA most frequently occurs with non-small cell carcinoma of the lung and less often with pulmonary metastases or other tumours; it is also reported with a variety of other pulmonary, cardiac, hepatic and intestinal disorders, most of which are benign.

The patient complains of pain, tenderness and swelling over the affected bones and joints. Examination shows clubbing and there may be induration and erythema over the affected bones and joints. X-ray examination shows periosteal reaction or periostitis. An isotopic bone scan shows abnormal uptake in the affected regions.

Treatment

Control of the underlying malignancy may produce marked improvement. Otherwise, treatment is symptomatic with NSAIDs. HOA is also reported to respond to bisphosphonate therapy.[17]

Bone metastases

Bone metastases are a major cause of pain and impaired function in patients with advanced cancer. The incidence of bone metastases varies with different tumour types, being most common (70–80%) in multiple myeloma, breast and prostate cancer. In practice, about three-quarters of bone metastases are due to cancers of the breast, lung and prostate.

Pathophysiology. Bone metastases usually develop by vascular spread, either arterial or via the vertebral and paravertebral venous plexuses. Metastases start in the vascular medullary cavity of the bone and progress to involve the cortex. Direct infiltration, seen with head and neck tumours and with rib invasion by intrathoracic malignancies, is less common.

Cancer cells cause bone destruction primarily by stimulation of osteoclast activity. A variety of substances are produced (including parathyroid hormone-related protein, transforming growth factors, prostaglandins and other cytokines) that stimulate osteoclast activity either directly or via an action on osteoblasts or immune cells. Except in purely lytic lesions such as those seen in myeloma, there is also increased osteoblast activity in bone metastases, and it is this osteoblastic activity that is responsible for abnormalities seen on an isotopic bone scan. If osteoclastic activity predominates, the lesions are lytic on x-ray; they appear sclerotic if osteoblastic activity predominates. Both lytic and sclerotic metastases may be seen in the same patient.

The mechanism by which bone metastases cause pain is incompletely understood and many patients are asymptomatic. In the initial phase, pain is probably caused by chemical stimulation of the endosteal nerve endings. With tumour progression there may be stretching and stimulation of the periosteal receptors. Reflex muscle spasm and extension of the tumour into adjacent soft tissues will cause pain. Pathological fracture causes an acute exacerbation of pain.

Clinical features. Bone metastases occur predominantly (80%) in the axial skeleton, which contains the more vascular red marrow. Metastases occur most frequently in the vertebrae, ribs, pelvis and femora with less frequent involvement of the pectoral girdle and skull.

Bone metastases cause local pain. Initially, this may be intermittent, aggravated by movement and perhaps more noticeable at night. Standing and walking aggravate pain in weight bearing bones. There may be local tenderness to pressure or percussion. Progression of the lesion leads to continuous pain. Bone metastases are associated with a number of other complications (Table 23.4).

Assessment. The diagnosis of bone metastases is by x-ray and isotopic bone scan. Plain x-rays are abnormal if more than half of the cancellous bone is destroyed. Lesions may be lytic, sclerotic or mixed in appearance. Bone scanning is much more sensitive for the detection of bone metastases but lacks specificity. Bone scanning can detect smaller metastases

(2mm) but may be negative in purely lytic lesions as occur in multiple myeloma. Bone scans will show abnormality wherever there is osteoblastic activity, as occurs with arthritis, infection, trauma and Paget's disease. Bone metastases can also be demonstrated on CT and MRI scans, the latter being the method of choice for examination of the vertebral column.

Table 23.4   Bone metastases: clinical features

Pain
Impaired mobility and function
Pathological fractures
Hypercalcaemia
Spinal cord compression
Nerve root compression
Impaired bone marrow function

Treatment

The aims of treatment are pain relief, preservation and restoration of function, skeletal stabilization, and local tumour control. In general, treatment is reserved for symptomatic disease, except for metastases in weight-bearing areas of the skeleton. The treatment options are summarized in Table 23.5.

Table 23.5   Treatment options for bone metastases

Analgesics	NSAIDs, corticosteroids, opioids
Adjuvant analgesic	bisphosphonates
Systemic therapy	hormonal, chemotherapy (sensitive tumours)
Radiotherapy	local, hemibody, radioisotopes
Surgery	prophylaxis and fixation of fractures
Physical	supports, mobility aids, physiotherapy

Analgesics. NSAIDs are the analgesics of choice for the treatment of mild to moderate bone pain by virtue of having less adverse effects than opioid drugs;[18–21] whether they are superior to opioid analgesics has not been established. NSAID therapy for bone pain showed more pain relief than placebo in two RCTs, but the difference was not statistically significant; a third trial of patients with bone pain taking oxycodone/acetaminophen showed significant improvement with the addition of ibuprofen (see Table 8.4). Continuous intravenous infusion of ketorolac has been reported to relieve intractable bone pain.[22] When given for some other indication, corticosteroids may greatly reduce bone pain. However, the side effects of prolonged therapy prohibit the routine use of corticosteroids for bone pain. For more severe pain, opioid drugs are used in addition to the NSAID.

Systemic therapy. Systemic therapy for sensitive tumours, if successful, will reduce bone pain.

Radiotherapy. Radiotherapy is the treatment of choice for bone pain due to metastases. Palliative radiotherapy will produce clinical improvement in the majority of patients, whatever the histological type or tissue of origin of the tumour.

A considerable number of different radiotherapy schedules has been advocated for the treatment of bone metastases.[23] A number of studies have shown that a single dose of 8 Gy produces equivalent results to longer courses of therapy (Table 23.6). Pain relief is reported in 50 to 80% of patients and lasts a median of 3 months; a significant proportion of patients remain pain free at the treated site for 12 months.[24] Retreatment is required more frequently with the 8 Gy dose, but this may reflect a readiness to give further treatment after a single fraction than after a longer course. A single dose of 4 Gy produced fewer responses, but the duration of pain relief was similar. The response to radiotherapy is usually manifest within 2 to 4 weeks of starting treatment. It may occur more rapidly, even within a day or two, with higher dose fractions.

Table 23.6 Radiotherapy for bone metastases: RCTs

Author	n	Intervention	Outcome
Single 8Gy fraction vs longer courses			
Price[25]	288	8Gy vs 30Gy	equivalent speed of onset and duration of analgesia
Nielsen[26]	241	8Gy vs 20Gy	equivalent frequency and duration of analgesia
Bone Pain Trial[27]	765	8Gy vs 20Gy or 30Gy	equivalent frequency, speed of onset and duration of analgesia; more retreatments with 8Gy
Steenland[28]	1171	8Gy vs 24Gy	equivalent frequency, speed of onset and duration of analgesia; more retreatments with 8Gy
Single 8Gy fraction vs lower doses			
Hoskin[29]	270	8Gy vs 4Gy	8Gy: 69 vs 44% pain relief at 4w (pS); fewer retreatments (pS)
Jeremic[30]	327	8Gy vs 6Gy vs 4Gy	onset: 8Gy more rapid (pS); frequency of analgesia: 4Gy inferior (pS); retreatment rate the same

Vertebral metastases associated with, or threatening, spinal cord compression may be better treated with longer courses of therapy. This is to avoid the acute oedema that can be associated with a large single fraction, and because the goal of treatment may be tumour shrinkage as well as pain control.

Hemibody irradiation (HBI). Hemibody irradiation can be considered for patients with widespread painful metastases. HBI involves a single treatment to the whole of the upper or lower half of the body and this can be followed, if indicated, with irradiation to the other half of the body four to six weeks later. It produces pain relief in days for 90% of patients.[31, 32] HBI does not prevent further local radiotherapy being given to local painful areas.

The toxicity of HBI is considerable and includes nausea, vomiting and diarrhoea, myelo-suppression, mucositis, pneumonitis and alopecia. HBI is therefore not appropriate for patients with significantly reduced blood counts, those in generally poor physical condition, or with a life expectancy of less than a few months.

Radiopharmaceuticals. The systemic administration of bone-seeking radioisotopes is effective in controlling pain related to bone metastases.[33, 34] Various isotopes have been used including [89]Strontium, [153]Samarium and [186]Rhenium (Table 23.7). The isotopes are preferentially taken up at sites of osteoblastic activity and cause only mild myelotoxicity. They are used to treat metastases that have increased osteoblastic activity, as evidenced by abnormality on bone scan. They are most effective for tumours that have markedly increased osteoblastic activity, with sclerotic changes on x-ray, as is seen with prostate and some breast cancers. Improved pain control is reported in up to 80% of patients. Responses are usually evident 2 to 3 weeks after treatment and last for 3 to 6 months. The degree and duration of analgesia after radioisotope therapy is equivalent to local or hemibody irradiation.[35,36] They are of benefit when used in addition to local radiotherapy; compared to local radiotherapy, they reduce the number of new pain sites for about four months following treatment.[36] Radioisotope therapy is well tolerated and the main side effect is myelosuppression, which is usually mild and not clinically significant. The main drawback of radioisotope therapy is the cost.

Table 23.7   Radioisotope therapy for painful bone metastases: RCTs

Author	n	Intervention	Outcome
[89]Strontium			
Lewington[37]	32	[89]Sr vs stable Sr	[89]Sr: ↑ pain relief (pS)
Porter[36]	126	local RT plus ^{89}Sr or stable Sr	[89]Sr: ↓ new pain sites (pS), ↑ QOL (pS)
Quilty[35]	284	local or hemibody RT vs [89]Sr	pain relief equivalent; [89]Sr: ↓ new pain sites (pS)
Sciuto[38]	70	[89]Sr + cisplatin vs [89]Sr	[89]Sr + cisplatin: ↑ pain relief, duration, ↓ new pain sites, ↓ progression of bone disease (all pS)
[153]Samarium			
Resche[39]	114	[153]Sm 0.5mCi/kg vs 1.0mCi/kg	higher dose: pain relief 70 vs 55% at 4 weeks (pS)
Serafini[40]	118	[153]Sm 0.5 vs 1.0mCi/kg vs placebo	higher dose: ↑ pain relief (pS)
Tian[41]	105	[153]Sm 37MBq/kg vs 18.5MBq/kg	pain relief (83%) and side effects independent of dose
[186]Rhenium			
Han[42]	111	[186]Re vs placebo	[186]Re: ↑ pain relief (pS)
Sciuto[43]	50	[89]Sr vs [186]Re	pain relief and duration equivalent; more rapid pain relief with [186]Re (pS)

Surgery. Surgery is employed for the prevention and treatment of pathological fractures. Prophylactic surgery is most frequently used for metastatic disease involving the region of the hip or the shaft of the femur. Radiographic assessment alone cannot adequately identify all lesions at high risk of fracture, but some general guidelines are listed in Table 23.8. Whether or not an individual patient should have surgery depends on the prognosis, fitness for surgery, and the degree of pain or functional loss.

Surgical fixation of fractures or potential fracture sites is best performed with curetting of the tumour, using methyl methacrylate bone cement to fill the defect created, in conjunction with internal fixation using a plate or rod. It is standard practice to give postoperative irradiation when the wound has healed although the value of such treatment, especially in patients with a short life expectancy, has not been documented. Surgical fixation provides prompt pain relief and allows early mobilization and rehabilitation.

Table 23.8 Bone metastases: indications for prophylactic surgery

Medullary lesion	>50% diameter of the bone
Cortical lesion	destruction of >50% of cortical width axial length > diameter of bone size >2-3 cm
Any lesion causing pain not relieved by radiotherapy	

Bisphosphonates. The bisphosphonate compounds are chemical analogues of pyrophosphate that inhibit bone resorption. They are effective in the treatment of hypercalcaemia associated with cancer and have been shown to reduce pain. They act by inhibiting osteoclast activity, blocking mineral dissolution, and may also have antitumour action.[44] The more recently introduced nitrogen-containing bisphosphonates (pamidronate, ibandronate, olpadronate and zoledronic acid) are more potent than the non-nitrogen-containing compounds etidronate and clodronate.

Systematic and Cochrane reviews of the many RCTs of bisphosphonate therapy indicate that it is effective in reducing pain and the incidence of skeletal-related events (SREs) in patients with bone metastases; SREs include pathological fracture, spinal cord compression, bone pain requiring radiotherapy, bone surgery, or hypercalcaemia.[45–51] There is no effect on survival. Guidelines for the use of bisphosphonates have been developed.[52–54]

The pain relief produced by bisphosphonate therapy occurs over time and there is insufficient evidence to recommend its use for immediate analgesia; bisphosphonates should be considered if analgesics and radiotherapy provide inadequate control.

Pamidronate has been shown to be effective in reducing pain and SREs related to lytic metastases or myeloma, but no significant benefits were seen with osteoblastic metastases from prostate cancer (Table 23.9). Pamidronate is given as an infusion each 4 weeks (90mg IV in

Table 23.9 Bisphosphonates and skeletal-related events (SREs): selected RCTs

Author	n	Intervention	Outcome
Breast cancer and myeloma			
Theriault[60]	371	breast cancer on hormone therapy: IV pamidronate vs placebo (2yr)	↓ % with SRE, ↑ time to SRE, less ↑ in pain scores, analgesic use (all pS)
Hortobagyi[61]	380	breast cancer on chemotherapy: IV pamidronate vs placebo (2yr)	↓ % with SRE, ↑ time to SRE, less ↑ in pain scores, analgesic use (all pS)
Berenson[62]	377	myeloma: IV pamidronate vs placebo (2yr)	↓ % with SRE, ↑ time to SRE (both pS)
Rosen[63]	1648	breast and myeloma: IV zoledronic acid vs pamidronate	% with SRE, time to SRE, pain scores – all equivalent
Berenson[55]	280	breast and myeloma: IV zoledronic acid (2 or 4mg) vs pamidronate	% with SRE, time to SRE, pain scores – all equivalent
Prostate cancer			
Lipton[64]	236	IV Pamidronate vs placebo	no significant benefits
Saad[57]	643	IV Zoledronic acid vs placebo	↓ % with SRE, ↑ time to SRE, less ↑ in pain scores (all pS)

500ml over 1–2 hours). The dose should be reduced or administered more slowly in patients with significant renal impairment. A few patients suffer mild nausea, bone pain or low-grade fever but there are no serious adverse effects and symptomatic hypocalcaemia is rare.

Zoledronic acid has been shown to be as effective as pamidronate for the treatment of lytic bone disease and has a similar adverse effect profile. It has the advantage of being given as a simple 15-minute injection. In addition, it has been shown to be effective in reducing pain and SREs related to osteoblastic metastases in prostate cancer (Table 23.9), and has activity against metastases from a range of primary tumours.[55-57] Olpadronate (given IV and PO) and ibandronate (given IV) are also reported to be effective in prostate cancer.[58, 59]

Terminal care

The treatment of bone metastases in the last days or week of life should be directed solely at patient comfort. Because of the uncertainty of estimating life expectancy, palliative radiotherapy needs to be considered if the pain is difficult to control and may be effective within days. Surgical procedures are usually not indicated. Splinting and skin traction may be of benefit. Adequate analgesia needs to be prescribed and extra doses must be available to be given before moving or turning the patient if such procedures cause increased pain.

References

1   Callen, J.P. (2000). Dermatomyositis. *Lancet* 355, 53–7.
2   Buchbinder, R., et al. (2001). Incidence of malignant disease in biopsy-proven inflammatory myopathy. A population-based cohort study. *Annals of Internal Medicine* 134, 1087–95.
3   Dalakas, M.C., et al. (1993). A controlled trial of high-dose intravenous immune globulin infusions as treatment for dermatomyositis. *New England Journal of Medicine* 329, 1993–2000.
4   Gottfried, I., et al. (2000). High dose intravenous immunoglobulin (IVIG) in dermatomyositis: clinical responses and effect on sIL-2R levels. *European Journal of Dermatology* 10, 29–35.
5   Wirtz, P.W., et al. (2002). Difference in distribution of muscle weakness between myasthenia gravis and the Lambert-Eaton myasthenic syndrome. *Journal of Neurology, Neurosurgery and Psychiatry* 73, 766–8.
6   Dalmau, J.O., et al. (1997). Paraneoplastic syndromes affecting the nervous system. *Seminars in Oncology* 24, 318–28.
7   Dropcho, E.J. and Soong, S.J. (1991). Steroid-induced weakness in patients with primary brain tumors. *Neurology* 41, 1235–9.
8   Siegal, T. (1991). Muscle cramps in the cancer patient: causes and treatment. *Journal of Pain and Symptom Management* 6, 84–91.
9   Man-Son-Hing, M. and Wells, G. (1995). Meta-analysis of efficacy of quinine for treatment of nocturnal leg cramps in elderly people. *British Medical Journal* 310, 13–17.
10   Quan, D., Teener, J.W. and Farrar, J.T. (2002). Neuromuscular dysfunction and palliative care. In *Principles and Practice of Palliative Care and Supportive Oncology* (ed. A.M. Berger, R.K. Portenoy and D.E. Weissman). Philadelphia, Lippincott, Williams and Wilkins.
11   Kita, M. and Goodkin, D.E. (2000). Drugs used to treat spasticity. *Drugs* 59, 487–95.
12   Brashear, A., et al. (2002). Intramuscular injection of botulinum toxin for the treatment of wrist and finger spasticity after a stroke. *New England Journal of Medicine* 347, 395–400.
13   Hagen, N. and Swanson, R. (1997). Strychnine-like multifocal myoclonus and seizures in extremely high-dose opioid administration: treatment strategies. *Journal of Pain and Symptom Management* 14, 51–8.
14   Mercadante, S., Villari, P. and Fulfaro, F. (2001). Gabapentin for opiod-related myoclonus in cancer patients. *Supportive Care in Cancer* 9, 205–6.

15 Martinez-Lavin, M., et al. (1993). Hypertrophic osteoarthropathy: consensus on its definition, classification, assessment and diagnostic criteria. *Journal of Rheumatology* 20, 1386–7.

16 Carsons, S. (1997). The association of malignancy with rheumatic and connective tissue diseases. *Seminars in Oncology* 24, 360–72.

17 Speden, D., et al. (1997). The use of pamidronate in hypertrophic pulmonary osteoarthropathy (HPOA). *Australian and New Zealand Journal of Medicine* 27, 307–10.

18 Pereira, J. (1998). Management of bone pain. In *Topics in Palliative Care* (ed. R. Portenoy and E. Bruera). New York, Oxford University Press.

19 Jenkins, C.A. and Bruera, E. (1999). Nonsteroidal anti-inflammatory drugs as adjuvant analgesics in cancer patients. *Palliative Medicine* 13, 183–96.

20 Mercadante, S., et al. (1999). Analgesic effects of nonsteroidal anti-inflammatory drugs in cancer pain due to somatic or visceral mechanisms. *Journal of Pain and Symptom Management* 17, 351–6.

21 Wallenstein, D.J. and Portenoy, R.K. (2002). Nonopioid and adjuvant analgesics. In *Principles and Practice of Palliative Care and Supportive Oncology* (ed. A.M. Berger, R.K. Portenoy and D.E. Weissman). Philadelphia, Lippincott, Williams and Wilkins.

22 Gordon, R.L. (1998). Prolonged central intravenous ketorolac continuous infusion in a cancer patient with intractable bone pain. *Annals of Pharmacotherapy* 32, 193–6.

23 McQuay, H.J., et al. (2000). Radiotherapy for the palliation of painful bone metastases (Cochrane Review). *Cochrane Database of Systematic Reviews* CD001793.

24 Brown, H.K. and Healey, J.H. (2001). Metastatic cancer to the bone. In *Cancer. Principles and Practice of Oncology. 6th edition* (ed. V.T. De Vita, S. Hellman and S.A. Rosenberg). Philadelphia, Lippincott, Williams and Wilkins.

25 Price, P., et al. (1986). Prospective randomised trial of single and multifraction radiotherapy schedules in the treatment of painful bony metastases. *Radiotherapy and Oncology* 6, 247–55.

26 Nielsen, O.S., et al. (1998). Randomized trial of single dose versus fractionated palliative radiotherapy of bone metastases. *Radiotherapy and Oncology* 47, 233–40.

27 Bone Pain Trial Working Party (1999). 8 Gy single fraction radiotherapy for the treatment of metastatic skeletal pain: randomised comparison with a multifraction schedule over 12 months of patient follow-up. *Radiotherapy and Oncology* 52, 111–21.

28 Steenland, E., et al. (1999). The effect of a single fraction compared to multiple fractions on painful bone metastases: a global analysis of the Dutch Bone Metastasis Study. *Radiotherapy and Oncology* 52, 101–9.

29 Hoskin, P.J., et al. (1992). A prospective randomised trial of 4 Gy or 8 Gy single doses in the treatment of metastatic bone pain. *Radiotherapy and Oncology* 23, 74–8.

30 Jeremic, B., et al. (1998). A randomized trial of three single-dose radiation therapy regimens in the treatment of metastatic bone pain. *International Journal of Radiation Oncology, Biology and Physics* 42, 161–7.

31 McSweeney, E.N., et al. (1993). Double hemibody irradiation (DHBI) in the management of relapsed and primary chemoresistant multiple myeloma. *Clinical Oncology* 5, 378–83.

32 Salazar, O.M., et al. (2001). Fractionated half-body irradiation (HBI) for the rapid palliation of widespread, symptomatic, metastatic bone disease: a randomized Phase III trial of the International Atomic Energy Agency (IAEA). *International Journal of Radiation Oncology, Biology and Physics* 50, 765–75.

33 Robinson, R.G., et al. (1995). Strontium 89 therapy for the palliation of pain due to osseous metastases. *Journal of the American Medical Association* 274, 420–4.

34 Berger, A.M. and Koprowski, C. (2002). Bone pain:assessment and management. In *Principles and Practice of Palliative Care and Supportive Oncology* (ed. A.M. Berger, R.K. Portenoy and D.E. Weissman). Philadelphia, Lippincott, Williams and Wilkins.

35 Quilty, P.M., et al. (1994). A comparison of the palliative effects of strontium-89 and external beam radiotherapy in metastatic prostate cancer. *Radiotherapy and Oncology* 31, 33–40.

36 Porter, A.T., et al. (1993). Results of a randomized phase-III trial to evaluate the efficacy of strontium-89 adjuvant to local field external beam irradiation in the management of endocrine resistant metastatic prostate cancer. *International Journal of Radiation Oncology, Biology and Physics* 25, 805–13.

37 Lewington, V.J., et al. (1991). A prospective, randomised double-blind crossover study to examine the efficacy of strontium-89 in pain palliation in patients with advanced prostate cancer metastatic to bone. *European Journal of Cancer* 27, 954–8.

38 Sciuto, R., et al. (2002). Effects of low-dose cisplatin on 89Sr therapy for painful bone metastases from prostate cancer: a randomized clinical trial. *Journal of Nuclear Medicine* 43, 79–86.

39 Resche, I., et al. (1997). A dose-controlled study of 153Sm-ethylenediaminetetramethylenephosphonate (EDTMP) in the treatment of patients with painful bone metastases. *European Journal of Cancer* 33, 1583–91.

40 Serafini, A.N., et al. (1998). Palliation of pain associated with metastatic bone cancer using samarium-153 lexidronam: a double-blind placebo-controlled clinical trial. *Journal of Clinical Oncology* 16, 1574–81.

41 Tian, J.H., et al. (1999). Multicentre trial on the efficacy and toxicity of single-dose samarium-153-ethylene diamine tetramethylene phosphonate as a palliative treatment for painful skeletal metastases in China. *European Journal of Nuclear Medicine* 26, 2–7.

42 Han, S.H., et al. (1999). 186Re-etidronate in breast cancer patients with metastatic bone pain. *Journal of Nuclear Medicine* 40, 639–42.

43 Sciuto, R., et al. (2001). Metastatic bone pain palliation with 89-Sr and 186-Re-HEDP in breast cancer patients. *Breast Cancer Research and Treatment* 66, 101–9.

44 Green, J.R. (2003). Antitumor effects of bisphosphonates. *Cancer* 97, 840–7.

45 Bloomfield, D.J. (1998). Should bisphosphonates be part of the standard therapy of patients with multiple myeloma or bone metastases from other cancers? An evidence-based review. *Journal of Clinical Oncology* 16, 1218–25.

46 Goudas, L., et al. (2001). *Management of cancer pain*. Rockville, MD: Agency for Healthcare Research and Quality. <www.ahrq.gov>

47 Carr, D., et al. (2002). *Management of Cancer Symptoms: Pain, Depression, and Fatigue. Evidence Report/Technology Assessment No. 61.* Rockville, MD: Agency for Healthcare Research and Quality. <www.ahrq.gov>

48 Body, J.J. and Mancini, I. (2002). Bisphosphonates for cancer patients: why, how, and when? *Supportive Care in Cancer* 10, 399–407.

49 Djulbegovic, B., et al. (2002). Bisphosphonates in multiple myeloma (Cochrane Review). *Cochrane Database of Systematic Reviews* CD003188.

50 Major, P.P. and Cook, R. (2002). Efficacy of bisphosphonates in the management of skeletal complications of bone metastases and selection of clinical endpoints. *American Journal of Clinical Oncology* 25, S10–8.

51 Wong, R. and Wiffen, P.J. (2002). Bisphosphonates for the relief of pain secondary to bone metastases (Cochrane Review). *Cochrane Database of Systematic Reviews* CD002068.

52 Mannix, K., et al. (2000). Using bisphosphonates to control the pain of bone metastases: evidence-based guidelines for palliative care. *Palliative Medicine* 14, 455–61.

53 Hillner, B.E., et al. (2000). American Society of Clinical Oncology guideline on the role of bisphosphonates in breast cancer. American Society of Clinical Oncology Bisphosphonates Expert Panel. *Journal of Clinical Oncology* 18, 1378–91.

54 Berenson, J.R., et al. (2002). American Society of Clinical Oncology clinical practice guidelines: the role of bisphosphonates in multiple myeloma. *Journal of Clinical Oncology* 20, 3719–36.

55 Berenson, J.R., et al. (2001). Zoledronic acid reduces skeletal-related events in patients with osteolytic metastases. *Cancer* 91, 1191–200.

56 Rosen, L., Harland, S.J. and Oosterlinck, W. (2002). Broad clinical activity of zoledronic acid in osteolytic to osteoblastic bone lesions in patients with a broad range of solid tumors. *American Journal of Clinical Oncology* 25, S19–24.

57 Saad, F., et al. (2002). A randomized, placebo-controlled trial of zoledronic acid in patients with hormone-refractory metastatic prostate carcinoma. *Journal of the National Cancer Institute* 94, 1458–68.

58 Pelger, R.C., et al. (1998). Effects of the bisphosphonate olpadronate in patients with carcinoma of the prostate metastatic to the skeleton. *Bone* 22, 403–8.

59 Heidenreich, A., Elert, A. and Hofmann, R. (2002). Ibandronate in the treatment of prostate cancer associated painful osseous metastases. *Prostate Cancer and Prostatic Disease* 5, 231–5.

60 Theriault, R.L., et al. (1999). Pamidronate reduces skeletal morbidity in women with advanced breast cancer and lytic bone lesions: a randomized, placebo-controlled trial. Protocol 18 Aredia Breast Cancer Study Group. *Journal of Clinical Oncology* 17, 846–54.

61 Hortobagyi, G.N., et al. (1998). Long-term prevention of skeletal complications of metastatic breast cancer with pamidronate. Protocol 19 Aredia Breast Cancer Study Group. *Journal of Clinical Oncology* 16, 2038–44.

62 Berenson, J.R., et al. (1998). Long-term pamidronate treatment of advanced multiple myeloma patients reduces skeletal events. Myeloma Aredia Study Group. *Journal of Clinical Oncology* 16, 593–602.

63 Rosen, L.S., et al. (2001). Zoledronic acid versus pamidronate in the treatment of skeletal metastases in patients with breast cancer or osteolytic lesions of multiple myeloma: a phase III, double-blind, comparative trial. *Cancer Journal* 7, 377–87.

64 Lipton, A. (2003). Bisphosphonates and metastatic breast carcinoma. *Cancer* 97, 848–53.

24

Dermatological

Cutaneous manifestations of cancer

There are many cutaneous manifestations of internal malignancy, occurring with variable frequency.[1–3] The significance of these clinical signs in the setting of palliative care is that their recognition may allow the patient to be reassured and, in some cases, symptomatic treatment applied.

Xerosis. Dry, fine scaling of the skin is common in patients with advanced cancer. Treatment is symptomatic with topical moisturizing medication.

Acquired ichthyosis. Ichthyosis appearing during adult life has a strong association with malignancy, particularly Hodgkin's disease. The entire skin is dry with the trunk and limbs most affected. The skin has a 'fish-scale' appearance being divided into rhomboidal areas by criss-crossing transverse lines. The palms and soles may be hyperkeratotic. Treatment is with emollients to keep the skin as moist as possible; if scaling is severe, a keratolytic such as 2% salicylic acid can be added to the emollient.

Acanthosis nigricans. The development of velvety brown hyperkeratotic plaques in the flexures of the axillae, groins and neck has a strong association with internal malignancy. It can also involve the periareolar and periumbilical area.

Hypertrichosis lanuginosa. This is characterized by the development of fine, silky lanugo-like hair ('malignant down'), first affecting the face and later the entire body surface.

Dermatomyositis. Dermatomyositis is the association of progressive proximal muscle weakness with a violaceous or erythematous rash symmetrically involving the periorbital skin, with blotch patches on the cheeks and nose and over the knuckles and elbows. It has a strong association with internal malignancy. It sometimes improves with control of the underlying tumour or may respond to corticosteroids or immunosuppression.

Pigmentation. Patients with advanced cancer frequently develop a sallow yellow waxy skin colour, the cause of which is unknown. Diffuse hyperpigmentation may occur with ectopic ACTH production and in adrenal insufficiency. Certain chemotherapy drugs, notably busulphan and bleomycin, may also produce hyperpigmentation. A few patients with disseminated melanoma develop a generalized slate-grey discolouration, often associated with very dark urine, due to pigment deposition.

Erythema ab igne. Areas of reticulated (lace-net-like) brown discolouration are seen commonly in patients with advanced cancer, due to the frequent self-application of hot water bottles or heating pads to relieve pain.

Seborrhoeic keratosis. Seborrhoeic keratoses are benign skin tumours that are common, especially in the elderly. The sudden and rapid development of large numbers of seborrhoeic keratoses can occur in association with internal malignancy and is known as the Leser-Trélat sign.

Pruritus

Pruritus or itch is 'an unpleasant cutaneous sensation which provokes the desire to scratch'.[4] Generalized itching or pruritus is not common in patients with advanced cancer but, if severe, can be both distressing and debilitating.

Pathophysiology. Pruritus may be caused by a variety of mechanisms, both peripheral and central, and involving histamine, serotonin (5HT), and opioid receptors (Table 24.1).[4,5] Stimulation of itch-specific nerve endings in the skin leads to impulses being conveyed via the dorsal horn and spinothalamic tract to the thalamus, and then on to the somatosensory cortex. Similar to pain, the peripheral sensation of itch can be modified by other effects in the CNS, including psychological factors. The nerve endings are sensitive to histamine released from dermal mast cells and to other pruritogens; other substances and cytokines may either promote the release of histamine or sensitize the nerve endings to it. This effect is blocked by H_1-antihistamines.

Other causes of pruritus do not involve peripheral nerve stimulation and are not relieved by H_1-antihistamines. The pruritus of cholestasis is associated with increased endogenous opioid production by the liver and increased plasma levels of enkephalins, and is relieved by opioid antagonists. Opioid-induced pruritus is also reversed by opioid antagonists. In uraemia, there are increased histamine levels in the skin and plasma, but H_1-antihistamines

Table 24.1 Classification of pruritus[4]

Pruritoceptive
stimulation of itch-specific fibres in the skin by histamine or other pruritogens
e.g. cutaneous infection, inflammation, urticaria
Neuropathic
damage to the afferent pathway
e.g. pruritus associated with postherpetic neuralgia, multiple sclerosis
Neurogenic
centrally mediated, without neural damage
e.g. cholestasis, exogenous opioids
Psychogenic
e.g. parasitophobia

are ineffective. Ultraviolet B (UVB) therapy, which reduces both the number of mast cells in the skin and the concentrations of divalent ions (calcium, magnesium, and phosphate), is effective; reports of the effect of opioid antagonists are conflicting.

Cause. The causes of pruritus are listed in Table 24.2. In palliative care, pruritus occurs most frequently as a consequence of intra- or extra-hepatic biliary obstruction by malignant disease. Drug induced cholestasis may occur with oestrogens, androgenic and anabolic steroids, and antibiotics including erythromycin, amoxycillin/clavulanic acid and flucloxacillin; similar reactions occur less commonly with a range of other drugs. Infective or drug related hepatitis usually cause only mild pruritus. Pruritus occurs frequently in polycythaemia vera and Hodgkin's disease, less commonly with other haematological malignancies, and rarely with solid tumours. A considerable number of drugs have been reported to cause a pruritic skin rash. Patients treated with opioids, particularly by the intraspinal route, may complain of pruritus. Dry skin (xerosis) is common in patients with cancer and in older people and may be associated with mild pruritus.

Pruritus is usually aggravated by heat; cold has the opposite effect. It may be made worse by psychological factors such as anxiety, and improved by relaxation or distraction.

Measurement. Like pain, itch is subjective and cannot be objectively quantified. Serial measurements on a visual analogue scale will provide subjective comparisons. Measurements of scratching activity, which may be difficult to standardize, provide a means of objective assessment against which new therapies should be judged.

Table 24.2   Causes of pruritus

Skin disease	Malignancy
drug reactions	polycythaemia vera
radiotherapy reactions	other myeloproliferative disorders
xerosis, ichthyosis	Hodgkin's disease
infections: scabies, candida	other lymphomas
atopic dermatitis	solid tumours
urticaria	Endocrine
Cholestasis	hyperthyroidism
malignant obstruction	hypothyroidism
drugs	carcinoid syndrome
hepatitis	diabetes (cutaneous candida)
Renal failure	Iron deficiency
Opioids	

Treatment

Therapy is symptomatic and, if possible, by treatment of the underlying cause. Primary skin disorders are treated appropriately.

General measures. A range of general measures aimed to keep the skin cool can be used to reduce or relieve pruritus. A cool or air-conditioned environment will reduce sweating and lessen itch. Hot baths and substances that cause vasodilatation (alcohol and hot or spicy foods and drinks) should be avoided. Dry skin is treated by the liberal use of moisturizing lotions and bath oils, and by avoiding soaps or applications containing alcohol which cause drying. Loose-fitting cotton clothing is less likely to cause sweating and irritation than woollen or synthetic materials. The nails should be short and cotton gloves used if scratching and excoriation are a problem.

Topical therapy. A large number of topical preparations are available for the treatment of pruritus. Preparations containing menthol or phenol produce a cooling sensation; calamine lotion contains 0.5% phenol. Topical antihistamines and local anaesthetics can be of benefit for localized pruritus but can cause contact dermatitis. Topical capsaicin is effective but is not suitable for generalized pruritus.

Systemic therapy. Antihistamines (H_1-receptor antagonists) are effective for histamine-mediated itching but are frequently ineffective for pruritus secondary to cholestasis, uraemia, opioid therapy and cancer. Sedating antihistamines may be more effective than non-sedating drugs, perhaps by virtue of an anxiolytic effect. Cimetidine, an H_2-receptor antagonist, augments the action of H_1-antihistamines for chronic urticaria.[4] The tricyclic antidepressant, doxepin, is a potent H_1- and H_2-receptor antagonist and may be of benefit in patients with chronic urticaria.[4] Ondansetron, a $5HT_3$ receptor antagonist, and opioid antagonists are effective in treating the pruritus of opioid therapy and cholestasis. The serotonin reuptake inhibitor, paroxetine, is reported to be effective for various types of pruritus.[4, 6] Mirtazapine, a new antidepressant with H_1-, $5HT_2$- and $5HT_4$-receptor antagonist activity, is reported to relieve the pruritus associated with cholestasis, uraemia and Hodgkin's disease.[7] The role of systemic corticosteroids in the treatment of pruritus is not defined. They may be effective in patients with cholestasis or lymphoproliferative disorders. A trial of corticosteroids (prednisolone 25–50 mg/d) can be considered in patients with severe or intractable pruritus not responding to other therapy.

Cholestasis. Extrahepatic obstruction is treated by stent insertion, bypass surgery or radiotherapy; intra-hepatic obstruction due to tumour may improve with corticosteroids. Drugs suspected of causing cholestasis should be stopped and treatment with corticosteroids considered. The opioid antagonists, naloxone and naltrexone, are effective in relieving cholestatic itch,[8, 9] but this is rarely feasible in palliative care where most patients are taking opioids for pain. Ondansetron has been reported to be of benefit.[10, 11] Other agents reported to be effective include rifampicin,[12, 13] androgens,[4, 14] and thalidomide. Cholestyramine is not recommended because it is unpalatable and may cause diarrhoea and malabsorption of other drugs and fat-soluble vitamins.

Uraemia. Pruritus associated with uraemia responds to dialysis, treatment with erythropoietin,[15] ultraviolet B (UVB) therapy,[4] and thalidomide.[16] Ondansetron was ineffective in RCTs.[17, 18] Two RCTs of opioid antagonists gave conflicting results, and it has been suggested that they are effective only in patients with severe pruritus.[19, 20]

Malignancy. Pruritus associated with polycythaemia vera may improve with disease control. Low-dose aspirin [21] and paroxetine [22] are reported to be effective. There are anecdotal reports of cimetidine reducing pruritus in some patients with polycythaemia vera or Hodgkin's disease. Cimetidine is of benefit to some patients with polycythaemia although the mechanism is not understood. Pruritus associated with Hodgkin's disease and other lymphomas improves with disease control and may respond to corticosteroids. Pruritus associated with solid tumours may respond to paroxetine.[4, 6]

Spinal opioids. Pruritus associated with intraspinal opioid therapy can be treated with ondansetron[23,24] or carefully titrated opioid antagonists.[25]

Herpes zoster

Herpes zoster or shingles results from reactivation of latent varicella zoster virus (VZV) from sensory nerve root ganglia, where it has remained dormant following varicella or chicken pox earlier in life. It occurs more frequently in people over the age of fifty and in those with compromised immunity.[26, 27]

Clinical features. Herpes zoster presents as a unilateral vesicular rash in a dermatomal distribution. It occurs most commonly in the thoracic region and on the face and neck. Pain in a dermatomal distribution can precede the appearance of the rash by one or two days. Herpes zoster is associated with pain (acute herpetic neuralgia) that can be severe, leading to the description 'a belt of roses from Hell'. The rash normally dries and crusts in 7 to 10 days but may take a month to heal; resolution may be slower in patients with lowered immunity. Herpes zoster of the face involves the ophthalmic divisions of the trigeminal nerve and can be complicated by keratitis and uveitis. Prophylactic therapy for the eye needs to be given and assessment by an ophthalmologist is advisable. Herpes zoster may progress and cause disseminated infection. Cutaneous dissemination causes a rash similar to varicella or chickenpox; the presence of a few skin lesions outside the primary or adjacent dermatomes is not unusual or important. Visceral dissemination can manifest as encephalitis, transverse myelitis, hepatitis or pneumonitis. Patients with herpes zoster are infective to persons who have not had varicella or chickenpox, until such time as all the lesions have dried.

Postherpetic neuralgia. Pain persisting for more than a month after the onset of the rash is referred to as postherpetic neuralgia (PHN). The incidence increases with age, but it is not more frequent in those with compromised immunity.[28] Other risk factors for PHN are the occurrence of prodromal pain before the appearance of the rash, more severe acute neuralgia, and involvement of the ophthalmic nerves. Most patients report a constant burning or aching pain, often associated with allodynia (pain provoked by otherwise trivial stimuli), and episodes of lancinating (electric shock-like) pain. PHN may last months or years and can be severe and debilitating.

Treatment

Antiviral therapy. Antiviral therapy (Table 24.3), started within 48–72 hours of the onset of the rash, is now standard treatment. The agents are well tolerated; all require dose reduction for renal impairment. The first of the antiviral drugs, aciclovir, is usually given orally but should be administered intravenously in severe cases (involvement of multiple dermatomes, signs suggestive of dissemination, and patients with compromised immunity). Valaciclovir, a prodrug of aciclovir, produces serum aciclovir levels three to five times as high as oral aciclovir. Famciclovir, a prodrug of penciclovir, has similarly high bioavailability.

Treatment with oral aciclovir improved the rate of healing and reduced the severity of acute pain in RCTs.[26] Meta-analysis of these studies showed a reduction in the incidence and duration of PHN.[29] Comparison of valaciclovir and aciclovir showed equivalent rates of cutaneous healing, and the incidence and duration of PHN was significantly less in the patients treated with valaciclovir.[30] Famciclovir was superior to placebo and equivalent to valaciclovir in its effects on the acute disease and PHN.[31, 32]

Corticosteroids. In two RCTs, the addition of prednisolone (40–60mg/d, tapered over 21 days) to aciclovir produced a moderate but significant improvement in the rate of cutaneous

Table 24.3 Herpes zoster: antiviral therapy

Aciclovir	800mg PO, 5 times daily, for 7–10 days or 10mg/kg IV q8h for 7–10 days
Valaciclovir	1g PO q8h for 7 days
Famciclovir	500mg PO q8h for 7 days

healing and alleviation of acute pain, but there was no effect on the incidence or duration of PHN.[33, 34] Prednisolone, in conjunction with an antiviral agent, should be considered for older patients with moderate or severe pain for whom corticosteroids are not contraindicated.

Analgesics. Acute herpetic neuralgia may be severe and require opioid analgesics. Topical aspirin is reported to be effective and superior to oral aspirin or other topical NSAIDs. [35–37]

Topical therapy. Topical treatment of the rash is symptomatic and includes saline-soaked gauze pads or Burow's solution (aluminium acetate) for early, weeping lesions and calamine lotion for pruritic, healing lesions. Secondary infection should be treated appropriately. Herpes zoster involving the eye requires therapy with topical aciclovir and corticosteroids [38] and should be assessed by an ophthalmologist.

Postherpetic neuralgia

Despite antiviral therapy during the acute phase, approximately 20% of patients over the age of 50 will suffer PHN.[39] Low-dose amitriptyline given during the acute phase may reduce the incidence of PHN, although the antiviral therapy part of this study was not controlled.[40, 41] Zoster immune globulin is reported to lower the incidence of PHN. Corticosteroids do not protect against PHN.

The treatment of established postherpetic neuralgia (Table 24.4) includes topical applications and oral analgesics.[42] Topical local anaesthetics may provide relief and lidocaine 5% patches have been shown to be safe and effective in RCTs.[43] Topical capsaicin,[42, 44] and aspirin[35, 36] are also effective.

Tricyclic antidepressants (TCAs) and anticonvulsants are effective for a proportion of patients.[42, 45] A comparison of TCAs and opioids showed equivalent response rates, although response to one class of drug did not predict response to the other in individual patients.[46] Nortriptyline is as effective as amitriptyline and may have fewer adverse effects.[47] There is no evidence that newer antidepressants (SSRIs) are more effective than TCAs.[45] Gabapentin produces pain relief for some patients with PHN,[48, 49] and whilst there is no evidence that it is superior to standard anticonvulsants,[45] it may have a more favorable adverse effect profile. Long-standing and intractable PHN has been successfully treated with intrathecal methylprednisolone.[50] Antiviral therapy, given to test the hypothesis that pain is due to continuing viral replication, had no effect on PHN.[51]

Table 24.4 Treatment of postherpetic neuralgia

Preventive therapy during acute phase
antiviral therapy
amitriptyline 25mg/d PO
zoster immune globulin
Topical therapy
lignocaine (lidocaine) or lignocaine and prilocaine (EMLA) creams
lidocaine 5% patches
capsaicin cream
topical aspirin
counterirritants: TENS, ethylchloride spray, cold packs
Systemic therapy
analgesics: nonopioids, opioids
antidepressant e.g. amitriptyline, nortriptyline
anticonvulsant e.g. carbamazepine, gabapentin

Fungating tumours

Fungation of cancer through the skin can cause disfigurement, pain and odour.[52] The physical appearance of fungating tumour or the odour associated with it may cause considerable psychological distress for patients and their carers. Fungation occurs most commonly with cancers of the breast and the head and neck.

Patients with fungating tumours are usually acutely aware of how unsightly and smelly their lesions are. The manner in which dressings are approached is very important and they should be performed in the most sensitive and tactful way.

Treatment

Anticancer treatment. Palliative radiotherapy is considered for all fungating lesions and can produce significant tumour shrinkage and relief of symptoms. Hormonal treatment or chemotherapy may be of benefit for patients with sensitive tumours.

Miltefosine. Miltefosine is a novel anticancer agent, which probably interacts with the cancer cell membrane rather than DNA. Topical application leads to regression of skin lesions in a proportion of women with breast cancer.[53] It is applied daily for the first week, then twice daily for eight weeks, and is most effective for small superficial lesions. Side effects are generally mild and include pruritus and erythema.

Topical therapy. Fungating tumours require frequent and regular dressings, the aim being to keep the area clean, dry and free of infection. This often relieves both odour and pain. The dressing is soaked off with warm water or in the bath. If the surface is clean, it is simply washed with normal saline. Dead and sloughing tissue is removed with a dilute solution of hydrogen peroxide and saline or debrided with an enzymatic preparation. Obvious infection is treated by topical application of sulfadiazine, povidone-iodine or similar antiseptic. If debridement or antiseptic solutions are used, care must be taken not to damage normal or healing tissues.[54] Bleeding is less likely if alginate dressings are used, and can be controlled by local pressure or the application of gauze soaked in adrenaline 1:1000. The lesion is dressed with a melonin or other nonadherent dressing, which needs to be sufficiently absorbent to soak up any exudate. The dressing is held in place with tubular elastic netting.

Odour control. The application of metronidazole gel will control anaerobic infection and reduce odour.[55, 56] If unsuccessful, systemic metronidazole (400mg PO, 8-hourly or 1g PR, 8–12 hourly) is frequently of benefit. An alternative to metronidazole is clindamycin (250mg PO, 6-hourly). Antibiotic therapy may lead to a significant reduction in pain. Charcoal pads placed under the netting holding the dressing are only effective for a few hours. A layer of cling film over the dressing can provide an extra barrier to odour.

Pain control. Nonopioid or opioid analgesics are prescribed as required. Dressing changes that are painful require premedication with appropriate analgesia. The topical application of morphine (morphine 1mg/ml in Intrasite gel, q12h) is reported to be effective for painful malignant wounds.[57, 58]

Pressure sores

Pressure sores occur in about 20% of patients with advanced cancer and can greatly detract from the quality of life. Damage to the skin and underlying tissues by pressure, friction or other irritation leads to the development of a pressure sore. If the skin is broken it may be termed a pressure ulcer, but the term pressure sore is preferred as it includes the precursor lesions in which the skin remains intact but which deserve energetic treatment. The terms bedsore and decubitus ulcer are also used but refer only to patients confined to bed and neglects the need and importance of pressure care for other patients including those in wheelchairs.

Pressure sores are caused by tissue ischaemia due to pressure, usually over bony prominences.[59] Further skin damage is caused by shearing forces or friction and by other irritants such as urine or faeces. Secondary infection will compound the damage. A considerable number of other factors predispose to the development of pressure sores (Table 24.5). Poor nursing care can contribute to tissue damage, such as sheet burns from dragging rather than lifting patients, improper use of heat and ultraviolet lamps, or giving injections at vulnerable sites. The ability of the skin to withstand injury and repair itself depends on the patient's nutritional state, although the use of dietary supplements that aid ulcer healing in other situations (protein, vitamin C and zinc) is probably of little benefit to patients with advanced cancer. Pressure sores are more likely to develop if there is immobility or reduced sensation causing a diminished response to pain or irritation.

Table 24.5 Causes of pressure sores

Tissue damage
    pressure
    friction, shearing forces
    urine, faeces, excess moisture
    infection
    direct tissue injury: burns, injections, crumpled bed clothes
    restlessness

Tissue fragility/poor repair
    weight loss, emaciation
    old age
    malnourishment: protein, vitamin C, zinc
    anaemia, vascular insufficiency, oedema
    corticosteroids
    chemotherapy, radiotherapy

Immobility
    weakness, paralysis, general debility
    sedation or impaired consciousness
    positioning for treatment of other pressure areas

Diminished response to pain or irritation
    hypoaesthesia, anaesthesia
    analgesics
    sedation or impaired consciousness

Pressure sores commonly occur over bony prominences. Various staging classifications have been proposed, which have common features.[60] A classification based on the visible depth of tissue damage provides a logical basis for treatment (Table 24.6), although it is important to remember that even in the earliest stages, when the skin is still intact, there is damage to all the underlying tissues down to bone.

Table 24.6   Pressure sores

Stage 1	skin intact blanching or non-blanching erythema soft tissue swelling and induration
Stage 2	skin broken shallow ulceration or skin loss involving epidermis or dermis abrasion, blister
Stage 3	ulceration involving subcutaneous fatty tissue necrotic tissue, eschar formation common
Stage 4	ulceration involving fascia, muscle or bone necrotic tissue

Treatment

Whilst theoretically preventable, the development of pressure sores in some terminally ill patients is unavoidable and does not reflect inadequate nursing care. The combination of immobility, emaciation, poor nutrition and incontinence can make the prevention of pressure sores almost impossible. Surveys of palliative care patients show them to be at high or very high risk of developing pressure sores.[61, 62] For the same reasons, all but superficial pressure sores may be difficult to heal in the terminally ill.

Preventive. The treatment of pressure sores is, wherever possible, preventive. Patients at risk of developing pressure sores should be identified and a range of preventive measures initiated (Table 24.7). Predictive scales have been developed to identify patients at risk, including the Braden and Norton scales in the USA[63] and the Waterlow score in the UK.[62] The skin is kept clean and dry; dry skin is treated with a moisturizer, wet skin with aluminium acetate

Table 24.7   Prevention of pressure sores

Identify patients at risk	
General hygiene	keep skin clean and dry
Avoid trauma	pat or blow skin dry, avoid rubbing avoid vigorous massage lift patients, avoid dragging avoid wet clothes, bedding avoid contamination with urine, faeces avoid rough garments, bedding avoid excess heat (lamps) avoid crumpled bedclothes avoid harsh soaps, alcohol rubs
Protective measures	sheepskin mats and boots to reduce friction
Relief of pressure	frequent turning, repositioning correct positioning special mattresses
General	optimize nutrition avoid corticosteroids, sedation, excess analgesics

(Burow's) solution or blown dry. The skin is protected from trauma or corrosion. Sheepskin mats and boots effectively protect against friction or shear but do not significantly affect pressure. The most important measure is the relief and prevention of pressure. This involves frequent (2- to 4-hourly) repositioning or turning. Correct positioning distributes the body weight over the largest possible area. A number of pressure relieving aids are available but they do not replace the need for turning and repositioning. These include polystyrene fibre and bead mattresses laid over the ordinary mattress, foam mattresses, air mattresses (Ripple, Roho) and water beds. Inflatable rubber rings or doughnuts need to be avoided as they reduce blood flow to the tissue inside the circle. Patients in wheelchairs need regular repositioning and may be helped by inflatable cushions.

Active treatment. The treatment of pressure sores needs to be appropriate to the stage of the patient's disease. Energetic therapy may be warranted for superficial lesions and for patients with a prognosis of months. For patients with shorter life expectancy or extensive ulceration, energetic therapy may stand little, if any, chance of healing the lesion. A balance must be found between the anticipated morbidity from the lesion and the inconvenience of treatment (Table 24.8).

A Cochrane review of the trials conducted to determine the optimum surface for the prevention and treatment of pressure sores concluded that it may not be possible to answer the question. However, there was good evidence of the effectiveness of high specification foam over standard hospital foam in prevention, and of air-fluidized and low air loss devices for treatment.[64] Other Cochrane reviews found no evidence to support the use of ultrasound or electromagnetic therapies in the treatment of pressure sores.[65, 66]

Table 24.8 Treatment of pressure sores

Relieve and prevent pressure	
Local hygiene	saline topical antiseptics (short term only)
Debridement	moist dressings enzymatic e.g. collagenase, Elase, Varidase hydrophilic substances e.g. dextranomer (Debrisan) surgical
Promote healing	superficial: semipermeable membrane (e.g. Opsite) deeper: impermeable hydrocolloid dressing (e.g. Duoderm)
Systemic antibiotics	for cellulitis, osteomyelitis
Analgesics	as required for pain
Reduce odour	topical metronidazole gel, charcoal dressings

The relief and avoidance of pressure until a sore heals is mandatory. This should be 4 hours for blanching erythema, 48 hours for non-blanching erythema, and longer if there is ulceration.

The use of topical antiseptics is controversial. The goal is to lower bacterial counts to facilitate healing. Ulcers not containing necrotic material can usually be cleansed with saline. Antiseptics such as povidone-iodine, hydrogen peroxide and sodium hypochlorite may impair healing and some are toxic to the surrounding skin. They need to be applied with care and their use discontinued as soon as the ulcer base is clean.

Necrotic tissue can be removed using one of the enzymatic debriding agents such as collagenase/fibrinolysin/deoxyribonuclease (Elase) or streptokinase/ streptodornase (Varidase Topical). These are not often required and will cause damage to healing tissue if continued after an ulcer is clean.

The healing of superficial ulceration, once clean, is aided by maintaining a moist environment. The ulcer is covered with a semipermeable membrane such as Opsite or Tegederm. The healing of deeper ulcers is aided by using an impermeable hydrocolloid dressing such as Duoderm or Comfeel. The inner hydrocolloid layer absorbs exudate and forms a soft moist gel inside the wound and promotes healing. Calcium alginate dressings are useful if there is considerable exudate. Surgery has little role in the management of pressure ulcers in patients with advanced cancer but can be considered for patients with extensive tissue necrosis whose life expectancy is several months or more. Systemic antibiotics are used if there is evidence of cellulitis or osteomyelitis.

Analgesics are used as required for pain control, particularly when dressings are changed. Two randomized pilot studies have reported positive results with topical opioids (Table 24.9).[67, 68]

Table 24.9 Topical opioids for painful ulcers: RCTs

Author	n	Intervention	Outcome
Flock[67]	7	diamorphine gel vs placebo	diamorphine: ↓ pain scores (pS)
Zeppetella[68]	5	morphine gel vs placebo	morphine: ↓ pain scores (pS)

Terminal care

The treatment of pressure sores in the terminally ill is purely symptomatic. Frequent turning and other measures designed to allow healing are irrelevant, especially if movement causes pain.

Radiotherapy skin reactions

Radiotherapy skin reactions occur more frequently with higher doses, treatment delivered more rapidly, and in normally moist areas such as the perineum, axilla or inframammary fold.[69, 70] The RTOG/EORTC grading system for radiation skin reactions is shown in Table 24.10.

Table 24.10 RTOG/EORTC grading criteria for radiation skin reactions[71, 72]

Acute
0   no change
1   faint erythema, dry desquamation, epilation, decreased sweating
2   tender or bright erythema, patchy moist desquamation, moderate oedema
3   confluent moist desquamation other than skin folds, pitting oedema
4   ulceration, haemorrhage, necrosis

Chronic
0   none
1   slight atrophy, pigmentation change, some hair loss
2   patchy atrophy, moderate telangiectasia, total hair loss
3   marked atrophy, gross telangiectasia
4   ulceration

Acute. In the acute stage there will be erythema and oedema associated with pruritus. This is followed by desquamation, alopecia and loss of sweating (anhidrosis). These changes usually resolve spontaneously over several months. During the acute phase, care should be taken to avoid any mechanical, chemical or thermal injury to the affected skin (Table 24.11).

Table 24.11 Management of acute radiation skin reactions

General	loose, soft, non-synthetic clothing (e.g. cotton)
	wash gently in lukewarm water, dry gently
	avoid perfumes, soaps, powders, lotions or deodorants
	use an electric shaver, not a razor
	protection from sun with sunscreens
Dry reaction	baby oil, lanolin ointment or non-irritating moisturizing cream
	hydrocortisone 1% cream if severe
Moist reaction	keep clean and dry, treat secondary infection
	bathe with aluminium acetate (Burow's solution)
	povidone-iodine or silver sulfadiazine for infected areas

Chronic. In the chronic phase, the skin is thin and atrophic and there may be hypo- or hyper-pigmentation and cutaneous telangiectasia. In more severe cases there may be necrosis and ulceration. Care should be taken to avoid sunburn in the treated area.

Radiation recall phenomenon. Acute skin reactions may occur in previously irradiated areas following the administration of chemotherapy drugs. The exact explanation is unknown. Treatment is as for acute skin reactions.

Chemotherapy reactions

Alopecia. Alopecia occurs frequently with certain drugs and is usually temporary.

Nail changes. Various nail changes including pigmentation, transverse lines or ridging, brittleness, slow growth and onycholysis (partial separation of the nail plate from the nail bed) may occur with a variety of chemotherapy agents. The drugs most commonly associated with these reactions are cyclophosphamide, doxorubicin, bleomycin, fluorouracil and mitozantrone. The patient should be reassured. Care with local hygiene is important to prevent secondary infection.

Photosensitivity. Increased skin sensitivity to the sun or to ionizing radiation may occur after chemotherapy, especially involving methotrexate and fluorouracil. The patient should be reassured and given the appropriate advice about protection from the sun.

Pigmentation. Generalized hyperpigmentation may occur after chemotherapy, notably after treatment with bleomycin or busulfan. Localized pigmentation may occur in areas previously subjected to radiotherapy or sunburn. Pigmentation may also occur along the course of veins used for chemotherapy.

Radiation recall. See Radiotherapy reactions (above).

Hand-foot syndrome. Marked swelling and erythema of the palms and soles occasionally occurs after chemotherapy treatment, most frequently with capecitabine or fluorouracil.[73] Treatment is with reassurance, analgesia and topical corticosteroids; there is anecdotal evidence that pyridoxine lessens the skin reactions caused by capecitabine. If severe, the chemotherapy may need to be stopped or changed.

Phlebitis. Phlebitis may occur with almost any of the anticancer drugs given intravenously, but it is more likely to occur with the drugs that are also vesicants. The patient may complain of soreness and tenderness of the superficial vein if it is thrombosed. Treatment is with analgesia and reassurance; heparinoid cream (Hirudoid) may be of benefit. The risk of phlebitis can be lessened by giving the drug more slowly, in a dilute solution, and into a larger vein.

References

1   Cohen, P.R. and Kurzrock, R. (1997). Mucocutaneous paraneoplastic syndromes. *Seminars in Oncology* 24, 334–59.

2   Fearfield, L. and Bunker, C. (1999). Cutaneous paraneoplastic syndromes—Part 1. *European Journal of Palliative Care* 6, 82–86.

3   Fearfield, L. and Bunker, C. (1999). Cutaneous paraneoplastic syndromes—Part 2. *European Journal of Palliative Care* 6, 117–20.

4   Twycross, R., et al. (2003). Itch: scratching more than the surface. *Quarterly Journal of Medicine* 96, 7–26.

5   Yosipovitch, G., Greaves, M.W. and Schmelz, M. (2003). Itch. *Lancet* 361, 690–4.

6   Zylicz, Z., Smits, C. and Krajnik, M. (1998). Paroxetine for pruritus in advanced cancer. *Journal of Pain and Symptom Management* 16, 121–4.

7   Davis, M.P., et al. (2003). Mirtazapine for pruritus. *Journal of Pain and Symptom Management* 25, 288–91.

8   Wolfhagen, F.H., et al. (1997). Oral naltrexone treatment for cholestatic pruritus: a double-blind, placebo-controlled study. *Gastroenterology* 113, 1264–9.

9   Bergasa, N.V., et al. (1999). Oral nalmefene therapy reduces scratching activity due to the pruritus of cholestasis: a controlled study. *Journal of the American Academy of Dermatology* 41, 431–4.

10 Schworer, H., Hartmann, H. and Ramadori, G. (1995). Relief of cholestatic pruritus by a novel class of drugs: 5-hydroxytryptamine type 3 (5-HT3) receptor antagonists: effectiveness of ondansetron. *Pain* 61, 33–7.

11 Muller, C., et al. (1998). Treatment of pruritus in chronic liver disease with the 5-hydroxytryptamine receptor type 3 antagonist ondansetron: a randomized, placebo-controlled, double-blind cross-over trial. *European Journal of Gastroenterology and Hepatology* 10, 865–70.

12 Ghent, C.N. and Carruthers, S.G. (1988). Treatment of pruritus in primary biliary cirrhosis with rifampin. Results of a double-blind, crossover, randomized trial. *Gastroenterology* 94, 488–93.

13 Price, T.J., Patterson, W.K. and Olver, I.N. (1998). Rifampicin as treatment for pruritus in malignant cholestasis. *Supportive Care in Cancer* 6, 533–5.

14 McCormick, P.A., et al. (1994). Thalidomide as therapy for primary biliary cirrhosis: a double-blind placebo controlled pilot study. *Journal of Hepatology* 21, 496–9.

15 De Marchi, S., et al. (1992). Relief of pruritus and decreases in plasma histamine concentrations during erythropoietin therapy in patients with uremia. *New England Journal of Medicine* 326, 969–74.

16 Silva, S.R., et al. (1994). Thalidomide for the treatment of uremic pruritus: a crossover randomized double-blind trial. *Nephron* 67, 270–3.

17 Balaskas, E.V., et al. (1998). Histamine and serotonin in uremic pruritus: effect of ondansetron in CAPD-pruritic patients. *Nephron* 78, 395–402.

18 Murphy, M., et al. (2003). A randomized, placebo-controlled, double-blind trial of ondansetron in renal itch. *British Journal of Dermatology* 148, 314–17.

19 Peer, G., et al. (1996). Randomised crossover trial of naltrexone in uraemic pruritus. *Lancet* 348, 1552–4.

20 Pauli-Magnus, C., et al. (2000). Naltrexone does not relieve uremic pruritus: results of a randomized, double-blind, placebo-controlled crossover study. *Journal of the American Society of Nephrology* 11, 514–19.

21 Jackson, N., et al. (1987). Skin mast cells in polycythaemia vera: relationship to the pathogenesis and treatment of pruritus. *British Journal of Dermatology* 116, 21–9.

22 Tefferi, A. and Fonseca, R. (2002). Selective serotonin reuptake inhibitors are effective in the treatment of polycythemia vera-associated pruritus. *Blood* 99, 2627.

23 Borgeat, A. and Stirnemann, H.R. (1999). Ondansetron is effective to treat spinal or epidural morphine-induced pruritus. *Anesthesiology* 90, 432–6.

24 Kyriakides, K., Hussain, S.K. and Hobbs, G.J. (1999). Management of opioid-induced pruritus: a role for 5-HT3 antagonists? *British Journal of Anaesthesia* 82, 439–41.

25 Kjellberg, F. and Tramer, M.R. (2001). Pharmacological control of opioid-induced pruritus: a quantitative systematic review of randomized trials. *European Journal of Anaesthesiology* 18, 346–57.

26 Gnann, J.W., Jr. and Whitley, R.J. (2002). Clinical practice. Herpes zoster. *New England Journal of Medicine* 347, 340–6.

27 Johnson, R.W. and Dworkin, R.H. (2003). Treatment of herpes zoster and postherpetic neuralgia. *British Medical Journal* 326, 748–50.

28 Kost, R.G. and Straus, S.E. (1996). Postherpetic neuralgia—pathogenesis, treatment, and prevention. *New England Journal of Medicine* 335, 32–42.

29 Wood, M.J., et al. (1996). Oral acyclovir therapy accelerates pain resolution in patients with herpes zoster: a meta-analysis of placebo-controlled trials. *Clinical Infectious Diseases* 22, 341–7.

30 Beutner, K.R., et al. (1995). Valaciclovir compared with acyclovir for improved therapy for herpes zoster in immunocompetent adults. *Antimicrobial Agents and Chemotherapy* 39, 1546–53.

31 Tyring, S., et al. (1995). Famciclovir for the treatment of acute herpes zoster: effects on acute disease and postherpetic neuralgia. A randomized, double-blind, placebo-controlled trial. Collaborative Famciclovir Herpes Zoster Study Group. *Annals of Internal Medicine* 123, 89–96.

32 Tyring, S.K., et al. (2000). Antiviral therapy for herpes zoster: randomized, controlled clinical trial of valacyclovir and famciclovir therapy in immunocompetent patients 50 years and older. *Archives of Family Medicine* 9, 863–9.

33 Wood, M.J., et al. (1994). A randomized trial of acyclovir for 7 days or 21 days with and without prednisolone for treatment of acute herpes zoster. *New England Journal of Medicine* 330, 896–900.

34 Whitley, R.J., et al. (1996). Acyclovir with and without prednisone for the treatment of herpes zoster. A randomized, placebo-controlled trial. The National Institute of Allergy and Infectious Diseases Collaborative Antiviral Study Group. *Annals of Internal Medicine* 125, 376–83.

35 De Benedittis, G. and Lorenzetti, A. (1996). Topical aspirin/diethyl ether mixture versus indomethacin and diclofenac/diethyl ether mixtures for acute herpetic neuralgia and postherpetic neuralgia: a double-blind crossover placebo-controlled study. *Pain* 65, 45–51.

36 Bareggi, S.R., Pirola, R. and De Benedittis, G. (1998). Skin and plasma levels of acetylsalicylic acid: a comparison between topical aspirin/diethyl ether mixture and oral aspirin in acute herpes zoster and postherpetic neuralgia. *European Journal of Clinical Pharmacology* 54, 231–5.

37 Balakrishnan, S., et al. (2001). A randomized parallel trial of topical aspirin-moisturizer solution vs. oral aspirin for acute herpetic neuralgia. *International Journal of Dermatology* 40, 535–8.

38 Marsh, R.J. and Cooper, M. (1991). Double-masked trial of topical acyclovir and steroids in the treatment of herpes zoster ocular inflammation. *British Journal of Ophthalmology* 75, 542–6.

39 Cunningham, A.L. and Dworkin, R.H. (2000). The management of post-herpetic neuralgia. *British Medical Journal* 321, 778–9.

40 Bowsher, D. (1997). The effects of pre-emptive treatment of postherpetic neuralgia with amitriptyline: a randomized, double-blind, placebo controlled trial. *Journal of Pain and Symptom Management* 13, 327–31.

41 Hugler, P., et al. (2002). Prevention of postherpetic neuralgia with varicella-zoster hyperimmune globulin. *European Journal of Pain* 6, 435–45.

42 Volmink, J., et al. (1996). Treatments for postherpetic neuralgia—a systematic review of randomized controlled trials. *Family Practice* 13, 84–91.

43   Galer, B.S., et al. (2002). The lidocaine patch 5% effectively treats all neuropathic pain qualities: results of a randomized, double-blind, vehicle-controlled, 3-week efficacy study with use of the neuropathic pain scale. *Clinical Journal of Pain* 18, 297–301.

44   Bernstein, J.E., et al. (1989). Topical capsaicin treatment of chronic postherpetic neuralgia. *Journal of the American Academy of Dermatology* 21, 265–70.

45   Collins, S.L., et al. (2000). Antidepressants and anticonvulsants for diabetic neuropathy and postherpetic neuralgia: a quantitative systematic review. *Journal of Pain and Symptom Management* 20, 449–58.

46   Raja, S.N., et al. (2002). Opioids versus antidepressants in postherpetic neuralgia: a randomized, placebo-controlled trial. *Neurology* 59, 1015–21.

47   Watson, C.P., et al. (1998). Nortriptyline versus amitriptyline in postherpetic neuralgia: a randomized trial. *Neurology* 51, 1166–71.

48   Rowbotham, M., et al. (1998). Gabapentin for the treatment of postherpetic neuralgia: a randomized controlled trial. *Journal of the American Medical Association* 280, 1837–42.

49   Rice, A.S. and Maton, S. (2001). Gabapentin in postherpetic neuralgia: a randomised, double blind, placebo controlled study. *Pain* 94, 215–24.

50   Kotani, N., et al. (2000). Intrathecal methylprednisolone for intractable postherpetic neuralgia. *New England Journal of Medicine* 343, 1514–19.

51   Acosta, E.P. and Balfour, H.H., Jr. (2001). Acyclovir for treatment of postherpetic neuralgia: efficacy and pharmacokinetics. *Antimicrobial Agents and Chemotherapy* 45, 2771–4.

52   Naylor, W. (2003). Palliative management of fungating wounds. *European Journal of Palliative Care* 10, 93–97.

53   Leonard, R., et al. (2001). Randomized, double-blind, placebo-controlled, multicenter trial of 6% miltefosine solution, a topical chemotherapy in cutaneous metastases from breast cancer. *Journal of Clinical Oncology* 19, 4150–9.

54   Moyle, J. (1998). The management of malodour. *European Journal of Palliative Care* 5, 148–51.

55   Bower, M., et al. (1992). A double-blind study of the efficacy of metronidazole gel in the treatment of malodorous fungating tumours. *European Journal of Cancer* 28A, 888–9.

56   Finlay, I.G., et al. (1996). The effect of topical 0.75% metronidazole gel on malodorous cutaneous ulcers. *Journal of Pain and Symptom Management* 11, 158–62.

57   Krajnik, M., et al. (1999). Potential uses of topical opioids in palliative care—report of 6 cases. *Pain* 80, 121–5.

58   Twillman, R.K., et al. (1999). Treatment of painful skin ulcers with topical opioids. *Journal of Pain and Symptom Management* 17, 288–92.

59   Walker, P. (1998). The pathophysiology and management of pressure ulcers. In *Topics in Palliative Care* (ed. R. Portenoy and E. Bruera). New York, Oxford University Press.

60   Bergstrom, N. (1995). Treatment of Pressure Ulcers. AHCPR Clinical Guideline Number 15. Washington DC: AHCPR.

61   Hatcliffe, S. and Dawe, R. (1996). Monitoring pressure sores in a palliative care setting. *International Journal of Palliative Nursing* 2, 182–6.

62   Galvin, J. (2002). An audit of pressure ulcer incidence in a palliative care setting. *International Journal of Palliative Nursing* 8, 214–21.

63   Bergstrom, N. and al, e. (1992). Pressure Ulcers in Adults: Prediction and Prevention. AHCPR Clinical Practice Guideline Number 3. Washington D.C.: AHCPR.

64   Cullum, N., et al. (2000). Beds, mattresses and cushions for pressure sore prevention and treatment (Cochrane Review). *Cochrane Database of Systematic Reviews* CD001735.

65   Flemming, K. and Cullum, N. (2000). Therapeutic ultrasound for pressure sores (Cochrane Review). *Cochrane Database of Systematic Reviews* CD001275.

66   Flemming, K. and Cullum, N. (2001). Electromagnetic therapy for the treatment of pressure sores (Cochrane Review). *Cochrane Database of Systematic Reviews* CD002930.

67   Flock, P. (2003). Pilot study to determine the effectiveness of diamorphine gel to control pressure ulcer pain. *Journal of Pain and Symptom Management* 25, 547–54.

68 Zeppetella, G., Paul, J. and Ribeiro, M.D. (2003). Analgesic efficacy of morphine applied topically to painful ulcers. *Journal of Pain and Symptom Management* 25, 555–8.

69 Hellman, S. (2001). Radiation Therapy. In *Cancer. Principles and Practice of Oncology. 6th edition* (ed. V.T. De Vita, S. Hellman and S.A. Rosenberg). Philadelphia, Lippincott, Williams and Wilkins.

70 Kirkbride, P. and Bezjak, A. (2002). Palliative radiation therapy. In *Principles and Practice of Palliative Care and Supportive Oncology* (ed. A.M. Berger, R.K. Portenoy and D.E. Weissman). Philadelphia, Lippincott, Williams and Wilkins.

71 Radiation Therapy Oncology Group (RTOG) (2000). Acute Radiation Morbidity Scoring Criteria. <www.rtog.org/members/toxicity/acute.html>

72 Radiation Therapy Oncology Group (RTOG)/European Organisation for Research and Treatment of Cancer (EORTC) (2000). RTOG/EORTC Late Radiation Morbidity Scoring Schema. <www.rtog.org/members/toxicity/late.html>

73 Abushullaih, S., et al. (2002). Incidence and severity of hand-foot syndrome in colorectal cancer patients treated with capecitabine: a single-institution experience. *Cancer Investigation* 20, 3–10.

25

Neurological

Cerebral metastases
Recurrent cerebral tumours
Spinal cord compression
Meningeal tumour infiltration
Seizures
Delirium

Terminal restlessness
Dementia
Insomnia
Paraneoplastic syndromes
Eye problems

Cerebral metastases

Cerebral metastases occur in 20–40% of patients with cancer. It is usually a manifestation of advanced disease and most patients have evidence of metastatic disease at other sites. The resulting neurological disabilities, particularly of cognitive and motor function, can have a profound effect on the quality of life.[1, 2]

The majority of cerebral metastases originate from lung and breast cancers and malignant melanoma. Certain tumours are associated with a high incidence of cerebral metastases, occurring in up to two-thirds of patients with malignant melanoma and small cell lung cancer.

About 80% of cerebral metastases are supratentorial, this being equivalent to the proportion of the brain mass above the tentorium. Cerebral metastases are usually multiple; single metastases are reported in one-quarter to one third of patients but autopsy studies suggest the incidence is less.

Clinical features

Symptoms and signs of cerebral metastases are due to focal disruption of neurological function, mechanical pressure and displacement of tissue, and raised intracranial pressure. More than two-thirds of patients with cerebral metastases will develop clinical symptoms or signs (Table 25.1). Headache is the most common symptom and is typically generalized and aggravated by coughing or any other manoeuvre that increases intracranial pressure; for some patients, it is noticeably worse in the mornings. Seizures occur in about 20% of patients and are usually tonic-clonic in type; they may be preceded by focal (Jacksonian) features or followed by transient motor weakness (Todd's paresis).

Metastases to specific areas of the brain are associated with particular clinical features. Frontal lobe metastases produce changes in affect, personality and behaviour. Parietal lobe

Table 25.1 Clinical features of cerebral metastases

Symptoms	Signs
headache	cognitive impairment
weakness: focal or hemiparetic	hemiparesis
mental state changes	sensory loss: focal or unilateral
seizures	loss of co-ordination, ataxia
loss of co-ordination, ataxia	papilloedema
sensory disturbance	aphasia
speech problems	behavioural, personality changes

metastases result in motor weakness and sensory loss. Temporal lobe metastases produce hallucinations. Occipital lobe metastases are associated with visual disturbances. Cerebellar metastases are associated with ataxia. Brain stem metastases are associated with cranial nerve palsies and abnormalities of co-ordination. Whilst focal signs may suggest the site of metastatic disease, there may also be false localizing signs, caused by compression or shifting of other parts of the brain secondary to raised intracranial pressure.

The clinical features of cerebral metastases usually develop insidiously over a number of weeks; in about one-quarter of patients the clinical onset is abrupt. The clinical features will depend on the site, size, number and rate of growth of the metastases. If tumours grow slowly, various compensatory changes occur that reduce the effect of raised intracranial pressure, including reduction of the cerebral vascular, extracellular and CSF fluid volumes. If growth occurs quickly, these mechanisms are less effective. Secondary haemorrhage or the development of hydrocephalus due to obstruction of the flow of CSF will cause rapid progression of the clinical signs. Cerebral herniation, in which acute or asymmetric increases in intracranial pressure cause significant displacement of brain tissue from its normal position, leads to profound obtundation and coma with pupillary and long tract signs within hours. Herniation is usually caused by haemorrhage or the performance of a lumbar puncture in the presence of raised intracranial pressure.

The natural history of cerebral metastases is progressive neurological deterioration with a median life expectancy of 1 to 2 months.

Assessment

The diagnosis is made on CT or MRI scanning, the latter being more sensitive. Cerebral metastases appear as discrete rounded lesions, surrounded by oedema, which enhance after the administration of intravenous contrast. If there has been central haemorrhage or necrosis they may appear cystic and resemble the appearance of abscesses. For patients with documented metastases at other sites, multiple focal lesions on scan strongly suggest cerebral metastases. The differential diagnosis of a single lesion includes a metastasis, primary brain tumour, abscess, haemorrhage or area of radiation necrosis; biopsy has occasionally to be considered, especially if there is no evidence of metastatic disease elsewhere.

Lumbar puncture and CSF examination are never indicated in an assessment for cerebral metastases. Cytological examination of the CSF will be positive only in the small proportion of patients that also have meningeal infiltration and, unless raised intracranial pressure has been excluded by cerebral scanning, lumbar puncture may cause cerebral herniation (coning) and death.

Treatment

The goal of treatment is to restore and maintain neurological function or at least to minimize deterioration.[3] The treatment options are listed in Table 25.2.

Table 25.2 Treatment for cerebral metastases

Specific therapy	Symptomatic care
corticosteroids	anticonvulsants
radiotherapy	physical therapy
surgery	psychological therapy
systemic therapy (sensitive tumours)	

Treatment must be appropriate to the stage of the patient's disease and prognosis

Corticosteroids. Corticosteroids will produce clinical improvement in 60–80% of patients with cerebral metastases, presumably by reduction of the peritumoral oedema. Improvement is usually seen within the first 24 hours, with 2 to 3 days taken for maximal effect. Corticosteroids are more effective against the generalized neurological symptoms and signs (e.g. headaches, confusion) than against focal neurological dysfunction (e.g. hemiparesis). Patients without significant neurological symptoms and signs can be treated without corticosteroids, avoiding the adverse effects that tend to increase with time.[4]

The corticosteroid most frequently used is dexamethasone, which has less mineralocorticoid effect than prednisolone and causes less fluid retention. It is usually started at 16 mg/d for the first few days or week and then slowly weaned, although a single small RCT reported that 4mg/d may have the same benefits with fewer side effects.[5] If there is neurological improvement, the dose is tapered slowly (by 2–4mg every few days) to the lowest effective dose. About 20% of patients have a neurological deficit that is at least partly reversible with corticosteroids and which prevents complete withdrawal of the drug. Corticosteroids lessen the side effects of radiotherapy and may need to be withdrawn more slowly in patients proceeding with irradiation. Patients not responding to standard doses may have a trial of a higher dose, but the chances of a clinically meaningful response are small. If there is no improvement with corticosteroids after 7 days, it should be rapidly tapered to the lowest possible dose.

Dexamethasone increases the metabolic clearance of phenytoin. Starting or increasing the dose of dexamethasone may lower phenytoin levels and lead to seizures; reducing the dose may lead to phenytoin toxicity. Phenytoin similarly induces the metabolism of dexamethasone and may reduce its clinical effectiveness.[1] The median survival of patients with cerebral metastases treated with corticosteroids is 2 to 3 months.

Radiotherapy. Patients with cerebral metastases are treated with radiotherapy, provided the state of their systemic disease and the degree of neurological dysfunction make such therapy appropriate. The clinical features that predict a beneficial response are performance status, absence of active disease at other sites, and age.[6] Patients responding well to corticosteroids are also more likely to benefit, as the initial response indicates that more of the neurological features were due to reversible oedema or raised intracranial pressure than to irreversible destruction of brain tissue. It is customary to give whole brain or cranial irradiation because of the high incidence of multiple metastases. The optimal schedule of radiotherapy has not been defined, but it is usual to give shorter courses than for primary brain tumours.[1] It is reported that about two-thirds of patients will show clinical improvement,[1] although much lower response rates are reported.[7] The median survival of patients treated with standard radiotherapy is 3 to 6 months.

Radiosurgery is a technique of stereotactic external irradiation that uses multiple convergent beams to deliver a high single dose of radiation to a small volume. Either x-rays from a linear accelerator or gamma rays from a gamma knife are used.[8, 9] Radiosurgery produces better local control and involves much less radiation to normal brain. It has been used successfully to treat metastases that have recurred after whole brain irradiation.[10] More recently, an RCT of radiosurgery given as an adjuvant to whole brain irradiation for patients with two to four metastases showed considerable improvement in local tumour control (Table 25.3).[11]

Surgery. For younger patients with a surgically accessible solitary metastasis, a good performance status and stable extracranial disease, surgery has been shown to prolong survival, reduce the risk of neurological relapse, and more often allows the discontinuation of corticosteroid therapy.[1] Surgery should be followed by whole brain irradiation, which significantly reduces the risk of recurrent neurological disease (Table 25.3).[12] Surgery may also be required for the relief of obstructive hydrocephalus by the insertion of a ventriculo-peritoneal shunt.

Systemic antitumour treatment. Hormonal therapy is indicated for patients with hormone-sensitive tumours and may be effective in controlling cerebral disease. Chemotherapy for cerebral metastases has generally disappointing results as the agents do not freely cross the blood-brain barrier; responses are seen in about one-third of patients with breast and non-small cell lung cancer.[13] Temozolomide, which has activity against melanoma and primary brain tumours and which is known to cross the blood-brain barrier more efficiently, significantly improved the response to whole brain irradiation in patients with breast and lung cancers (Table 25.3).[14]

Table 25.3 Radiotherapy for cerebral metastases: selected RCTs

Author	n	Intervention	Outcome
Kondziolka[11]	27	whole brain RT ± radiosurgery	combined therapy: local recurrence 8 vs 100% (pS); survival 11 vs 7.5mo. (pNS)
Patchell[12]	95	surgery (single met.) ± wholebrain RT	combined therapy: local recurrence 10 vs 46% (pS), brain recurrence 18 vs 70% (pS). Survival similar.
Antonadou[14]	52	whole brain RT ± temozolomide	combined therapy: responses 96 vs 67% (pS), ↑ neurological recovery. Survival similar.

Anticonvulsants. About 20% of patients with cerebral metastases will suffer seizures and should receive anticonvulsant therapy. A meta-analysis of patients with brain tumours (primary and metastatic) given prophylactic anticonvulsants did not show a significant effect on seizure incidence or seizure-free survival, although 42% of patients who suffered a seizure whilst taking anticonvulsants had subtherapeutic levels.[15] One-quarter of patients taking prophylactic anticonvulsants had adverse effects severe enough to warrant changing or stopping the medication. The relatively low incidence of seizures, the high rate of adverse effects, and the lack of demonstrated benefit argue against the use of prophylactic anticonvulsants for patients with cerebral metastases. The potential drug interaction between dexamethasone and phenytoin is described above (see Corticosteroids).

Physical therapy. Patients with motor or sensory deficits or problems of co-ordination require appropriate physiotherapy and rehabilitation. The patient and family need help adjusting to neurological deficits and the use of physical aids and modifications to the patient's immediate environment at home are important.

Psychological therapy. Patients with cerebral metastases may have labile mood, personality alteration, depression and anxiety, as well as impairment of cognitive function. Treatment includes the appropriate use of anxiolytics, antidepressants, tranquillizers and hypnotics, as well as supportive counselling for both the patient and the family.

Treatment of herniation. Emergency measures to control raised intracranial pressure and prevent cerebral herniation are only appropriate if it is considered that active therapy for the underlying cerebral metastatic disease will result in significant clinical benefit. Measures include elevation of the patient's head, high dose dexamethasone (24mg IV), mannitol (25-100g IV), and mechanical hyperventilation to reduce cerebral blood flow by reducing the pCO_2.

Terminal care

Patients whose life expectancy is very short because of progression of extracranial disease are appropriately treated with analgesics and antiemetics. Corticosteroids may prolong the dying process but should be considered if seizures or headache are difficult to control. Radiotherapy is not indicated for terminally ill patients. Patients lapsing into coma can have their corticosteroids discontinued; continued parenteral administration is only indicated for patients with seizures that are difficult to control.

Recurrent cerebral tumours

Patients with recurrent primary brain tumours present similar clinical features to those with cerebral metastases from other tumours but can be considerably more difficult to manage. Patients with recurrent tumours are more likely to have significant physical disability, cognitive impairment and psychological disturbance, due to the combined effects of recurrent tumour and previous radiotherapy.[16] There is usually no evidence of metastatic disease outside the CNS. The patients are frequently severely Cushingoid from chronic corticosteroid administration. Recurrent primary brain tumours may progress only slowly and the period of time for which these patients require palliative care is often much longer than patients with cerebral metastases.

Treatment

Therapy is symptomatic and the options are few. Surgery is rarely indicated unless obstructive hydrocephalus develops. The patients are often receiving substantial doses of corticosteroids and increasing the dose is usually of limited clinical benefit. These tumours do not respond to hormonal therapy and the response to chemotherapy is limited. Further radiotherapy is usually not feasible, the maximum tolerable dose having been given at the time of initial treatment; localized radiosurgery can be considered if it is available. Treatment is with analgesics and antiemetics, psychological counselling and the appropriate use of psychotropic medications, physiotherapy and physical supports, delivered as part of a co-ordinated overall plan of supportive care for the patient and the family.

Spinal cord compression

Spinal cord compression (SCC), untreated, leads to permanent paralysis, sensory loss and loss of sphincter control, which greatly complicates patient care and severely compromises the quality of life. Early diagnosis and treatment are imperative, as the single most important determinant of neurological outcome is the degree of neurological impairment at the time of starting therapy.[17, 18]

SCC with neurological dysfunction develops in approximately 5% of patients with cancer. However, myelography or scanning of patients with abnormal plain x-rays of the spine, but without neurological symptoms or signs, will show epidural involvement in about 30%.[19]

About half of the patients with SCC have primary cancers of the breast, lung and prostate. Other frequent causes are less common tumours with a predilection for vertebral metastases including lymphoma, melanoma, and multiple myeloma.

The site of SCC is cervical in 10%, thoracic in 70% and lumbosacral in 20%. MRI studies show multiple sites of compression in about one-third of patients; in two-thirds of these, the lesions are non-contiguous and affect different regions of the spine.[20, 21]

Pathology. SCC nearly always occurs secondary to metastatic involvement of a vertebral body, where continued tumour growth leads to extension into the extradural space, causing anterior compression of the spinal cord. If there is pathological fracture of the vertebra, bone fragments may contribute to the cord compression as well as tumour. Rarely, SCC occurs secondary to epidural or intraspinal metastases, or by extension of a paraspinal tumour through the intervertebral foramen; in these situations, there may be no evidence of bone disease. Compression of the spinal cord causes oedema and impaired venous drainage, leading to neurological dysfunction. Rapid onset or progression of spinal cord signs over a period of several hours, with complete loss of neurological function, is usually due to cord infarction and is irreversible.

Clinical features

Pain is the initial symptom in more than 90% of patients and can precede the development of neurological deficit by days or months. Vertebral involvement causes local central back pain that is constant and progressive. It is described as dull or aching and is associated with local tenderness to percussion. Nerve root irritation produces unilateral or bilateral radicular pain, which is often intermittent or shooting and may be associated with numbness or tingling. Pain due to either vertebral or nerve root involvement is aggravated by movement, coughing, straining, or lying down, and can often be provoked by gentle neck flexion or straight leg raising. Pain that is made worse by lying down suggests metastatic disease, whilst pain due to disc disease is usually relieved.

SCC produces progressive weakness and sensory loss, as well as constipation and urinary retention. At presentation, about 50% of patients are ambulatory, 35% are paretic and non-ambulatory, and 15% are plegic or paralysed.[18] Examination shows objective signs of sensory loss and motor weakness. Anal tone is reduced or absent and the bladder may be distended.

Subclinical spinal cord compression. Recent studies of patients with prostate cancer and vertebral metastases, but without any evidence of neurological deficit, have demonstrated that one-third have subclinical cord compression on MRI scans.[19] Compared to patients with overt SCC, many of these patients did not have back pain. Treatment of subclinical disease with radiotherapy results in all patients remaining ambulatory.[22] In the future it is likely that more patients with vertebral metastases will be screened by MRI scanning before they develop pain, let alone neurological symptoms.

Assessment

Plain x-rays show evidence of vertebral involvement in more than 80% of patients with SCC and back pain. Patients with compression not secondary to vertebral involvement may have normal x-rays.

MRI scanning is the investigation of choice. It is non-invasive and avoids the neurological deterioration associated with lumbar puncture in some patients with spinal cord compression. It allows visualization of the whole spinal cord and is superior to CT myelography in the detection of multiple sites of compression when there is a complete block on myelography. It distinguishes extradural from intradural disease and is better able to define additional bone disease or a paraspinal mass. It is contraindicated in patients with a cardiac pacemaker.

MRI studies show multiple sites of compression in about one-third of patients; in two-thirds of these, the lesions affect different regions of the spine, which has important implications for treatment planning.[20, 21]

CT myelography should be performed if MRI is unavailable or contraindicated. Raised intracranial pressure (due to cerebral metastases) should be excluded by clinical examination and CT scanning before a lumbar puncture is performed for myelography. If the myelogram shows a partial block, the upper limit of the lesion can be defined and other epidural deposits excluded. If there is a complete block, a cervical or cisternal myelogram needs to be considered to define the upper limit of the lesion and to exclude multiple lesions.

Treatment

SCC is regarded as a medical emergency because delay in treatment may lead to permanent paralysis and loss of sphincter control. The need for early diagnosis and rapid treatment is emphasized by the neurological outcome of therapy, whatever treatment modalities are used (Table 25.4).[18] Loss of ambulation is associated with shorter survival.

Table 25.4 Neurological outcome after treatment for SCC

Pretreatment condition	Ambulatory post treatment (%)
ambulatory	75–80
paretic, non-ambulatory	30–50
plegic, paralysed	10

The primary aim of treatment is to maximize the recovery of neurological function. Secondary to this are the goals of local tumour control, pain control and spinal stability.[23] There is insufficient data to define the optimal treatment of SCC and therapy is individualized for each patient. The clinical features that are important in making decisions regarding radiotherapy and surgery are summarized in Table 25.5. In the palliative care setting, it is important that treatment is appropriate to the stage of the patient's disease and prognosis.

Corticosteroids. Dexamethasone will relieve pain and improve or maintain neurological function. It should be given as soon as a diagnosis of spinal cord compression is made or suspected, particularly if there are neurological signs. The conventional dose is 16-24 mg/day but

Table 25.5 Spinal cord compression

Favour radiotherapy	Favour surgery
diagnosis established	diagnosis uncertain
no previous radiotherapy	previously irradiated area
radiosensitive tumour	radioresistant tumour
no spinal instability	spinal instability
paralysis >72h*	paralysis <48-72h
rapid complete paralysis*	not rapid complete paralysis
	deterioration during RT

Treatment must be appropriate to the stage of the patient's disease and prognosis

* RT is for local pain or tumour control; neurological recovery most unlikely

the optimal dose and schedule have not been defined. Higher doses (100mg/day) have been recommended, based on animal models and the results of a single RCT that compared high dose dexamethasone to no dexamethasone (Table 25.6). Higher doses are associated with an increased risk of serious toxicity, particularly gastrointestinal haemorrhage and perforation.[24] Patients with no neurological deficit may not require treatment with dexamethasone.

Table 25.6 Dexamethasone for spinal cord compression

Author	n	Intervention	Outcome
Vecht[25]	37	dexamethasone 100mg vs 10mg IV, then 16mg/d	no difference in pain control or neurological outcome
Sorensen[26]	57	dexamethasone 96mg/d for 4d, then tapered vs no dexamethasone	dexamethasone: 81 vs 63% ambulant post therapy (pS); 3 serious toxicities

Surgery. Indications for surgery include doubt about the diagnosis, deterioration during radiotherapy, a known radioresistant tumour, relapse at a previously irradiated site, and pathological vertebral fracture with spinal instability. Previous standard practice involved posterior laminectomy with removal of the vertebral spines, allowing cord decompression. However, epidural tumour is most frequently found anterior to the cord and posterior laminectomy may not permit adequate tumour removal and can contribute to spinal instability. For these reasons, selected patients with anterior compression due to crush fractures are now treated with anterior vertebral body resection and replacement with methylmethacrylate bone cement and spinal stabilization with metal fixtures. This procedure is limited to selected patients with a solitary lesion, good performance status, good neurological status before treatment, and either no or controllable disease at other sites. It is reported to provide better decompression, spinal stability and local pain control.[27] The neurological outcome is similar to radiotherapy, although perioperative mortality and morbidity have to be taken into account.[28] Surgery performed following radiotherapy is associated with a significantly higher complication rate.[29] Posterior laminectomy remains the standard emergency treatment for patients showing rapid neurological deterioration. It is customary to follow surgical decompression with radiotherapy and rapid mobilization is encouraged.

Surgery is not indicated for patients with established paraplegia (>72 hours), those in whom complete paralysis developed rapidly over a few hours due to cord infarction, or those who are severely debilitated or have restricted mobility.

Radiotherapy. Radiotherapy is the standard treatment for malignant cord compression. It reduces tumour mass and relieves pain and nerve root compression. A considerable number of different treatment plans have been reported, but no particular dose or fractionation schedule has been shown to be superior.[28, 30] Treatment for patients with limited life expectancy should be given in the least time consuming way (e.g. 30Gy in 10 treatments).[31] Hypofractionated therapy (8Gy x 2, 7d apart) is reported to produce equivalent results to longer courses in patients with prostate cancer.[32] This warrants further study as shorter courses are likely to have less impact on the patient's quality of life.

Treatment fields are defined by the results of myelography or scanning. If there is a second area of subclinical asymptomatic cord compression, this should also be irradiated. In a study of patients with a second subclinical area of cord compression, none of 14 patients relapsed following radiotherapy to the second lesion, compared to 3 of 23 who did not receive treatment to the second lesion.[33]

Radiotherapy may cause minor worsening of neurological signs due to reactive oedema and this is treated with full doses of dexamethasone (24mg/d) and carefully monitored; continued deterioration is an indication for surgery.

Retreatment with radiotherapy for spinal cord compression in areas that have received previous irradiation raises concerns about spinal cord tolerance and myelopathy. However, such therapy is reported to produce the same benefits in terms of neurological outcome as in patients not previously irradiated, and the incidence of myelopathy with normally fractionated irradiation (daily treatments) is very low.[34, 35]

Systemic therapy. Hormonal therapy or chemotherapy can be given to patients with sensitive tumours but cannot be relied upon to produce neurological improvement, and do not replace the need for radiotherapy or surgery in the acute situation.

Paraplegia. Patients with permanent paralysis require a programme of rehabilitation and supportive care. This includes bowel, bladder and skin care as well as physiotherapy and the use of physical aids including a wheel chair. Physical alterations to the patient's home environment are frequently necessary.

Preventive treatment. Treatments that inhibit the development or progression of bone metastases might be expected to lead to a reduction in the incidence of SCC. Local radiotherapy, treatment with radioactive strontium (^{89}Sr), and bisphosphonate therapy are all reported to reduce the incidence of SCC in men with hormone-refractory prostate cancer.[22, 36]

Terminal care

Patients who are terminally ill before the onset of SCC do not benefit from active intervention. Treatment with corticosteroids may be of symptomatic benefit. Radiotherapy can be considered for pain control. The development of paralysis will compromise the quality of life for these patients but the morbidity may well be less than they would experience with hospitalization, investigations, surgery and radiotherapy.

Meningeal tumour infiltration

Diffuse or multifocal infiltration of the meninges occurs infrequently with solid tumours but is relatively common with haematological malignancies. It occurs in about 4% of patients with solid tumours, the most common being carcinomas of the breast and lung, and the condition is referred to as carcinomatous meningitis.[37] It occurs much more frequently in patients with malignant lymphoma and acute lymphocytic leukaemia, when it is termed lymphomatous or leukaemic meningitis.

Meningeal tumour infiltration produces a diffuse, sheet-like covering over the surface of the brain and the spinal cord, which is nodular in areas. It causes entrapment of nerve roots and blood vessels and can obstruct normal CSF flow, leading to hydrocephalus. Progressive and clinically significant infiltration is most likely to occur over the base of the brain and in the lumbosacral region.

Meningeal tumour infiltration characteristically produces neurological dysfunction at multiple levels. Cerebral features include headache, nausea and vomiting, lethargy, confusion and mental state changes, and a few patients suffer seizures. Cranial nerve lesions are common and frequently multiple. Spinal features include back pain, neck stiffness, motor weakness and unsteadiness, radicular pain, numbness, and autonomic dysfunction with loss of bowel and bladder function; the spinal features may mimic extradural spinal cord compression. The natural history of carcinomatous meningitis is one of rapidly progressive neurological deterioration with a life expectancy of 1 to 2 months.

The imaging investigation of choice is a gadolium-enhanced MRI scan,[38] which may show meningeal thickening or nodularity, particularly in the region of the basal cisterns; hydrocephalus without evidence of a mass lesion is another common finding. A spinal MRI scan or CT myelogram characteristically show meningeal thickening around nerve roots and multiple meningeal nodules.

Examination of the CSF usually shows increased pressure, a lymphocytic pleocytosis, an elevated protein and a reduced glucose level. Cytological examination for malignant cells is positive in most patients, although multiple examinations may be necessary.

Treatment

Haematological malignancies causing meningeal infiltration may respond well to intrathecal chemotherapy and radiation. In contrast, meningeal infiltration by solid tumours usually occurs when there are signs of progressive disease at other sites, and treatment is largely palliative and symptomatic.[37] The exception is the patient who presents with a good performance status, no serious neurological deficit or CSF obstruction, and stable systemic disease, for whom more intensive therapy of the type used for haematological malignancies might be considered, including systemic and intrathecal chemotherapy and craniospinal irradiation.

Radiotherapy to the whole neuroaxis (craniospinal irradiation) may lead to neurological improvement, but is associated with significant toxicity (particularly myelosuppression) and requires a number of weeks to administer. Careful consideration is needed before embarking on craniospinal irradiation for patients with solid tumours, as the median survival after therapy may be only a few weeks.[39] Local radiotherapy given to areas of symptomatic or bulky disease may improve neurological function.

Intrathecal chemotherapy, given by lumbar puncture or via an Ommaya reservoir, will produce improvement in only one third of patients with chemosensitive solid tumours such as breast and small cell lung cancers; the response rate for other solid tumours is even lower. Intrathecal chemotherapy given in conjunction with radiotherapy does not improve response rates and is associated with significant extra toxicity including leukoencephalopathy.[40] Systemic hormonal therapy may be effective in controlling meningeal infiltration caused by sensitive tumours.

Corticosteroids will improve symptoms related to raised intracranial pressure and radiotherapy, but are unlikely to have a significant effect on any neurological deficits. Obstructive hydrocephalus can be relieved by the insertion of a shunt.

Terminal care

Meningeal infiltration in the terminally ill is treated symptomatically with analgesics, antiemetics and supportive care to accommodate any neurological deficit. Dexamethasone may improve the quality of life by lessening pain, nausea, vomiting and confusion but it is unlikely to produce significant neurological improvement.

Seizures

Generalized seizures or convulsions occur in about 1% of patients with disseminated cancer. Seizures are reported to occur in 20–50% of patients with primary cerebral tumours, 20% of those with cerebral metastases, and less commonly in patients with meningeal involvement. Seizures can also occur with metabolic disturbances, infection, and haemorrhage or as a result of drug therapy (Table 25.7).

Table 25.7   Causes of seizures

Tumour	primary, metastatic, meningeal infiltration
	obstructive hydrocephalus
	haemorrhage
Infection	bacterial, fungal, parasitic, viral
Metabolic	hepatic encephalopathy, uraemia
	hyponatraemia, hypocalcaemia, hypoglycaemia
Drug toxicity	opioids, particularly pethidine (meperidine)
	tricyclic antidepressants, phenothiazines
	local anaesthetics
Drug withdrawal	alcohol, benzodiazepines, barbiturates

The clinical features of generalized seizures in patients with cancer are no different from those of patients with epilepsy. The tonic-clonic phase can be preceded by focal (Jacksonian) features that may be progressive, starting with twitching in the hand, foot or face, progressing centrally and culminating in a typical tonic-clonic seizure.

The investigations performed depend on the clinical circumstances. For a patient with documented cerebral metastases, investigations may be considered unnecessary. If there is no known CNS disease, a brain scan should be performed. Other appropriate investigations are performed if a metabolic cause is suspected.

Treatment

Drug therapy. Treatment with a benzodiazepine is given following a generalized seizure to reduce the risk of a second convulsion (Table 25.8). However, the anticonvulsant action is short lived and other therapy should be instituted promptly. Phenytoin is the most frequently used anticonvulsant and the dose should be adjusted according to blood levels.

Alternatively, if therapy is likely to be short term, blood levels need only be checked if the patient has more seizures or there are signs of toxicity.

The toxicity of phenytoin includes sedation, cognitive impairment, ataxia, dysarthria and nystagmus. Elderly and debilitated patients and those with impaired liver function are at increased risk of toxicity. Dexamethasone increases the metabolic clearance of phenytoin: starting dexamethasone or increasing the dose can lower the phenytoin levels and lead to seizures; alternatively, reducing the dose of dexamethasone can cause phenytoin toxicity [1]. A number of other drugs can affect phenytoin metabolism and lead to either toxicity or recurrent seizures. An increased incidence of erythema multiforme and Stevens-Johnson syndrome has been reported with phenytoin and cranial irradiation, although rashes may occur before radiation starts[2].

Table 25.8 Management of seizures

Immediate therapy
    diazepam 10mg IV or PR (rectal enema), repeat after 15 min if not settled, *or*
    clonazepam 1mg IV (at 0.5mg/min), repeat after 15 min if not settled, *or*
    midazolam 10mg IV or SC, repeat after 15 min if not settled

Standard anticonvulsant therapy with phenytoin

loading dose	1000mg (or 15–20mg/kg) PO in divided doses over 24h
maintenance	300–400mg/d (or 5–6mg/kg/d) PO, adjusted according to blood levels
adverse effects	sedation, cognitive impairment, ataxia, dysarthria, nystagmus
drug interactions	common
alternatives	carbamazepine, sodium valproate, clonazepam

Status epilepticus
    diazepam 10–20mg IV (at 5mg/min), *or*
    clonazepam 1mg IV (at 0.5mg/min), *followed by*
    phenytoin 15–20mg/kg IV (at 50mg/min), *or*
    phosphenytoin 15mg(PE)/kg IV (at 100–150mg(PE)/min)

Treatment for patients unable to take oral medications
    midazolam 10–30mg/24h CSCI and titrate, *or*
    clonazepam 0.5–2mg/d SL drops or 1–2mg/24h CSCI and titrate, *or*
    diazepam 10mg PR q12h and titrate

Alternatives to phenytoin include carbamazepine, sodium valproate and clonazepam. The side effects of the different drugs are similar, with gastric intolerance (nausea and vomiting), sedation, ataxia, dizziness and confusion being the most common. Carbamazepine may also cause leucopenia.

Patients requiring continuing anticonvulsant therapy who are unable to take oral medication can be treated with midazolam by subcutaneous infusion, sublingual clonazepam drops, or rectal diazepam.

Status epilepticus. Patients who do not recover consciousness between seizures are treated as a medical emergency. Treatment is with intravenous diazepam or clonazepam followed by phenytoin (Table 25.8). Phosphenytoin is a pro-drug of phenytoin and can be given more rapidly; the dose is expressed as phenytoin equivalent (PE). If seizures continue, phenobarbital (100mg SC or 20mg/kg IV at 50mg/min) or general anaesthesia with thiopentone or propofol should be considered.

Focal seizures. Cerebral metastases can cause focal seizures, consisting of episodes of twitching in one limb or the face, which may be distressing to patients. Treatment is with an anticonvulsant.

Counselling. Patients suffering seizures require counselling as for any patient with epilepsy. A seizure may be the first sign of progressive or metastatic disease and cause considerable anxiety for the patient and family. Patients with cerebral metastases who have suffered a seizure need to be instructed not to drive a motor vehicle, both for reasons of safety and because most insurance policies are invalid should an accident occur.

Terminal care

At some stage during the terminal phase, patients will no longer be able to take oral anticonvulsant medication. For patients who have had no recent seizures, the medication should be stopped. Patients requiring continuing therapy are treated with sublingual clonazepam drops or midazolam or clonazepam by CSCI.

Table 25.9 Causes of delirium

Intracranial pathology
  tumour: primary, metastatic, meningeal, secondary hydrocephalus
  haemorrhage: related to tumour, systemic bleeding diathesis, hyperviscosity
  encephalopathy: radiation, chemotherapy
  infection: abscess, meningitis, encephalitis
  paraneoplastic syndromes
  post seizure
  cerebrovascular disease, stroke

Metabolic
  respiratory failure: hypoxia, hypercapnia
  liver failure, hepatic encephalopathy
  renal failure
  acidosis, alkalosis
  electrolyte disturbance: sodium, calcium
  hyperglycaemia, hypoglycaemia
  adrenal, thyroid, pituitary dysfunction

Infection, fever

Circulatory
  dehydration, hypovolaemia, heart failure, shock, hyperviscosity, anaemia

Nutritional
  general malnutrition, vitamin B_1, B_6 and B_{12} deficiency

Drug withdrawal
  alcohol, benzodiazepine, barbiturate, opioids, nicotine

Drug adverse effects
  alcohol, anticholinergics, anticonvulsants, antidepressants, antiemetics (phenothiazines, metoclopramide, nabilone), antihistamines, antiparkinsonian, antipsychotics, anxiolytics and hypnotics (benzodiazepines, barbiturates), corticosteroids, NSAIDs, opioid analgesics, stimulants (amphetamine, methylphenidate, cocaine) and, less frequently, many other drugs

Delirium

Delirium is an organic brain syndrome characterized by the acute onset of disordered attention and cognition, usually accompanied by disturbances of psychomotor behaviour and perception. It causes significant distress for patients, relatives and staff,[41] interferes with optimal pain and symptom management,[42, 43] and is associated with shorter survival.[44,45] A number of recent reviews have been published.[42, 43, 46–51]

Delirium is reported to occur in about 30–40% of patients with advanced cancer and the incidence in terminally ill patients has been reported to be as high as 88%.[52] The incidence may be increasing, reflecting an increasingly elderly patient population.[42]

The more frequent causes of delirium in patients with advanced cancer are listed in Table 25.9, many of which are at least potentially reversible. Delirium is reported to be due to more than one cause in two-thirds of patients.[53] The adverse effects of drugs, psychoactive and opioid medications in particular, are a frequent cause of delirium.[54] This is more likely to occur in patients who are elderly, debilitated, or have renal impairment. The practice of polypharmacy, or the prescription of a number of drugs for an individual patient, also predisposes to adverse effects.

In addition to the causes listed in Table 25.9, there are a number of risk factors that make patients more vulnerable to the development of delirium, which are listed in Table 25.10. Patients with pre-existing dementia are particularly prone to develop delirium.

Table 25.10   Delirium: pre-existing risk factors

Increasing age	Renal impairment
Advanced disease, general debility	Depression
Dementia, cognitive impairment	Pain, discomfort
Altered environment, hospitalization	Sleep deprivation

Clinical Features. The criteria for the diagnosis of delirium from the American Psychiatric Association's Diagnostic and Statistical Manual of Mental Disorders, Fourth Edition (DSM-IV)[55] are listed in Table 25.11. The DSM-IV criteria characterize delirium as primarily a disorder of arousal (attention) and cognition, and place less emphasis on the characteristic associated phenomenon such as psychomotor behavioural changes and perceptual disturbances.

Table 25.11   DSM-IV criteria for delirium due to a general medical condition[55]

A.	Disturbance of consciousness (that is, reduced clarity of awareness of the environment) with reduced ability to focus, sustain, or shift attention.
B.	Change in cognition (such as memory deficit, disorientation, language disturbance, or perceptual disturbance) that is not better accounted for by a pre-existing, established or evolving dementia.
C.	The disturbance develops over a short period of time (usually hours to days) and tends to fluctuate during the course of the day.
D.	There is evidence from the history, physical examination, or laboratory findings of a general medical condition judged to be etiologically related to the disturbance.

Delirium may be hyperactive (agitated), hypoactive (lethargic), or a mixed type with alternating features of both. It is estimated that about two-thirds of deliria are of the hypoactive or mixed type, and the classical agitated delirious patient accounts for less than half of deliria that occur.[42]

The clinical features of delirium are numerous and variable (Table 25.12). The onset may be acute or subacute, developing over hours or days. The first signs include restlessness with periods of confusion, daytime drowsiness and insomnia at night, or subtle changes in mood and personality. Inability to write one's name and address has been suggested as a simple screening test.[56] The cardinal sign is that there has been a change in the patient's mental state from a short time previously. Delirium characteristically fluctuates and almost invariably deteriorates in the evening and at night.

Table 25.12 Clinical features of delirium

Attention/arousal
    altered conscious state: reduced awareness
        hypoactive: lethargic, drowsy, stupor
        hyperactive: agitated
    reduced attention
    poor concentration, easily distractible, unresponsive
    disturbance of sleep–wake cycle

Cognition
    disorientation for time, place, person
    impaired memory
    impaired thinking, reasoning
    speech: rambling, incoherent
    perception: misperceptions, illusions, delusions, hallucinations

Affect
    irritability, anger, anxiety, hypomania
    dysphoria, depression, withdrawn
    terrified, euphoric

Psychomotor
    hypoactive: withdrawn, lethargic, stupor
    hyperactive: restless, irritable, aggressive, noisy; repetitive semi-purposeful activity

Assessment. This is outlined in Table 25.13 and includes general physical, neurological and mental state examinations. Mental state examination includes assessment of the patient's mood and affect, orientation, thought content, short-term memory and other intellectual functions. The Folstein Mini-Mental State Examination (MMSE) (Table 25.15) is a useful screening tool for cognitive impairment.[57] A patient's subjective self-reports of cognitive function may differ from the results of objective assessment.[58]

Some of the clinical features of delirium may also be seen in other psychiatric conditions, including dementia, depression and psychosis. Some of the differences between delirium and dementia are listed in Table 25.14. The cognitive impairment in dementia is usually much more gradual in onset and the patients are alert and do not display the alteration in consciousness that is the hallmark of delirium. Patients with depression or mania usually have normal consciousness and do not show the severe cognitive impairment typical of delirium.

Table 25.13 Assessment of acute confusion or delirium

Knowledge of
  previous mental state
  previous psychiatric disorder
  previous alcohol or drug abuse

Examination
  physical, neurological, mental

Assess recent and current drug administration

Laboratory tests
  electrolytes, renal function, liver function, calcium, sugar
  arterial blood gases and pH
  coagulation profile and platelet count
  microbiological studies

CT or MRI scan

CSF examination (after exclusion of raised intracranial pressure)

Investigation should be appropriate to the stage of the patient's disease and prognosis

Table 25.14 Differences between delirium and dementia

	Delirium	**Dementia**
Onset	acute or subacute	gradual
Conscious state	usually impaired	alert
Cognitive impairment	global	memory loss before other changes
Attention deficit	always	sometimes
Mood (affect)	released	reduced
Impaired perception	common	uncommon
Hallucinations	common	rare
Incoherent speech	common	uncommon
Course	fluctuating, worse at night	slowly progressive
Reversibility	often reversible	rarely reversible

Other investigations can be considered (Table 25.13) if clinical assessment suggests the possibility of a reversible cause. Patients earlier in the course of advanced cancer usually warrant thorough investigation, as they are more likely to have a reversible cause that can be treated.[42, 53] Delirium in the terminally ill is less likely to be amenable to effective therapy, although care must be taken not to overlook easily reversible causes.[47]

Measurement. A number of different instruments have been used to diagnose and rate delirium.[42, 49, 59] The Folstein Mini-Mental State Examination (MMSE) [57] (Table 25.15) is used to detect cognitive impairment, but does not distinguish delirium from dementia. It also has limitations related to the patient's educational level and physical condition. For example, patients who are poorly receptive because of deafness, limited intellectual ability, or advanced debility should not be classified as having an organic brain syndrome. It has also been criticized because serial use in palliative care patients suffering progressive cognitive decline may be distressing to the patient.[60] The Confusion Assessment Method (CAM) is a 9-item scale for diagnosing delirium.[61] The Delirium Rating Scale (DRS) and the 1998 revision (DRS-R-98) are used to both diagnose and rate the severity of delirium but require a trained rater.[62, 63] The Memorial Delirium Assessment Scale (MDAS) is also used for diagnosis and severity rating of delirium.[64, 65] The severity rating instruments are valuable in the research setting but have not been widely used in clinical practice. Outside the research setting, there is need for a simpler instrument that can be used by any member of the team to screen for delirium. The Bedside Confusion Scale, which comprises an assessment of alertness and a test of attention (a timed recitation of the months of the year in reverse order), may meet this need.[66]

Table 25.15   The Folstein Mini-Mental State Examination[57]

Question	Scoring	Max. score
Where are you (state, county, city, hospital, ward)?	1 pt for each	5
What is the (day, date, month, season, year)?	1 pt for each	5
Name 3 objects. Ask patient to repeat them.	1 pt for each	3
Serial 7s (count backwards from 100) or spell 'world' backwards	1 pt for each	5
Recall the 3 words given in Q3.	1 pt for each	3
Ask patient to name 'watch', then 'pencil'	1 pt for each	2
Ask patient to repeat 'No ifs, ands or buts'	1 pt if correct	1
3-stage command: Take this paper in your right hand, fold it in half and put it on the floor	1 pt for each	3
Ask patient to read and obey 'CLOSE YOUR EYES'	1 pt if correct	1
Ask patient to write a sentence	1 pt if correct	1
Ask patient to copy design (two overlapping pentagons)	1 pt if correct	1
Total Score 24–30: no impairment; 18–23: mild impairment; 0–17: severe impairment		

Treatment

The underlying cause should be identified and treated, where possible and appropriate. If medications are believed to be the cause of delirium, they should be reduced or stopped, or an alternative drug employed, providing good symptom and pain control are maintained. All non-essential medications should be withheld. If delirium is caused by alcohol or drug withdrawal a case can be made, especially in the terminally ill, for allowing the patient to continue to take the offending agent; nicotine withdrawal can be treated with nicotine skin patches.

Dehydration may contribute to delirium, but the evidence that rehydration is of benefit is equivocal. The state of consciousness was not improved by artificial hydration in one study;[67] the reported reduction in the incidence of agitated delirium associated with the more frequent use of subcutaneous hydration in another may be explained by simultaneous implementation of early opioid rotation.[68] A recently published RCT reported no improvement in cognitive function or delirium after 48 hours of subcutaneous hydration.[69]

Treatment of the underlying cause will lead to the resolution of delirium in between one-half and two-thirds of patients.[42, 52, 53]

General measures. The provision of an appropriate physical environment and good nursing care are the cornerstone of management of most patients with mild delirium and may be the only measures used for the terminally ill. The patient's room needs to be quiet and well lit; a night-light should be available. Repeated calm reassurance and explanation, minimizing the number of different staff having contact with the patient, the presence of a family member or trusted friend, avoidance of disruptive disturbances, and the development of a regular daily routine may all lessen, or at least not aggravate, a patient's delirium. A delirious patient should not be moved from familiar surroundings unless absolutely necessary. Hallucinations, nightmares and misperceptions may reflect unresolved fears and anxieties, and allowing discussion of these may be beneficial for the patient.

Physical restraints are avoided if possible. Restless patients can be allowed to ambulate if accompanied; habitual smokers should be allowed to smoke with supervision.

The family and patient need to be reassured that the delirium is due to organic disease.[70] There are usually lucid intervals, which may help calm both the patient and the family. A delirious patient should be treated in the same manner and with the same respect as one who is not delirious.

Drug Therapy. Haloperidol is the neuroleptic drug most frequently used for delirium in medically ill patients.[42, 71] Chlorpromazine and levomepromazine are alternatives, but are more likely to cause hypotension and sedation. Treatment with one of the neuroleptic drugs is usually effective in controlling the symptoms of delirium and improving cognitive function in both the hypoactive and hyperactive types of delirium.[42, 72] The initial dose is determined by the patient's age and weight, and the severity of the symptoms. If symptoms are mild, haloperidol can be given orally (1–2mg PO) and titrated against effect. If agitation is severe, haloperidol should be given by injection (5mg IV, IM or SC), and repeated each 30 minutes until the patient is calm. After the initial titration, maintenance therapy is continued at a dose that effectively controls symptoms.

Benzodiazepines should not be used as the sole treatment for delirium, as they compound cognitive impairment by causing sedation and may worsen the delirium.[72] The exception is the delirium associated with alcohol withdrawal, for which a benzodiazepine is the drug of choice. For severely agitated patients, or in the terminal care setting where sedation may be desirable, a benzodiazepine can be given in conjunction with the neuroleptic drug; haloperidol and midazolam can be given together as a continuous subcutaneous infusion.

Psychostimulants have been used for the treatment of hypoactive delirium.[73]

The new antipsychotic drugs that have dopamine-blocking effects, such as risperidone and olanzapine, are reported to be effective in the treatment of delirium, but are only available as oral preparations.[42] A trial of olanzapine for delirium in patients with cancer reported it to be effective in 76% of cases. No patient suffered extrapyramidal reactions and sedation was the only significant adverse effect. Olanzapine was less effective in hypoactive delirium or severe hyperactive delirium and in patients who were older, had cerebral metastases, dementia or hypoxia.[74]

Terminal restlessness

Terminal restlessness is an agitated delirium that occurs in some patients during the last few days of life.[42, 48, 75]

The clinical features (Table 25.16) include agitation and restlessness, muscle twitching, multifocal myoclonus and occasionally seizures, usually in a patient with impaired conscious state. Moaning, grunting or crying out is common. The syndrome does not include restlessness due to anxiety or fear, unrelieved pain, urinary retention or faecal impaction, or substance withdrawal.

Table 25.16 Terminal restlessness

Agitation, restlessness	Seizures
Muscle twitching	Impaired conscious state
Multifocal myoclonus	Distressed vocalizing

Treatment

Remediable causes should be sought and treated appropriately. The use of opioid analgesics should be reviewed, as they may cause or aggravate myoclonus in terminally ill patients with deteriorating renal function.

After appropriate discussions with staff and the patient's family, treatment is by sedation with a benzodiazepine (Table 25.17). Benzodiazepines are preferred to neuroleptic drugs because they are effective for myoclonus and have anticonvulsant activity; neuroleptic drugs may lower the seizure threshold. Clonazepam is effective when given by the sublingual or subcutaneous route and is particularly useful for myoclonus. Midazolam is quick acting and is usually given as a subcutaneous infusion. Diazepam can be given rectally (by suppository or injection into a rectal catheter) or intravenously if a line is in place for other reasons. Sublingual lorazepam is effective but short acting.

Table 25.17 Treatment of terminal restlessness

Exclude restlessness due to	anxiety, fear unrelieved pain urinary retention, faecal impaction drug, alcohol or nicotine withdrawal
Review opioid use	
Benzodiazepines	
clonazepam	0.5mg SL, SC or IV q12h, or 1–2mg/24h CSCI and titrate
midazolam	2.5–10mg SC q2h, or 20–60mg/24h CSCI and titrate
diazepam	5–10mg IV or 10–20mg PR, q6–8h and titrate
lorazepam	1–2.5mg SL, q2–4h and titrate
For benzodiazepine failure	
haloperidol	5mg SC, followed by 20–30mg/24h CSCI and titrate
levomepromazine	12.5–50mg SC q4–8h and titrate; continue as 24h CSCI
phenobarbitone	100–200mg SC q4–8h and titrate; continue as 24h CSCI
propofol	10mg/h IV; increase by 10mg/h q15min

If benzodiazepine therapy is unsuccessful, haloperidol or levomepromazine can be added; the sedation caused by levomepromazine may be of benefit. Phenobarbitone can be used although it occasionally produces paradoxical agitation; it can be given as a subcutaneous infusion but, unlike the benzodiazepines, is not compatible in the same syringe with morphine.[76] The short acting anaesthetic, propofol, has also been used for terminal sedation.[42]

Dementia

Dementia is characterized by cognitive impairment that is sufficiently severe to interfere with the activities of daily living.

Dementia in patients with cancer is unrelated to the cancer or treatment in most cases (Table 25.18). A small proportion will have dementia due to a potentially reversible cause. Treatment with thalidomide can cause a reversible dementia.[77]

Table 25.18 Causes of dementia

Unrelated to cancer or treatment	Related to cancer or treatment
Alzheimer's disease	malignant infiltration
alcoholic dementia	radiotherapy
cerebrovascular disease	chemotherapy
hydrocephalus	infection
thyroid dysfunction	paraneoplastic syndromes
vitamin deficiency	obstructive hydrocephalus

A small number of patients with cancer will develop dementia of relatively rapid onset. This can occur with malignant infiltration, infection, obstructive hydrocephalus, or one of the paraneoplastic syndromes. High doses of radiotherapy are associated with dementia, which develops months or years after treatment.

Table 25.19 Dementia: clinical features

Onset	insidious
Course	slowly progressive, little fluctuation
Conscious state	alert
Attention	normal except in severe cases
Affect	limited
Memory	impaired
Thinking	impaired
Judgement	impaired
Orientation	variably impaired
Hallucinations	uncommon
Speech	stereotyped, limited
Insight	often unaware

The clinical features of dementia are outlined in Table 25.19 and the features that distinguish it from delirium are shown in Table 25.14. Patients with dementia are more prone to develop delirium if subject to any of the causes or contributing factors shown in Tables 25.9 and 25.10.

Early dementia must be distinguished from depression. A diagnosis of depression is suggested by an acute onset, poor self-image, guilt, withdrawal and apathy. On examination, the depressed patient can produce answers, whereas the truly demented cannot.

Treatment

A potentially treatable cause for dementia should always be considered. Treatment of infection or malignant infiltration of the central nervous system occasionally leads to improvement. There is no specific treatment for the paraneoplastic syndromes.

Patients with dementia will fare better in familiar surroundings, which should be simplified as much as possible to reduce demands on them. They are not kept in hospital unless necessary and their neuropsychiatric condition may improve after discharge home. Patients incapable of self-care need varying amounts of assistance. The condition needs to be explained to the patient and the family and reassurance given that the disorder has an organic basis, to counteract any possible sense of shame.[78]

Delirium and psychosis in patients with dementia are treated with haloperidol, although a Cochrane review reported a significant improvement in aggressive behaviour but not other aspects of agitation.[79] The newer antipsychotic agents, risperidone and olanzapine, are effective for the treatment of psychosis and behavioural disturbances, notably aggression, in patients with dementia.[80–82]

Insomnia

Patients with advanced cancer commonly suffer insomnia for a variety of reasons (Table 25.20). Insomnia is frequently multifactorial.[83–86]

Table 25.20 Causes of insomnia

Physical	Drug related
pain	Drugs causing insomnia
dyspnoea, hypoxia, cough	corticosteroids
fevers, sweats, pruritus	amphetamine, methylphenidate, cocaine
nocturia, polyuria, diarrhoea	xanthines
fear of urinary, faecal incontinence	caffeine
restless legs	Drug withdrawal causing insomnia
Psychological, psychiatric	benzodiazepines
anxiety, depression	barbiturates
psychosis, mania	alcohol
delirium	nicotine
fear of dying	Environmental factors

Treatment

The management of insomnia should not simply be by the prescription of sedatives and hypnotics (Table 25.21). Physical factors related to the disease that may be preventing or disturbing sleep, particularly pain, need to be assessed and treated. The patient's medications and caffeine consumption are assessed, and note made of any drugs recently ceased. Psychological and psychiatric factors need to be assessed and treated appropriately. Some patients with advanced cancer have a great fear of dying in their sleep and need to discuss these fears and anxieties and be reassured. Good psychological support and relaxation training can be of great benefit. Environmental factors that prevent or disturb sleep such as noise, need for a night-light, bed comfort, and hospital routines are managed appropriately.

Table 25.21 Treatment of insomnia

Treat any factors related to physical disease causing or aggravating insomnia
Assess the patient's medications
Treat any psychological or psychiatric factors causing or aggravating insomnia
Control environmental disturbances and discomforts
Prescribe benzodiazepines *e.g.* temazepam 10–20mg at night

If nocturnal sedation is required, a benzodiazepine should be used. There are no trials to support this choice,[87] but they are safe and effective and possible physical dependence is not of concern for patients with advanced cancer. Temazepam has an intermediate half-life of 8–10 hours, does not produce metabolites that may cause cumulative toxicity, and is preferred to shorter or longer acting drugs. Patients unable to take oral medication can be treated with sublingual lorazepam or subcutaneous midazolam. Patients with insomnia related to delirium are treated with haloperidol or levomepromazine.

Paraneoplastic syndromes

The neurological paraneoplastic syndromes are an uncommon and heterogeneous group of disorders that are remote or nonmetastatic effects of cancer on the nervous system.[88–90] The neuropathies are the only syndromes commonly seen. In some cases, the neurological syndrome may be more disabling than the underlying cancer.

The paraneoplastic syndromes may precede, follow or coincide with the diagnosis of cancer. In most cases the syndromes run a course independent of the progression (or regression, with treatment) of the primary tumour.

The mechanisms by which the paraneoplastic syndromes produce neurological damage remain largely unknown. Mechanisms that have been proposed include tumour-associated toxins, tumour-associated antibodies directed against nervous system tissue, and opportunistic viral infections.

Recognition of the neurological paraneoplastic syndromes may allow better explanation of a patient's symptoms and can be important therapeutically. Some of these syndromes respond to anticancer, corticosteroid or immunosuppressive treatment, and specific therapy is available for patients with the myasthenic syndrome.

Subacute cerebellar degeneration. This syndrome frequently precedes the diagnosis of cancer and has a strong association with small cell carcinoma of the lung and ovarian cancer. Progressive cerebellar ataxia develops over a few weeks or months. The upper limbs are usually as badly affected as the legs and severe dysarthria is common. Dementia may develop. There are occasional reports of improvement with successful treatment of the primary tumour, corticosteroids or plasmapheresis, consistent with an immune aetiology. However, it is usually progressive and unresponsive to treatment.

Limbic encephalitis. This rare syndrome involves degenerative changes in the thalamus and medial temporal lobes with changes in behaviour, mood and memory, leading to dementia. It is usually associated with small cell carcinoma of the lung. There is no effective therapy and treatment of the primary tumour usually has no effect.

Opsoclonus myoclonus syndrome. The syndrome of opsoclonus (rapid, irregular eye movements) and myoclonus, with or without cerebellar ataxia, is associated with neuroblastoma and small cell carcinoma. Treatment is rarely effective.

Progressive multifocal leukoencephalopathy. This syndrome is due to a papovavirus infection and occurs in immunosuppressed patients with leukaemia and lymphoma. It is characterized by progressive dementia and focal neurological signs. It does not respond to treatment.

Subacute necrotising myelopathy. This rare syndrome consists of rapidly ascending sensory and motor loss, usually to the mid-thoracic level, resulting in a clinical picture similar to acute transverse myelitis. There is no effective therapy.

Subacute motor neuropathy. This is characterized by subacute, progressive, patchy lower motor neurone weakness involving the legs. It occurs in patients with lymphoma and is rarely severe or incapacitating. It may spontaneously stabilize or improve.

Subacute sensory neuropathy. This syndrome involves sensory loss, with ataxia and areflexia, which progresses over days to weeks to involve all four limbs and ascends to involve the trunk and face. It has a strong association with small cell lung cancer. It does not improve with therapy.

Sensorimotor polyneuropathy. Distal sensorimotor neuropathy is relatively common in patients with cancer, and is usually attributable to neurotoxic chemotherapy, metabolic abnormalities or nutritional problems. A rare sensorimotor neuropathy is associated with lung cancer; it may follow a chronic course but is unaffected by therapy.

Ascending acute polyneuropathy. The Guillain-Barré syndrome occurs in patients with cancer, particularly those with lymphoma, and the clinical course is similar to that of patients without malignant disease. It is uncertain whether this is a true paraneoplastic effect of cancer or whether the occurrence is coincidental.

Autonomic neuropathy. This syndrome, most commonly associated with small cell carcinoma of the lung, produces predominantly autonomic effects with orthostatic hypotension, neurogenic bladder and paralytic ileus.

Myasthenic (Lambert-Eaton) syndrome. This is discussed in Chapter 23.

Eye problems

Conjunctivitis

Conjunctivitis is acute inflammation of the conjunctivae due to infection, allergy or other toxic reaction (Table 25.22). The patient complains of mild discomfort associated with watering, itching and a gritty feeling in the eye. Vision is well preserved. Examination shows diffuse inflammation of the conjunctivae. Treatment is with regular saline washes. Topical antibiotics can be used if there is significant discharge. If there is worsening of the condition or lack of resolution, bacteriological and viral swabs are taken and ophthalmological opinion sought. Treatment of viral conjunctivitis is symptomatic using washes and topical lubricants; antiviral agents are reserved for corneal disease (see below). The treatment of allergic conjunctivitis is symptomatic.

Table 25.22   Conjunctivitis

Infection	bacterial
	viral: adenovirus, herpes virus
Drug reaction	fluorouracil, methotrexate, cytarabine
Radiotherapy	acute inflammation; chronic dryness
Loss of blinking	VIIth nerve palsy, proptosis
Allergy	

Keratitis

Keratitis or inflammation of the cornea is characterized by conjunctivitis with pain, photophobia, and watering of the eye. There is usually some blurring of vision. In patients with cancer it is most commonly due to infection or an inability to close the eye, leading to traumatic keratitis with secondary infection (Table 25.23). Infection with herpes simplex virus (HSV) is usually associated with signs of nasolabial infection and dendritic ulceration is seen on ophthalmological examination; treatment is with topical aciclovir. Corneal infection with the varicella zoster virus (VZV) occurs in association with herpes zoster of the ophthalmic nerves. Corneal ulceration is seen on examination and treatment is with a combination of oral and topical aciclovir. Bacterial and fungal keratitis are less common but may occur in immunosuppressed patients. Bacterial infection may occur secondary to traumatic keratitis caused by inability to close the eye, as occurs with proptosis or VIIth nerve palsy. Treatment is with topical antibiotics and lubricants (artificial tears). Surgical tarsorrhaphy to allow proper closure of the eye should be considered if the condition is chronic.

Table 25.23   Keratitis

Infection	HSV, VZV, bacterial, fungal
Traumatic	VIIth nerve palsy, proptosis
Radiotherapy	acute inflammation; chronic dryness
Immune	keratoconjunctivitis sicca

Uveitis

Uveitis or intra-ocular inflammation presents different clinical patterns depending on whether the inflammation is anterior, posterior or involving the whole globe. Anterior uveitis or iritis will present with a painful red eye; posterior uveitis may be painless. In patients with cancer, uveitis may be due to infection (CMV, herpes viruses and toxoplasmosis), radiotherapy and tumour infiltration. Uveitis requires formal ophthalmological assessment. The treatment is that of the underlying disorder.

Glaucoma

Closed angle glaucoma may present as a painful red eye with diminished visual acuity and raised intra-ocular pressure. Closed angle glaucoma can be precipitated or aggravated by anticholinergic drugs and drugs with anticholinergic effects including phenothiazines, tricyclic antidepressants, and antihistamines. By contrast, open angle glaucoma presents as a painless deterioration of vision. Chronic administration of corticosteroids, either topically or systemically, can produce a similar syndrome. Intra-ocular tumour, primary or metastatic, may present as glaucoma.

Impaired vision

Blurred vision can occur in patients with keratitis, uveitis, optic neuritis or glaucoma.[91] Drugs that may cause blurred vision include anticholinergic agents and corticosteroids. Blurred vision can be due to cataract formation, which occurs more frequently after chronic corticosteroid use and invariably after radiotherapy to the eye.

Loss of part of the visual field to one or both eyes implies abnormality of the optic nerve or an intracerebral lesion. The pattern of visual field loss will help locate the responsible lesion. Intracerebral lesions are often associated with visual hallucinations. Patients with hemianopia require their immediate environment to be organized so that visitors and personal items are on the side with intact vision.

Blindness in one eye occurs with retinal vascular occlusion (as may occur in the hyperviscosity syndromes) or following tumour-related secondary haemorrhage into the vitreous. Intra-ocular tumour should be treated with local radiotherapy before secondary haemorrhage and visual impairment occur.

Diplopia or double vision is due either to cranial nerve involvement or to orbital metastases. Orbital metastases usually cause proptosis and pain as well as diplopia. Treatment is with corticosteroids, local radiotherapy, and treatment of the underlying tumour. Wearing a patch reduces the distress of diplopia.

Exophthalmos

Protrusion of the eye is a distressing symptom for patients. It can be caused by orbital infection but is more commonly due to malignant infiltration. If due to tumour, treatment is with corticosteroids and local radiotherapy. If proptosis is severe and the eye cannot be closed, topical lubricants (artificial tears) should be used regularly.

References

1   Wen, P.Y., Black, P.M. and Loeffler, J.S. (2001). Metastatic brain cancer. In *Cancer. Principles and Practice of Oncology. 6th edition* (ed. V.T. De Vita, S. Hellman and S.A. Rosenberg). Philadelphia, Lippincott, Williams and Wilkins.

2   Ziai, W.C. and Hagen, N.A. (2002). Headache and other neurologic complications. In *Principles and Practice of Palliative Care and Supportive Oncology* (ed. A.M. Berger, R.K. Portenoy and D.E. Weissman). Philadelphia, Lippincott, Williams and Wilkins.

3   Edwards, A. and Gerrrd, G. (1998). The management of cerebral metastases. *European Journal of Palliative Care* 5, 7–11.

4   Hempen, C., Weiss, E. and Hess, C.F. (2002). Dexamethasone treatment in patients with brain metastases and primary brain tumors: do the benefits outweigh the side-effects? *Supportive Care in Cancer* 10, 322–8.

5   Vecht, C.J., et al. (1994). Dose-effect relationship of dexamethasone on Karnofsky performance in metastatic brain tumors: a randomized study of doses of 4, 8, and 16 mg per day. *Neurology* 44, 675–80.

6   Gaspar, L.E., et al. (2000). Validation of the RTOG recursive partitioning analysis (RPA) classification for brain metastases. *International Journal of Radiation Oncology, Biology and Physics* 47, 1001–6.

7   Bezjak, A., et al. (2002). Symptom response after palliative radiotherapy for patients with brain metastases. *European Journal of Cancer* 38, 487–96.

8   Pollock, B.E., et al. (1999). The Mayo Clinic gamma knife experience: indications and initial results. *Mayo Clinic Proceedings* 74, 5–13.

9   Sims, E., et al. (1999). Stereotactically delivered cranial radiation therapy: a ten-year experience of linac-based radiosurgery in the UK. *Clinical Oncology* 11, 303–20.

10 Noel, G., et al. (2001). Radiosurgery for re-irradiation of brain metastasis: results in 54 patients. *Radiotherapy and Oncology* 60, 61–7.

11 Kondziolka, D., et al. (1999). Stereotactic radiosurgery plus whole brain radiotherapy versus radiotherapy alone for patients with multiple brain metastases. *International Journal of Radiation Oncology, Biology and Physics* 45, 427–34.

12 Patchell, R.A., et al. (1998). Postoperative radiotherapy in the treatment of single metastases to the brain: a randomized trial. *Journal of the American Medical Association* 280, 1485–9.

13 Robinet, G., et al. (2001). Results of a phase III study of early versus delayed whole brain radio-therapy with concurrent cisplatin and vinorelbine combination in inoperable brain metastasis of non-small-cell lung cancer: Groupe Francais de Pneumo-Cancerologie (GFPC) Protocol 95-1. *Annals of Oncology* 12, 59–67.

14 Antonadou, D., et al. (2002). Phase II randomized trial of temozolomide and concurrent radio-therapy in patients with brain metastases. *Journal of Clinical Oncology* 20, 3644–50.

15 Glantz, M.J., et al. (2000). Practice parameter: anticonvulsant prophylaxis in patients with newly diagnosed brain tumors. Report of the Quality Standards Subcommittee of the American Academy of Neurology. *Neurology* 54, 1886–93.

16 Brajtman, S., et al. (2002). Malignant brain tumours and palliative care. *European Journal of Palliative Care* 9, 16–19.

17 Fuller, B.G., Heiss, J.D. and Oldfield, E.H. (2001). Spinal cord compression. In *Cancer. Principles and Practice of Oncology. 6th edition* (ed. V.T. De Vita, S. Hellman and S.A. Rosenberg). Philadelphia, Lippincott, Williams and Wilkins.

18 Weinstein, S.M. (2002). Management of spinal cord and cauda equina compression. In *Principles and Practice of Palliative Care and Supportive Oncology* (ed. A.M. Berger, R.K. Portenoy and D.E. Weissman). Philadelphia, Lippincott, Williams and Wilkins.

19 Bayley, A., et al. (2001). A prospective study of factors predicting clinically occult spinal cord com-pression in patients with metastatic prostate carcinoma. *Cancer* 92, 303–10.

20 Cook, A.M., et al. (1998). Magnetic resonance imaging of the whole spine in suspected malignant spinal cord compression: impact on management. *Clinical Oncology* 10, 39–43.

21 Husband, D.J., Grant, K.A. and Romaniuk, C.S. (2001). MRI in the diagnosis and treatment of suspected malignant spinal cord compression. *British Journal of Radiology* 74, 15–23.

22 Maranzano, E., et al. (1997). Short-course radiotherapy (8 Gy x 2) in metastatic spinal cord com-pression: an effective and feasible treatment. *International Journal of Radiation Oncology, Biology and Physics* 38, 1037–44.

23 Hillier, R. and Wee, B. (1997). Palliative management of spinal cord compression. *European Journal of Palliative Care* 4, 189–92.

24 Heimdal, K., et al. (1992). High incidence of serious side effects of high-dose dexamethasone treatment in patients with epidural spinal cord compression. *Journal of Neurooncology* 12, 141–4.

25 Vecht, C.J., et al. (1989). Initial bolus of conventional versus high-dose dexamethasone in metasta-tic spinal cord compression. *Neurology* 39, 1255–7.

26 Sorensen, S., et al. (1994). Effect of high-dose dexamethasone in carcinomatous metastatic spinal cord compression treated with radiotherapy: a randomised trial. *European Journal of Cancer* 1, 22–7.

27 Yen, D., et al. (2002). Long-term outcome of anterior decompression and spinal fixation after placement of the Wellesley Wedge for thoracic and lumbar spinal metastasis. *Journal of Neurosurgery* 96, 6–9.

28 Loblaw, D.A. and Laperriere, N.J. (1998). Emergency treatment of malignant extradural spinal cord compression: an evidence-based guideline. *Journal of Clinical Oncology* 16, 1613–24.

29   Ghogawala, Z., Mansfield, F.L. and Borges, L.F. (2001). Spinal radiation before surgical decompression adversely affects outcomes of surgery for symptomatic metastatic spinal cord compression. *Spine* 26, 818–24.

30   Janjan, N.A. (1996). Radiotherapeutic management of spinal metastases. *Journal of Pain and Symptom Management* 11, 47–56.

31   Rades, D., Karstens, J.H. and Alberti, W. (2002). Role of radiotherapy in the treatment of motor dysfunction due to metastatic spinal cord compression: comparison of three different fractionation schedules. *International Journal of Radiation Oncology, Biology and Physics* 54, 1160–4.

32   Maranzano, E., et al. (1998). Comparison of two different radiotherapy schedules for spinal cord compression in prostate cancer. *Tumori* 84, 472–7.

33   Helweg-Larsen, S., Hansen, S.W. and Sorensen, P.S. (1995). Second occurrence of symptomatic metastatic spinal cord compression and findings of multiple spinal epidural metastases. *International Journal of Radiation Oncology, Biology and Physics* 33, 595–8.

34   Schiff, D., Shaw, E.G. and Cascino, T.L. (1995). Outcome after spinal reirradiation for malignant epidural spinal cord compression. *Annals of Neurology* 37, 583–9.

35   Wong, C.S., et al. (1994). Radiation myelopathy following single courses of radiotherapy and retreatment. *International Journal of Radiation Oncology, Biology and Physics* 30, 575–81.

36   Soerdjbalie-Maikoe, V., et al. (2002). Strontium-89 (Metastron) and the bisphosphonate olpadronate reduce the incidence of spinal cord compression in patients with hormone-refractory prostate cancer metastatic to the skeleton. *European Journal of Nuclear Medicine* 29, 494–8.

37   Grossman, S.A. and Krabak, M.J. (1999). Leptomeningeal carcinomatosis. *Cancer Treatment Reviews* 25, 103–19.

38   Singh, S.K., Leeds, N.E. and Ginsberg, L.E. (2002). MR imaging of leptomeningeal metastases: comparison of three sequences. *American Journal of Neuroradiology* 23, 817–21.

39   Hermann, B., Hultenschmidt, B. and Sautter-Bihl, M.L. (2001). Radiotherapy of the neuroaxis for palliative treatment of leptomeningeal carcinomatosis. *Strahlentherapie und Onkologie* 177, 195–9.

40   Bokstein, F., Lossos, A. and Siegal, T. (1998). Leptomeningeal metastases from solid tumors: a comparison of two prospective series treated with and without intra-cerebrospinal fluid chemotherapy. *Cancer* 82, 1756–63.

41   Breitbart, W., Gibson, C. and Tremblay, A. (2002). The delirium experience: delirium recall and delirium-related distress in hospitalized patients with cancer, their spouses/caregivers, and their nurses. *Psychosomatics* 43, 183–94.

42   Breitbart, W. and Cohen, K. (2000). Delirium in the terminally ill. In *Handbook of Psychiatry in Palliative Medicine* (ed. H.M. Chochinov and W. Breitbart). New York, Oxford University Press.

43   Ingham, J. and Caraceni, A. (2002). Delirium. In *Principles and Practice of Palliative Care and Supportive Oncology* (ed. A.M. Berger, R.K. Portenoy and D.E. Weissman). Philadelphia, Lippincott, Williams and Wilkins.

44   Lawlor, P.G., et al. (2000). Delirium as a predictor of survival in older patients with advanced cancer. *Archives of Internal Medicine* 160, 2866–8.

45   Caraceni, A., et al. (2000). Impact of delirium on the short term prognosis of advanced cancer patients. Italian Multicenter Study Group on Palliative Care. *Cancer* 89, 1145–9.

46   Macleod, A.D. (1997). The management of delirium in hospice practice. *European Journal of Palliative Care* 4, 116–20.

47   Fainsinger, R.L. (2000). Treatment of delirium at the end of life: medical and ethical issues. In *Topics in Palliative Care* (ed. R.K. Portenoy and E. Bruera). New York, Oxford University Press.

48   Breitbart, W. (2001). Diagnosis and management of delirium in the terminally ill. In *Topics in Palliative Care* (ed. E. Bruera and R.K. Portenoy). New York, Oxford University Press.

49   Brown, S. and Degner, L. (2001). Delirium in the terminally-ill cancer patient: aetiology, symptoms and management. *International Journal of Palliative Nursing* 7, 266–72.

50   Casarett, D.J. and Inouye, S.K. (2001). Diagnosis and management of delirium near the end of life. *Annals of Internal Medicine* 135, 32–40.

51 Caraceni, A. and Grassi, L. (2003). *Delirium. Acute Confusional States in Palliative Medicine*. Oxford, Oxford University Press.

52 Lawlor, P.G., et al. (2000). Occurrence, causes, and outcome of delirium in patients with advanced cancer: a prospective study. *Archives of Internal Medicine* 160, 786–94.

53 Tuma, R. and DeAngelis, L.M. (2000). Altered mental status in patients with cancer. *Archives of Neurology* 57, 1727–31.

54 Lawlor, P.G. (2002). The panorama of opioid-related cognitive dysfunction in patients with cancer: a critical literature appraisal. *Cancer* 94, 1836–53.

55 American Psychiatric Association (1994). *Diagnostic and Statistical Manual of Mental Disorders, Fourth Edition*. Washington, D.C., American Psychiatric Association.

56 Macleod, A.D. and Whitehead, L.E. (1997). Dysgraphia and terminal delirium. *Palliative Medicine* 11, 127–32.

57 Folstein, M.F., Folstein, S.E. and McHugh, P.R. (1975). 'Mini-mental state'. A practical method for grading the cognitive state of patients for the clinician. *Journal of Psychiatric Research* 12, 189–98.

58 Klepstad, P., et al. (2002). Self-reports are not related to objective assessments of cognitive function and sedation in patients with cancer pain admitted to a palliative care unit. *Palliative Medicine* 16, 513–19.

59 Smith, M.J., Breitbart, W.S. and Platt, M.M. (1995). A critique of instruments and methods to detect, diagnose, and rate delirium. *Journal of Pain and Symptom Management* 10, 35–77.

60 Grealish, L. (2000). Mini-Mental State Questionnaire: problems with its use in palliative care. *International Journal of Palliative Nursing* 6, 298–302.

61 Inouye, S.K., et al. (1990). Clarifying confusion: the confusion assessment method. A new method for detection of delirium. *Annals of Internal Medicine* 113, 941–8.

62 Trzepacz, P.T. (1999). The Delirium Rating Scale. Its use in consultation-liaison research. *Psychosomatics* 40, 193–204.

63 Trzepacz, P.T., et al. (2001). Validation of the Delirium Rating Scale-revised-98: comparison with the delirium rating scale and the cognitive test for delirium. *Journal of Neuropsychiatry and Clinical Neuroscience* 13, 229–42.

64 Breitbart, W., et al. (1997). The Memorial Delirium Assessment Scale. *Journal of Pain and Symptom Management* 13, 128–37.

65 Lawlor, P.G., et al. (2000). Clinical utility, factor analysis, and further validation of the memorial delirium assessment scale in patients with advanced cancer: Assessing delirium in advanced cancer. *Cancer* 88, 2859–67.

66 Stillman, M.J. and Rybicki, L.A. (2000). The bedside confusion scale: development of a portable bedside test for confusion and its application to the palliative medicine population. *Journal of Palliative Medicine* 3, 449–56.

67 Waller, A., Hershkowitz, M. and Adunsky, A. (1994). The effect of intravenous fluid infusion on blood and urine parameters of hydration and on state of consciousness in terminal cancer patients. *American Journal of Hospice and Palliative Care* 11, 22–7.

68 Bruera, E., et al. (1995). Changing pattern of agitated impaired mental status in patients with advanced cancer: association with cognitive monitoring, hydration, and opioid rotation. *Journal of Pain and Symptom Management* 10, 287–91.

69 Cerchietti, L., et al. (2000). Hypodermoclysis for control of dehydration in terminal-stage cancer. *International Journal of Palliative Nursing* 6, 370–4.

70 Gagnon, P., et al. (2002). Delirium in advanced cancer: a psychoeducational intervention for family caregivers. *Joournal of Palliative Care* 18, 253–61.

71 Mazzocato, C., et al. (2000). Psychopharmacology in supportive care of cancer: a review for the clinician: II. Neuroleptics. *Supportive Care in Cancer* 8, 89–97.

72 Breitbart, W., et al. (1996). A double-blind trial of haloperidol, chlorpromazine, and lorazepam in the treatment of delirium in hospitalized AIDS patients. *American Journal of Psychiatry* 153, 231–7.

73 Morita, T., et al. (2000). Successful palliation of hypoactive delirium due to multi-organ failure by oral methylphenidate. *Supportive Care in Cancer* 8, 134–7.

74 Breitbart, W., Tremblay, A. and Gibson, C. (2002). An open trial of olanzapine for the treatment of delirium in hospitalized cancer patients. *Psychosomatics* 43, 175–82.

75 Burke, A.L. (1997). Palliative care: an update on 'terminal restlessness'. *Medical Journal of Australia* 166, 39–42.

76 Stirling, L.C., Kurowska, A. and Tookman, A. (1999). The use of phenobarbitone in the management of agitation and seizures at the end of life. *Journal of Pain and Symptom Management* 17, 363–8.

77 Morgan, A.E., Smith, W.K. and Levenson, J.L. (2003). Reversible dementia due to thalidomide therapy for multiple myeloma. *New England Journal of Medicine* 348, 1821–2.

78 Ahronheim, J.C., et al. (2000). Palliative care in advanced dementia: a randomised controlled trial and descriptive analysis. *Journal of Palliative Medicine* 3, 265–73.

79 Lonergan, E., Luxenberg, J. and Colford, J. (2002). Haloperidol for agitation in dementia (Cochrane Review). *Cochrane Database of Systematic Reviews* CD002852.

80 De Deyn, P.P., et al. (1999). A randomized trial of risperidone, placebo, and haloperidol for behavioral symptoms of dementia. *Neurology* 53, 946–55.

81 Katz, I.R., et al. (1999). Comparison of risperidone and placebo for psychosis and behavioral disturbances associated with dementia: a randomized, double-blind trial. Risperidone Study Group. *Journal of Clinical Psychiatry* 60, 107–15.

82 Street, J.S., et al. (2000). Olanzapine treatment of psychotic and behavioral symptoms in patients with Alzheimer disease in nursing care facilities: a double-blind, randomized, placebo-controlled trial. The HGEU Study Group. *Archives of General Psychiatry* 57, 968–76.

83 Kupfer, D.J. and Reynolds, C.F., 3rd (1997). Management of insomnia. *New England Journal of Medicine* 336, 341–6.

84 Savard, J. and Morin, C.M. (2001). Insomnia in the context of cancer: a review of a neglected problem. *Journal of Clinical Oncology* 19, 895–908.

85 Sanna, P. and Bruera, E. (2002). Insomnia and sleep disturbances. *European Journal of Palliative Care* 9, 8–12.

86 Davidson, J.R., et al. (2002). Sleep disturbance in cancer patients. *Social Science and Medicine* 54, 1309–21.

87 Hirst, A. and Sloan, R. (2002). Benzodiazepines and related drugs for insomnia in palliative care (Cochrane Review). *Cochrane Database of Systematic Reviews* CD003346.

88 Hinton, R.C. (1996). Paraneoplastic neurologic syndromes. *Hematology/Oncology Clinics of North America* 10, 909–25.

89 Dalmau, J.O. and Posner, J.B. (1997). Paraneoplastic syndromes affecting the nervous system. *Seminars in Oncology* 24, 318–28.

90 Arnold, S.M., et al. (2001). Paraneoplastic syndromes. In *Cancer. Principles and Practice of Oncology. 6th edition* (ed. V.T. De Vita, S. Hellman and S.A. Rosenberg). Philadelphia, Lippincott, Williams and Wilkins.

91 Saita, L., Polastri, D. and De Conno, F. (1999). Visual disturbances in advanced cancer patients: clinical observations. *Journal of Pain and Symptom Management* 17, 224–6.

Psychiatric

A degree of psychological distress occurs inevitably in patients with cancer, most frequently at the time of diagnosis, treatment failure, or disease progression. It usually manifests as depressive symptoms and anxiety. For most, it is transient and resolves with time and general supportive care, and is considered a normal response to the crisis or stress. For others, the degree or duration of distress is greater than would be considered normal and these patients are categorized as having an adjustment disorder with depressed or anxious mood, which may also be termed reactive depression or anxiety. The distinction between these two groups is inexact and a matter of clinical judgment. Whilst it is disputed that reactive anxiety and depression should be considered abnormal or psychiatric in patients who are medically ill, they are considered in this chapter together with other causes of the affective and anxiety disorders. The recently advanced demoralization syndrome is of particular relevance to the palliative care population. Other aspects of the psychological response to the disease and treatment are dealt with in Chapter 30.

Depression

Significant symptoms of depression are reported to occur in about 25% of patients with advanced cancer.[1, 2] The incidence is probably higher in patients with advancing disease, increasing physical disability, or troublesome pain.[3, 4] In palliative care, the evidence suggests that many patients with depression are not diagnosed or treated appropriately, or that they are started on antidepressants during the last few weeks of life when there is insufficient time for the medication to have any therapeutic effect.[5]

Diagnostic criteria

The symptoms upon which a diagnosis of depression is made in physically healthy individuals are shown in Table 26.1. According to the DSM-IV criteria,[6] a patient must have at least one of two core symptoms—depressed mood and anhedonia (decreased interest or pleasure)—together with at least four other symptoms from the list. Each symptom needs to be severe (most of the day, nearly every day), durable (more than two weeks), be judged to cause clinically significant distress or impairment, and not be attributable to the patient's medical condition or therapy.

Table 26.1 DSM-IV criteria for major depressive episode[6]

Depressed mood	
Anhedonia	markedly diminished interest or pleasure in activities
Weight change	unintentional weight gain or loss (>5% body weight in a month)
Sleep disturbance	insomnia or hypersomnia
Psychomotor problems	agitation or retardation
Lack of energy	fatigue or loss of energy
Excessive guilt	feelings of worthlessness or inappropriate guilt
Poor concentration	diminished ability to think or concentrate, indecisiveness
Suicidal ideation	recurrent thoughts of death or suicide, or suicide attempt

In patients with advanced cancer, the significance of the somatic symptoms is questionable as all may be attributable to the disease or treatment; they might be considered significant if clearly out of proportion to the physical illness. Other criteria that have been advocated as indicators of depression in the terminally ill are listed in Table 26.2.[7]

Table 26.2 Indicators of depression in terminally ill patients

Psychological symptoms	Other indicators
Dysphoria	Intractable pain or other symptoms
Depressed mood	Excessive somatic preoccupation
Sadness	Disproportionate disability
Tearfulness	Poor cooperation or refusal of treatment
Lack of pleasure	History related indicators
Hopelessness	History of depression
Helplessness	History of alcoholism or substance abuse
Worthlessness	Pancreatic cancer
Social withdrawal	
Guilt	
Suicidal ideation	

Reproduced with permission from Block S.D. for the ACP-ASIM End-of-Life Care Consensus Panel: Assessing and Managing Depression in the Terminally Ill Patient. Annals of Internal Medicine 2000; 132: 209–218.

Clinical spectrum

Symptoms of depression can occur as part of the normal response to a crisis, in reactive depression, as part of a major affective illness, or in association with an organic brain syndrome (Table 26.3).

Normal depressive symptoms. Symptoms of depression and anxiety can occur as part of a normal psychological stress response at times of crisis such as treatment failure or disease progression. These reactions last one to two weeks during which there may be significant symptoms of anxiety and depression. They resolve spontaneously with time and appropriate supportive care from family, friends and the treatment team.

Table 26.3 Depressive symptoms in patients with cancer

Normal depressive symptoms
    part of transient normal response to crises, stress

Adjustment disorder with depressed mood (reactive depression)
    mild or short lived episodes of depression

Major depressive disorder

Organic brain syndromes
    acute confusional state or delirium
    dementia
    adverse effects of drugs

Adjustment disorder with depressed mood. Reactive depression differs from the normal self-limited stress response in either degree or duration. The depressive response is maladaptive and greater than would be expected as a normal reaction. The symptoms last longer than expected (more than two weeks) and may be more severe or intense, causing more disruption and interference with daily functioning, social activities, and relationships with others. Reactive depression is frequently associated with some degree of anxiety, and the patient may demonstrate an obsessive concern with symptoms.

Major depressive disorder. Serious depression occurs in a small proportion of patients with advanced cancer. Compared to reactive depression, the symptoms are usually more severe and the mood is incongruent with the disease outlook and does not respond to support, understanding, caring or distraction. Delusional thoughts and hallucinations, features of psychotic depression, are rare except in patients with organic brain syndromes. The risk of developing severe depression is greater if there is a past history of depression and is more likely to occur in patients with advanced disease and significant physical limitations. A strong correlation has been found between depression and a desire for death in the palliative care population.[8–10]

Organic brain syndromes. Patients with acute confusional states (delirium) or early dementia may exhibit features of depression. Examination of the patient's mental state including memory, concentration and attention, orientation, thinking and comprehension will reveal evidence of organic brain dysfunction and appropriate investigations are carried out to determine the cause (see Chapter 25). A number of drugs used in oncology and palliative care have been associated with depressive symptoms, including interferon, tamoxifen, corticosteroids, amphotericin and metoclopramide. However, attributing depression to a particular medication is difficult if there is an underlying depression associated with the disease itself. Cranial irradiation is also linked to depressive symptoms.

Assessment

The structured clinical interview is the gold standard for the diagnosis of depression.[1,7]

There are a number of screening tools that have been employed in palliative care and found to be useful when compared to the results of a psychiatric interview.[1, 11, 12] These include the Hospital Anxiety and Depression Scale (HADS),[13–15] the Edinburgh Postnatal Depression Scale (EPDS) (chosen because it does not contain any somatic-type symptoms),[16] and the short form of the Beck Depression Inventory (BDI-SF).[17] The use of a single question 'Are you depressed?' correctly identified the eventual diagnostic outcome in 197 palliative care patients.[17] A trial of a visual analogue scale (VAS) for mood showed good correlation with HADS.[18]

The assessment of depressive symptoms in patients with cancer depends on the duration and severity of the symptoms and needs to be carried out in the context of the patient's overall illness and prognosis (Table 26.4).

Table 26.4 Assessment of patients with cancer and depression or anxiety

Exclude organic brain syndrome
  acute confusional state, dementia, adverse effects of drugs

Assess the state of physical disease, prognosis

Assess other potential causative or aggravating factors
  pain, other physical symptoms, social, cultural, spiritual

Assess other psychological factors
  understanding of medical situation
  insight into illness
  impact of illness
  concurrent life stresses
  past losses and how they coped
  history of anxiety or other psychiatric illness
  history of alcoholism, substance abuse

Suicide. Cancer patients have twice the risk of committing suicide as the general population and suicidal ideation requires careful assessment.[3, 8] Risk factors for suicide are listed in Table 26.5.[3, 19, 20]

Table 26.5 Suicide risk factors in patients with cancer

Related to mental state	Related to history
severe depression	previous attempted suicide
suicidal ideation	few social supports, social isolation
definite plans for suicide	previous psychiatric illness
confusion, delirium	history of alcoholism or substance abuse
hopelessness	recent death of a relative or close friend
Related to cancer	
advanced disease, poor prognosis	
unrelieved pain	

Treatment

If an organic brain syndrome is present it is treated appropriately (see Chapter 25). Treatment of other problems causing or aggravating depression, particularly pain, can be of great benefit. Optimal therapy includes supportive counselling and psychotherapy in addition to antidepressant medications (Table 26.6).

Normal depressive symptoms. Patients with transient depression occurring in response to acute crises usually require only good general supportive care (Table 26.6). Temporary use of a hypnotic at night and an anxiolytic by day is of benefit in severe cases. Psychotherapy is not usually required although relaxation training may be helpful if anxiety is pronounced.

Psychotherapy. Patients with more severe depression, reactive or endogenous, require more intensive therapy with both psychotherapy and antidepressants. Psychotherapy should be of

Table 26.6 Treatment of depression

Diagnose and treat organic brain syndrome, if present

Treat any causative or aggravating factors
    pain, other physical symptoms, social, cultural, spiritual

General support
    caring and empathy
    reassurance of continued care and interest
    provision of information about illness
    explore patients' understanding and fears about illness, prognosis
    encourage, strengthen family and social supports

Brief, supportive psychotherapy
    resolution of issues regarding disease, treatment, future, coping, etc.
    family, group therapy
    behavioural techniques

Antidepressants (see Table 26.7)

Other drugs: hypnotics, anxiolytics, neuroleptics

short duration (4 to 6 weeks), supportive, and aim for conflict resolution or acceptance. It is directed at clarification and resolution of problems pertaining to the patient's medical situation, the goals and expectations of treatment, and fears about suffering and death. It is designed to improve coping skills and previously successful coping mechanisms are reinforced. Behavioural techniques such as relaxation therapy may reduce anxiety and allow the patient to have some sense of being in control.[21] This type of brief psychotherapy should include family members and will provide them with appropriate support as well as a better insight into the patient's situation.

Table 26.7 Antidepressants classified by principal actions[22]

SNRIs – serotonin and noradrenaline (norepinephrine) re-uptake inhibitors
    TCAs: amitriptyline, imipramine, dothiepin
    venlafaxine

SSRIs – selective serotonin re-uptake inhibitors
    fluoxetine, paroxetine, sertraline, citalopram

NRIs - noradrenaline (norepinephrine) re-uptake inhibitors
    TCAs: desipramine, nortriptyline
    reboxetine
    maprotiline

NaSSA – noradrenergic and specific serotoninergic antidepressant
    mirtazapine

Serotonin $5HT_2$ receptor antagonists
    trazadone, nefazodone, mianserin

Mono-amine oxidase inhibitors
    non-selective MAOIs: isocarboxazide, phenelzine
    RIMAs – reversible inhibitor of mono-amine oxidase-A: moclobemide

Psychostimulants: methylphenidate, dextroamphetamine

Tricyclic antidepressants (TCAs). Antidepressant medication is considered for any patient with significant depression although adverse effects are common and can be clinically troublesome, especially in elderly or frail patients. The various TCAs differ in their sedative, anticholinergic and cardiovascular effects and different drugs are more suited to certain situations. Patients with agitation or insomnia are treated with a sedating antidepressant such as amitriptyline or doxepin; patients with psychomotor slowing require a less sedating drug such as desipramine; and patients with problems related to intestinal motility or urinary retention need a drug with less anticholinergic effect such as desipramine or nortriptyline. TCAs are usually started at a dose of 25–50 mg at night and increased gradually over several weeks. A period of 2 to 4 weeks is required for clinical response. Most adults without physical illness require doses of 150–300 mg/d, but elderly or debilitated patients with cancer may only be able to tolerate much lower doses.

A systematic review of RCTs of TCAs given at low dose (<100mg/d) compared to placebo or standard doses indicates these drugs are effective at lower doses when compared to placebo, and that increasing to standard doses did not improve the response rate but did produce more adverse effects.[23]

There are few RCTs of antidepressant therapy in patients with advanced cancer (Table 26.8).[24]

Table 26.8   Antidepressant therapy in advanced cancer: RCTs

Author	n	Intervention	Outcome
Costa[25]	73	mianserin vs placebo (4w)	mianserin effective (pS) and safe (Hamilton Depression Rating Scale)
Holland[26]	40	desipramine vs fluoxetine (6w)	no difference in efficacy (Hamilton Depression Rating Scale)
Theobold[27]	20	mirtazapine 15 vs 30mg	depression score improved with both doses (pS) (Zung Self-Rating Depression Scale)

Heterocyclic antidepressants. Mianserin is a heterocyclic antidepressant that is moderately sedating but has few anticholinergic or cardiac effects. It has been shown to be safe and effective for the treatment of depression in patients with advanced cancer (Table 26.8).[25] Maprotiline reduces the seizure threshold and is of limited use in palliative care. Amoxapine has dopamine-blocking activity and may increase the risk of dyskinesia in patients taking other dopamine blockers such as haloperidol or metoclopramide.

Selective serotonin re-uptake inhibitors (SSRIs). These drugs have little sedative, anticholinergic or cardiac side effects but can cause transient anxiety, insomnia, nausea and diarrhoea during the first few weeks of treatment. Sertraline is possibly the best drug to use in patients with physical illness; paroxetine is more likely to cause drug interactions and fluoxetine has a slow onset of action.

There is no evidence with which to answer the question whether palliative care patients are better treated with TCAs or SSRIs. A Cochrane review of the use of antidepressants in patients with medical illness suggested that TCAs might be more effective than SSRIs but were associated with more adverse effects.[28] As there is no dramatic difference in efficacy, the challenge is to select a drug with acceptable adverse effects with which the patient will comply.[20, 22]

Mono-amine oxidase inhibitors (MAOIs). Non-selective MAOIs should not be used in palliative care because of the need for dietary restrictions and the frequency of interactions with other drugs. The safety profile of the reversible inhibitor of mono-amine oxidase-A, moclobemide, is better, but drug interactions occur and there is little to recommend its use in palliative care.

Mirtazapine. This noradrenergic and serotoninergic receptor antagonist reduced depression scores in a small trial of patients with advanced disease (Table 26.8). It acts more quickly than traditional TCAs. The main adverse effects are sedation, dry mouth and weight gain.

Venlafaxine. This noradrenaline and serotonin re-uptake inhibitor does not have the sedative, anticholinergic or cardiac effects of amitriptyline and acts more quickly. It is a good alternative to amitriptyline (although much more expensive) and is available as a slow-release preparation. The main adverse effects are dizziness, dry mouth, nausea and insomnia.

Lithium. Patients treated with lithium carbonate before the diagnosis of cancer can be continued on it but require careful monitoring. The dose will need to be reduced if there is deterioration in renal function. Care must be taken when administering other potentially nephrotoxic agents such as platinum or aminoglycosides.

Psychostimulants. Methylphenidate has been used to treat depression in patients with advanced cancer and a life expectancy of weeks to a few months.[29-31] It is effective in the majority of patients and serious adverse effects are uncommon. It should be given earlier in the day (5mg PO at 0800 and 1200h) to avoid insomnia. The effect is often seen within two to three days and it has the beneficial side effects of counteracting opioid-related sedation, improving appetite and cognitive function, counteracting the feelings of weakness and fatigue, and promoting a sense of general well being.[1, 7, 31]

Electroconvulsive therapy (ECT). ECT has an extremely limited place in the treatment of severe depression in patients with advanced cancer. It requires that they have no evidence of brain metastases and that they are medically fit for general anaesthesia. It should be reserved for patients with severe depression and a high risk of suicide who are unresponsive to optimal antidepressant medication.

St John's wort. This extract of *Hypericum perforatum* is a popular over-the-counter antidepressant. Some studies report activity equivalent to other antidepressants with fewer adverse effects.[32-34] However, there are three RCTs that report it to have no superiority over placebo.[35]

Other drugs. The use of a hypnotic at night and an anxiolytic during the day can be useful adjuvant therapy. Patients with depression and psychotic symptoms or an acute confusional state are treated with a neuroleptic drug such as haloperidol or chlorpromazine.

Demoralization syndrome

Demoralization is a prominent form of existential distress in which meaninglessness, hopelessness and helplessness predominate and which may lead to a desire to die.[36, 37] It is associated with chronic physical illness, disability, bodily disfigurement, fear of loss of dignity, social isolation, and feelings of greater dependency on others or the perception of being a burden. The diagnostic criteria are listed in Table 26.9. It can be distinguished from depression by the absence of anhedonia—the demoralized patients can enjoy the present, their lack of hope being confined to the future. In the past, the features of this syndrome have probably been regarded as subclinical depression.

The demoralization syndrome can be actively treated with cognitive behavioural therapy to counter the sense of pessimism and promote the setting of goals, meaning-based therapy that explores continued role and purpose, and supportive therapies to reduce feelings of isolation and dependence.

Table 26.9   Diagnosis of the demoralization syndrome

Symptoms of existential distress: meaninglessness, pointlessness, hopelessness

Sense of pessimism, helplessness, loss of motivation to cope differently, desire to die

Associated social isolation, alienation or lack of support

Phenomena persist over more than two weeks

Anxiety

Anxiety is a normal and universal emotion. Symptoms of anxiety may occur in different situations in patients with cancer and should be regarded as a continuous clinical spectrum ranging from normal to psychiatric. The characteristics that distinguish abnormal from adaptive anxiety include anxiety out of proportion to the stress, persistence of symptoms for more than two weeks, severe physical symptoms or recurrent panic attacks, and disruption to normal functioning.[3, 38, 39]

Normal anxiety. Anxiety occurs normally in response to the stress and crises associated with cancer and its treatment and is more frequent in the terminal phases of the disease (Table 26.10).

Table 26.10   Causes of anxiety

Normal anxiety
    transient anxiety in response to stress, crises

Adjustment disorder with anxious mood (reactive anxiety)
    mild or short lived episodes of anxiety

Anxiety disorder
    generalized anxiety, panic, phobias

Organic anxiety syndromes
    uncontrolled pain
    hypoxia, respiratory distress
    hypoglycaemia
    any uncontrolled or severe physical symptoms
    acute confusional state or delirium
    drug adverse effects: corticosteroids, metoclopramide, bronchodilators
    drug withdrawal: opioids, barbiturates, benzodiazepines, alcohol, nicotine

Anxious adjustment disorder. If anxiety lasts longer than expected (more than 2 weeks) and exceeds the level that is regarded as normal and adaptive, patients may be classified as having an adjustment disorder with anxious mood. Reactive anxiety follows a defined incident or stress. Depressive symptoms frequently coexist.

Generalized anxiety disorder. Generalized anxiety, panic disorders and various phobias may be precipitated or aggravated by cancer and its treatment. A generalized anxiety disorder is characterized by chronic unrealistic worries with autonomic hyperactivity, apprehension and hypervigilance. The anxiety is more pervasive and persistent, occurring in many different situations. These patients have more severe and disabling symptoms, which appear inappropriate or out of proportion to the medical situation.

Panic disorder. Patients repeatedly suffer sudden, unpredictable attacks of intense fear and physical discomfort. The attacks follow a crescendo pattern, reaching a maximum in a few minutes, and may occur in many different situations.

Phobic anxiety. Anxiety is provoked by exposure to a specific feared object or situation, and usually results in an avoidance response.

Organic anxiety syndromes. Anxiety occurs with any severe or unrelieved physical symptoms, particularly uncontrolled pain or respiratory distress. Acute confusion or delirium is usually associated with anxiety. Anxiety is an adverse effect of certain drugs and occurs after the withdrawal of others (Table 26.10).

Clinical features

The physical symptoms and signs of anxiety are numerous (Table 26.11). The patient describes fear, apprehension or panic, which may be nonspecific and not particularly associated with other features of the illness. More commonly for patients with cancer, the fear relates to the uncertainty of the future, bodily dysfunction, unrelieved pain or other symptoms, or to the fear of death itself. Patients with severe anxiety may exhibit panic attacks or phobic anxiety. Significant depression is often present in patients with severe anxiety, treatment of which may relieve the anxiety disorder.

Table 26.11 Clinical features of anxiety

Cognitive	non-specific fear, fear of dying, fear of 'going crazy' poor attention and concentration
Cardiovascular	palpitations, tachycardia, systolic hypertension, chest pain
Autonomic	flushing, sweating, dry mouth
Respiratory	breathlessness, hyperventilation, feeling of choking
Neurological	dizziness, feeling faint, trembling and shaking, paraesthesiae weakness, exhaustion, insomnia
Gastrointestinal	anorexia, nausea, indigestion, diarrhoea, difficulty swallowing
General	mentally tense, keyed up, worried, restless, irritable

Assessment

The assessment of patients with anxiety is described in Table 26.4. Instruments that have been used to screen for anxiety and to measure progress with therapy include the Hospital Anxiety and Depression Scale (HADS)[13] and the State-Trait Anxiety Inventory (STAI).[39] In a prospective observational study, these instruments showed reasonable correlation with the results of psychiatric interview; patients with anxiety disorders also had impaired cognitive and emotional function as measured by the EORTC Quality of Life Questionnaire-C30.[40]

Treatment

The treatment of anxiety is summarized in Table 26.12. The control of pain and other causative or aggravating factors are of particular importance.

Normal anxiety. Patients with normal anxiety responses do not require special therapy except for good supportive care. Temporary use of a hypnotic at night and an anxiolytic by day is appropriate if the symptoms are severe.

Table 26.12   Treatment of anxiety in patients with cancer

Treat the cause of organic anxiety syndrome, if present
Treat other factors that may cause or aggravate anxiety   pain, other physical symptoms, social, cultural, spiritual
Treat depression, if present
General support (see Table 26.6)
Brief, supportive psychotherapy (see Table 26.6)
Psychological behavioural therapies   relaxation training, hypnosis, cognitive-behavioural therapy, biofeedback
Distraction therapies   music therapy, art therapy, socialization
Drug therapy: anxiolytics, hypnotics, antidepressants, neuroleptics

Severe anxiety. Patients with more severe reactive anxiety benefit from treatment with hypnotics and anxiolytics. Depression is frequently present and the use of antidepressants should be considered, as treatment of the depression may resolve the anxiety. Brief supportive psychotherapy aimed at clarification of anxiety-provoking issues, such as the fear of treatment or treatment failure, is frequently beneficial. Behavioural techniques including distraction, relaxation therapy (isometric and deep breathing) and stress management techniques are of benefit to some patients and may give them a sense of being in control. Hypnosis helps some patients. More frequently, treatment is by a combination of anxiolytic medication, supportive counselling, and behavioural and relaxation therapy.

Patients with long standing anxiety disorders, which are aggravated by the cancer or its treatment, are more difficult to manage. Longer term cognitive behavioural therapy may not be feasible for patients with advanced cancer and treatment with anxiolytic and antidepressant drugs is usual.

Benzodiazepines. Benzodiazepines are the drugs used most frequently to treat anxiety (Table 26.13). Drugs with short and intermediate half-lives are preferred to longer acting drugs such as diazepam. Lorazepam has the advantage that it can be given sublingually. Midazolam can be given by subcutaneous injection as a continuous subcutaneous infusion.

The side effects of benzodiazepines include drowsiness, incoordination and confusion, which are dose related and reversible. Approximately one third of patients taking benzodiazepines will experience difficulty withdrawing from the drug, but considerations of

Table 26.13   Anxiolytic drugs

Benzodiazepines	
short acting	midazolam 2-5mg SC q1-2h or 24h CSCI
intermediate	alprazolam 0.25-0.5mg PO q6-8h and titrate
	lorazepam 1-2mg PO or SL q6-8h and titrate
	oxazepam 15-30mg PO q8-12h and titrate
long acting	diazepam 5-10mg PO or PR q8-12h and titrate
Non-benzodiazepine	
	buspirone 5-10mg PO q8h

dependency and withdrawal are unimportant in patients with advanced and terminal cancer. The exception is the patient who is not terminally ill but can no longer take oral medications, who needs to be observed carefully for any signs of withdrawal. If appropriate, a benzodiazepine is administered by another route.

Other anxiolytics. The non-benzodiazepine drug, buspirone, has been shown to be effective in the treatment of anxiety and does not cause significant sedation, but takes 5 to 10 days to be effective.

Other drugs. A hypnotic such as temazepam is often helpful in the management of anxiety. Antidepressants can be used if there are significant depressive symptoms and may be useful in the management of panic disorders. Neuroleptic drugs (haloperidol, chlorpromazine) are indicated for the management of severe anxiety or agitation not controlled with a benzodiazepine, in patients with features of psychosis, and where anxiety is part an agitated delirium.

References

1   Wilson, K.G., et al. (2000). Diagnosis and management of depression in palliative care. In *Handbook of Psychiatry in Palliative Care* (ed. H.M. Chochinov and W. Breitbart). Oxford, Oxford University Press.

2   Stiefel, R., et al. (2001). Depression in palliative care: a pragmatic report from the Expert Working Group of the European Association for Palliative Care. *Supportive Care in Cancer* 9, 477–88.

3   Payne, D.K. and M.J., M. (2002). Depression and anxiety. In *Principles and Practice of Palliative Care and Supportive Oncology* (ed. A.M. Berger, R.K. Portenoy and D.E. Weissman). Philadelphia, Lippincott, Williams and Wilkins.

4   Chochinov, H.M. (2003). Depression in the terminally ill: prevalence and measurement issues. In *Issues in Palliative Care Research* (ed. R. Portenoy and E. Bruera). New York, Oxford University Press.

5   Lloyd-Williams, M., Friedman, T. and Rudd, N. (1999). A survey of antidepressant prescribing in the terminally ill. *Palliative Medicine* 13, 243–8.

6   American Psychiatric Association (1994). *Diagnostic and Statistical Manual of Mental Disorders. Fourth Edition.* Washington D.C.,

7   Block, S.D. (2000). Assessing and managing depression in the terminally ill patient. ACP-ASIM End-of-Life Care Consensus Panel. American College of Physicians—American Society of Internal Medicine. *Annals of Internal Medicine* 132, 209–18.

8   Rosenfeld, B., et al. (2000). Suicide, assisted suicide, and euthanasia in the terminally ill. In *Handbook of Psychiatry in Palliative Care* (ed. H.M. Chochinov and W. Breitbart). Oxford, Oxford University Press.

9   Kelly, B., et al. (2003). Factors associated with the wish to hasten death: a study of patients with terminal illness. *Psychological Medicine* 33, 75–81.

10 Chochinov, H.M., et al. (1995). Desire for death in the terminally ill. *American Journal of Psychiatry* 152, 1185–91.

11 Hotopf, M., et al. (2002). Depression in advanced disease: a systematic review Part 1. Prevalence and case finding. *Palliative Medicine* 16, 81–97.

12 Lloyd-Williams, M., Spiller, J. and Ward, J. (2003). Which depression screening tools should be used in palliative care? *Palliative Medicine* 17, 40–3.

13 Hopwood, P., Howell, A. and Maguire, P. (1991). Screening for psychiatric morbidity in patients with advanced breast cancer: validation of two self-report questionnaires. *British Journal of Cancer* 64, 353–6.

14 Le Fevre, P., et al. (1999). Screening for psychiatric illness in the palliative care inpatient setting: a comparison between the Hospital Anxiety and Depression Scale and the General Health Questionnaire-12. *Palliative Medicine* 13, 399–407.

15 Lloyd-Williams, M., Friedman, T. and Rudd, N. (2001). An analysis of the validity of the Hospital Anxiety and Depression scale as a screening tool in patients with advanced metastatic cancer. *Journal of Pain and Symptom Management* 22, 990–6.

16 Lloyd-Williams, M., Friedman, T. and Rudd, N. (2000). Criterion validation of the Edinburgh postnatal depression scale as a screening tool for depression in patients with advanced metastatic cancer. *Journal of Pain and Symptom Management* 20, 259–65.

17 Chochinov, H.M., et al. (1997). 'Are you depressed?' Screening for depression in the terminally ill. *American Journal of Psychiatry* 154, 674–6.

18 Lees, N. and Lloyd-Williams, M. (1999). Assessing depression in palliative care patients using the visual analogue scale: a pilot study. *European Journal of Palliative Care* 9, 220–23.

19 Massie, M.J., Gagnon, P. and Holland, J.C. (1994). Depression and suicide in patients with cancer. *Journal of Pain and Symptom Management* 9, 325–40.

20 Peveler, R., Carson, A. and Rodin, G. (2002). Depression in medical patients. *British Medical Journal* 325, 149–52.

21 Sloman, R. (2002). Relaxation and imagery for anxiety and depression control in community patients with advanced cancer. *Cancer Nursing* 25, 432–5.

22 Kent, J.M. (2000). SNaRIs, NaSSAs, and NaRIs: new agents for the treatment of depression. *Lancet* 355, 911–18.

23 Furukawa, T.A., McGuire, H. and Barbui, C. (2002). Meta-analysis of effects and side effects of low dosage tricyclic antidepressants in depression: systematic review. *British Medical Journal* 325, 991.

24 Ly, K.L., et al. (2002). Depression in palliative care: a systematic review. Part 2. Treatment. *Palliative Medicine* 16, 279–84.

25 Costa, D., Mogos, I. and Toma, T. (1985). Efficacy and safety of mianserin in the treatment of depression of women with cancer. *Acta Psychiatry Scandinavia* 72 (Suppl 30), 85–92.

26 Holland, J.C., et al. (1998). A controlled trial of fluoxetine and desipramine in depressed women with advanced cancer. *Psychooncology* 7, 291–300.

27 Theobald, D.E., et al. (2002). An open-label, crossover trial of mirtazapine (15 and 30 mg) in cancer patients with pain and other distressing symptoms. *Journal of Pain and Symptom Management* 23, 442–7.

28 Gill, D. and Hatcher, S. (2000). Antidepressants for depression in medical illness (Cochrane Review). *Cochrane Database of Systematic Reviews* CD001312.

29 Homsi, J., et al. (2000). Methylphenidate for depression in hospice practice: a case series. *American Journal of Hospice and Palliative Care* 17, 393–8.

30 Homsi, J., et al. (2001). A phase II study of methylphenidate for depression in advanced cancer. *American Journal of Hospice and Palliative Care* 18, 403–7.

31 Rozans, M., et al. (2002). Palliative uses of methylphenidate in patients with cancer: a review. *Journal of Clinical Oncology* 20, 335–9.

32 Kim, H.L., Streltzer, J. and Goebert, D. (1999). St. John's wort for depression: a meta-analysis of well-defined clinical trials. *Journal of Nervous and Mental Disorders* 187, 532–8.

33 Gaster, B. and Holroyd, J. (2000). St John's wort for depression: a systematic review. *Archives of Internal Medicine* 160, 152–6.

34 Linde, K. and Mulrow, C.D. (2000). St John's wort for depression (Cochrane Review). *Cochrane Database of Systematic Reviews* CD000448.

35 Hypericum Depression Trial Study Group (2002). Effect of Hypericum perforatum (St John's wort) in major depressive disorder: a randomized controlled trial. *Journal of the American Medical Association* 287, 1807–14.

36 Kissane, D.W., Clarke, D.M. and Street, A.F. (2001). Demoralization syndrome—a relevant psychiatric diagnosis for palliative care. *Journal of Palliative Care* 17, 12–21.

37 Clarke, D.M. and Kissane, D.W. (2002). Demoralization: its phenomenology and importance. *Australian and New Zealand Journal of Psychiatry* 36, 733–42.

38 Payne, D.K. and Massie, M.J. (2000). Anxiety in palliative care. In *Handbook of Psychiatry in Palliative Care* (ed. H.M. Chochinov and W. Breitbart). Oxford, Oxford University Press.
39 House, A. and Stark, D. (2002). Anxiety in medical patients. *British Medical Journal* 325, 207–9.
40 Stark, D., et al. (2002). Anxiety disorders in cancer patients: their nature, associations, and relation to quality of life. *Journal of Clinical Oncology* 20, 3137–48.

27

Endocrine and metabolic

Hypercalcaemia	Hyperglycaemia
Hypocalcaemia	Hypoglycaemia
Hyperphosphataemia	Hypomagnesaemia
Hypophosphataemia	Adrenal insufficiency
Hypernatraemia and diabetes insipidus	Tumour lysis
Hyponatraemia and SIADH	Carcinoid syndrome
Hyperkalaemia	Islet cell carcinomas
Hypokalaemia and ectopic ACTH	Gynaecomastia

Hypercalcaemia

Hypercalcaemia occurs in 8–10% of patients with cancer, with an incidence as high as 40% in patients with breast cancer and multiple myeloma.[1, 2]

Cause

Cancer can cause hypercalcaemia by humoral or local effects or by a combination of the two. A number of other factors, unrelated to the tumour, can either cause hypercalcaemia or precipitate its occurrence in patients at risk (Table 27.1).

Humoral hypercalcaemia. In the majority of patients with solid tumours, hypercalcaemia is due to secretion of parathyroid hormone-related protein (PTHrP) by the tumour. PTHrP stimulates osteoclastic bone resorption with mobilization of skeletal calcium; it also increases calcium reabsorption in the distal renal tubule. Secretion of PTHrP explains the occurrence of hypercalcaemia in patients with no bone metastases, but increased levels are also found in patients with breast cancer with widespread osteolytic metastases and hypercalcaemia. In these patients, hypercalcaemia is presumably due to a combination of local bone destruction and the renal and skeletal effects of PTHrP.

Local osteolytic hypercalcaemia. Local bone destruction is mediated by a range of cytokines produced by tumour cells that act as osteoclast activating factors (OAFs). Interleukins, prostaglandins, tumour growth factors and others are variously involved. In myeloma there may also be renal tubular damage related to the myeloma proteins, which inhibits the excretion of a calcium load. In patients with bone metastases due to breast cancer or other solid tumours, the skeletal and renal effects of PTHrP may compound the effects of local bone destruction.

Table 27.1 Causes of hypercalcaemia

Associated with cancer	Not due to cancer
humoral (PTHrP)	immobilization
bone destruction	excess ingestion of calcium, vitamins A or D
	milk alkali syndrome
	thiazide diuretics
	primary hyperparathyroidism

Clinical features

The symptoms and signs associated with hypercalcaemia are shown in Table 27.2. The common presenting symptoms are fatigue, lethargy, nausea and polyuria; the combination of nausea and polyuria can lead to dehydration and worsening of the hypercalcaemia. The severity of the symptoms depends on the level of ionized calcium (free or not protein-bound) and the speed with which the level rises. The serum calcium result is adjusted according to the serum albumin in patients with significant hypoalbuminaemia. Coexistent acidosis increases the ionized calcium level and can precipitate symptoms; alkalosis has the opposite effect.

Table 27.2 Clinical features of hypercalcaemia

General	dehydration, polydipsia, polyuria, pruritus, weight loss
Gastrointestinal	anorexia, nausea, vomiting, constipation, ileus
Neurological	fatigue, lethargy, muscle weakness, hyporeflexia confusion, psychosis, seizure, drowsiness, coma
Cardiac	bradycardia, prolonged P-R, shortened Q-T, wide T-waves, arrhythmias

Treatment

Given the efficacy and lack of toxicity of bisphosphonate therapy, all patients who are symptomatic of hypercalcaemia warrant a trial of therapy, regardless of the stage of their disease. Correction of hypercalcaemia will not affect the prognosis but may greatly improve symptoms in patients with advanced cancer.

General measures. There are a number of general measures that are useful in the treatment of mild hypercalcaemia or in the maintenance of normocalcaemia after bisphosphonate therapy (Table 27.3). Low calcium diets are unpalatable and probably have no effect on hypercalcaemia related to malignancy. The underlying disease is treated, where possible and appropriate.

Rehydration. The treatment of severe hypercalcaemia is initially by intravenous rehydration with normal saline (Table 27.4). The addition of frusemide may increase calcium excretion but should not be used until the patient is fully rehydrated.

Bisphosphonates. Treatment with a bisphosphonate compound is now standard therapy for the hypercalcaemia of malignancy (Table 27.4). The bisphosphonates are chemical analogues of

Table 27.3 Hypercalcaemia: general measures

Maintain mobility, avoid immobilization
Increased fluid intake: 2-3L/d
Stop thiazide diuretics

Dietary
    stop calcium or vitamin supplements, excess milk or antacids
    normal calcium diet

Treatment of underlying disease, where possible

Table 27.4 Hypercalcaemia: drug therapy

Rehydration with normal saline ± frusemide	

Bisphosphonate
    pamidronate
    zoledronic acid
	
	60–90mg IV in 500ml saline or dextrose over 2–4h
	4mg IV over 15min

Calcitonin	100–200 units IM, SC
Gallium nitrate	200mg/m2/24h IV x 5d
Prednisolone	50mg/d PO
Oral phosphate	1–3g/d PO

pyrophosphate and inhibit bone resorption. The more recently introduced nitrogen-containing bisphosphonates (pamidronate, ibandronate, olpadronate and zoledronic acid) are more potent than the non-nitrogen-containing compounds etidronate and clodronate. The studies of regular pamidronate therapy in patients with lytic bone disease that demonstrate a significant reduction in skeletal events show a reduced incidence of hypercalcaemia in breast cancer but not multiple myeloma (Table 27.5). Studies of zoledronic acid show it may be more effective than pamidronate.

Table 27.5 Bisphosphonates and prevention of hypercalcaemia: selected RCTs

Author	n	Intervention	Outcome
Theriault[3]	371	Breast cancer on hormone therapy: IV pamidronate vs placebo (2yr)	pamidronate : hypercalcaemia in 4 vs 10% (pS)
Hortobagyi[4]	380	Breast cancer on chemotherapy: IV pamidronate vs placebo (2yr)	pamidronate : hypercalcaemia in 7 vs 15% (pS)
Berenson[5]	377	Myeloma: IV pamidronate vs placebo (2yr)	no difference in incidence of hypercalcaemia
Rosen[6]	766	Breast and myeloma: IV zoledronic acid vs pamidronate	less hypercalcaemia with zoledronic acid (pNS)

Pamidronate will restore normocalcaemia in 60–75% of patients with hypercalcaemia. It is less effective in patients without bone metastases and with elevated levels of PTHrP.[1,7] It is given as an infusion over 2 hours, more slowly in patients with renal impairment. The effect of pamidronate is usually evident within 1 to 2 days but, unless treatment can be given to control the underlying disease, further therapy is often required within 2 to 4 weeks. Repeated therapy may produce lesser responses, particularly where the hypercalcaemia is predominantly humoral in patients without bone metastases.[8] Mild nausea and fever are the only frequently reported adverse effects. Symptomatic hypocalcaemia is rare.

Zoledronic acid is reported to be more potent than pamidronate in preclinical studies. It is given as a five-minute injection and is reported to correct hypercalcaemia in 87% of patients.[7] Compared to pamidronate, it has a higher response rate, a more rapid onset and longer duration of action, and a similar adverse effect profile (Table 27.6). It was equally effective in patients with and without bone metastases; it may be less effective in patients with elevated PTHrP levels.

Ibandronate is reported to be effective in about 75% of patients with hypercalcaemia.[9]

Table 27.6 Pamidronate (P) and zoledronic acid (Z) for hypercalcaemia: RCTs

Author	n	Intervention	Outcome
Major[7]	275	IV Z 4mg & 8mg vs IV P 90mg	Z: response (day 10): 87 vs 70%; more rapid response; median duration response: 32 & 43 vs 18d; (all pS)

Other drugs. Calcitonin can be used for the rapid correction of severe hypercalcaemia and its effect is usually seen within 2 to 3 hours. The duration of response is increased by concurrent use of a corticosteroid. Tachyphylaxis occurs within a few days due to down-regulation of the calcitonin receptors in osteoclasts, and its role is probably in the rapid correction of severe hypercalcaemia in conjunction with a bisphosphonate. The anticancer agent, gallium nitrate, is effective in controlling hypercalcaemia with response rates similar to bisphosphonates. However, it has to be given as a continuous infusion over 5 days and can cause nephrotoxicity. Corticosteroids are frequently advocated in the treatment of malignant hypercalcaemia but are only of use in patients with corticosteroid-sensitive tumours including myeloma, lymphoma and a few patients with breast cancer. Treatment is started at a higher dose, such as prednisolone 50 mg/day, and tapered according to response. Oral phosphate may be useful in maintaining normocalcaemia. It acts by raising the serum phosphate level, causing a secondary lowering of the serum calcium, and cannot be used in patients with renal failure or hyperphosphataemia. The main side effects are diarrhoea and nausea, which are dose-limiting and a frequent cause for patient noncompliance. The prostaglandin synthetase inhibitors, aspirin and the NSAIDs, have no role in the treatment of hypercalcaemia: the frequency of response is negligible and they may impair renal function and aggravate hypercalcaemia.

Hypocalcaemia

Hypocalcaemia occurs as frequently as hypercalcaemia in patients with cancer but is rarely symptomatic. The causes of hypocalcaemia are shown in Table 27.7. Hypoalbuminaemia is the most frequent cause of hypocalcaemia but is usually asymptomatic as the level of ionized calcium is maintained. Hypomagnesaemia causes functional hypoparathyroidism with hypocalcaemia unresponsive to calcium therapy. Neck surgery can cause transient hypocalcaemia; it is permanent after parathyroidectomy. Hyperphosphataemia associated with oral phosphate therapy or renal failure can cause hypocalcaemia. Severe alkalosis may precipitate symptoms of hypocalcaemia by decreasing the level of ionized calcium.

Table 27.7 Causes of hypocalcaemia

Hypoalbuminaemia	Tumour lysis
Hypoparathyroidism	Treatment of hypercalcaemia
hypomagnesaemia	Major transfusion
neck surgery, irradiation	Acute pancreatitis
Hyperphosphataemia	Severe alkalosis
iatrogenic	hyperventilation
renal failure	prolonged nasogastric drainage

The clinical features of hypocalcaemia are those of progressive neuromuscular irritability (Table 27.8).[10] The severity of symptoms depends on the serum calcium and whether or not there is a coexistent alkalosis. There may be paraesthesiae, muscle cramps and tetany (carpopedal spasm). Chvostek's sign is twitching of the facial muscles after percussion of the facial nerve. Trousseau's sign is spasm of the hand after 3 to 4 minutes exercise with a blood pressure cuff inflated to between diastolic and systolic pressure.

Table 27.8 Clinical features of hypocalcaemia

Paraesthesiae of face, hands, feet	Laryngospasm
Muscle spasm, cramps	Weakness, lethargy
Tetany (carpopedal spasm)	Poor memory
Chvostek's sign	Cerebral irritation, seizures
Trousseau's sign	Diarrhoea

Treatment. Treatment depends on the degree of hypocalcaemia and the presence or absence of symptoms. Hypocalcaemia associated with a low albumin level is asymptomatic and requires no treatment. Treatment of hypocalcaemia secondary to alkalosis or hyperphosphataemia is that of the cause. Severe hypocalcaemia caused by surgery or the treatment of hypercalcaemia, and that secondary to hypomagnesaemia, requires parenteral therapy (Table 27.9). The symptoms and signs of hypocalcaemia secondary to hypomagnesaemia will not improve unless the magnesium level is also corrected. Treatment is with intravenous calcium chloride and, if the serum magnesium is unknown or likely to be low, magnesium sulfate is also given. Treatment may need to be continued for several days. Hypocalcaemia secondary to parathyroidectomy is treated with vitamin D and calcium supplements.

Table 27.9 Treatment of severe hypocalcaemia

Calcium: 10% calcium chloride 1g (10ml) IV over 10 min
repeat q15-20 min if tetany persists
follow with 1g in 500-1000 ml fluid q6-8h, and titrate
Magnesium: 50% magnesium sulfate 1g (2ml) IV
or 5g (10ml) IV by 24 hour infusion (requires separate IV line)

Hyperphosphataemia

The causes of hyperphosphataemia are shown in Table 27.10. Hyperphosphataemia causes hypocalcaemia and tetany. It can lead to the precipitation of calcium phosphate in tissues, which may cause renal failure [11].

Table 27.10 Causes of hyperphosphataemia

Oral phosphate supplements	Hypoparathyroidism
Renal failure	surgery
Tumour lysis syndrome	hypomagnesaemia

Treatment. Treatment is directed at avoiding renal damage and the correction of hypocalcaemia. Phosphate supplements should be stopped and an aluminium hydroxide-containing antacid, which will precipitate phosphate in the intestine, is given every 2 to 6 hours. Adequate hydration and urine output need to be maintained.

Hypophosphataemia

Hypophosphataemia may occur as a result of decreased intake, decreased absorption (aluminium hydroxide-containing antacids), or abnormal renal losses as occur in multiple myeloma. Severe hypophosphataemia may cause anorexia, dizziness and generalized weakness.[11] Hallucinations may occur and hypophosphataemia is thought to be associated with the hallucinations that occur in delirium tremens and chronic hepatic encephalopathy. Treatment is directed at the underlying cause and with phosphate supplements.

Hypernatraemia and diabetes insipidus

Hypernatraemia may result from inadequate fluid intake or increased fluid losses (Table 27.11).[17] Diabetes insipidus is caused by a deficiency of antidiuretic hormone (ADH) due to infiltration of the pituitary or hypothalamus.

Table 27.11 Causes of hypernatraemia

Decreased fluid intake (relative or absolute)
bedridden, semiconscious, aphagia
Increased fluid loss
gastrointestinal: vomiting, diarrhoea, fistulas, nasogastric drainage
renal: diuretic therapy, hyperglycaemia
diuresis following correction of renal failure or obstruction
diabetes insipidus
skin: fever, sweating, hot environment
pulmonary: hyperventilation, dry atmosphere
third space fluid collection: bowel obstruction, pancreatitis, peritonitis

The significant clinical features relate to cerebral dehydration, which progressively causes lethargy, weakness, restlessness, irritability, muscle twitching, seizures, coma, and death. Polyuria occurs with diabetes insipidus. The diagnosis of diabetes insipidus is made by the measurement of the serum sodium level and the serum and urine osmolality. The blood osmolality will be elevated above 280 mmol/kg and the urine osmolality rarely exceeds 200 mmol/kg.

Treatment

Treatment consists of repletion of total body water, matching any continuing losses, and treating the underlying cause. Body water needs to be replaced gradually to avoid cerebral oedema.

Diabetes insipidus. Diabetes insipidus is treated by hormone replacement with vasopressin (the natural human hormone, made synthetically) or desmopressin (a synthetic analogue with a longer duration of action). Initial therapy for a seriously ill patient is with vasopressin, given by intramuscular or subcutaneous injection. The dose is 5 to 10 units and subsequent doses can be given after 6 to 8 hours if polyuria recurs. Intranasal desmopressin is used for continuing therapy. The average daily dose is 10–40 µg/d, given as two divided doses. Chlorpropamide and carbamazepine, if employed for other reasons, may increase the secretion of ADH and require reduction of the dose of desmopressin.

Hyponatraemia and SIADH

The causes of hyponatraemia in patients with cancer are listed in Table 27.12.[13] Appropriate clinical assessment will usually reveal the cause, to which treatment is directed. The detection of significant hyponatraemia in a patient with cancer should raise the possibility of inappropriate antidiuretic hormone secretion, which is potentially life threatening and requires special treatment.

Table 27.12 Causes of hyponatraemia

Excess water drinking
Oedematous states   cardiac, renal, hepatic failure
Hypothyroidism
Salt wasting states   mineralocorticoid or corticosteroid deficiency, diuretics, chronic renal failure
Gastrointestinal losses (without adequate sodium replacement)   vomiting, diarrhoea, fistulas
Excess ADH for diabetes insipidus
Pseudohyponatraemia   paraproteinaemia, hyperglycaemia

Syndrome of inappropriate ADH (SIADH)
    tumours — small cell lung cancer, others
    neurological — primary or metastatic tumour, post neurosurgery
    pulmonary — pneumonia, abscess, TB
    drugs — vincristine, cyclophosphamide
    carbamazepine, antidepressants (TCAs, SSRIs)

Syndrome of inappropriate antidiuretic hormone secretion (SIADH)

This syndrome is characterized by the excessive and inappropriate secretion of antidiuretic hormone (ADH) either by a tumour or as the result of other influences acting on the posterior pituitary gland (Table 27.12). There is a strong association with small cell carcinoma of the lung and SIADH occurs less commonly with a variety of other tumours. In SIADH there is reduced renal excretion of water, leading to a state of water intoxication with hyponatraemia and hypotonicity of the plasma.

The signs and symptoms of SIADH depend on the severity of the hyponatraemia and the rapidity of onset. Symptoms are uncommon until the serum sodium falls below 125 mmol/l or the plasma osmolality below 250 mmol/kg. The initial symptoms are nonspecific and include anorexia, nausea and general malaise. With progressive hyponatraemia and hypotonicity, signs and symptoms of cerebral oedema develop with headache, lethargy, confusion and agitation, leading to obtundation, seizures and coma, which can be fatal.

Table 27.13 Diagnosis of SIADH

	SIADH	Normal
Serum sodium	<125mmol/L	135-145 mmol/L
Plasma osmolality	<270 mmol/L	280-300 mmol/L
Urine osmolality	usually >500mmol/L	50-1200 mmol/L

The diagnosis of SIADH is made on the basis of a low serum sodium, low plasma osmolality, and a urine osmolality reflecting inappropriately concentrated urine. Other conditions may occasionally produce a similar picture and it is customary to exclude the presence of dehydration or hepatic, cardiac, renal, adrenal and thyroid dysfunction.

Treatment

Treatment depends on the severity of the syndrome, the cause and the stage of the patient's disease. Mild cases usually respond well to fluid restriction. The antibiotic, demeclocycline,

Table 27.14 Management of SIADH

Correct or treat cause, where possible
Demeclocycline 300-600mg PO q12h

Fluid management
    se Na >120 mmol/L and asymptomatic
        fluid restriction: 500-1000 ml/d
    se Na 110 120 mmol/L without serious symptoms
        fluid restriction: 500 ml/d
        frusemide 40-80mg PO or IV q6h
        replacement of urinary electrolyte losses (IV saline)
    se Na <110 mmol/L or serious symptoms
        3% hypertonic saline 1l q6-8h
        frusemide 40-80mg IV q6-8h
        cardiac failure: additional frusemide, decrease infusion rate
        neurological deterioration: dexamethasone 4-20mg IV, mannitol 25-50g IV

is particularly useful for patients in whom fluid restriction is otherwise undesirable, and for those patients with SIADH due to recurrent cancer which is unlikely to respond to further anticancer therapy. More severe SIADH requires special management of fluids (Table 27.14).

Hyperkalaemia

Hyperkalaemia in patients with cancer is most frequently due to renal impairment but can occur for other reasons (Table 27.15). Hyperkalaemia predisposes to cardiac arrhythmias that can be fatal. Treatment is that of the cause. Serum potassium levels can be reduced by administration of intravenous glucose and insulin; bicarbonate is also given if acidosis is present. The cation exchange resin sodium polystyrene sulfonate (15–60g PO or PR) will help control hyperkalaemia.

Table 27.15 Causes of hyperkalaemia

Renal impairment	renal disease, obstruction
Reduced aldosterone	adrenal failure, aminoglutethimide
Potassium-sparing diuretics	spironolactone, amiloride, triamterene
Tumour lysis syndrome	
Haemolysis	improper specimen collection

Hypokalaemia and ectopic ACTH

Causes of hypokalaemia relevant to patients with advanced cancer are shown in Table 27.16. Hypokalaemia causes muscle weakness and cramps and, if severe, constipation and paralytic ileus. More importantly, it predisposes to cardiac arrhythmias that can be life threatening. Treatment is with oral or parenteral supplements in addition to therapy directed at the underlying cause.

Table 27.16 Causes of hypokalaemia

Inadequate intake, malnutrition	Mineralocorticoid excess
Gastrointestinal losses	hyperaldosteronism
vomiting, nasogastric drainage	mineralocorticoid administration
intestinal fistulas, diarrhoea	Corticosteroid excess
Renal losses	Cushing's syndrome
diuretics	ectopic ACTH production
osmotic diuresis (hyperglycaemia)	corticosteroid administration
antibiotics, corticosteroids	

Ectopic ACTH

The secretion of adrenocorticotrophic hormone (ACTH) by tumours will cause excess cortisone secretion by the adrenal gland, leading to a type of Cushing's syndrome. Ectopic ACTH secretion is characteristically associated with small cell carcinoma of the lung and less often with other tumours. Ectopic ACTH secretion produces a syndrome of hypokalaemia, profound muscle weakness, hyperglycaemia, weight loss and oedema; hypertension is sometimes present. The characteristic physical features of Cushing's syndrome including truncal obesity, cutaneous striae and Cushingoid (moon) facies, are usually absent.

The diagnosis of ectopic ACTH production is made on the findings of hypokalaemic alkalosis, increased cortisol levels without diurnal variation, and increased levels of ACTH that do not suppress with dexamethasone administration.

Treatment. Treatment is primarily directed at the underlying tumour. If the tumour is not amenable to therapy, or whilst such treatment is being initiated, the use of drugs that suppress adrenal function can be of value. Ketoconazole (400–1200mg/d) is the drug of choice and produces symptomatic and biochemical improvement in the majority of patients[14]. Alternatives are aminoglutethimide and metyrapone, both of which may cause troublesome toxicity in the doses required. Doses are adjusted according to urinary cortisol excretion. If adrenal suppression is achieved, patients will require corticosteroid replacement at physiological dosage. Ectopic ACTH production can sometimes be inhibited by the somatostatin analogue, octreotide.[15, 16]

Hyperglycaemia

Hyperglycaemia occurs in diabetes mellitus and the condition may be unmasked or aggravated by the administration of corticosteroids or diuretics (Table 27.17). Hyperglycaemia is characteristic of ectopic ACTH secretion and can also be caused by substances secreted by rare endocrine tumours including glucagonomas and somatostatinomas. In addition, a significant proportion of patients with cancer have reduced glucose tolerance for reasons that are not fully understood.

Treatment. Treatment is directed at the cause, where possible, and significant hyperglycaemia is managed with either oral hypoglycaemic agents or insulin.

Table 27.17 Causes of hyperglycaemia

Diabetes mellitus

Corticosteroid excess
    administration of corticosteroids
    ectopic ACTH secretion
Uncommon endocrine tumours

Diuretics : frusemide, thiazides, chlorthalidone, ethacrynic acid
Glucose intolerance (cancer related)

Hypoglycaemia

Hypoglycaemia occurs as a result of malnutrition or too much insulin (Table 27.18). Tumour-related hypoglycaemia occurs with large retroperitoneal or intrathoracic tumours, most often a soft tissue sarcoma, mesothelioma or hepatoma. These tumours are thought to produce insulin growth factor (IGF II), which both promotes the utilization of glucose and inhibits the compensatory processes designed to restore the blood level to normal.[17] Patients with extensive hepatic infiltration can develop hypoglycaemia, possibly related to lack of glucagon reserves or to the mechanism described above.

Table 27.18 Causes of hypoglycaemia

Starvation
Excess insulin: iatrogenic, insulinomas
Tumour related hypoglycaemia: soft tissue sarcoma, mesothelioma, hepatoma
Extensive liver metastases

Hypoglycaemic attacks may be heralded by tremor, hunger and sweating. More commonly, they present with weakness, fatigue, dizziness, confusion and somnolence. Seizures and coma can occur in severe cases.

Treatment. Treatment of tumour-related hypoglycaemia is primarily directed at the tumour. Symptomatic management involves the regular ingestion of food or sugar. Corticosteroids may suppress tumour production of IGF II. In severe or resistant cases, treatment with glucagon, octreotide or growth hormone can be tried.[17] Diazoxide, which inhibits insulin secretion, and octreotide are used for patients with insulinomas.[18]

Hypomagnesaemia

Hypomagnesaemia occurs in patients with cancer because of poor intake or abnormal losses from the renal or gastrointestinal tracts (Table 27.19). Hypomagnesaemia causes muscle weakness, cramps and paraesthesiae.[11] The importance of hypomagnesaemia is that it often causes hypocalcaemia and is frequently associated with hypokalaemia. Hypocalcaemia that is secondary to hypomagnesaemia is unresponsive to therapy with calcium until the magnesium deficit is corrected. Similarly, recalcitrant hypokalaemia may be secondary to hypomagnesaemia and will resolve after magnesium replacement.

Table 27.19 Causes of hypomagnesaemia

Poor intake	malnutrition
Gastrointestinal	prolonged nasogastric drainage, malabsorption, diarrhoea
Renal loss	platinum drugs, diuretics, aminoglycosides, amphotericin

Adrenal insufficiency

Adrenal insufficiency or failure occurs in patients with advanced cancer more frequently than has previously been recognized. Causes include metastatic infiltration, therapy with aminoglutethimide or metyrapone, or the sudden withdrawal of corticosteroids after treatment lasting more than one or two weeks. Typical clinical features include weakness and fatigue, anorexia, hyperpigmentation, and postural hypotension. The symptoms and signs of adrenal insufficiency can be precipitated by infection or other stress. Investigations show hyponatraemia and hyperkalaemia. If appropriate, the diagnosis can be established by an ACTH stimulation test. Treatment is by adequate physiological corticosteroid replacement (cortisone acetate 25mg in the morning,12.5mg in the early evening). Mineralocorticoid replacement (fludrocortisone 0.05–0.1mg/d) is also required for patients with no effective adrenal function. Physiological doses of dexamethasone or prednisolone do not provide adequate mineralocorticoid coverage and should be accompanied by fludrocortisone.

Tumour lysis syndrome

The tumour lysis syndrome occurs when effective chemotherapy is given to certain chemosensitive tumours. It characteristically occurs with acute leukaemia, Burkitt's lymphoma and occasionally with other lymphoproliferative diseases. Within hours of receiving chemotherapy, massive tumour cell lysis causes hyperkalaemia, hyperphosphataemia, hyperuricaemia and hypocalcaemia. Untreated, the tumour lysis syndrome is usually fatal due to cardiac arrhythmias and renal failure. Treatment is by vigorous intravenous hydration and correction of the various metabolic abnormalities.

Carcinoid syndrome

Carcinoid tumours most frequently occur in the ileum and appendix with a small proportion occurring in the colon and rectum; about 10% of primary carcinoid tumours are pulmonary. The carcinoid syndrome occurs when tumour products are released into the systemic circulation by pulmonary tumours or from the hepatic metastases of gastrointestinal tumours.[19, 20]

The carcinoid syndrome comprises cutaneous flushing, diarrhoea, wheezing and right heart failure. The metabolic symptoms are caused by serotonin as well as a host of other substances released from the tumours including kallikrein, substance P and other neuropeptides, prostaglandins, histamine and catecholamines. Pulmonary carcinoid tumours, but not those from the gastrointestinal tract, may also secrete ACTH and ADH. The cardiac disease involves a characteristic deposition on the valves of the right side of the heart, causing tricuspid incompetence and pulmonary stenosis. The carcinoid syndrome has usually been present for more than five years before carcinoid heart disease becomes clinically evident.

Treatment

Therapy of the carcinoid syndrome (Table 27.20) includes inhaled salbutamol for wheezing anxd standard therapy for diarrhoea. Various antiserotonin agents have been used for the treatment of the flushing and diarrhoea. Cyproheptadine is reported to lessen diarrhoea, but not flushing. Flushing is attributed to the release of histamine and some patients benefit from treatment with antihistamines. The 5HT$_3$ receptor antagonist, ondansetron, can be effective for diarrhoea and nausea, but rarely affects the flushing.[20]

Table 27.20 Treatment of carcinoid syndrome

Standard therapy
    diarrhoea: loperamide, diphenoxylate
    bronchospasm: salbutamol, theophylline

Blocking agents
    cyproheptadine 4mg PO q8h
    antihistamines
    ondansetron 8mg PO q8h

Somatostatin analogues
    octreotide   0.1mg SC q8-12h, and titrate
    octreotide LAR 20mg IM q4w, and titrate
    lanreotide SR   30mg IM q14d, and titrate

Somatostatin analogues. The introduction of the somatostatin analogue, octreotide, greatly improved the treatment of the carcinoid syndrome. About 80% of patients have improvement in flushing and diarrhoea with doses of 400μg/d. Most patients will show response for more than a year, and one-third for more than two years. When symptoms recur, increasing the dose is sometimes effective. The only common adverse effect is transient pain at the injection site. Insulin-dependent diabetics may require less insulin. A long acting preparation of octreotide (octreotide LAR) and of another somatostatin analogue, lanreotide (lanreotide SR), give equivalent biochemical and symptomatic control and are considerably easier to administer.[20] Chronic therapy is associated with an increased incidence of gallstones.

Carcinoid crisis. Carcinoid crisis is a potentially life-threatening event that occurs in patients with the carcinoid syndrome, usually associated with stress such as general anaesthesia. There is a severe and persistent flush associated with abdominal pain and diarrhoea. There can be severe hypotension or hypertension and CNS depression. Intravenous octreotide usually reverses this syndrome promptly; it is recommended that all patients with carcinoid tumours should be treated with octreotide for at least 24 hours before surgery or anaesthesia.

Islet cell carcinomas

Pancreatic islet cell carcinomas are rare tumours, a proportion of which will recur, metastasize and prove fatal.[18] They produce a range of active hormonal substances, which produce a variety of different clinical syndromes (Table 27.21). Insulinomas may be treated with diazoxide, which inhibits the release of insulin; octreotide therapy is successful in a proportion of patients. The Zollinger-Ellison syndrome (abdominal pain, severe peptic ulcer disease) is treated with high doses of H_2-receptor antagonists or a proton pump inhibitor. Octreotide is frequently effective with tumours secreting glucagon or vasoactive intestinal polypeptides (VIP), although the responses may not be durable. The treatment of the other syndromes listed is dealt with elsewhere in this chapter.

Table 27.21 Clinical features of pancreatic islet cell carcinomas

Hormone	Clinical syndrome
insulin	hypoglycaemia
gastrin	Zollinger-Ellison syndrome
glucagon	diabetes, rash, muscle weakness
vasoactive intestinal polypeptide	watery diarrhoea
parathyroid hormone	hypercalcaemia
serotonin	carcinoid syndrome
adrenocorticotrophic hormone	ectopic ACTH syndrome
antidiuretic hormone	SIADH
somatostatin	diabetes, cholelithiasis, steatorrhoea

Gynaecomastia

Male patients are sometimes quite concerned about gynaecomastia. Examination shows unilateral, or more often bilateral, tenderness and breast swelling with firm plaque-like subareolar tissue.

Gynaecomastia can be caused by a deficiency of androgens or a relative or absolute excess of oestrogens. Some of the causes encountered in men with cancer are shown in Table 27.22. If a drug is suspected, the offending agent should be stopped, if possible; however, most of the causes are not reversible and treatment is by reassurance.[21]

Table 27.22 Gynaecomastia

Diminished androgen	Drugs (various mechanisms)
orchidectomy	digoxin
decreased synthesis	spironolactone
old age	cimetidine
oestrogens, progestogens, GnRH analogues	ranitidine
decreased action: antiandrogens	ketoconazole
Increased oestrogen	antidepressants (TCAs)
oestrogen therapy	antihypertensives
oestrogen secreting tumours	omeprazole
gonadotrophin secreting tumours	simvastatin
liver disease	

References

1   Warrell, R.P. (2001). Metabolic emergencies. In *Cancer. Principles and Practice of Oncology. 6th edition* (ed. V.T. De Vita, S. Hellman and S.A. Rosenberg). Philadelphia, Lippincott, Williams and Wilkins.

2   Morton, A.R. and Ritch, P.S. (2002). Hypercalcemia. In *Principles and Practice of Palliative Care and Supportive Oncology* (ed. A.M. Berger, R.K. Portenoy and D.E. Weissman). Philadelphia, Lippincott, Williams and Wilkins.

3   Theriault, R.L., et al. (1999). Pamidronate reduces skeletal morbidity in women with advanced breast cancer and lytic bone lesions: a randomized, placebo-controlled trial. Protocol 18 Aredia Breast Cancer Study Group. *Journal of Clinical Oncology* 17, 846–54.

4   Hortobagyi, G.N., et al. (1998). Long-term prevention of skeletal complications of metastatic breast cancer with pamidronate. Protocol 19 Aredia Breast Cancer Study Group. *Journal of Clinical Oncology* 16, 2038–44.

5   Berenson, J.R., et al. (1998). Long-term pamidronate treatment of advanced multiple myeloma patients reduces skeletal events. Myeloma Aredia Study Group. *Journal of Clinical Oncology* 16, 593–602.

6   Rosen, L.S., et al. (2001). Zoledronic acid versus pamidronate in the treatment of skeletal metastases in patients with breast cancer or osteolytic lesions of multiple myeloma: a phase III, double-blind, comparative trial. *Cancer J* 7, 377–87.

7   Major, P., et al. (2001). Zoledronic acid is superior to pamidronate in the treatment of hypercalcemia of malignancy: a pooled analysis of two randomized, controlled clinical trials. *Journal of Clinical Oncology* 19, 558–67.

8   Body, J.J., Louviaux, I. and Dumon, J.C. (2000). Decreased efficacy of bisphosphonates for recurrences of tumor-induced hypercalcemia. *Supportive Care in Cancer* 8, 398–404.

9   Ralston, S.H., et al. (1997). Dose-response study of ibandronate in the treatment of cancer-associated hypercalcaemia. *British Journal of Cancer* 75, 295–300.

10 Bushinsky, D.A. and Monk, R.D. (1998). Electrolyte quintet: Calcium. *Lancet* 352, 306–11.

11 Weisinger, J.R. and Bellorin-Font, E. (1998). Magnesium and phosphorus. *Lancet* 352, 391–6.

12 Adrogue, H.J. and Madias, N.E. (2000). Hypernatremia. *New England Journal of Medicine* 342, 1493–9.

13 Adrogue, H.J. and Madias, N.E. (2000). Hyponatremia. *New England Journal of Medicine* 342, 1581–9.

14 Winquist, E.W., et al. (1995). Ketoconazole in the management of paraneoplastic Cushing's syndrome secondary to ectopic adrenocorticotropin production. *Journal of Clinical Oncology* 13, 157–64.

15 Woodhouse, N.J., et al. (1993). Acute and long-term effects of octreotide in patients with ACTH-dependent Cushing's syndrome. *American Journal of Medicine* 95, 305–8.

16 Vignati, F. and Loli, P. (1996). Additive effect of ketoconazole and octreotide in the treatment of severe adrenocorticotropin-dependent hypercortisolism. *Journal of Clinical Endocrinology and Metabolism* 81, 2885–90.

17 Ford-Dunn, S., Smith, A. and Sykes, N. (2002). Tumour-induced hypoglycaemia. *Palliative Medicine* 16, 357–8.

18 Alexander, H.R. and Jensen, R.J. (2001). Pancreatic endocrine tumours. In *Cancer. Principles and Practice of Oncology. 6th edition* (ed. V.T. De Vita, S. Hellman and S.A. Rosenberg). Philadelphia, Lippincott, Williams and Wilkins.

19 Kulke, M.H. and Mayer, R.J. (1999). Carcinoid tumors. *New England Journal of Medicine* 340, 858–68.

20 Jensen, R.J. and Doherty, G.M. (2001). Carcinoid tumors and the carcinoid syndrome. In *Cancer. Principles and Practice of Oncology. 6th edition* (ed. V.T. De Vita, S. Hellman and S.A. Rosenberg). Philadelphia, Lippincott, Williams and Wilkins.

21 Braunstein, G.D. (1993). Gynecomastia. *New England Journal of Medicine* 328, 490–5.

28

Constitutional

Anorexia	Dehydration
Cachexia	Fever and sweating
Asthenia	Hormonal flushes

Anorexia

Anorexia, or a reduced desire to eat, occurs at some stage in all patients with advanced cancer. Diminished food intake predisposes to weight loss, but it is only one contributing factor in the cachexia syndrome, which includes a number of metabolic disturbances (see Cachexia).

Centres in the hypothalamus are responsible for coordinating the various stimuli related to hunger and appetite. Under normal circumstances appetite is stimulated by gustatory, olfactory and visual stimuli, and reduced by a full stomach. The centres are also sensitive to the arteriovenous gradient of blood sugar, a high gradient and a low gradient causing suppression and stimulation of appetite, respectively. There is also input from cortical centres, reflecting emotional and psychological influences.

The causes of anorexia are listed in Table 28.1. Patients with advanced cancer frequently have multiple causes. In some patients anorexia is due to the presence of the cancer *per se* and it has been shown that some tumour products and tumour necrosis factor (TNF) can have a profound anorectic effect. Aversion to certain foods should be distinguished from true anorexia in which there is aversion to all food.

Treatment

Treatment of anorexia is important for two reasons. First, having a reasonable appetite and eating well improves the patient's morale and reduces the anxiety of family members. Second, the preservation of optimal nutrition will improve tolerance of any anticancer treatment and may delay the onset of cachexia.

Treatment of cause. Wherever possible, treatment is directed at the cause and many of those listed in Table 28.1 are amenable to some degree of palliation.

General measures. There are a number of general measures that can be taken which may improve appetite (Table 28.2). The patient's medications are reviewed. Pain control needs to be adequate. The assistance of a dietician may be invaluable, particularly for those patients who have developed perversions of appetite and for those with particular religious or cultural

Table 28.1 Causes of anorexia

Cancer	
Pain	
Intracranial disease	metastases, radiotherapy
Abnormal taste, smell	cancer
	stomatitis
	malodorous ulcer or fungating tumour
	radiotherapy, chemotherapy, other drugs
Stomatitis	mucositis, infection
	chemotherapy, radiotherapy
Gastrointestinal	oesophagitis, dysphagia
	small stomach: gastrectomy, linitis plastica
	gastric compression: hepatomegaly, splenomegaly, ascites
	gastric distension, delayed gastric emptying
	bowel obstruction, constipation
	hepatic metastases
Metabolic	electrolyte imbalance: sodium, calcium, sugar
	organ failure: liver, kidney, adrenal
Infections	
Drugs	
Psychological	anxiety, depression, disinterest
	intolerance of institutional food, unappetizing food
Religious or cultural	

Table 28.2 Management of anorexia

Treat or palliate the underlying cause
Activity, exercise
Dietary
dietary advice (dietician)
small frequent meals
what they want, when they want it
tasty, visually appealing food
eat sitting at a table, in a room free of odours
Appetite stimulants
alcohol
prokinetic agent: metoclopramide 10mg q6h
corticosteroid: prednisolone 15-30mg/d
progestogen: megestrol acetate 160-800mg/d
cannabinoid: dronabinol 5mg/d
Explanation, counselling

customs. For other patients, simple measures including small frequent meals, being served what they want and when they want it, eating sitting up in a room free of odours, and the provision of tasty, visually appealing food can be beneficial. Activity, even passive exercise, can help appetite.

Appetite stimulants. The use of appetite stimulants can be of benefit. However, with the exception of progestogens and dronabinol, they have no effect on the development or progression of cachexia. A small amount of alcohol taken before or with meals may stimulate appetite as well as improving mood and providing a few calories. The prokinetic drugs, metoclopramide and cisapride, will improve anorexia related to delayed gastric emptying and gastroparesis. Other appetite stimulants found to be not significantly superior to placebo in RCTs include cyproheptadine,[1] hydrazine,[2] pentoxifylline,[3] and fish oil.[4]

Corticosteroids will stimulate appetite and improve well being in the majority of patients, although the effect may last only a few weeks. Prednisolone 30 mg/d or dexamethasone 4 mg/d is given for 5 to 7 days; the dose can be doubled for a further trial period if there is no response or when the initial response wanes.

Treatment with megestrol acetate leads to improved appetite and weight gain, although there may be no improvement in quality of life measures or survival.[5,6] There is a dose-response effect up to doses of 800 mg/d[7] (Table 28.3). A comparison of dexamethasone and megestrol showed similar improvements in appetite and non-fluid weight gain.[8] Adverse effects of megestrol include fluid retention, hypertension and thrombophlebitis, which are dose dependent.

The cannabinoid, dronabinol, has been reported to improve appetite and weight in patients with cancer.[9] In a comparative study, megestrol produced significantly more improvement of appetite and weight gain than dronabinol, and the combination of the two treatments did not confer any additional benefit over megestrol alone (Table 28.3).[10] Adverse effects of dronabinol, including sedation, dizziness and dysphoria, may be troublesome in elderly or frail patients.

Table 28.3 Treatment of anorexia: selected RCTs

Author	n	Intervention	Outcome
Loprinzi[7]	342	megestrol 160 vs 480 vs 800 vs 1280mg/d	improved appetite dose-related (pS)
Bruera[11]	84	megestrol 480mg/d vs placebo	megestrol: increased appetite (pS)
Loprinzi[8]	475	megestrol 800mg vs dexamethasone 3mg	similar increase in appetite (pNS)
Jatoi[10]	469	megestrol 800mg vs dronabinol 5mg vs both	megestrol: appetite superior to dronabinol (pS); no additional benefit with combination

Counselling. Anorexia and poor nutritional intake frequently cause much distress for patients and families and require careful discussion and explanation. Family members have to be dissuaded from trying to force patients to eat more than they want, as this simply causes more physical and psychological distress for the patient. When anorexia is primarily due to advanced and progressing cancer, it may need to be explained that enteral or parenteral nutrition will not affect the patient's anorexia or the progression of cachexia.

Cachexia

Cachexia is the progressive wasting seen in patients with advancing cancer. It is not simply a form of starvation and intensive nutritional therapies, including enteral and parenteral nutrition, do not reverse or prevent it. It is primarily due to alterations in protein, carbohydrate and lipid metabolism caused by inflammatory cytokines released by the tumour or in response to it (Table 28.4).[12–14] The role of malnutrition is minor except for patients with gastrointestinal obstruction or dysfunction. The nutritional requirements of the tumour also make a minor contribution.

Table 28.4   Causes of cachexia

Metabolic abnormalities caused by cytokines released by tumour   TNF, interleukin-1and -6, interferon-γ

Malnutrition
    poor intake due to anorexia (see Table 28.1)
    functional blockage: mouth, oesophagus, stomach
    malabsorption
    vomiting, diarrhoea, fistulas
    protein loss: ulceration, haemorrhage, repeated paracenteses
    general effects of surgery, radiotherapy, chemotherapy

Tumour metabolism

The clinical features of cachexia are well known (Table 28.5). General weakness, ill-fitting dentures, or early satiety will further compromise nutritional intake. Progressive cachexia is often associated with anxiety or depression, for both patient and family. The maintenance of social relationships may become increasingly difficult.

Table 28.5   Clinical features of cachexia

Weight loss	Pallor, anaemia
Lethargy	Oedema (hypoalbuminaemia)
Muscle wasting, asthenia	Poor wound healing
Loss of body fat	Pressure sores

Treatment

The treatment options are listed in Table 28.6. Where possible and appropriate, causes of anorexia or malnutrition are corrected or palliated. Systemic therapy for sensitive tumours, if successful, may halt the progression of cachexia.

Dietary. Dietary and nutritional therapy may improve a patient's psychological state and reduce family anxieties. A patient will feel more cared for if concern is expressed about nutritional intake and dietary advice given. General measures include providing small frequent meals, of what the patient wants and when they want it. Liquid nutritional supplements containing most of the dietary requirements of protein and carbohydrate are commercially available. The use of a multivitamin supplement will do no harm and may be appreciated by the patient and family.

Table 28.6 Treatment of cachexia

Correct or palliate cause of malnutrition, anorexia
Treat tumour, where feasible
Drug treatment of cachexia progestogen: megestrol 160-800mg/d cannabinoid: dronabinol 5mg/d
Dietary measures general measures dietary supplements enteral nutrition parenteral nutrition
Management of the psychosocial consequences

Drug therapy. There is no satisfactory drug therapy for cachexia. Corticosteroids, alcohol and metoclopramide may reduce anorexia but have no effect on the metabolic abnormalities of cachexia. The progestogens may exert an anabolic effect, increasing lean body mass and fat, but a significant effect on survival has not been demonstrated (Table 28.7).[7, 15] The cannabinoid, dronabinol, has been reported to lead to weight gain in cancer patients.[9] In a comparative study, megestrol produced significantly more weight gain than dronabinol, and the combination of the two treatments did not confer any additional benefit over megestrol alone.[10] Treatment with thalidomide, which suppresses tumour necrosis factor-alpha (TNF-α), led to increased weight and lean body mass in a small group of patients with advanced cancer.[16]

A number of other treatments are under investigation for the management of cachexia, including human growth hormone and anabolic steroids.[17] Treatment with an omega-3 fatty acid derived from fish oil, eicosapentaenoic acid (EPA), ameliorated some of the biochemical changes associated with cachexia in patients with advanced cancer,[18, 19] but was not shown to be of clinical value in an RCT.[4] Treatment with infusions of adenosine 5-triphosphate (ATP) prevented weight loss in a small RCT of patients with advanced lung cancer.[20] Treatment with a combination of nutrients designed to reduce protein catabolism and increase synthesis—hydroxymethylbutyrate (HMB), L-arginine, and L-glutamine—led to increased weight and fat free mass in a small RCT of patients with advanced cancer.[21] In an RCT of melatonin and supportive care compared to supportive care alone, patients treated with melatonin were reported to have a significantly lower incidence of cachexia.[22]

Table 28.7 Treatment of cachexia: selected RCTs

Author	n	Intervention	Outcome
Loprinzi[7]	342	megestrol 160 vs 480 vs 800 vs 1280mg/d	weight gain dose-related (pNS)
Vaddell[15]	150	megestrol 480mg/d vs 160mg/d vs placebo	megestrol 480mg/d: ≠ weight compared to 160mg/d or placebo (pS)
Jatoi[10]	469	megestrol 800mg vs dronabinol 5mg vs both	megestrol: more weight gain (pS); no additional benefit with combination

Enteral feeding. Enteral feeding via a nasogastric tube or gastrostomy has little place in the management of patients with advanced cancer, with the exception of patients with gastrointestinal obstruction or dysfunction who may otherwise suffer starvation. For other patients, enteral feeding will not reverse or prevent cachexia. The adverse effects of enteral feeding include fluid overload, abdominal cramps and diarrhoea.

Parenteral nutrition. For patients with advanced cancer, total parenteral nutrition (TPN) is not effective in improving either survival or the response to anticancer treatment and is associated with significant complications and cost. The exception is a patient who will be temporarily unable to eat for two weeks or more because of cancer treatment, for whom TPN would be entirely appropriate.

Counselling. The compassionate management of the psychological and social consequences of cachexia is difficult but important. For both the patient and the family, progressive cachexia represents progression of the cancer and counselling and discussions may facilitate acceptance and understanding. Family members need to be dissuaded from trying to force the patient to eat, as this will only cause physical and psychological distress for the patient. They need to be helped to show love to the patient by means other than feeding them or pressuring them to eat.

Asthenia: weakness and fatigue

Asthenia is generalized weakness associated with fatigue and lethargy. It is one of the most common symptoms in patients with advanced cancer, with profound effects on the quality of life.[23] It is most frequently associated with progression of the cancer although other causes (Table 28.8) need to be considered, as some are amenable to treatment or palliation. Asthenia occurs most frequently in patients with advanced disease who have lost a significant amount

Table 28.8 Causes of generalized weakness and asthenia

Neuromuscular	cachexia-related loss of muscle mass
	cachexia-related muscular dysfunction
	myasthenic syndrome (Lambert-Eaton)
	polymyositis
	overactivity, prolonged immobility
	polyneuropathy: carcinomatous or independent of cancer
	intracranial tumour, paraneoplastic encephalopathies
	acute confusion or delirium
Metabolic	electrolyte imbalance, dehydration
	renal, hepatic failure
Endocrine	adrenal insufficiency, ectopic ACTH secretion, diabetes
Malnutrition	inanition, malabsorption
Anaemia	
Infection	
Psychological	anxiety, depression, dependency, boredom, insomnia
Anticancer therapy	radiotherapy, chemotherapy, interferon
Drugs	opioids, tranquillizers, sedatives, antidepressants, diuretics, others

of weight and muscle mass. Muscular weakness may also occur in patients without weight loss due to cachexia-related changes in skeletal muscle.

All patients with advanced cancer suffer asthenia to some degree at some stage of their illness. The patient tires easily and is progressively less able to perform activities.

Assessment. A patient's weakness and lethargy, or lack of it, are usually recorded as their performance score. The two scales most commonly used are the Karnofsky and the Eastern Cooperative Oncology Group scales (Table 28.9). The grading criteria for treatment-related fatigue are listed in Table 28.10.

Table 28.9 Performance status scales

ECOG score	description	Karnofsky score	description
0	fully active	100	normal
		90	able to carry on normal activity
1	ambulatory, capable of light or sedentary work	80	normal activity with effort
		70	cares for self, unable to do normal activity, work
2	ambulatory >50% of waking hours capable of self-care, not work	60	requires occasional assistance, able to care for most of own needs
		50	requires considerable assistance
3	confined to bed or chair >50% of waking hours capable of only limited self-care	40	disabled, requires special care and assistance
		30	severely disabled death not imminent
4	completely disabled capable of no self-care totally confined to bed or chair	20	very sick, hospitalization indicated death not imminent
		10	moribund, fatal processes progressing rapidly

There are a number of instruments that measure cancer-related fatigue, which can be used to compare patients, or to measure changes with therapy or disease progression.[25, 26] Unidimensional instruments such as visual analogue scales (VAS) and verbal descriptor scales can be employed. Multidimensional instruments that measure the psychological and quality of life correlates of fatigue provide more information. These include the Brief Fatigue

Table 28.10 NCI CTC grading criteria for treatment-related fatigue[24]

0	none
1	increased fatigue, but not altering normal activities
2	moderate (e.g. ↓ 1 ECOG level or 20% Karnofsky), or difficulty performing activities
3	severe (e.g. ↓ ≥2 ECOG levels or 40% Karnofsky), or inability to perform some activities
4	disabling, bedridden

Inventory (BFI),[27] the Functional Assessment of Cancer Therapy-Fatigue scale (FACT-F),[28] the fatigue subscale of the EORTC Quality of Life Questionnaire C30 (QLQ-C30),[29] and the Multidimensional Fatigue Inventory (MFI).[30]

Treatment

Treatment is that of the cause, where possible. Correction of some of the uncommon metabolic disturbances listed in Table 28.8 may lead to significant improvement. Transfusion will be of benefit for patients who are severely anaemic but, unless there has been recent active blood loss, the response is often suboptimal and transient. The use of epoetin is of benefit to some patients with advanced cancer and may counteract weakness and fatigue (see Table 22.5, Chapter 22).

For other patients, management of weakness and fatigue requires a multidisciplinary approach involving the setting of realistic goals, education and counselling, together with pharmacological and nonpharmacological therapies.[26, 31–33]

Drug therapy. Corticosteroids will provide symptomatic improvement in the majority of patients but the effect may only last a few weeks. The mechanism of action is unknown, but is probably due to an improvement in the patient's general feeling of well being. Corticosteroids need to be used with care in treating asthenia because of the risk of proximal myopathy with continued therapy. Methylphenidate produces symptomatic improvement in fatigue for a proportion of patients with advanced cancer,[34–37] presumably by a central mechanism. Patients with advanced cancer treated with melatonin are reported to have significantly less asthenia.[22]

Physical therapy. When weakness is mild, exertion and activity are encouraged, within the patient's physical limitations. Physiotherapy can be of benefit, both physically and psychologically. Programs of exercise are of benefit in the treatment of fatigue for cancer patients earlier in the course of their disease,[26, 38] but the experience with the palliative care population is limited.[39]

As weakness progresses, activities providing diversion from a patient's feeling of weakness and helplessness are encouraged, including music, reading, games and hobbies they enjoy. As disability increases further, the patient will need assistance with the activities of daily living. Physical aids including walking frames, wheelchairs and support rails need to be considered. Reorganization of the patient's immediate environment to accommodate reduced mobility will help maintain a feeling of independence. Continued physical exercises and physiotherapy may be of benefit in maintaining dwindling muscle strength.

Counselling. For most patients, progressive weakness is a reflection of advancing disease and there are no correctable or treatable underlying causes. Management consists of physical and psychological supportive therapy to enable them to adjust and cope as well as possible. Psychological adaptation to progressive weakness is the more difficult and the patient and family usually have to redefine goals and expectations.

Dehydration

The inability of some patients with advanced cancer to drink normal amounts may lead to requests from relatives or staff for intravenous or subcutaneous fluids.

Dehydration in patients not terminally ill

Patients unable to take or retain adequate fluids who have signs or symptoms of dehydration should be managed with parenteral fluids.

Dehydration in terminally ill patients

Whether or not terminally ill patients benefit from intravenous or subcutaneous fluid administration is controversial. Decisions have to be individualized and depend very much on how close the patient is to death. A bedridden patient will not suffer the weakness and postural hypotension experienced by a patient still ambulatory.

Proponents of artificial hydration claim dehydration causes a dry mouth, thirst and impaired cognitive function, but the evidence that rehydration is of benefit is equivocal. The state of consciousness was not improved by artificial hydration in one study;[40] the reported reduction in the incidence of agitated delirium associated with the more frequent use of subcutaneous hydration in another may be explained by simultaneous implementation of early opioid rotation.[41] A recently published RCT reported no improvement in cognitive function or delirium after 48 hours of subcutaneous hydration.[42] Dying patients do not complain of thirst and a dry mouth is well palliated with topical therapy.

Alternatively, it can be argued that dehydration is a natural part of the dying process and may be of benefit. Reduced urine output requires less movement needed to void and incontinence is less likely; less gastrointestinal secretions can reduce nausea, vomiting and diarrhoea; less respiratory secretions reduce dyspnoea and terminal congestion; oedema and effusions may be less troublesome and reduced oedema around tumours may aid pain control.

Artificial hydration might have the opposite effect and worsen the patient's situation. There is also the possibility that it will contribute to a lingering or prolonged death. It may give an ambiguous signal or false hope to a patient or family who were otherwise well prepared for the impending death. The equipment necessary for artificial hydration can inhibit physical closeness with family members at a time when such is important, and staff may be more intent on the fluid balance chart than on the patient. Anxious relatives who demand artificial hydration for the terminally ill need to be counselled that it may be of no benefit and that it might even increase the patient's suffering. Decisions about artificial hydration need to be individualized, taking into account each patient's particular clinical circumstances.

Fevers and sweating

The causes of fever in patients with cancer are listed in Table 28.11. Tumour-related fever is due to the release of inflammatory cytokines (interleukin-1 and –6, tumour necrosis factor, and interferon), either by the tumour or in response to it, which act on the temperature regulating centre in the hypothalamus. Cancer-related fevers and sweats occur frequently with renal cell carcinoma, hepatoma, and malignant lymphomas, and less often with a wide variety of other tumours.

Table 28.11 Causes of fever and sweats

Infection
Cancer
Environmental factors
Drug reactions
Transfusion reactions

Treatment

Treatment of fever is that of the cause, where possible. If present, infection is treated, if that is clinically appropriate. Control of disease-related fever is best achieved by control of the tumour. If this is not feasible, minor environmental changes (fewer bedclothes, fan, tepid sponging) may be of benefit. Treatment with paracetamol or one of the NSAIDs is effective for some patients. Treatment with corticosteroids (prednisolone 15–30mg/d) can be considered.[43]

Excessive sweating may respond to NSAIDs, anticholinergic medication (hyoscine hydro-bromide or butylbromide), or thioridazine.[44] A beta-blocker such as propranolol is effective for the sweating associated with anxiety.

Fever with rigors (involuntary shivering) caused by non-haemolytic transfusion reactions, drug infusions (e.g. amphotericin), or related to the disease itself, may respond to pethidine (meperidine) (25mg IV slowly).[45]

Hormonal or hot flushes

Hot flushes ('hot flashes' in American parlance) occur in most women with ovarian failure of whatever cause. Similar symptoms occur in men treated with oestrogens, GnRH analogues or by orchidectomy; they are uncommon with antiandrogen therapy.

Hot flushes are described as starting with a discomfort in the lower abdomen or epigastrium, followed quickly by an intense hot feeling ascending towards the head. There is redness of the skin and sweating, often involving the face and head. The episode is short lived and may be followed by a feeling of exhaustion. Hot drinks and meals, alcohol, a warm room or bed, and emotional upset can precipitate hot flushes.

Treatment

Treatment with oestrogen or combined hormone replacement therapy (HRT) is highly effective for most menopausal women.[46] If oestrogen therapy is poorly tolerated or there is an oestrogen-sensitive tumour, treatment is with a progestogen (megestrol 20mg twice daily); this is equally effective for men who have undergone androgen deprivation therapy (Table 28.12).[47] Other therapies found to be not statistically superior to placebo in RCTs include clonidine,[48, 49] soy phytoestrogen preparations,[50, 51] and black cohosh.[52] Vitamin E produced minor improvements, of questionable clinical significance.[53] Research into the management of hot flushes is complicated by a high placebo response rate.[54, 55] Venlafaxine is effective at higher doses, although adverse effects of anorexia and nausea can be troublesome (Table 28.12).[56] Fluoxetine showed modest benefit.[57] Paroxetine was effective in a pilot study.[58]

Table 28.12 Treatment of hot flushes: selected RCTs

Author	n	Intervention	Outcome
Loprinzi[47]	97F 66M	Megestrol 40mg/d vs placebo	Megestrol: ≥50% ↓ in hot flushes in 74 vs 20% (pS)
Loprinzi[56]	191	Venlafaxine vs placebo	Venlafaxine: ↓ hot flush scores by 60 vs 27% at 4w (pS)
Loprinzi[57]	81	Fluoxetine 20mg/d vs placebo	Fluoxetine: ↓ hot flush scores in 50 vs 36% at 4w (pS)

References

1   Kardinal, C.G., et al. (1990). A controlled trial of cyproheptadine in cancer patients with anorexia and/or cachexia. *Cancer* 65, 2657–62.

2   Loprinzi, C.L., et al. (1994). Randomized placebo-controlled evaluation of hydrazine sulfate in patients with advanced colorectal cancer. *Journal of Clinical Oncology* 12, 1121–5.

3   Goldberg, R.M., et al. (1995). Pentoxifylline for treatment of cancer anorexia and cachexia? A randomized, double-blind, placebo-controlled trial. *Journal of Clinical Oncology* 13, 2856–9.

4   Bruera, E., et al. (2003). Effect of fish oil on appetite and other symptoms in patients with advanced cancer and anorexia/cachexia: a double-blind, placebo-controlled study. *Journal of Clinical Oncology* 21, 129–34.

5   Jatoi, A., et al. (2000). On appetite and its loss. *Journal of Clinical Oncology* 18, 2930–2.

6   Maltoni, M., et al. (2001). High-dose progestins for the treatment of cancer anorexia-cachexia syndrome: a systematic review of randomised clinical trials. *Annals of Oncology* 12, 289–300.

7   Loprinzi, C.L., et al. (1993). Phase iii evaluation of four doses of megestrol acetate as therapy for patients with cancer anorexia and/or cachexia. *Journal of Clinical Oncology* 11, 762–7.

8   Loprinzi, C.L., et al. (1999). Randomized comparison of megestrol acetate versus dexamethasone versus fluoxymesterone for the treatment of cancer anorexia/cachexia. *Journal of Clinical Oncology* 17, 3299–306.

9   Bagshaw, S.M. and Hagen, N.A. (2002). Medical efficacy of cannabinoids and marijuana: a comprehensive review of the literature. *Journal of Palliative Care* 18, 111–22.

10 Jatoi, A., et al. (2002). Dronabinol versus megestrol acetate versus combination therapy for cancer-associated anorexia: a North Central Cancer Treatment Group study. *Journal of Clinical Oncology* 20, 567–73.

11 Bruera, E., et al. (1998). Effectiveness of megestrol acetate in patients with advanced cancer: a randomized, double-blind, crossover study. *Cancer Prevention and Control* 2, 74–8.

12 Bruera, E. and Higginson, I. (ed.) (1996). *Cachexia-Anorexia in Cancer Patients*. Oxford, Oxford University Press.

13 Jatoi, A. and Loprinzi, C.L. (2002). Anorexia/weight loss. In *Principles and Practice of Palliative Care and Supportive Oncology* (ed. A.M. Berger, R.K. Portenoy and D.E. Weissman). Philadelphia, Lippincott, Williams and Wilkins.

14 Strasser, F. and Bruera, E. (2002). Mechanism of cancer cachexia: progress on disentangling a complex problem. *Progress in Palliative Care* 10, 161–67.

15 Vadell, C., et al. (1998). Anticachectic efficacy of megestrol acetate at different doses and versus placebo in patients with neoplastic cachexia. *American Journal of Clinical Oncology* 21, 347–51.

16 Khan, Z.H., et al. (2003). Oesophageal cancer and cachexia: the effect of short-term treatment with thalidomide on weight loss and lean body mass. *Alimentary Pharmacology & Therapeutics* 17, 677–82.

17 Basaria, S., Wahlstrom, J.T. and Dobs, A.S. (2001). Clinical review 138: Anabolic-androgenic steroid therapy in the treatment of chronic diseases. *Journal of Clinical Endocrinology and Metabolism* 86, 5108–17.

18 Gogos, C.A., et al. (1998). Dietary omega-3 polyunsaturated fatty acids plus vitamin e restore immunodeficiency and prolong survival for severely ill patients with generalized malignancy: a randomized control trial. *Cancer* 82, 395–402.

19 Barber, M.D., et al. (2001). Effect of a fish oil-enriched nutritional supplement on metabolic mediators in patients with pancreatic cancer cachexia. *Nutrition and Cancer* 40, 118–24.

20 Agteresch, H.J., et al. (2002). Beneficial effects of adenosine triphosphate on nutritional status in advanced lung cancer patients: a randomized clinical trial. *Journal of Clinical Oncology* 20, 371–8.

21 May, P.E., et al. (2002). Reversal of cancer-related wasting using oral supplementation with a combination of beta-hydroxy-beta-methylbutyrate, arginine, and glutamine. *American Journal of Surgery* 183, 471–9.

22   Lissoni, P. (2002). Is there a role for melatonin in supportive care? *Supportive Care in Cancer* 10, 110–16.

23   Curt, G.A. (2001). Fatigue in cancer. *British Medical Journal* 322, 1560.

24   National Cancer Institute Cancer Therapy Evaluation Program (1998). Common toxicity criteria, version 2.0. <http://ctep.cancer.gov/reporting/ctc.html>

25   Richardson, A. (1998). Measuring fatigue in patients with cancer. *Supportive Care in Cancer* 6, 94–100.

26   Miaskowski, C.A. and Portenoy, R. (2002). Assessment and management of cancer-related fatigue. In *Principles and Practice of Palliative Care and Supportive Oncology* (ed. A.M. Berger, R.K. Portenoy and D.E. Weissman). Philadelphia, Lippincott, Williams and Wilkins.

27   Mendoza, T.R., et al. (1999). The rapid assessment of fatigue severity in cancer patients: use of the brief fatigue inventory. *Cancer* 85, 1186–96.

28   Yellen, S.B., et al. (1997). Measuring fatigue and other anemia-related symptoms with the functional assessment of cancer therapy (FACT) measurement system. *Journal of Pain and Symptom Management* 13, 63–74.

29   Aaronson, N.K., et al. (1993). The European Organization for Research and Treatment of Cancer QLQ-C30: a quality-of-life instrument for use in international clinical trials in oncology. *Journal of the National Cancer Institute* 85, 365–76.

30   Smets, E.M., et al. (1995). The multidimensional fatigue inventory (MFI): psychometric qualities of an instrument to assess fatigue. *Journal of Psychosomatic Research* 39, 315–25.

31   Barnes, E.A. and Bruera, E. (2002). Fatigue in patients with advanced cancer: a review. *International Journal of Gynecological Cancer* 12, 424–8.

32   Coackley, A., et al. (2002). Assessment and management of fatigue in patients with advanced cancer: developing guidelines. *International Journal of Palliative Nursing* 8, 381–8.

33   Wessely, S.C. (2003). Studying nonpharmacological interventions for fatigue. In *Issues in Palliative Care Research* (ed. R. Portenoy and E. Bruera). New York, Oxford University Press.

34   Meyers, C.A., et al. (1998). Methylphenidate therapy improves cognition, mood, and function of brain tumor patients. *Journal of Clinical Oncology* 16, 2522–7.

35   Homsi, J., et al. (2001). A phase II study of methylphenidate for depression in advanced cancer. *American Journal of Hospice and Palliative Care* 18, 403–7.

36   Sarhill, N., et al. (2001). Methylphenidate for fatigue in advanced cancer: a prospective open-label pilot study. *American Journal of Hospice and Palliative Care* 18, 187–92.

37   Sugawara, Y., et al. (2002). Efficacy of methylphenidate for fatigue in advanced cancer patients: a preliminary study. *Palliative Medicine* 16, 261–3.

38   Dimeo, F., Rumberger, B.G. and Keul, J. (1998). Aerobic exercise as therapy for cancer fatigue. *Medicine and Science in Sports and Exercise.* 30, 475–8.

39   Porock, D., et al. (2000). An exercise intervention for advanced cancer patients experiencing fatigue: a pilot study. *Journal of Palliative Care* 16, 30–6.

40   Waller, A., Hershkowitz, M. and Adunsky, A. (1994). The effect of intravenous fluid infusion on blood and urine parameters of hydration and on state of consciousness in terminal cancer patients. *American Journal of Hospice and Palliative Care* 11, 22–7.

41   Bruera, E., et al. (1995). Changing pattern of agitated impaired mental status in patients with advanced cancer: association with cognitive monitoring, hydration, and opioid rotation. *Journal of Pain and Symptom Management* 10, 287–91.

42   Cerchietti, I., et al. (2000). Hypodermoclysis for control of dehydration in terminal-stage cancer. *International Journal of Palliative Nursing* 6, 370–4.

43   Johnson, M. (1996). Neoplastic fever. *Palliative Medicine* 10, 217–24.

44   Hami, F. and Trotman, I. (1999). The treatment of sweating. *European Journal of Palliative Care* 6, 184–87.

45   Johnson, M.J. (1994). Pethidine for the treatment of disease related rigors. *Palliative Medicine* 8, 339–40.

46   Maclennan, A., Lester, S. and Moore, V. (2001). Oral oestrogen replacement therapy versus placebo for hot flushes (Cochrane Review). *Cochrane Database of Systematic Reviews* CD002978

47   Loprinzi, C.L., et al. (1994). Megestrol acetate for the prevention of hot flashes. *New England Journal of Medicine* 331, 347–52.

48   Goldberg, R.M., et al. (1994). Transdermal clonidine for ameliorating tamoxifen-induced hot flashes. *Journal of Clinical Oncology* 12, 155–8.

49   Loprinzi, C.L., et al. (1994). Transdermal clonidine for ameliorating post-orchiectomy hot flashes. *Journal of Urology* 151, 634–6.

50   Quella, S.K., et al. (2000). Evaluation of soy phytoestrogens for the treatment of hot flashes in breast cancer survivors: a North Central Cancer Treatment Group trial. *Journal of Clinical Oncology* 18, 1068–74.

51   van Patten, C.L., et al. (2002). Effect of soy phytoestrogens on hot flashes in postmenopausal women with breast cancer: a randomized, controlled clinical trial. *Journal of Clinical Oncology* 20, 1449–55.

52   Jacobson, J.S., et al. (2001). Randomized trial of black cohosh for the treatment of hot flashes among women with a history of breast cancer. *Journal of Clinical Oncology* 19, 2739–45.

53   Barton, D.L., et al. (1998). Prospective evaluation of vitamin E for hot flashes in breast cancer survivors. *Journal of Clinical Oncology* 16, 495–500.

54   Davis, S.R. (2001). Phytoestrogen therapy for menopausal symptoms? *British Medical Journal* 323, 354–5.

55   Stearns, V. and Hayes, D.F. (2002). Cooling off hot flashes. *Journal of Clinical Oncology* 20, 1436–8.

56   Loprinzi, C.L., et al. (2000). Venlafaxine in management of hot flashes in survivors of breast cancer: a randomised controlled trial. *Lancet* 356, 2059–63.

57   Loprinzi, C.L., et al. (2002). Phase iii evaluation of fluoxetine for treatment of hot flashes. *Journal of Clinical Oncology* 20, 1578–83.

58   Weitzner, M.A., et al. (2002). A pilot trial of paroxetine for the treatment of hot flashes and associated symptoms in women with breast cancer. *Journal of Pain and Symptom Management* 23, 337–45.

29

Adverse effects of anticancer therapy

Radiotherapy
Bone marrow transplantation
Chemotherapy

Biologic therapy
Hormonal therapy

Awareness of the adverse effects of various anticancer therapies is important in palliative care. Patients may still be receiving anticancer treatment when they are first seen by a palliative care service, or such therapy may be considered for the palliation of symptoms. A knowledge of the adverse effects and long term complications of treatments given months or years earlier is also relevant, as they may only become clinically evident during the period the patient is receiving palliative care and in some cases may be mistaken for progression of the cancer.

Radiotherapy

Radiotherapy, or the treatment of cancer with ionizing radiation, is used in three different situations. First, it may be given with curative intent, in which case higher doses will be given and more adverse effects will be expected and considered acceptable. Second, palliative treatment may be given to improve life expectancy. Third, it may be given to patients with advanced disease to relieve symptoms, using the lowest effective dose in the least number of treatment fractions, and following which adverse effects should be uncommon.[1–3]

Adverse effects. The acute effects of radiotherapy occur within days or weeks of treatment and are due to inflammation, oedema and cell death (Table 29.1). Patients receiving radiotherapy, particularly to the head or abdomen, often develop a mild form of radiation sickness with tiredness, fatigue, nausea and anorexia; depression may occur secondarily. The delayed effects of radiotherapy appear months or years after treatment and are predominantly caused by fibrosis

Table 29.1 Adverse effects of radiotherapy

Acute (days/weeks)	Chronic (months/years)
Inflammation	Fibrosis
Oedema	Ischaemia
Cell death	Carcinogenesis

and ischaemia. The other long-term consequence of radiotherapy, carcinogenesis, is of limited relevance in palliative care. Many reviews of the toxicity of radiotherapy have been published.[4, 5] Standardized criteria for grading radiation toxicity have been produced by the Radiation Therapy Oncology Group (RTOG) and the NCI Cancer Therapy Evaluation Program.[6-8]

The severity of the adverse effects of radiotherapy depends on factors pertaining to both the treatment and the patient (Table 29.2). The most important are the volume of tissue irradiated and the effects of irradiation on normal tissues within the treatment field.

Table 29.2 Severity of adverse effects of radiotherapy

Treatment factors	Patient factors
Volume irradiated	General condition, performance status
Body site irradiated	Condition of area to be treated
Total dose	Radiosensitivity of normal tissues in treatment field
Dose per fraction	Other concurrent treatment
Dose rate	surgery
Energy of radiation	chemotherapy

The adverse effects of radiotherapy are summarized in Table 29.3. Most are included in the chapters dealing with specific organ systems involved.

Gastrointestinal

Irradiation of the epigastrium is frequently accompanied by significant nausea and vomiting. Gastritis, mucosal ulceration and haemorrhage may occur. Treatment is with antiemetics (e.g. ondansetron), antacids and dietary advice.

Acute radiation enteritis causes nausea and vomiting, anorexia, colicky abdominal pain, diarrhoea and, less commonly, haemorrhage. Treatment is with analgesics, antiemetics, antidiarrhoeals and dietary modification. Chronic radiation enteritis is due to mucosal and submucosal fibrosis and may present with malabsorption, bowel obstruction, perforation, or enteric fistulas.

Radiation colitis causes diarrhoea and bleeding. Radiation proctitis causes tenesmus, bleeding, and pain. Measures to prevent radiation proctitis are discussed in Chapter 19 (see Table 19.64). Proctitis is treated with stool softeners and a low residue diet, analgesics and antispasmodics, and topical corticosteroids. If there is recurrent tumour in the perirectal or perivesical tissues, rectovaginal or rectovesical fistulas can develop.

The liver is particularly sensitive to radiation. Acute radiation hepatitis with malaise, nausea, anorexia, fever and hepatitic liver function tests occurs after doses of 20–24 Gy. The radiotherapy should be stopped and treatment is symptomatic. Liver failure due to chronic radiation hepatitis should not occur with proper treatment planning.

Stomatitis, xerostomia and oesophagitis are discussed in Chapter19.

Genitourinary

Kidney. Acute radiation nephritis may be asymptomatic. Chronic radiation nephritis causes proteinuria, hypertension and uraemia, which are irreversible.

Bladder. Acute radiation cystitis causes frequency, nocturia, urgency, dysuria, and haematuria. A bladder relaxant medication may improve symptoms (see Table 20.7). Secondary infection is common and is treated appropriately. Sterile dysuria may improve with phenazopyridine (100–200mg PO 8-hourly). Haemorrhagic cystitis can develop (see

Table 29.3 Adverse effects of radiotherapy

	Acute	Delayed
General	radiation sickness	
Skin	erythema, oedema desquamation alopecia, anhidrosis	hypo-, hyper-pigmentation alopecia, anhidrosis telangiectasia, ulceration
Oropharynx	mucositis xerostomia altered taste	xerostomia altered taste dental decay
Oesophagus	oesophagitis	stricture

Stomach	gastritis
	    ulceration, haemorrhage
		chronic gastritis
		    ulceration, haemorrhage

Small bowel	enteritis
	    diarrhoea, haemorrhage
		chronic enteritis
		    malabsorption, stricture

Colon	colitis	stricture

Rectum	proctitis
	    tenesmus, pain, bleeding
		chronic proctitis
		    fistulas, stricture

Liver	hepatitis	liver failure

Kidney	acute nephritis
	    often asymptomatic
		chronic nephritis
		    proteinuria, hypertension,
		    renal failure

Bladder	acute cystitis
	    haemorrhage
		chronic cystitis
		    fibrosis, haemorrhage

Vagina	acute vaginitis
	    secondary infection
		atrophic vaginitis
		    fibrosis, fistulas

Lung	acute pneumonitis	pulmonary fibrosis
Heart	acute pericarditis	chronic pericarditis, constriction
Arteries		accelerated atherosclerosis
Lymphatics		lymphoedema
Brain	radiation sickness somnolence syndrome	brain necrosis, dementia
Spinal cord	acute myelitis Lhermitte's syndrome	transverse myelopathy (Brown-Sèquard syndrome)
Eye	conjunctivitis, keratitis	dry eyes, retinal failure, cataracts
Bone		osteonecrosis
Bone marrow	pancytopenia	aplasia
Thyroid		hypothyroidism
Ovaries		amenorrhoea, menopausal symptoms

Chapter 20). Chronic cystitis with frequency, urgency and nocturia is due to contracture and fibrosis of the bladder. Treatment is symptomatic and, in severe cases, surgical urinary diversion and ileal conduit formation may need to be considered.

Vagina. Irradiation will cause acute vaginitis with pain, discharge and bleeding, frequently complicated by secondary infection. Management is symptomatic, including the treatment of infection. Some patients will subsequently develop atrophic vaginitis with fibrosis and stenosis causing dyspareunia and predisposing to infection. Treatment is with lubricants, topical oestrogen creams and vaginal dilatation.

Neurological

Brain. Cranial irradiation produces tiredness, nausea and headache in the acute phase. It is usually associated with oral mucositis and some patients develop transient deafness. The clinical symptoms and signs may deteriorate after the first few doses of radiotherapy, consistent with increased oedema; treatment is with corticosteroids. Some patients develop a 'somnolence syndrome' with tiredness, anorexia and irritability, starting a few weeks to a few months after treatment and lasting a similar period of time. It is self-limiting and is due to inflammation secondary to the radiotherapy. High dose treatment can cause radiation necrosis, which presents with the signs and symptoms of a mass lesion and may be difficult to differentiate from recurrent tumour. Treatment is symptomatic.

Spinal cord. Irradiation of the spinal cord may cause worsening of symptoms and signs after the first few treatments, related to increased oedema, which should be treated with increased doses of corticosteroids. Shortly after the completion of treatment, the patient may complain of electric shock-like sensations shooting down the spine or into the limbs, occurring on neck flexion. This is known as Lhermitte's syndrome and is a transient manifestation of radiation myelitis. It is almost always self-limited and the patient should be reassured. Higher doses, usually due to the inadvertent overlapping of two treatment fields, cause symptoms and signs of transverse myelitis (Brown-Sèquard syndrome).

Eye. Irradiation of the orbit will cause acute conjunctivitis and keratitis. If infection is present, it should be treated appropriately; if there is no evidence of infection, corticosteroid drops may be of benefit. In the chronic phase, the patient will have dry eyes and should use artificial tears. Cataract formation in the lens is inevitable following irradiation, but does not usually develop for several years after treatment.

Radiotherapy and surgery

Surgery performed in a previously irradiated area has a much higher risk of local complications because of the compromised vascularity of irradiated tissues. Surgery performed in a recently irradiated area where the tissues are inflamed and friable is even more hazardous. Anastomoses are more prone to break down, suture lines will take significantly longer to heal, and local infection occurs more frequently.

Bone marrow transplantation

Bone marrow transplantation is increasingly used in the treatment of both haematological malignancies and solid tumours. Bone marrow transplantation may be either allogeneic or autologous. In allogeneic transplantation, the donor is usually an HLA-matched sibling and the pre-transplant conditioning programme consists of high doses of chemotherapy, with or without total body irradiation. Autologous bone marrow transplantation involves the use of high doses of chemotherapy, followed by reinfusion of the patient's own bone marrow or peripheral blood stem cells, previously harvested.

The side effects of bone marrow transplantation include the toxicity of the conditioning regimen, infection in the immediate post-transplant period and, in the case of allogeneic transplantation, graft versus host (GVH) disease. The conditioning regimen uniformly produces profound myelosuppression and severe stomatitis. Other acute toxicities include veno-occlusive disease of the liver, myocarditis, interstitial pneumonitis and leucoencephalopathy. Delayed side effects which may be seen months later include cytopenias, cataracts, gonadal failure in both sexes, and impaired cardiac and pulmonary function.

Acute GVH disease, occurring shortly after transplantation, usually presents with a rash, abdominal pain, diarrhoea, and liver dysfunction. It can usually be well controlled with prednisolone and cyclosporin. Chronic GVH disease is seen in 30–50% of patients and usually occurs three to fifteen months after transplantation. It has many of the features of a collagen vascular disease with scleroderma-like skin lesions, keratoconjunctivitis, arthralgia, stomatitis, chronic liver disease, general wasting, and pulmonary insufficiency due to obliterative bronchiolitis. Treatment is with prednisolone and cyclosporin.

Chemotherapy

Chemotherapy is employed in different clinical situations, with different goals and toxicity. Given with curative intent, the treatment schedule is intensive and the toxicity significant. Chemotherapy may also be given to patients who cannot be cured, but for whom treatment may significantly improve their survival or quality of life. It may also be used for symptom control in the palliative care setting, where the treatment should be designed to have minimal or no adverse effects.

Adverse effects. Chemotherapy drugs may cause damage by either a direct toxic action of the chemical or by a cytotoxic action on rapidly dividing normal tissues. Examples of direct chemical toxicity are vomiting caused by stimulation of the chemoreceptor trigger zone, tissue necrosis following drug extravasation, and hepatic or renal impairment. Myelosuppression, mucositis, alopecia and amenorrhoea are due to the effect on rapidly dividing normal tissues. The toxicity of chemotherapy depends on factors relating to the drug, to the organ or tissue in question, and to the patient's general condition (Table 29.4). The common adverse effects and the drugs most likely to cause them are summarized in Tables 29.5 and 29.6. The toxicity in most cases is dose-dependent and the frequencies shown in Table 29.6 refer to standard doses used in oncology.

Drug extravasation

Extravasation of chemotherapy drugs into the tissues outside a vein will cause local tissue damage. The reaction is mild in the case of many drugs, but vesicant drugs will cause local tissue necrosis that may lead to ulceration. The vesicant chemotherapy drugs are doxorubicin, daunorubicin, epirubicin, actinomycin, mitomycin, and the vinca alkaloids. The reaction takes weeks or months to settle and may require surgical debridement and grafting.

The treatment is primarily preventive by using good veins, with good technique and by giving drugs slowly. In addition, extravasation should be detected as early as possible by asking the patient to report pain and discomfort and by regular observation of the cannulation

Table 29.4 Factors related to the toxicity of chemotherapy

Drug	Patient	Organ or tissue

specific drug
dose
route of administration
rate of administration
frequency of administration
drug metabolism, excretion
    hepatic, renal dysfunction
	age
	performance status
	psychological state
		pre-treatment function
		other adverse influences
		    previous chemotherapy
		    previous radiation
		    malignant infiltration
		    metabolic abnormalities
		    infection

Table 29.5 Summary of adverse effects of chemotherapy

	Acute	Chronic
Allergic	hypersensitivity, anaphylaxis	
Bladder	haemorrhagic cystitis	bladder fibrosis, cancer
Carcinogenic		second malignancies
Cardiac	arrhythmias	cardiomyopathy, cardiac failure
Gastrointestinal	nausea, vomiting stomatitis, mucositis diarrhoea ileus, constipation (vincristine)* pancreatitis (asparaginase)*	
Endocrine	hyperglycaemia (asparaginase)*	gonadal failure, infertility
Extravasation	acute inflammation	ulceration
Haematological	myelosuppression	bone marrow impairment
Hepatic	hepatocellular damage	cirrhosis, liver failure
Neurological	polyneuropathy tinnitus, high frequency deafness (cisplatin)*	chronic neuropathy leukoencephalopathy (methotrexate + radiation)*
Pulmonary	pneumonitis acute respiratory failure	pulmonary fibrosis respiratory failure
Renal	impaired renal function	chronic renal impairment
Skin	alopecia nail changes photosensitivity pigmentation radiation recall foot/hand syndrome phlebitis	permanent pigmentation photosensitivity

* For adverse effects unique to a particular drug, the responsible agent is shown in brackets

Table 29.6 Cytotoxic chemotherapy: frequency of common adverse effects

	Allergy	Marrow	Nausea, vomiting	Stomatitis	Diarrhoea	CNS	Peripheral neuropathy	Liver	Kidney	Lung	Heart	Skin	Alopecia
Altretamine		•	•		○	○	•	○					
Amsacrine		•	•	•	•						•	○	•
Asparaginase	•		•	○									
Bleomycin	○		•	•						•		•	○
Busulfan		•	○	○	○			○		○		•	
Capecitabine		•	•	•	•		•	○				•	
Carboplatin		•	•	•	○	○	○	○	○				○
Carmustine		•	•	○	○					○		•	
Cisplatin		•	•			•	•		•				
Cyclophosphamide		•	•	○	○			○				○	•
Cytarabine		•	•	○	○	○	○	•		○		○	○
Dacarbazine		•	•				•					•	•
Dactinomycin		•	•	•	○	•						•	•
Daunorubicin		•	•	•	○			○			•	○	•
Docetaxel	•	•	•	•	•		○			•	•	•	•
Doxorubicin		•	•	•	•						•	○	•
Epirubicin		•	•	•	•						•	○	•
Etoposide	○	•	•	○	○								•
Fludarabine		•	○	○	○	○	•			•	○	•	○
Fluorouracil		•	•	•	•							•	•
Fotemustine		•	•		○	○		•	○				
Gemcitabine		•	•	•	•			•	•	•		•	•
Ifosfamide		•	•	•	•	•	○	○				○	•
Irinotecan		•	•	•	•					•		•	•
Lomustine		•	•	•	○	○	○			○		○	○
Methotrexate		•	•	•	○			○	•	○		○	○
Mitomycin		•	•	○	○		○	○	○	○		○	○
Mitoxantrone		•	•	•	•	○		•	○		○	○	•
Oxaliplatin		•	•	•	•	○	•	•	•			•	•
Paclitaxel	•	•	•	•	•		•	•			•		•
Raltitrexed		•	○		•			•				○	○
Temozolomide		•	•		○	○	○				○	○	○
Topotecan		•	•	•			○			○			○
Vinblastine		•	•	○	○	○							•
Vincristine			○			○	○				○	○	•
Vinorelbine		•	•				•						•

• *occurs in >10% of cases*   ○ *occurs in 1-10% of cases.*

site. If extravasation occurs, the infusion is stopped. Before removing the cannula, an attempt should be made to aspirate the drug through it. Vinca extravasation is treated by injection of 150 IU hyaluronidase into the site and warm compresses. Extravasation of other vesicant drugs is treated by topical application of dimethylsulfoxide (DMSO) (8-hourly for 7 days) in conjunction with cold compresses (for 1h, q8h for 3 days). If extravasation is severe, an early surgical consultation should be sought.

Biologic therapy

Interferon

Interferons are used in the treatment of a variety of malignancies. Treatment is by subcutaneous injection, usually given three times weekly. The adverse effects (Table 29.7) are dose related and reversible. When treatment is started there is invariably a flu-like illness with fever, fatigue, chills, myalgia, and headache. This may be self-limiting or respond to treatment with anti-inflammatory drugs; dose modification is required if symptoms are severe. The usual dose limiting toxicity consists of fatigue, weakness, anorexia, and weight loss. These adverse effects can suggest progression of a patient's malignant disease and, if doubt exists, it may be necessary to reduce or temporarily discontinue therapy.

Table 29.7 Adverse effects of interferon therapy

General	flu-like illness: fever, fatigue, chills, myalgia, headache malaise, weakness, weight loss
Cardiovascular	hypotension
Dermatological	rashes, mild alopecia
Gastrointestinal	nausea, anorexia, alteration of taste, mild diarrhoea
Haematological	anaemia, neutropenia, thrombocytopenia
Hepatic	elevated transaminases
Neurological	headache, somnolence, confusion, cognitive impairment
Psychological	anxiety, depression, psychosis
Renal	proteinuria
Rheumatological	myalgia, arthralgia

Table 29.8 Adverse effects of interleukin-2 therapy

General	fever, chills, lethargy
Cardiovascular	myocarditis
Dermatological	diffuse erythroderma
Gastrointestinal	nausea, diarrhoea
Haematological	anaemia, thrombocytopenia, eosinophilia
Hepatic	elevated transaminases

Interleukin-2

The immunomodulating agent, interleukin-2 (IL-2), is commercially available and is used for the treatment of renal cell carcinoma and malignant melanoma. It has potential to cause severe toxicity (Table 29.8), and is only suitable for younger patients with a good performance status, normal organ function, and no evidence of cardiac disease.

Rituximab (Mabthera)

Rituximab (Mabthera) is the chimeric anti-CD20 monoclonal antibody used for the treatment of B-cell lymphoproliferative diseases. It is often associated with allergic or hypersensitivity reactions at the time of administration, but other adverse effects are usually mild and transient.

Trastuzumab (Herceptin)

Trastuzumab (Herceptin) is a recombinant humanized monoclonal antibody that recognizes the HER-2/*neu* receptor that is overexpressed on one-quarter of adenocarcinomas. Used with chemotherapy, it improves the response rate in women with breast cancer. Patients treated with trastuzumab have an increased risk of congestive cardiac failure, particularly if they have also received anthracyclines.[9]

Colony stimulation factors

Granulocyte (G-CSF, filgrastim, lenograstim) and granulocyte-macrophage (GM-CSF, sargramostim, molgramostim) colony stimulating factors are used for the prevention and treatment of chemotherapy-related neutropenia.[10] They are administered as a daily subcutaneous injection. Their use results in shorter periods of neutropenia with less fever, infection and mucositis. Mild to moderate medullary bone pain and mild fever are the only adverse effects frequently reported. G-CSF is now available as a long acting preparation, pegfilgrastim, which only needs to be given each 2 or 3 weeks.

Hormonal therapy

Corticosteroids

Corticosteroids are widely used in palliative care as adjuvant analgesics and for their anti-inflammatory effects. The adverse effects are listed in Table 13.4.

Table 29.9 Adverse effects of oestrogens

General	weight gain
Cardiovascular	sodium and fluid retention, oedema, hypertension venous thromboembolism
Dermatological	rash, chloasma
Endocrine	male: feminization, gynaecomastia, impotence female: menstrual irregularity, mastalgia, endometrial cancer
Hepatic	abnormal liver function tests, jaundice
Psychological	depression

Oestrogens

Oestrogen preparations were commonly used in the past for the treatment of advanced breast and prostate cancers. This was associated with an increased morbidity and mortality from cardiovascular and thromboembolic disease (Table 29.9). With the development of less toxic alternatives, oestrogens are no longer commonly used.

Antioestrogens

Tamoxifen and toremifene are used in the treatment of metastatic breast cancer. They have few severe adverse effects (Table 29.10).[11] There is a slightly increased risk of endometrial carcinoma in women taking tamoxifen and postmenopausal bleeding or vaginal discharge requires careful assessment.

Table 29.10 Adverse effects of antioestrogens

Cardiovascular	fluid retention thrombosis (slightly increased risk)
Endocrine	hot flushes, sweating
Gastrointestinal	nausea
Genitourinary	amenorrhoea, vaginal discharge, pruritus vulvae, endometrial cancer
Neurological	dizziness, light headedness
Psychological	depression

Aromatase inhibitors

The third generation aromatase inhibitors anastrozole, exemestane and letrozole are used for the treatment of metastatic breast cancer and have largely replaced aminoglutethimide.[12] They selectively inhibit the enzyme aromatase in peripheral tissues, blocking the conversion of androstenedione to oestrogen in postmenopausal or oophorectomized women. In contrast to aminoglutethimide, they are generally well tolerated with fewer adverse effects, and corticosteroid replacement therapy is not required (Table 29.11).

Table 29.11 Adverse effects of aromatase inhibitors

General	fatigue, weakness
Cardiovascular	oedema
Dermatological	alopecia/hair thinning
Endocrine	hot flushes, sweating
Gastrointestinal	nausea, vomiting, diarrhoea, anorexia
Neurological	insomnia, headache

Progestogens

Progestogens have progesterone-like action and are used for the treatment of breast and endometrial cancer, as well as for the management of cachexia. The two compounds most frequently used are megestrol acetate and medroxyprogesterone acetate. The adverse effects of progestogens (Table 29.12) are dose-related. At the higher doses advocated for the treatment of patients with cancer, the frequent dose-limiting side effects are nausea, weight gain, and fluid retention.

Table 29.12 Adverse effects of progestogens

General	appetite stimulation, weight gain
Cardiovascular	mild fluid retention
Genitourinary	menstrual irregularities, amenorrhoea
Hepatic	elevated enzymes
Neurological	weakness, lethargy
Psychological	depression

Antiandrogens

The antiandrogen drugs cyproterone acetate, bicalutamide, and flutamide are used for the treatment of prostate cancer and act by competitive inhibition at the androgen receptor. Adverse effects are generally mild with the exception that severe hepatotoxicity may occur (Table 29.13).

Table 29.13 Adverse effects of antiandrogens

General	weight gain, fatigue, lethargy
Endocrine	gynaecomastia, hot flushes, diminished libido
Gastrointestinal	nausea, anorexia
Hepatic	(rare) severe hepatotoxicity

Gonadorelin (GnRH) analogues

The gonadotrophin-releasing hormone (GnRH, gonadorelin) analogues, leuprorelin and goserelin, are used for the treatment of prostate cancer and premenopausal breast cancer. Regular use lowers the leuteinizing hormone levels and produces testosterone and oestrogen levels equivalent to castration. However, there is an initial period of stimulation during which

Table 29.14 Adverse effects of gonadorelin analogues

Tumour flare	increased pain, aggravation of other clinical features
General	weight gain
Endocrine	hot flushes, sweating men: gynaecomastia, diminished libido, impotence women: diminished libido, menopausal symptoms
Gastrointestinal	nausea, vomiting, diarrhoea
Neurological	headaches, dizziness, lethargy
Psychological	depression

testosterone and oestrogen levels may rise and cause a tumour flare. Men should be treated with an antiandrogen for three days before and three weeks after the initiation of GnRH analogue therapy. Women at risk of spinal cord compression should be carefully observed for the first few weeks of therapy. Long acting depot preparations are available that are administered by injection each three months. The adverse effects of gonadorelin analogues (Table 29.14) are primarily due to hormonal changes. Flushes, if severe, can be treated with low dose progestogen.

References

1   Hoskin, P. (1999). Radiotherapy fractionation in palliative care. *European Journal of Palliative Care* 6, 111–15.

2   Barton, R. and Kirkbride, P. (2000). Special techniques in palliative radiation oncology. *Journal of Palliative Medicine* 3, 75–83.

3   Jones, B., Cominos, M. and Dale, R.G. (2003). Application of biological effective dose (BED) to estimate the duration of symptomatic relief and repopulation dose equivalent in palliative radiotherapy and chemotherapy. *International Journal of Radiation Oncology, Biology and Physics* 55, 736–42.

4   Sutcliffe, S. and O'Sullivan, B. (1985). The toxicity of radiotherapy. *Clinics in Oncology* 4,

5   De Vita, V.T., et al. (2001). Adverse effects of treatment. In *Cancer. Principles and Practice of Oncology. 6th edition* (ed. V.T. De Vita, S. Hellman and S.A. Rosenberg). Philadelphia, Lippincott, Williams and Wilkins. (pp 2869–2976).

6   Radiation Therapy Oncology Group (2000). Acute Radiation Morbidity Scoring Criteria. <www.rtog.org/members/toxicity/acute.html>

7   Radiation Therapy Oncology Group and the European Organisation for Research and Treatment in Cancer (2000). RTOG/EORTC Late Radiation Morbidity Scoring Schema. <www.rtog.org/members/toxicity/late.html>

8   National Cancer Institute Cancer Therapy Evaluation Program (1998). Common Toxicity Criteria, version 2.0. <http://ctep.cancer.gov/reporting/ctc.html>

9   Seidman, A., et al. (2002). Cardiac dysfunction in the trastuzumab clinical trials experience. *Journal of Clinical Oncology* 20, 1215–21.

10   Griffin, J.D. (2001). Hematopoietic growth factors. In *Cancer. Principles and Practice of Oncology. 6th edition* (ed. V.T. De Vita, S. Hellman and S.A. Rosenberg). Philadelphia, Lippincott, Williams and Wilkins.

11   Day, R., Ganz, P.A. and Costantino, J.P. (2001). Tamoxifen and depression: more evidence from the National Surgical Adjuvant Breast and Bowel Project's Breast Cancer Prevention (P-1) Randomized Study. *Journal of the National Cancer Institute* 93, 1615–23.

12   Smith, I.E. and Dowsett, M. (2003). Aromatase inhibitors in breast cancer. *New England Journal of Medicine* 348, 2431–42.

Psychosocial aspects of care

... when death does come—
to them, their wives, their children, their friends—
catching them unawares and unprepared,
then what storms of passion overwhelm them,
what cries, what fury, what despair! ...

Michel de Montaigne (1533–92)

... peace for those who seek answers
about the meaning and purpose of life and death,
of suffering and pain,
not only of the physical body,
but of the whole person.

Elizabeth Kübler-Ross
To Live Until We Say Good-bye, 1978

To be successful, doctors have to know more about the sick person...
than just the name of the disease and its pathophysiology.

Eric J. Cassell
The Nature of Suffering and the Goals of Medicine, 1991

30

Psychological issues

The stress associated with advanced cancer inevitably causes emotional or psychological suffering. For some patients it may cause more distress and detract more from the quality of life than the physical disease itself. A lot has been written about the distress patients suffer but only recently has more attention focused on how patients adapt to minimize this suffering and how the health care team can facilitate these coping mechanisms.[1]

Psychological distress is intimately interrelated with the other aspects of suffering. Persistent or untreated problems related to other causes of suffering—pain, other physical symptoms, social problems, cultural factors and spiritual concerns—may all cause or aggravate psychological suffering (Figure 30.1). Treatment of these problems can lead to improvement or

Figure 30.1 The interrelationships between psychological problems and other causes of suffering. (a) Psychological distress may cause or aggravate other problems and may present solely as pain or other physical symptoms not responding to appropriate therapy. (b) Unresolved or untreated problems related to other causes of suffering may cause or aggravate psychological problems.

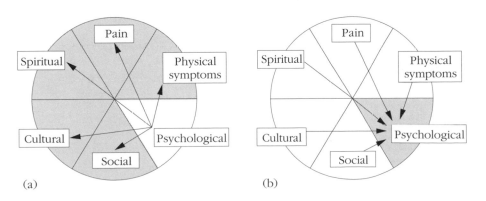

(a)　　　　　　　　　　　　　(b)

resolution of psychological distress. This relationship emphasizes that psychological care must be an integrated part of overall care. The opposite relationship, in which untreated psychological distress causes or aggravates other aspects of suffering, will be clinically manifest as pain or other symptoms unresponsive to appropriate treatment.

The management of psychological problems is primarily directed at facilitating the patient's adaptive and coping mechanisms in order to minimize suffering and maximize the quality of life. As each patient is a unique individual, with a unique set of problems and coping mechanisms, management needs to be individualized.

Psychological distress

Cause

The possible causes of psychological distress in patients with advanced cancer are legion and include matters related to the disease, the patient, the treatment and the treatment team (Table 30.1).

Table 30.1 Factors predisposing to psychological distress

Disease	Cultural
rapidly progressive	cultural differences
present, anticipated disabilities	language barriers
disfigurement	Spiritual
physical dependence	religious issues
long illness: psychological exhaustion	spiritual issues
Patient	remorse, guilt
fear of pain, dying, disfigurement	unfulfilled expectations
loss (or fear of loss) of control, independence, dignity	meaninglessness
helplessness, hopelessness	Treatment
insight regarding (or fear of) poor prognosis	diagnostic delays
loss of self esteem	multiple failed treatments
anxious personality	bureaucracy
neuroticism, hypochondriasis	financial cost
maladaptive perception of guilt	adverse effects of therapy
history of psychiatric illness	Team
Pain	poor communication
unrelieved pain	unhelpful, disinterested
Symptoms	lack of information
uncontrolled symptoms	lack of continuity of care
Social	exclusion of family, carers
loss (or fear of loss) of job, social position, family role	culturally insensitive
feels isolated (actual or perceived)	spiritual concerns not discussed
pre-existing family problems	
failure social supports, resources	
unfinished business: personal, interpersonal, financial	
financial hardship	
fears for family	
anticipatory grieving	

Clinical features

Psychological distress is often described in terms of anxiety or depression (see Chapter 26) but patients with advanced cancer suffer a range of other emotional problems. These do not necessarily or commonly reflect psychopathology and some, like denial, are best regarded as the clinical manifestations of coping mechanisms.[2] Coping means dealing with stress to prevent, avoid or control emotional distress; the term is usually reserved for dealing with difficult or unusual problems that require adaptation. In coping with advanced cancer a wide range of psychological reactions and physical symptoms may be manifest, all representing underlying psychological distress (Table 30.2).

Table 30.2 Some clinical features of psychological distress

Anxiety	Grief
Depression	Sadness, misery, remorse
Anger, frustration, irritability	Withdrawal, apathy
Hopelessness, despair	Passivity
Helplessness	Avoidance
Regression	Inappropriate compensation (joyful)
Denial	Lack of co-operation with carers
Guilt	Unresponsive pain or physical symptoms
Fear	

A number of different types of coping mechanisms have been described (Table 30.3). Most patients with advanced cancer will manifest some features of one or more coping mechanisms which, in most cases, should be regarded as a normal defence mechanism and not pathological. Used to excess, they are considered maladaptive and may be counter-productive in the treatment setting. Regression or reversion to an earlier developmental stage may attract increased support and relieve the patient of some responsibilities; in extreme cases, immature and demanding behaviour may lead to less or inappropriate care. Rationalization is a form of denial in which manifestations of cancer are attributed to something other than the disease. Intellectualization allows patients to distance themselves from reality by intellectualizing or theorizing. Distraction involves putting a lot of energy and time into matters unrelated to the disease. Repression is the unconscious suppression of painful memories; in extreme cases there may be a detached, emotionless acceptance.

Table 30.3 Some coping mechanisms

Regression	Distraction
Denial	Repression
Rationalization	Suppression
Intellectualization	Withdrawal

Withdrawal or avoidance reflects an individual's inability to come to terms with or take responsibility for what is happening.

Denial is the most frequently seen coping mechanism and is not necessarily abnormal or pathological. Denial allows patients time to come to terms with their situation; an alternative description is 'suppression of information' which emphasizes its protective function. Denial does not necessarily indicate that patients are unaware of their situation. It is common for patients exhibiting denial to the doctor and nurses to simultaneously confide in someone else that they have a realistic view of their condition. Each patient with advanced cancer is a unique individual and each must find their own level between denial and acceptance.

Studies have shown that the most effective strategies, in terms of reduced psychological distress, were an open acknowledgement of the disease and a willingness to deal with the illness and current problems according to realistic considerations; least effective strategies were those that emphasized retreat, avoidance, passivity or apathy.

The level of psychological distress depends on patients' ability to cope or the efficacy of their coping mechanisms. A number of factors have been defined which help identify those patients at increased risk of emotional distress when confronted with a major illness (Table 30.4). Not surprisingly, these indicate that previously emotionally stable individuals with good social supports and resources are likely to adjust and cope better. The age-related meaning of the disease to the patient is an important determinant of psychological suffering and is different for patients in the various age groups. These factors include the effects on interpersonal relationships, independence, goals, body image and existential concerns. Patients with religious beliefs or those maintaining some equivalent value system are likely to cope better. Cultural attitudes to serious disease vary greatly and have a profound impact on a patient's ability to cope and the psychological distress experienced.

Table 30.4 Predictive factors for poor coping

Personal
  anxious or pessimistic personality
  poor coping with previous illnesses, stresses
  inflexibility of coping
  adverse experiences with cancer in relatives or friends
  history of recent personal losses
  multiple family problems, obligations
  marital problems
  history of psychiatric illness
  personality disorder
  history of alcohol or substance abuse
  age-related interruptions to life cycle

Social
  few social supports, resources; isolated
  lower socioeconomic class

Cultural
  cultural traditions

Spiritual
  not religious; no alternative value system

In addition to these factors that predict an individual's risk of psychological distress, the stresses with which they have to cope increase as the disease advances. Advancing disease leads to progressive losses—loss of job, loss of social position, loss of mobility, loss of attractiveness, loss of independence, loss of control—until finally the patient is dependent on others for personal hygiene and toileting. Another major cause of emotional distress is the need to complete unfinished business, whether this be a religious or spiritual atonement, mending personal or family relationships, or concluding family and worldly affairs.

Treatment

The effective treatment of psychological distress in patients with advanced cancer may greatly improve the quality of life. The assessment and management of psychological distress requires the collaborative efforts of various members of the multidisciplinary team if all aspects of care are to be addressed. Patients likely to cope poorly and those predisposed to psychological distress need to be identified at the time of initial assessment and appropriate treatment measures included in their overall plan of care.

Management of psychological distress has to be tailored to the needs of each individual patient and can be broadly divided into general measures (Table 30.5) and psychological

Table 30.5   Psychological distress: general measures

General
  caring, considerate, unhurried approach
  good listening
  good communication
  providing information
  reassurance about continuing care
  respect for the person and individuality
  involvement in treatment and care, maintain sense of control
  allow discussion of fears regarding, future suffering, life expectancy

Pain
  control pain

Physical symptoms
  relieve physical symptoms

Social
  address social issues
  encourage available social supports
  provide support for family and carers
  facilitate use of social services
  assist with financial, legal issues

Cultural
  respect cultural differences
  use interpreters for language barriers
  involve ethnic support services

Spiritual
  address religious or spiritual concerns

approaches (Table 30.6). The literature on psychological and psychosocial interventions for patients with cancer is largely focused on patients earlier in the course of their disease,[3–7] although some generalizations from these studies are relevant to the management of patients with advanced disease. First, the incidence of psychological distress found on routine screening is significantly higher than is clinically apparent. Second, interventions applied early are likely to be more beneficial. Third, relatively brief, simple interventions can have a significant effect on psychological well being and quality of life.[8]

Table 30.6 Psychological distress: psychological approaches

General supportive counselling	Support groups
Relaxation therapy	Psychological therapies
deep breathing	coping skills training
progressive muscular relaxation	stress management techniques
autogenic relaxation	cognitive therapy
imagery	Psychotherapy
meditation	anxiolytics, antidepressants
Distraction	supportive psychotherapy
art, music, hobbies	Psychotherapeutic intervention
occupational therapy	for maladaptive responses
socialization	

Factors causing or aggravating psychological distress (Table 30.1) should be treated, if possible. The successful treatment of pain and other physical symptoms may greatly reduce anxiety and fear. Reassurance is given about continuing care. Good communication is required, including honest answers to questions posed by the patient. Unrealistic fears about future problems or disabilities need to be discussed. It is important to respect patients' individuality and to keep them as involved as possible in their own treatment.

The uncertainties, fears and anxieties of the patient's family and carers need to be addressed so as not to complicate the patient's management. The use of social and community resources can be encouraged and assistance given with financial and legal problems.

Cultural differences need to be respected or there may be an escalating misunderstanding between the health care team and the patient and family that causes more, not less, emotional distress.

Spiritual concerns, whether religious or relating to some other value system, need to be explored. Unresolved spiritual issues are a frequent cause of emotional distress.

Providing information. For many patients, their ability to cope depends on having adequate information about their situation and disease.[9] Information is presented in a sensitive and understandable manner, and how much is given depends on what the patient wants. Provision of information can help patients cope and engenders a feeling of being involved and having some control.

Support groups. A support group provides patients and their families with social and emotional support and allows expression of emotions. If a professional carer is included, the group can have an educative function with the provision and explanation of information. Groups can also have a therapeutic role with instruction about relaxation therapy and basic coping skills.

Relaxation. Relaxation therapy can be of benefit in the management of stress associated with advanced cancer. It will produce general calming and help the patient cope with crises.

A number of techniques of varying complexity are advocated. The simplest is deep breathing and control of respiration. Progressive muscular relaxation, with or without imagery, involves the tensing and relaxing of specific muscle groups, progressing sequentially across the body. Autogenic relaxation involves sequential relaxing of each area of the body and focusing on a feeling of warmth and heaviness. Imagery involves concentrating on a comfortable situation or on a particular aspect of the disease. Meditation is a state of detached observation during which a patient may focus either on a comfortable situation or some aspect of the disease, and by assessing different sensations as they occur, develop insight. Meditation with imagery is considered by some to be akin to self-hypnosis. Relaxation therapy is performed initially with a therapist and then continued by the patient alone.

Distraction. The benefits of pursuing interests in art, music and other hobbies are well known. A programme of occupational therapy, to emphasize patients' skills or help them adapt to physical disabilities, may restore some self-esteem and reduce psychological distress. Socializing with other patients, countering boredom and loneliness, will help patients cope.

Psychological therapies. Teaching patients coping skills and stress management techniques will help them deal with day to day stress. Cognitive therapy directed at thought and affect control will help them manage crises.[10] Realistic goals can be set. Difficulties can be viewed from a different perspective and overwhelming problems broken down into ones which are manageable.

Psychotherapy. Patients with significant anxiety or depression may benefit from anxiolytic or antidepressant medication. A few patients will need formal psychotherapy, which should be of short duration and focused on cognitive restructuring and coping skills.

Maladaptive coping. The different coping mechanisms present various clinical features, which need to be recognized and understood, but rarely require any specific treatment. However, normal psychological defence or coping mechanisms that become exaggerated or maladaptive cause increased problems for the patient and family as well as the professional carers. Patients may give up or regress, becoming withdrawn and apathetic when their physical death is not imminent; sensitive counselling and the encouragement of social contacts may improve the situation. A few patients will follow the oft-quoted exhortation and 'rage against the dying of the light'. Such anger is usually associated with severe anxiety and unresolved psychological problems, and treatment (if accepted by the patient) is with both psychotropic drugs and psychotherapy. Patients with gross denial or severe anger may become isolated from family and friends and require the intervention of a skilled psychological counsellor or psychiatrist as well as psychotropic medication.

Terminal care

How much is said about death and dying varies with every patient. The secret is to be in tune with the patient who determines how much discussion there is. Many patients do not wish to discuss death or, if they do, are selective with whom they share their feelings. Staff caring for terminally ill patients need to be able to respond if a patient does want to talk about death. The belief that all patients need and should be able to talk about death and dying is not true.

References

1   Vachon, M.L. (2003). The emotional problems of the patient in palliative medicine. In *Oxford Textbook of Palliative Medicine, 3rd edition* (ed. D. Doyle, G. Hanks, N. Cherny and K. Calman). Oxford, Oxford University Press.

2   Beeney, L.J., Buttow, P.N. and Dunn, S.M. (1997). 'Normal' adjustment to cancer: characteristics and assessment. In *Topics in Palliative Care* (ed. R. Portenoy and E. Bruera). New York, Oxford University Press.

3   Devine, E.C. and Westlake, S.K. (1995). The effects of psychoeducational care provided to adults with cancer: meta-analysis of 116 studies. *Oncology Nursing Forum* 22, 1369–81.

4   Meyer, T.J. and Mark, M.M. (1995). Effects of psychosocial interventions with adult cancer patients: a meta-analysis of randomized experiments. *Health Psychology* 14, 101–8.

5   Sheard, T. and Maguire, P. (1999). The effect of psychological interventions on anxiety and depression in cancer patients: results of two meta-analyses. *British Journal of Cancer* 80, 1770–80.

6   Luebbert, K., Dahme, B. and Hasenbring, M. (2001). The effectiveness of relaxation training in reducing treatment-related symptoms and improving emotional adjustment in acute non-surgical cancer treatment: a meta-analytical review. *Psychooncology* 10, 490–502.

7   Newell, S.A., Sanson-Fisher, R.W. and Savolainen, N.J. (2002). Systematic review of psychological therapies for cancer patients: overview and recommendations for future research. *Journal of the National Cancer Institute* 94, 558–84.

8   Spiegel, D., et al. (2000). Group psychotherapy and the terminally ill. In *Handbook of Psychiatry in Palliative Medicine* (ed. H.M. Chochinov and W. Breitbart). New York, Oxford University Press.

9   Jenkins, V., Fallowfield, L. and Saul, J. (2001). Information needs of patients with cancer: results from a large study in UK cancer centres. *British Journal of Cancer* 84, 48–51.

10. Turk, D.C. and Feldman, C.S. (2000). A cognitive-behavioral approach to symptom management in palliative care. In *Handbook of Psychiatry in Palliative Medicine* (ed. H.M. Chochinov and W. Breitbart). New York, Oxford University Press.

31

Social problems

Interpersonal
Family
Financial and legal

Patients with advanced cancer do not exist in social isolation; usually they have family and friends as well as social and financial responsibilities. Advanced cancer frequently has devastating effects on these relationships, requiring adjustment on a repeated or continuing basis as the disease progresses. The social difficulties most commonly encountered by patients with advanced cancer are problems with interpersonal relationships, problems relating to self-care, and the need for financial or legal assistance (Table 31.1). Family members may require assistance for similar difficulties in adjustment and coping. There are a number of

Table 31.1 Social problems

Problems with interpersonal relationships
    due to the patient's reaction to the illness
        anxiety, depression, fear, anger, guilt
        anticipatory grieving
    due to other person's reaction to the illness
        anxiety, depression, fear, anger, guilt
        anticipatory grieving
    exacerbation of pre-existing interpersonal problems
    marital problems
    disagreement about anticancer therapy

Family problems
    home care
    role shifts
    exhaustion
    family coping

Increased physical and psychological problems with disease progression

Financial and legal needs

reviews of the social problems related to advanced cancer.[1–7] The involvement of a social worker in the management of these problems is crucial.[8–11]

Social problems may be precipitated or aggravated by problems related to other causes of suffering (Figure 31.1), treatment of which may be necessary before the social difficulties can be addressed or resolved. Similarly, untreated or unresolved social problems may cause or aggravate other problems, and physical symptoms not responding to appropriate therapy should raise the possibility of unrecognized social difficulties.

Figure 31.1 The interaction of social problems with other causes of suffering. (a) Unresolved or untreated social problems may cause or aggravate problems related to other causes of suffering. (b) Unresolved or untreated problems related to other causes of suffering may cause or aggravate social difficulties.

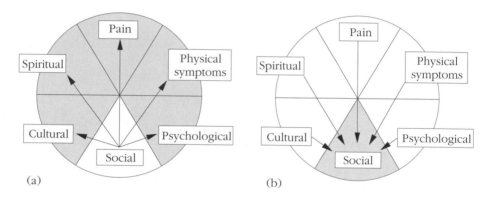

(a)　　　　　　　　　(b)

Interpersonal relationships

Relationships with other people, both family and friends, greatly influence a patient's ability to cope with advanced cancer. Without being overly protective, strong relationships form a buffer against the stress of the illness and provide additional coping reserves. They will also facilitate adjustment and adaptation by providing feedback to patients about the adequacy and acceptability of their coping mechanisms. Breakdown of these social supports may greatly compromise the patient's ability to cope and cause increased suffering.

Disruption of interpersonal relationships may occur as a result of a patient's reaction to the illness. As discussed in Chapter 30, patients exhibit a range of psychological reactions including anxiety, depression, fear and anger, which may lead to breakdown of relationships. Family and friends may experience just the same responses, usually to a lesser degree, but with similarly disruptive effects on relationships. Both may suffer anticipatory grieving (see Chapter 34). Problems with interpersonal relationships may be an exacerbation of pre-existing difficulties, in which case there may also be significant guilt.

The management of these problems is complex. The treatment of the patient's psychological problems is dealt with in Chapter 30. Problems experienced by family members or friends are addressed if they are causing difficulties with the clinical care of the patient or if there is a high risk of a pathological grief reaction. This may take the form of counselling by either a member of the treatment team or the person's own family physician. A meeting of the family members with the patient and a member of the treatment team will clarify the medical situation and help allay anxieties. Differences that may exist between the patient and the family regarding treatment can be resolved. Discussion or support groups, involving other patients and their families, can be helpful.

The strength of any marriage is severely tested by a terminal illness in one partner. If the marriage is unsound, it may disintegrate under the added stress of the illness. In contrast, it is not unusual for estranged couples to come back together when one is faced with a terminal illness. This may greatly reduce the patient's suffering and leave the surviving partner feeling that something positive and worthwhile was done. Even sound marriages can be the source of distress, and it is well recorded that one of the greatest concerns of both the patient and the healthy partner is to shield the other from upset and stress.

Conflict may occur between patients and their families or carers if they have received differing information about the disease, prognosis or treatment. If only the family members have been accurately apprised of the situation, there may be a conspiracy of silence that will blunt all communication. Alternatively, well informed patients who are at ease with their situation may be pressured by less informed relatives to adopt unrealistic views about prognosis or submit to what amounts to futile therapy. Issues of this nature are best resolved by discussion between members of the treatment team and the patient and family together. Better still, they can be avoided if family members or carers are included in consultations and discussions through the course of a patient's illness.

Family problems

The family of a patient with advanced cancer is subject to many strains and stresses, both physical and psychological. The degree of distress experienced by family members depends on many factors. Most important are the course of the patient's disease, whether it is rapid or relatively slow, and how much suffering the patient has. Also important are the family members' age, their physical and psychological health, their previous experience in dealing with stress, availability of their own social supports, and the degree to which the illness disrupts their own family and personal lives.

Home care. Managing terminally ill patients at home is potentially much more stressful for family carers but may be more satisfying for both. For the caregiver, the extra physical effort and emotional stress may be balanced by easier adjustment after the patient's death and a feeling of having done something worthwhile in making home care possible. However, the stresses can be considerable and the situation may arise where the family is more in need of attention than the patient.

When patients are nursed at home, family members will be responsible for many nursing tasks for which they need guidance and training. If family members are expected to change dressings, give injections or manage the patient's toileting, they should be shown how to do it by professional staff. Ideally, this should be done before the patient is discharged home. Family members are always anxious about what might go wrong and contingency plans should be made and rehearsed for any anticipated problems. The role of professional carers is to support and encourage the family and not to interpose between them and the patient. Family carers need to feel useful and helpful and deserve acknowledgement for their efforts. Volunteers who have experienced similar situations can be an important source of support.

Role shifts. As the patient's condition deteriorates the tasks they normally perform in the family will need to be carried out by someone else. This may involve any of the chores of family life, although the one that most frequently causes trouble is the management of the family finances. Families should be encouraged to discuss these matters, allowing patients to relinquish roles gradually and to act as mentor to the person assuming the task. This may help preserve patients' self-esteem and lessen the anxiety that the task can be performed satisfactorily. If patients refuse to relinquish tasks because of denial or because they see it as a sign of weakness, disorganization and chaos will result. Alternatively, patients stripped of their former roles are likely to feel useless, isolated and depressed.

Children. Children of a dying patient have special problems that need careful attention. The level of involvement in the illness experience will vary with their age, but children frequently have difficulty understanding or talking about what they see and hear. Adolescents who assume adult roles are easily overburdened with responsibility for their age and need extra support. Other issues that may need to be addressed include fears about the other parent dying and personal guilt about the cause of the parent's illness.

Exhaustion. Physical and psychological exhaustion occur frequently in family members of the terminally ill. All members of the health care team should be alert to the possibility and provide support as required. For patients nursed at home, temporary admission to hospital or hospice may be necessary to allow some respite for the carer, particularly if the illness is protracted. The possible need for, and the availability of, such admissions should be discussed before the patient is discharged home.

Family coping. As with the individual patient, families exhibit a range of coping mechanisms, some of which compound suffering rather than lessening it. Families that are supportive and cohesive and can resolve conflict effectively are likely to adapt well to the situation and cope better. These families have good communication and are able to share distress and provide mutual support. Interventions are not usually required and there is likely to be less psychological and social morbidity following the illness. Other families in which there is poor communication, limited expression, conflict or hostility are likely to cope poorly. Communication is inhibited and mutual support lacking. Poor flexibility or adaptability may lead to chaotic responses; there may be anger and hostility directed at the treatment team. The management of poor or maladaptive family coping includes family meetings with counselling to expose and resolve underlying issues. Teaching basic coping skills will help some family members. If possible, normal family rituals or routines are continued to provide a sense of stability, particularly if children are involved. Bereavement issues are discussed in Chapter 34.

Increasing problems with disease progression

A patient's continuing deterioration will heighten the normal psychological problems associated with a terminal illness, for both patient and family. The time at which patients become confined to bed and lose the ability to care for themselves is usually seen as a watershed or 'point of no return' and is associated with increased emotional distress for both patient and family. There will also be an increase in the need for physical nursing for patients being managed at home. Every effort is made to maximize the support, both professional and non-professional, available to families. Physical nursing aids need to be supplied and minor alterations to the home may be necessary. The use of available community services and resources is encouraged. If the physical care is demanding, the family may need help in organizing a roster of times and duties to avoid exhaustion; nevertheless, temporary admission of the patient to a hospital or hospice may still be necessary to allow some respite for the caregivers.

Financial and legal needs

A terminal illness may have devastating financial consequences for a family, particularly if the patient is the breadwinner. Advice regarding eligibility for social security benefits and assistance with financial planning may be required. Emergency financial relief from charitable sources is sometimes needed.

Problems relating to legal and business affairs must be addressed, particularly the making of a will. Patients may procrastinate about making a will if they see it as an admission of defeat; family members may not raise the matter for fear of upsetting the patient. Disordered worldly affairs and the lack of a will may cause additional chaos after the patient dies and every encouragement should be given to attend to these matters.

References

1. Kristjanson, L.J. (1997). The family as a unit of treatment. In *Topics in Palliative Care* (ed. R. Portenoy and E. Bruera). New York, Oxford University Press.
2. Kinsella, G., et al. (1998). A review of the measurement of caregiver and family burden in palliative care. *Journal of Palliative Care* 14, 37–45.
3. Loscalzo, M.F. and Zabora, J.R. (1998). Care of the cancer patient: response of family and staff. In *Topics in Palliative Care. Volume 2* (ed. E. Bruera and R. Portenoy). New York, Oxford University Press.
4. Borneman, T. and Ferrell, B. (2001). Care of the elderly with advanced diseases: caregiver issues. In *Topics in Palliative Care* (ed. E. Bruera and R. Portenoy). New York, Oxford University Press.
5. Scott, G., Whyler, N. and Grant, G. (2001). A study of family carers of people with a life-threatening illness 1: the carers' needs analysis. *International Journal of Palliative Nursing* 7, 290–1.
6. Ferrell, B. and Panke, J. (2003). Emotional problems in the family. In *Oxford Textbook of Palliative Medicine, 3rd edition* (ed. D. Doyle, G. Hanks, N. Cherny and K. Calman). Oxford, Oxford University Press.
7. Sheldon, F. (2003). Social impact of advanced metastatic cancer. In *Psychosocial Issues in Palliative Care* (ed. M. Lloyd-Williams). Oxford, Oxford University Press.
8. Sheldon, F.M. (2000). Dimensions of the role of the social worker in palliative care. *Palliative Medicine* 14, 491–8.
9. Oliviere, D. (2001). The social worker in palliative care—the 'eccentric' role. *Progress in Palliative Care* 9, 237–41.
10. Sheldon, F. (2001). Social work in palliative care: couselling and communicating. *Progress in Palliative Care* 9, 242–3.
11. Monroe, B. (2003). Social work in palliative medicine. In *Oxford Textbook of Palliative Medicine, 3rd edition* (ed. D. Doyle, G. Hanks, N. Cherny and K. Calman). Oxford, Oxford University Press.

32

Cultural factors

Culture
Culture-related problems
Culturally appropriate management

The continued expansion of the palliative care movement has brought it into contact with many and diverse cultures. In multicultural societies like Australia, the United Kingdom and America, the wider application of palliative care has necessitated an understanding and appreciation of the many European, Asian, African and Hispanic cultures. The establishment of palliative care services in countries with different cultures has required some modifications to make the services culturally appropriate to local tradition and custom.

Culture

An individual's culture is a complex reflection of a number of different factors (Table 32.1). In some societies the distinction between cultural and religious traditions is difficult, particularly with some of the Eastern religions that are more a way of life and culture than just a faith; in other situations, cultural factors may be completely independent of religious beliefs.

Table 32.1   Ingredients of a culture

History
Race
Language
Traditions
Beliefs
non-religious
religious
Customs, rituals
Family structure

A *trans-cultural* situation exists when cultural factors are transported into a different ethnic environment by immigration. The term *cross-cultural* is applied to the descendants of immigrants, born and educated in the adopted country, who may have a mixture of attitudes, some belonging to their parents and some to the adopted country. Cross-cultural phenomena are further complicated by a drift or erosion with time of some of the pure cultural attitudes inherited from the parents.

Cultural factors in palliative care

Variations in cultural attitudes to illness and death have long been known to have an enormous bearing on the degree of suffering associated with a terminal illness. People in societies in which there is a genuine appreciation and acceptance of the inevitability of death have less physical and mental suffering; this may have a religious basis, as with some Eastern religions, or be non-religious as occurs, for example, in some primitive communities.

Many reviews of the role of cultural factors in the planning and delivery of palliative care have been published.[1-5] Different models of care have evolved in different countries.[6-9] Difficulties are most likely with ethnic minorities in multicultural societies.[10-13]

Clinical problems related to cultural issues occur for a variety of reasons (Table 32.2). These occur in trans-cultural and cross-cultural situations and should not develop where a palliative care service has been established in a culturally distinct society and is culturally appropriate to it. Problems arise if there is lack of respect for an individual's cultural (and religious) background, or if the ethnic group to which the patient belongs is the subject of persecution. Inability to speak the local language may compromise the patient's understanding and make treatment more difficult. Different hierarchical family structures may complicate communication and treatment, especially in the situation where the male both answers and speaks for the female. Cultural and religious customs concerning the treatment of the

---

Table 32.2 Cultural problems in palliative care

Due to staff, society
  lack of respect for an individual's culture (or religion)
  persecution of an ethnic group

Due to cultural customs
  language
  family structure
  subordination of females
  treatment and disposal of the body after death

Due to patient's cultural attitudes to
  sickness, cancer
  pain
  death
  orthodox medical treatment
  hospitals, institutions
  philosophy of palliative care
  disclosure of the diagnosis
  discussion of the prognosis

---

body after death are particularly important, so much so that some ethnic groups withdraw their dying relatives from hospital or hospice for fear these traditions might be desecrated.

More varied and complex are the cultural attitudes to disease and treatment. Attitudes to disease, pain and death vary from stoic acceptance and detachment to anxiety and depression. Ethnic groups need extra explanation and reassurance in order to understand and not fear ordinary medical treatment and institutions.

The most vexing and unresolved questions arise from the attitude of different cultural groups to the philosophy of palliative care and particularly to the open discussion of the diagnosis and prognosis. The original palliative care philosophy was that patients were informed of their diagnosis and prognosis, spared further unnecessary treatment, and helped to come to terms with their situation. There is little doubt that this is culturally appropriate in those areas in the United Kingdom, America and Australia where palliative care has flourished, but it may not be appropriate in other situations. In practice, difficulty most often arises when the patient is an elderly migrant who speaks no English and whose adult children specifically prohibit discussion of the diagnosis or prognosis with the patient.

Cultural factors have a significant impact on other clinical features. Unresolved cultural issues may cause or aggravate problems related to other causes of suffering including pain, other physical symptoms, psychological, social and spiritual issues (Figure 32.1). On the other hand, cultural beliefs (particularly those relating to Eastern religions) may greatly reduce or ameliorate the physical and mental suffering caused by disease.

Figure 32.1 The interaction of cultural problems and other causes of suffering. (a) Cultural problems may exacerbate or ameliorate suffering due to other problems. (b) Unresolved physical or psychosocial problems may cause or aggravate problems related to cultural differences.

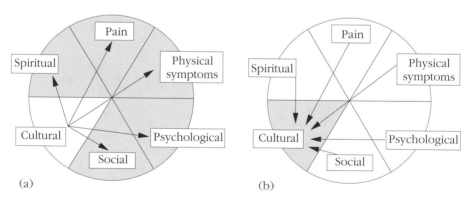

(a)   (b)

Management

The management of cultural issues in palliative care requires first and foremost that the patient's individual cultural (and religious) background is understood and respected. Palliative medicine must be conducted in a culturally appropriate and sensitive manner.[14] There remains a considerable need for professional education about the management of cultural issues in palliative care.[15]

How best to deal with the situation that arises when a family prohibits communication with the patient is unresolved. The problem is avoided if patients have guessed their diagnoses or require referral to a cancer centre for palliative therapy. The problem is less likely to occur if there has been an on-going partnership of care with open communication between the patient and family and the professional carers throughout the course of the illness. The advantages (and possible disadvantages) of disclosure need to be discussed with the family in a sensitive manner. Threats and coercion are unhelpful. One approach is confrontational and regards open communication as absolutely essential; the other is to do the best one can whilst the family maintains the patient in a cultural cocoon. Until there is objective evidence that these patients from whom the diagnosis is concealed have more mental or physical suffering, it is better for a palliative care service to be flexible and respect differences in attitude than to be confrontational.

Adapting services to meet multicultural needs

In addition to the unreserved acceptance and respect of cultural differences by staff, there may need to be some adaptation of the service itself in order to better meet the needs of patients in a multicultural society.

Language barriers may inhibit access to the service. This can be addressed by having information and literature about palliative care and hospice translated into the relevant languages and distributed appropriately.[16]

Cultural barriers may also inhibit access. A service must reach out to minority groups to learn more about their needs and to provide information and reassurance that the service is sensitive to the needs of patients of different ethnic or cultural backgrounds.[11, 13, 17] The inclusion of members of the ethnic community into the service's activities, whether as staff or volunteers or committee members, is often of great benefit in breaking down barriers. Targeting the general practitioners and health services that serve the ethnic population may also improve relations.

References

1   Firth, S. (1993). Cultural issues in terminal care. In *The Future for Palliative Care* (ed. D. Clark). Buckingham, Open University Press.

2   Hall, P., Stone, G. and Fiset, V.J. (1998). Palliative care: how can we meet the needs of our multicultural communities? *Journal of Palliative Care* 14, 46–9.

3   Oliviere, D. (1999). Culture and ethnicity. *European Journal of Palliative Care* 6, 53–6.

4   Hallenbeck, J.L. (2002). Cross-cultural issues. In *Principles and Practice of Palliative Care and Supportive Oncology* (ed. A.M. Berger, R.K. Portenoy and D.E. Weissman). Philadelphia, Lippincott, Williams and Wilkins.

5   Nyatanga, B. (2002). Culture, palliative care and multiculturalism. *International Journal of Palliative Nursing* 8, 240–6.

6   Brenneis, C. and Bruera, E. (2001). Models for the delivery of palliative care: the Canadian model. In *Topics in Palliative Care. Volume 5* (ed. E. Bruera and R.K. Portenoy). New York, Oxford University Press.

7   Centeno, C. and Gomez-Sancho, M. (2001). Models for the delivery of palliative care: the Spanish model. In *Topics in Palliative Care. Volume 5* (ed. E. Bruera and R.K. Portenoy). New York, Oxford University Press.

8   Wenk, R. and Bertolini, M. (2001). Models for the delivery of palliative care in developing countries: the Argentine model. In *Topics in Palliative Care. Volume 5* (ed. E. Bruera and R.K. Portenoy). New York, Oxford University Press.

9   Fainsinger, R.L., Nunez-Olarte, J.M. and Demoissac, D.M. (2003). The cultural differences in perceived value of disclosure and cognition: Spain and Canada. *Journal of Palliative Care* 19, 43–8.

10 Chan, A. and Woodruff, R.K. (1999). Comparison of palliative care needs of English- and non-English-speaking patients. *Journal of Palliative Care* 15, 26–30.

11 Jack, C.M., Penny, L. and Nazar, W. (2001). Effective palliative care for minority ethnic groups: the role of a liaison worker. *International Journal of Palliative Nursing* 7, 375–80.

12 Goldstein, D., Thewes, B. and Butow, P. (2002). Communicating in a multicultural society. II: Greek community attitudes towards cancer in Australia. *Internal Medicine Journal* 32, 289–96.

13 Randhawa, G., et al. (2003). Communication in the development of culturally competent palliative care services in the UK: a case study. *International Journal of Palliative Nursing* 9, 24–31.

14 Crawley, L.M., et al. (2002). Strategies for culturally effective end-of-life care. *Annals of Internal Medicine* 136, 673–9.

15 McNamara, B., et al. (1997). Palliative care in a multicultural society: perceptions of health care professionals. *Palliative Medicine* 11, 359–67.

16 Lasch, K.E., et al. (2000). Using focus group methods to develop multicultural cancer pain education materials. *Pain Management Nursing* 1, 129–38.

17 Karim, K., Bailey, M. and Tunna, K. (2000). Nonwhite ethnicity and the provision of specialist palliative care services: factors affecting doctors' referral patterns. *Palliative Medicine* 14, 471–8.

Spiritual or existential concerns

Spiritual care should be an integral part of comprehensive palliative care afforded to every patient, but is probably the least understood and the most often neglected.[1, 2] The most frequent misunderstanding is to equate spirituality with religious beliefs; while some people express their spirituality through an organized religion, there are many who do not. Spiritual care, as described below, has much wider application. Use of the term 'existential' (meaning pertaining to existence) instead of spiritual emphasizes the universality of these issues and that they are not necessarily dependent on any religion or religious practice.

Spirituality

Every human being, be they religious or not, possesses spirituality. Spirituality encompasses the purpose and meaning of an individual's existence and involves relationships with, and perceptions of, people and all other things and events. Spirituality is unique to each person. It is founded in cultural, religious and family traditions, and is modified by life experiences; it is the basis for an individual's attitudes, values, beliefs, and actions. It may or may not be expressed through a formal belief structure or religion.

Questions pertaining to spiritual and existential issues may arise as the result of any life event, but occur most frequently (probably invariably) in response to terminal illness.

For patients who observe particular religious practices and customs, spirituality is usually encompassed within their religion. Some aspects of various religious beliefs are dealt with in the second part of this chapter.

Spiritual and existential distress

Most, if not all, patients with a terminal illness will experience spiritual or existential distress. Spiritual and existential problems, whether recognized or not, are an important source of clinical suffering; they may cause or aggravate pain and psychosocial problems, or may cause an anguish all their own. Recognition and successful management of spiritual and existential problems may be of great benefit to the patient. There is a strong inverse correlation between spiritual well being and both depression and the desire to hasten death in the terminally ill,[3-5] which underlines the need for research into spirituality-based interventions.

Spiritual and existential problems

Spiritual and existential problems encountered by the terminally ill can be broadly grouped as relating to the past, the present and the future (Table 33.1). Patients may have painful memories or shame about things past, may question the value or meaning of their life, the worth of relationships, and there may be guilt about failures and objectives not achieved. Contemplation of the present brings questions about meaning—both the meaning of their life and the meaning of suffering. There is continued need for identity, respect, and self-esteem in the face of physical, psychological, and social changes associated with progressive disease. Questions pertaining to the future may include the hope of understanding life and death, the hope to love and be loved, and the hope that those left behind will prosper. Death anxiety, with concerns or fears about impending death, is common.

Religious beliefs may be the cause of spiritual distress, and such problems are more likely to be openly voiced. There may be questions about the existence of God or a life after death. People who have let their religious practices lapse for many years may wish to reaffirm their beliefs. Others may consider their disease as a punishment or feel betrayed, and have difficulty continuing their practices.

Table 33.1 Spiritual and existential distress

Relating to the past
    value and meaning of a person's life
    worth of relationships
    value of previous achievements
    painful memories or shame
    guilt about failures, unfulfilled aspirations

Relating to the present
    disruption of personal integrity
        physical, psychological and social changes
        increased dependency
    meaning of a person's life
    meaning of suffering

Relating to the future
    impending separation
    hopelessness
    meaninglessness
    concerns about death

Relating to religion
    existence of after-life
    disease as a punishment

Clinical features

Spiritual or existential suffering most often manifests as physical or psychological problems. As with each of the other causes of suffering, unresolved spiritual or existential problems may cause or aggravate pain or other physical symptoms or psychosocial distress

(Figure 33.1). These may be the only manifestation of spiritual or existential suffering, and pain or other symptoms unresponsive to appropriate therapy should alert the clinician to the possibility of unrecognized spiritual or existential problems. A few patients will ask direct questions relating to their spiritual concerns. It is possible that many of the patients classified as withdrawn and depressed are really suffering spiritual or existential distress. The clinical expression of spiritual or existential suffering is frequently overshadowed by other clinical problems and is often not apparent until other physical and psychosocial problems are controlled.

Figure 33.1 The interrelationship between spiritual concerns and other causes of suffering. (a) Unresolved spiritual problems, non-religious and religious, may cause or aggravate other problems; equally importantly, religious beliefs may ameliorate or control physical and mental suffering. (b) Unresolved problems related to other causes of suffering may aggravate spiritual or religious problems.

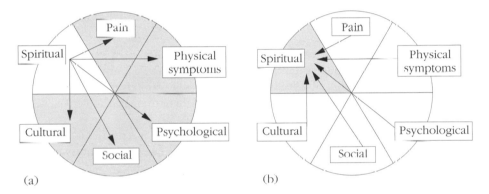

Treatment

Patients vary greatly in their desire to pursue issues related to either existential concerns or their spirituality: some will not discuss it, some just need the presence of a sympathetic person to listen, and others may wish to pursue matters in greater depth.

Spiritual care is person-centred and begins at the level of the patients' own insight.[6, 7] They must be accepted exactly as they are, in a caring and non-judgmental way. The pastoral care worker's views, particularly religious beliefs, never enter into the discussion unless specifically requested by the patient.

Issues relating to the past can be addressed and the aim of therapy is to help re-establish a sense of personal meaning and worth (Table 33.2). Cognitive techniques allow the patient to modify appraisal of things past, with emphasis on those things that are positive and meaningful. A more formal life review may bring to attention those issues causing distress and about which they may need to talk. The carer supporting a life review needs to be non-judgmental, supporting and helping patients explore their own spiritual or existential issues. If successful, feelings of being unworthy or having meaningless lives may resolve.

Therapy of problems related to the present is directed at the maintenance of dignity and self-esteem. Reversible physical, psychological and social problems are addressed. Cosmetic and functional supports are used to maintain the patient's appearance and independence. Cognitive therapy allows them to modify their appraisal of the current situation. Insight-directed therapy can allow the patient to acknowledge there are meaningful and fulfilling tasks to be done and restore a sense of purpose.

Table 33.2 Therapy for spiritual or existential distress

Past events
> cognitive restructuring, reappraisal
> life review

Present
> treatment of reversible physical, psychological, social problems
> maintenance of appearance, dignity, independence
> cognitive therapy, reappraisal of current situation
> insight-directed therapy to re-establish sense of purpose

Future
> cognitive therapy
> setting achievable short-term goals
> address fears associated with death
> address religious issues

Spiritual or existential problems related to the future are addressed in a similar manner. Hopelessness and futility require cognitive re-structuring focused on realistic and achievable short-term goals. Restoration of a feeling of purpose will counter meaninglessness. Fears about death need to be discussed. The appropriate chaplain or minister should deal with specific religious problems.

Successful treatment of spiritual and existential suffering will help patients' acceptance of their situation. It will allow them to concentrate more on the quality than the quantity of life remaining and there may be much less pain, anxiety and depression.

Religious care

Religion is the relationship between an individual and God, characterized by belief in, reverence for, and desire to please that God. For patients who profess a religious faith, their spirituality is usually closely allied with their religion, and they are less likely to have unmet spiritual concerns if their religious needs are met.

In palliative care, religious care is of great importance. Lack of respect for an individual's religious beliefs or needs may cause problems between the patient and staff. As with other spiritual problems, unresolved issues may cause or aggravate other problems including pain, physical and psychosocial symptoms (Figure 33.1). Equally important is the effect that religious beliefs, particularly Eastern religions, may have in lessening the physical and mental suffering associated with terminal illness.

The management of religious issues is both simple and complex. First, there should be unreserved respect for an individual's religious beliefs and practices. This does not require knowledge of the customs of all the different religions or denominations, but does necessitate that the patient or family be asked about religious matters including prayer, diet, and routines of personal hygiene; rituals of washing have religious importance for some people. Secondly, the manner in which individuals practise their religion must be respected. This means that a patient's religious needs are assessed on an individual basis and not by their denomination or religion. No two Christians are likely to have the same religious needs, and so it is with people of other faiths.

Some knowledge of the basic customs and practices of the common religions is helpful, and provides a background to develop a programme of religious care for an individual patient. The brief descriptions of the major religions that follow are to be regarded as very general and are focused on the areas pertinent to palliative care. They do not replace the need to ask each patient and family about individual practices and observances.

Conflict most often arises not through disrespect but because the patient's religious practices such as fasting may prevent proper care or pain control. These matters have to be negotiated with the patient and the involvement of the appropriate minister or priest may be helpful. In most religions there is provision for the seriously ill to waive certain practices. The final decision on these matters will, however, rest with the patient.

Buddhism

The discipline of Buddhism is based on the four truths of Buddha. These are that suffering and human existence are strongly linked; that suffering is caused by selfishness and the desire for pleasure that make knowledge and insight difficult; and that correction of these will eliminate suffering. The fourth teaches the noble eightfold path: that right understanding, aspiration, speech, action, livelihood, effort, thought and meditation will lead to the end of the state of suffering. In Buddhism, there is rebirth of the soul after death. Each life builds on past experiences, gradually progressing toward perfect freedom and peace without suffering, or *nirvana*.

Customs. Many Buddhists are vegetarian and few drink alcohol. There may be strict rules for hygiene, including washing after urination and defaecation, with which a terminally ill patient may need assistance.

Terminal care. Buddhists approach death in a calm and accepting manner [8]. They require the opportunity to meditate without interruption at various times through the day. They may appreciate a visit from a Buddhist monk or *bhikku*, although there are no religious last rites. Buddhists are reluctant to take analgesics or any drugs that may cause mental clouding and interfere with their ability to meditate; meditating upon one's own death influences the next reincarnation.

After death, the body is wrapped in a plain sheet. Buddhists customarily request cremation.

Christianity

Christianity is the religion of the followers of Jesus Christ, the Son of God, whom they believe to have been both human and divine, and through whom they approach God himself. Christians believe in a loving, just and personal God and that the salvation of mankind lies in following the teachings of Jesus as recorded in the Holy Bible. There are three main divisions in the Christian Church—Roman, Protestant and Orthodox—beyond which are many different denominations and the variety of beliefs and practices is considerable.

Customs. There are no dietary or other customs observed by all Christians that influence care in a palliative care setting, although some sects and individuals may observe certain dietary restrictions or abstain from alcohol.

Terminal care. Christian teaching is of the existence of an afterlife, either in Heaven or Hell. Contemplation of being condemned to Hell may be the source of fear and anxiety for some patients, but belief in the confession and absolution of sins will provide comfort. This is normally performed by a minister or priest as the Sacrament of the Sick (formerly known as the Last Rites), which is administered not only to those who are terminally ill and is not just a preparation for death. The person will make an act of confession, receive absolution for sins, take Holy Communion and be anointed with the oil of the sick. The involvement of a minister or chaplain may also be of considerable comfort and support to the family.

After death, there are no particular Christian rules that need to be observed.

Hinduism

Hinduism is a very ancient religion that has many gods and goddesses, although most Hindus believe they are manifestations of one God. Hindus believe in reincarnation and death is seen as a rebirth, the soul of a person moving on to be incorporated in another living being. An important element of Hinduism is to learn to withstand pain and suffering through the practice of detachment and meditation. Pain and suffering are regarded both as inevitable and as mental processes. It should be possible, therefore, to train the mind to be detached from physical pain and suffering; when the mind is attached to God it is easy to forget physical suffering.

Customs. There is no standard form of worship. Some Hindus meditate, some pray, and some combine meditation and prayer with physical exercises as in some forms of yoga. Modesty is important, especially for Hindu women, who may be unwilling to co-operate with male nurses and doctors.

Diet. Most Hindus are vegetarian. Anything derived from the cow, which is sacred, is forbidden.

Terminal care. With the Hindu philosophy of life and reincarnation, anger and fear of death are uncommon.[9] The patient needs time and space to pray and meditate, undisturbed. The attendance of a Hindu priest or *pandit* will assist the patient in these philosophical and psychological adjustments. Routines of personal hygiene that may require assistance include rinsing the mouth with water before and after every meal and washing the anal region after every bowel action. Hindus bathe daily and this is a necessary part of their devotions and prayers; running water is desirable and a shower is preferred to a bath. A drop or two of water from the holy River Ganges may be placed in the patient's mouth just before or soon after death.

After death, ritual washing of the body is performed by the family. The eldest son is involved, even if he is young. Some Hindu women wear a gold nuptial thread around their neck, which can only be removed after death and only by the husband. The dark red linear mark in the centre of the forehead is not washed off. Some men wear a sacred thread around their arm, as a sign of religious maturity, which is left in place.

Hindus are cremated. It is the duty of the eldest son to light the funeral pyre, although this may have to be done symbolically in western societies. Some of the ash or small pieces of bone may be sent away to be immersed in the holy River Ganges.

Islam

The word Islam means submission and Muslims submit themselves to the will of God (Allah) and follow the teaching of the great prophet Mohammed as recorded in the Koran. The spiritual leader or minister is an Imam, the place of worship a mosque. There is a large number of different Muslim sects including Sunni, Shi'ite and Ismaili, which differ in various ways but there is generally strict adherence to Islamic law.

Customs. Special prayers or *salah* are said five times a day, facing towards Mecca. Before praying, a Muslim must perform a ritual washing of the face, feet, hands and arms in running water. There is also ritual washing of the anogenital region with running water after urination or defaecation, and a Muslim cannot pray unless this is done. Muslims fast from dawn to sunset during the festival of Ramadan and this may include any medications. The strong tradition of modesty makes it desirable, whenever possible, that male patients be attended by male doctors and nurses, and female patients by females; many Muslim women are reluctant to be undressed or examined in the presence of any man other than their husband. Female patients should be addressed in the presence of the husband whose opinion and consent they may require; wives of patients should be addressed in the presence of the husband or the eldest family male.

Diet. Forbidden are pork or any pig products and alcohol. Other meat is acceptable if it is killed according to Islamic law *(halal)*. Most patients will follow a vegetarian diet unless they are certain that other food has been prepared appropriately.

Dress. Females are traditionally clothed from head to foot except for their faces. They are also fully dressed at night and may expect to remain so in hospital or hospice.

Terminal care. A Muslim patient does not usually have great difficulty facing death because it is God's will and there is belief in a life after death.[10] Religious rituals are important and patients may wish to continue normal praying as long as possible. They will require assistance with washing (pouring water from a jug) and positioning so they may face Mecca. Even terminally ill patients may attempt to fast during Ramadan. If medications are included in the fast, conflict may develop between staff and patient if it allows recurrence of pain or other symptoms. The intervention of an Imam may be of assistance as there is provision for the seriously ill to be excluded from these practices. There may be an apparently stoical acceptance of pain, if it is regarded by the patient as God's will. Special prayers are said for the dying by family and friends. There are no religious last rites or confession. If possible, a dying Muslim should be positioned so they face Mecca.

After death, the body should not be touched by non-Muslims, nor washed.[11] Family members or friends perform ritual washing. Females are washed by women, males by men. The head should be turned to the right shoulder, to be buried facing Mecca. Muslims are buried, never cremated, and this takes place as soon as possible, usually within 24 hours.

Judaism

Judaism involves belief in one God and the teaching and laws laid down in the Torah and Talmud. A Jewish chaplain is a Rabbi, the place of worship a synagogue. There is great variation in the degree to which the laws are observed, ranging from strict Orthodoxy to more liberal groups who preserve what they regard as the important parts of the law but do not observe other rituals.

Customs. The Jewish Sabbath begins before sunset on Friday and ends at sunset on Saturday. The Sabbath is a day of rest and no work should be done. When praying, a Jewish male wears a skullcap or *yarmulke* and prayer shawl or *tallith*.

Diet. Forbidden foods include pork, any pig products and shellfish. Orthodox Jews require a kosher diet which involves the killing and preparation of food according to strict religious laws and the crockery and cutlery used must be kept separate from that used for non-kosher food; in addition, meat and milk may not be taken at the same meal. Patients may elect to have vegetarian food if kosher food is not available.

Terminal care. Two basic tenets of Jewish law, relating to the sanctity of life and the preservation of hope, might be interpreted as indicating that the principles of palliative care are contrary to Jewish values.[12] This is not necessarily so as, whilst active measures to hasten a death are strictly forbidden, there is no obligation to prolong a futile existence. A balance between hope and acceptance can usually be achieved. The prayers for the Day of Atonement, which may be used by the dying as a means of confession, may allow hope to be maintained.

Whilst there is belief in an afterlife, the emphasis in Judaism is very much on this life and the living. Eating is seen as a hold on this life, which explains why relatives may become more concerned about an unwillingness or inability to eat than anything else. The family and rabbi may recite prayers, but there are no religious last rites.

After death, the eyes are closed, the limbs straightened, the jaw bandaged and the body wrapped in a plain sheet. To leave the body unattended is disrespectful and a 'watcher' may stay with the body, reciting psalms, until burial. Washing and ritual purification are performed by special members of the Jewish community or *chevra kaddisha*. For Orthodox Jews, only burial is allowed and it is completed as soon as possible. Cremation is contrary to Orthodox law but is practised by some more liberal communities.

Sikhism

Sikhism is based on the teaching of ten sixteenth century gurus, as recorded in the Granth Sahib, and incorporates many features of Hinduism and Islam. Like Muslims, Sikhs are completely monotheistic; like Hindus, they believe in reincarnation. Sikhs have a strict code of discipline in which they must be truthful, helpful and kind to others. The Sikh temple is called the *gurdwara, which* also functions as a community centre; there are no Sikh ministers or priests.

Customs. Sikh custom is to rise early and bathe prior to prayers, which should be said at sunrise; prayers are repeated at sunset and bedtime.

Dress. A male Sikh wears a number of objects of great religious significance, called the 5Ks, which should not be removed. They are the *kesh* or uncut hair, a *kangha* or small comb worn in the hair which is covered by a turban, a *kara* or steel bangle worn on the right wrist, a *kirpan* or dagger (now usually symbolic), and the white shorts or *kaccha* which are worn as underwear. The *kaccha* have come to be a symbol of modesty and morality and may be worn constantly, including in the shower.

Diet. The only dietary restriction laid down by the gurus was that meat slaughtered according to Islamic law is forbidden. Alcohol and smoking are prohibited.

Terminal care. Because of the doctrine of reincarnation, few Sikhs are fearful of death. Time and privacy for prayers are important. There may be readings from the scriptures by family and friends and playing of the psalm of peace. Daily bathing, an important religious ritual, may require assistance; the tradition of using running water makes a shower preferable to a bath. At no time should any of the 5Ks be taken from a patient.

After death, washing of the body is performed by the family. Cremation is performed, preferably within 24 hours. Men are cremated wearing their 5Ks. The ashes are collected and scattered in a river or the sea or may be taken back to the holy River Sutlej in the Punjab.

References

1   Cobb, M. (2001). *The Dying Soul. Spiritual Care at the End of Life*. Buckingham, Open University Press.
2   Rumbold, B. (ed.) (2002). *Spirituality and Palliative Care*. Oxford, Oxford University Press.
3   Breitbart, W. (2002). Spirituality and meaning in supportive care: spirituality- and meaning-centered group psychotherapy interventions in advanced cancer. *Supportive Care in Cancer* 10, 272–80.
4   Nelson, C.J., et al. (2002). Spirituality, religion, and depression in the terminally ill. *Psychosomatics* 43, 213–20.
5   McClain, C.S., Rosenfeld, B. and Breitbart, W. (2003). Effect of spiritual well being on end-of-life despair in terminally-ill cancer patients. *Lancet* 361, 1603–7.

6   Rousseau, P. (2000). Spirituality and the dying patient. *Journal of Clinical Oncology* 18, 2000–2.

7   Lo, B., et al. (2002). Discussing religious and spiritual issues at the end of life: a practical guide for physicians. *Journal of the American Medical Association* 287, 749–54.

8   Sibley, D. (1997). Caring for dying Buddhists. *International Journal of Palliative Nursing* 3, 26–30.

9   Sharma, K. (2000). A question of faith for the Hindu patient. *European Journal of Palliative Care* 7, 99–100.

10. Gatrad, A.R. and Sheikh, A. (2002). Palliative care for Muslims and issues before death. *International Journal of Palliative Nursing* 8, 526–31.

11. Gatrad, R. and Sheikh, A. (2002). Palliative care for Muslims and issues after death. *International Journal of Palliative Nursing* 8, 594–7.

12. Neuberger, J. (1999). Judaism and palliative care. *European Journal of Palliative Care* 6, 166–68.

34

Grief and bereavement

Palliative care includes the management of grief and bereavement. Careful and honest consideration of family members during the patient's terminal illness will lessen grieving. The involvement of a social worker, psychologist or psychiatrist in a palliative care team will help predict bereavement problems and provide support and treatment, if required.

Bereavement is the loss of a close or loved person; bereavement reactions are the psychological, physiological or behavioural reactions to that loss. Grief is the psychological response or feeling resulting from the loss. Mourning is the social expression of grief and includes the mourning rituals and behaviours that are specific to each culture and religion.

In the great majority of cases, support from family and friends, and time, are all that is required for successful bereavement. A person working in palliative care needs to know what constitutes normal and abnormal bereavement, so that help or counselling can be provided if required. However, there are so many religious, cultural and individual variations that the definition of what is normal or abnormal is difficult. Many reviews of grief and bereavement have been published.[1–5]

Phases of normal grief

The compartmentalization of the grief reaction is artificial and there is an infinite range of reactions that are not necessarily abnormal. However, a conceptual framework facilitates identification of those in need of specialized help.

Anticipatory grief

During the terminal phase of an illness such as cancer, when it becomes obvious or undeniable that death is going to occur, relatives may demonstrate signs of grieving such as anxiety, anger, or other emotional responses to the impending loss. This is more likely to occur if the patient is being nursed at home. Whether or not anticipatory grieving lessens the severity of the grief response after death is debated, but it should be associated with less shock and acute reaction. There is some evidence that relatives who are adequately forewarned and have time for some anticipatory grieving may adjust more easily after the death. A strong case can be made for making certain that the family are completely and honestly informed of the patient's prognosis, and not surprised with the truth when the patient is transferred to a hospice or palliative care service.

Anticipatory grieving is more likely to occur with a protracted terminal illness and may be problematic if it is severe or occurs too early. The relatives may withdraw from the patient who may suffer a feeling of emotional abandonment. It is particularly troublesome if the patient's condition temporarily improves, requiring the relatives to re-establish a relationship with the patient to whom, from an emotional point of view, they have already said goodbye.

Acute grief

The immediate reaction to the death of a family member varies from stoical acceptance to hysteria. Noisy lamentation is the required behaviour in some cultures but is considered less acceptable in others.

The acute grief reaction begins within hours or days. It may be delayed of necessity (the need to recover physically from nursing the dying patient or the need to organize and be in charge) or because a person may wish to grieve privately after the funeral is completed. Delayed grieving, beginning more than two weeks after the death, is more likely to be severe and become chronic.

The acute grief reaction is often preceded by a period of shock or numbness during which the person may intellectually accept what has happened but feels nothing. This frequently enables the relatives to cope with all the necessary practicalities and may help carry them through the ordeal of the funeral. A variety of clinical features may follow (Table 34.1). There may be anxiety (due to loss of the loved one, loss of security, or change in the daily routine of life), agitation and restlessness (with purposeless activity and inability to do anything constructive), or inactivity, apathy and withdrawal. Depressive symptoms, including guilt, are common. There may be preoccupation with the deceased, associated with pining and searching for them. Anger is not uncommon and may be directed at either the deceased or at the carers and institutions responsible for the patient's treatment. Fatigue and tiredness by day and insomnia by night are common. Other somatic symptoms may occur including anorexia, diarrhoea, palpitations and the bereaved may complain of similar symptoms to those experienced by the deceased.

Table 34.1 Acute grief reactions

Shock, 'numbness', unreality	Crying
Anxiety	Anorexia
Agitation	Diarrhoea
Aimless activity, inactivity	Palpitations
Anger	Fatigue
Preoccupation	Insomnia
Depressive symptoms, including guilt	Symptoms similar to the deceased

The acute phase usually lasts about six weeks but may be longer without being abnormal. No specific treatment is warranted although short-term night time sedation may be helpful.

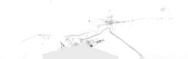

During this phase, care is supportive and it is important that the grieving person understands that it is acceptable to grieve and to be seen to be grieving.

Chronic phase of normal grief

There usually follows a period lasting a few months (up to two years) characterized by reducing signs of acute grief and during which the person is likely to be apathetic, socially withdrawn, sad and depressed. Anxiety and insomnia may persist. The person lacks direction or a sense of purpose. Management is supportive and needs to be non-judgmental to allow the true expression of feelings. Involvement in bereavement groups and receiving support from other widows or widowers the same age may be beneficial during the latter part of this phase. As important as it is to encourage people to grieve in the acute phase, it is sometimes necessary to give them encouragement and permission to stop grieving; this can usually be addressed, at the appropriate time, by suggesting that the deceased would not have expected them to remain in perpetual mourning.

Resolution phase

The start of recovery is marked by a phase of reorganization during which the physical and psychological symptoms diminish and tasks are tackled with purpose. Memories of the deceased can be recalled without sadness and new relationships can be formed without guilt or anxiety. Many bereaved feel that the normal grieving process leads to an increased emotional and psychological maturity and to personal growth.

Abnormal bereavement reactions

Grief reactions that last longer, are more severe, or differ in some other way, are considered to be abnormal. However, as there are no definitions of the normal, their characterization is subjective. There are a number of risk factors that identify persons at increased risk of abnormal bereavement or poor bereavement outcome (Table 34.2). [3, 6, 7]

Inhibited bereavement

Inhibited grief reactions in adults, in which there is little outward sign of bereavement, are usually abnormal. It may result in an altered lifestyle in which any reminders of the deceased are avoided and previous social ties are broken; it is often associated with anxiety, irritability and depression. Therapy should be by counselling rather than medications. The bereaved is taken through a programme of guided mourning in which they are helped to think about the deceased, to review the lost relationship, however painful that may be, and to express any anger or guilt; involvement of other family members in the programme is helpful.

Distorted bereavement

The two common types of distorted bereavement involve extreme anger and extreme guilt. Anger is likely if the bereaved was very dependent on the deceased or if there is a strong sense of desertion. In the case of guilt, the whole bereavement process is taken up by continuing guilty ruminations and self-blame.

Chronic bereavement

Chronic grief, also called unresolved grief, is characterized by the persistence of the signs and symptoms of acute grief that do not resolve with time. There are a number of defined risk factors for chronic grief (Table 34.2). The patient may exhibit anxiety and hypochondriasis but depressive symptoms usually predominate. A small proportion of patients will present with progressive symptoms suggesting major depression, sometimes with suicidal tendencies. For other patients, deciding when their reaction is pathological is a matter of clinical judgment.

Table 34.2 Risk factors for poor bereavement outcome

High initial distress with depressive symptoms

Unanticipated death

Death of a child

Inhibited grief

High dependency on the deceased

Other concurrent significant stresses

Poor social supports

Poor response to previous losses

History of psychiatric illness, depression

Treatment

Most bereaved people require no special assistance and recover satisfactorily with the support of family and friends, and time.

Before death

Bereavement care begins before the patient's death. The relatives need an honest appraisal of the patient's situation and life expectancy, in order that they are prepared for the death and so that tasks may be completed. As grieving is a family affair, a family meeting with the health care professionals may be appropriate. Individuals or families considered to be at increased risk of bereavement difficulties can be counselled. A program of family focused grief therapy for selected families, identified as being at increased risk of morbid grief, is the subject of an on-going RCT.[3]

At the time of death

When a patient's death is anticipated, the family are informed and encouraged to be present. Being present at the time of death or seeing the deceased assists acceptance of the reality of the death. The bereaved need support to stay with the dead person for a while, to be encouraged to talk or to touch, or to just sit quietly. Some relatives will wish to assist in the laying out process. With death from progressive cancer, the situation can usually be honestly described as a release from further suffering and this is often of comfort to the family. When appropriate, the bereaved are complimented on their care for the deceased, especially if the patient was managed at home. The bereaved should be given an open invitation to make contact in the future if they have any unresolved problems or questions.

After death

Follow up contact should always be made. This may be by letter or phone call and gives the bereaved a sense of being cared for and helps detect those with abnormal bereavement

responses. If the bereaved request help, they are referred to an experienced grief counsellor or psychiatrist, as appropriate. Bereavement self-help groups may also be useful. In other situations, it should be the responsibility of the bereaved's own doctor, who has often known the family for many years, to judge whether additional help is required. Memorial services conducted by palliative care units, held once or twice a year, may be an effective means of bereavement follow up.[8] A review of bereavement services provided by palliative care units showed considerable variation in what help was offered or available.[9] This underlines the need for a better understanding of the needs of families, as well as education and guidelines for the provision of bereavement services.

Bereaved children

Children, especially those of school age, require special attention at the time of death of a parent. The problem may be compounded if the surviving parent suffers a severe grief reaction. Anticipation of death sometimes allows better preparation of a child for the parent's death. Parents frequently seek advice about what their children should know and understand, and it is important that expert supportive counselling be available at this time. Bereavement reactions in children may take the form of behavioural or disciplinary problems and physical or somatic symptoms are common. Insecurity, anger and guilt occur as well. Follow up of bereaved children suggests an increase in maladaptive behaviour that may interfere with social and academic performance, in which case counselling may be appropriate and beneficial.

References

1   Katz, L. and Chochinov, H.M. (1998). The spectrum of grief in palliative care. In *Topics in Palliative Care* (ed. E. Bruera and R. Portenoy). New York, Oxford University Press.
2   Hockey, J., Katz, J. and Small, N. (ed.) (2001). *Grief, Mourning and Death Ritual.* Buckingham, Open University Press.
3   Kissane, D.W. and Bloch, S. (2002). *Family Focused Grief Therapy.* Buckingham, Open University Press.
4   Kissane, D.W. (2003). Bereavement. In *Oxford Textbook of Palliative Medicine. Third edition* (ed. D. Doyle, G. Hanks, K. Calman and N. Cherny). Oxford, Oxford University Press.
5   Payne, S. and Lloyd-Williams, M. (2003). Bereavement care. In *Psychosocial Issues in Palliative Care* (ed. M. Lloyd-Williams). Oxford, Oxford University Press.
6   Kelly, B., et al. (1999). Predictors of bereavement outcome for family carers of cancer patients. *Psychooncology* 8, 237–49.
7   Ringdal, G.I., et al. (2001). Factors affecting grief reactions in close family members to individuals who have died of cancer. *Journal of Pain and Symptom Management* 22, 1016–26.
8   Rawlings, D. and Glynn, T. (2002). The development of a palliative care-led memorial service in an acute hospital setting. *International Journal of Palliative Nursing* 8, 40–7.
9   Bromberg, M.H. and Higginson, I. (1996). Bereavement follow-up: what do palliative support teams actually do? *Journal of Palliative Care* 12, 12–17.

Complementary and alternative therapies

I know a maiden fair to see
Take care!
She an both false and friendly be,
Beware! Beware!

H.W. Longfellow (1807–82)

A perfect quack is a most obsequious sycophant—
his medicines are always exactly what the patients wants.
They are never disagreeable, and perfectly safe in all cases,
and always certain to cure.

Dan King
Quackery Unmasked, 1858

35

Complementary and alternative medicine (CAM)

CAM therapies claiming anticancer activity
Alternative systems of medical practice
Mind–body interventions
Biologic-based therapies
Manual healing methods
Energy therapies

Complementary and alternative medicine (CAM) encompasses a spectrum of different therapies not routinely used by conventional practitioners (Table 35.1). The majority of patients with advanced cancer will use some form of CAM,[1-5] and health care professionals need to be able to discuss the possible benefits and disadvantages of these therapies with patients. The National Council for Complementary and Alternative Medicine (USA) maintains an information website that provides detailed descriptions of many CAM therapies, including references to the relevant clinical trials and studies.[6]

Table 35.1   Classification of complementary and alternative medicine

Alternative medical systems	Biologic-based therapies
acupuncture	diets
Ayurveda	herbal medicines
homeopathy	hyperoxygenation therapies
traditional Chinese medicine	naturopathy
Mind-body interventions	supplements e.g. shark's cartilage
aromatherapy	vitamins and minerals
biofeedback	Manipulative and body-based methods
healing	chiropractic
hypnosis	massage
meditation	osteopathy
music, art therapy	Energy therapies
prayer	bioelectrical field manipulation
relaxation	radionics
visualization, guided imagery	reiki
yoga	therapeutic touch

The increasing popularity of CAM over the last few decades is a consumer-driven phenomenon, for which there may be a number of explanations.[7] Practitioners of alternative medicine often take a more holistic approach to care than do medical oncologists, with attention to psychological, social and spiritual matters, which patients may find more satisfying. The emphasis on diet and on the naturopathic principles that the body is capable of healing itself given the correct nutritional and psychological adjustments, allows patients to maintain hope, to feel involved in their own treatment, and satisfied that at least some form of active therapy is being pursued. In addition, the therapies are often referred to as 'natural', 'non-toxic', and 'can do no harm', even though serious and life-threatening adverse effects have occasionally been reported.

The use of CAMs increases with advancing disease, unmet patient needs, and helplessness.[8] Surveys of the reasons why cancer patients use CAMs—to feel hopeful, to improve quality of life, for the relief of symptoms, and to have greater control in the decision making process—are a salutary reminder of the shortcomings in the care these patients receive.[9]

The scientific evidence supporting the use of CAM therapies is scarce and mostly inadequate.[3, 10] Published studies are frequently small, non-randomized and non-blinded. Problems inherent in conducting proper clinical trials with CAMs include the establishment of proper control groups, adequate blinding, and using herbal-medication preparations that are not standardized.[11, 12]

In oncology and palliative care, CAM therapies can be broadly divided according to whether or not it is claimed the treatment will cause regression or cure of cancer. Most of the complementary therapies in use, for which no anticancer activity is claimed, appear to be of benefit, particularly in regard to anxiety and psychological distress. They are in general harmless and can be used at the same time as orthodox medical treatment.

CAM therapies claiming anticancer activity

These are offered as an alternative for patients not wishing to pursue, or having failed, conventional treatment (Table 35.2). They have been advertised as 'natural', 'non-toxic', and 'can do no harm', in contrast to the 'cutting, burning, and poisoning' of conventional treatment. None have been shown to be of benefit (with the possible exception of melatonin) and some

Table 35.2 Alternative anticancer therapies

Immunotherapy	Supplements
immunoaugmentative vaccines	hydrazine
Livingstone-Wheeler method	laetrile
bovine thymus extract	vitamin C
Dietary methods	Di Bella therapy
Gerson diet	shark and bovine cartilage
macrobiotic diets	coffee enemas
mono-diets	melatonin
Bristol Cancer Help Centre	
Herbal therapy	
mistletoe extract	
PC-SPES	
essiac	

cause harm. Claims of efficacy are often based on patient satisfaction and testimonials, but properly conducted clinical trials have shown them to be of no value.

Palliative care patients with progressive disease may experiment with these therapies or be pressured to do so by family and friends.

Immunotherapy

The possibility of eradicating cancer by augmenting the body's own immune system has long been the dream of cancer therapists. In conventional cancer research, a range of immune therapies have been used to this end but have never been shown to be effective, especially in patients with advanced cancer. A number of immunoaugmentative vaccines, some completely fraudulent, were marketed in the alternative medicine sector. Treatment often involved travelling long distances to the treatment centre, being separated from family and friends for weeks or months, and the financial cost of the therapy itself was considerable.

The Livingstone-Wheeler treatment involved an autogenous immune-enhancing vaccine, together with BCG, vegetarian diets and coffee enemas. A matched-pair comparison with patients receiving standard cancer therapy showed no improvement in survival and a poorer quality of life for the patients treated by the alternative method compared to those receiving conventional radiation and chemotherapy.[13]

Treatment with bovine thymus extracts has been reported to improve immune function, but a systematic review of RCTs reported no compelling evidence of clinical efficacy in the treatment of human cancers.[14]

Dietary therapy

More diets have been devised for the treatment of cancer than for any other disorder except obesity. Most are based on two principles that remain unproven. The first is based on the valid observation that a diet rich in fruit and vegetables, low in fat, and including antioxidants, is associated with a lower incidence of cancer. However, there is no scientific basis to believe that increasing the amounts of these ingredients in the diet will cure an existing cancer. The second, employed in naturopathy is that fasting or the use of a mono-diet allows 'detoxification' and the clearing of accumulated metabolic toxins, liberating the body's own curative forces.

The Gerson Diet and its derivatives. Dr Max Gerson (1881–1959) advocated radical dietary change as a means of curing cancer and a number of diets currently advocated are based on his recommendations. The diet comprises raw or freshly prepared fruits and vegetables, freshly pressed calf's liver juice, and coffee enemas. Juices must be prepared by pressing, not by a juice extractor, and aluminium utensils and microwave cooking are not permitted. A number of dietary supplements including vitamins, enzymes, royal jelly and liver injections may be included. Exclusions include salt, oils, fat, preservatives, caffeine and alcohol. The use of hair dyes, cosmetics and tobacco are prohibited. The Gerson Diet and its derivatives are expensive and time-consuming to prepare, and there is no scientific evidence that they are of benefit.

Macrobiotic diets. These consist largely of whole grains, cereals, and cooked vegetables. A significant proportion of cancer patients on a macrobiotic diet experience problems with weight loss.[15]

Mono-diets. Mono-diets, in which a patient eats only one food or food group for a number of days or weeks, are advocated as part of a 'detoxification' phase in the treatment of cancer. The Grape Diet and the Brown Rice Diet are two examples. These diets are nutritionally inadequate and may lead to accelerated weight loss.

Bristol Cancer Help Centre. Patients with cancer were treated with a special diet and a package of CAM modalities claimed to enhance the quality of life and foster a positive attitude to cancer. A comparison with patients treated in a cancer centre reported poorer survival in Bristol patients, but baseline differences between the two groups are a probable cause for this finding.[16]

Herbal therapy

Herbal medicine is as old as civilization and many drugs in use today have their origin in herbal medicine. Herbalism is used extensively in naturopathic practice and is a major component of ancient or traditional medical practices, such as those of China and India. Modern Western herbalism is focused more on the maintenance and restoration of normal function than treatment of specific pathology.

Herbal medicines can have toxic effects. Adverse effects that have been recorded include rashes, haemolytic anaemia, bleeding diatheses, blood dyscrasias, hepatitis, and neuropathy. Herbal preparations may also potentiate or counteract the effect of prescribed medications such as anticoagulants, anticonvulsants and insulin with potentially serious consequences.

Many cancer patients take herbal medicines as part of naturopathic therapy or a special cancer diet. Taken correctly, they may aid physiological function and provide alternatives to caffeine, alcohol and other substances excluded from special diets.

Mistletoe. Iscador is an extract made from the leafy twigs of the European mistletoe, *Biscum album*. It is reputed to have anticancer activity although reviews of published reports concluded that there was no reliable evidence to recommend its use.[3, 17, 18]

PC-SPES. This was marketed as a mixture of Chinese herbs and shown to be effective in the treatment of hormone-refractory prostate cancer.[19] It was withdrawn in 2002 after analysis revealed the presence of the synthetic drugs diethylstilboestrol, indomethacin, and warfarin.[20]

Essiac. This is a herbal mixture manufactured in Canada for which there is no published clinical evidence.[3]

Supplements

Hydrazine sulfate. Three RCTs have been conducted that showed no significant benefit from treatment with hydrazine.[5]

Laetrile. Amygdalin (laetrile, 'vitamin' B_{17}) is a cyanide-containing glycoside found in apricot kernels and other stone fruits. Its use for the treatment of cancer became extremely popular although a prospective study reported only one partial remission in 175 patients.[21] Laetrile has been associated with neuromyopathy and there are a number of documented deaths due to cyanide poisoning.

Vitamin C. After a number of uncontrolled studies reported high doses of vitamin C to be of benefit in the treatment of cancer, an RCT in patients with advanced cancer showed it to be of no value.[22] The proponents of vitamin C therapy claimed the results were due to prior chemotherapy, but a second RCT with patients who had received no chemotherapy similarly showed no benefit of vitamin C therapy.[23]

Di Bella therapy. Patients were treated with melatonin, bromocriptine, either somatostatin or octreotide, and retinoid solution (as well as cyclophosphamide and hydroxyurea in some cases). Eleven studies including 386 patients with advanced cancer, undertaken to assess the efficacy of the treatment, reported only three partial responses.[24] A retrospective matched-pair analysis showed significantly poorer survival for Di Bella's patients.[25]

Shark's cartilage. Shark's (or bovine) cartilage is widely used as a cure for cancer although there is no scientific evidence that it is effective. A trial of shark's cartilage in 60 patients with advanced cancer showed no complete or partial responses.[26] Molecules with anti-angiogenic activity have been isolated from cartilage, but it has been questioned whether these macromolecules would be absorbed from commercially available preparations.[3] Hypercalcaemia has been reported in cancer patients taking shark's cartilage.[27] Several molecules derived from cartilage that have shown anti-angiogenic activity are the subject of pre-clinical and clinical trials.

Coffee enemas. Coffee delivered per rectum is absorbed into the portal venous system where it is able to 'detoxify' the liver. There is no evidence for this and there are no clinical studies showing benefit. Patients taking coffee enemas experience a 'high' as one might after drinking several cups of strong coffee. The use of any coffee enemas, never mind every four hours, can only produce inconvenience and discomfort. Serious and life-threatening complications have been documented including colitis, septicaemia, cerebral abscess, and renal failure.[3]

Table 35.3 Melatonin in advanced cancer: RCTs

Author	n	Intervention	Outcome
Lissoni[28]	1440	supportive care ± melatonin	melatonin: ↓ incidence cachexia, asthenia; ↑ disease stabilization, 1-year survival (all pS)
Lissoni[28]	200	chemotherapy ± melatonin	melatonin: objective responses 33 vs 20% (pS); ↓ chemotherapy toxicity (pS)

Melatonin. The pineal hormone, melatonin (20mg/d, taken at night), is reported to have beneficial effects in patients with advanced cancer (Table 35.3).[28] These initial results await confirmation in independent RCTs.

Adverse effects

The disadvantages and dangers of alternative therapies must also be considered (Table 35.4). Alternative therapies may involve considerable time and expense, both of which the patient can ill afford. Rarely, patients with treatable cancer may refuse conventional therapy in favour of alternative treatments; similarly, patients admitting to receiving alternative therapies may be discriminated against by practitioners who cannot understand or tolerate why patients turn to such treatments. Patients using both conventional and alternative therapies may suffer fragmentation of their care. The alternative medicine industry is responsible for the perpetuation of a number of misconceptions that can make the treatment of other patients more difficult. The simplistic belief that cancer is caused by a dietary deficiency and can be cured by the administration of megadoses of the appropriate vitamin or mineral is scientific nonsense. In its extreme form, this has been referred to as 'holistic fundamentalism': if one eats the correct foods, takes enough vitamins, exercises, relaxes, meditates and thinks positively, any illness can be cured.

Some alternative therapies may cause serious physical injury and patient deaths have been recorded. In addition, they can cause significant psychological harm.[29] Patients practising meditation or taking complex diets may suffer guilt and depression when disease progression occurs, as it indicates they have not tried hard enough.

Table 35.4 Disadvantages and dangers of alternative therapies

Treatment
cost (in time and money)
fragmentation of care
refusal of conventional therapy
exclusion from conventional therapy

Physical adverse effects
cyanide toxicity (laetrile)
infection: hepatitis B (immune sera), septicaemia (coffee enemas)
electrolyte imbalance (coffee enemas)
chemical phlebitis (ozone)
neuropathy (excess pyridoxine)
renal calculi (excess vitamin C)
orange discolouration (excess ß-carotene)
malnutrition (exclusion diets)

Psychological adverse effects
guilt for having contracted the disease
increased guilt and depression at time of disease progression

Disinformation
simplistic relationship between diet and all types of cancer
'holistic fundamentalism'

Alternative systems of medical practice

Increasing attention is being given to traditional medical practices, particularly those from China and India. Although based on philosophies different from modern western medicine, these treatments have been in use for several thousand years.

Acupuncture

Acupuncture has been practised in China for at least 3,000 years. In its traditional form it is a holistic system of healing, based on the premise that health depends on a balance between opposing forces or vital energies, represented by *yin* and *yang*. The basis of acupuncture is that the body surface is covered by a network of pathways or meridians that are connected to internal organs and through which energy may pass; stimulation of these anatomically defined areas of skin with needles will correct an imbalance which may have occurred between the vital energies in a particular organ.

Other methods of acupuncture are also in use. Ear acupuncture or auricular therapy, which is of French rather than Oriental origin, relies on the fact that the organs and parts of the body are represented on the external ear. Acupuncture at these sites can be used to treat other parts of the body. Electro-acupuncture uses electrical stimulation of acupuncture needles to improve response. In laser acupuncture, a thin infra-red laser beam is applied to the standard acupuncture points. Acupressure involves digital pressure on acupuncture points and is used in Shiatsu therapy and may be useful for self-treatment of painful conditions. Moxibustion is the burning of rolled cones of dried herbs over acupuncture points.

Controlled trials of acupuncture are confounded by the problem of controlling for placebo effects. Systematic reviews and meta-analyses support the use of acupuncture for the treatment of nausea and vomiting.[3] In palliative care, there is anecdotal evidence that it may be helpful in the management of pain, and when used in its holistic form may lessen anxiety and provide a feeling of general well being.

The risks of acupuncture include infection, bleeding and pneumothorax but serious adverse effects should not occur with experienced practitioners.

Ayurveda

This ancient Indian 'science of life' originated in the third century BC. The essence of Ayurveda is a balance between all the constituents, qualities and energies, within and without. It has a strong mind–body component including yoga and meditation, and a sophisticated dietary system incorporating the use of herbs and spices.

Homeopathy

Homeopathy is a system of treatment developed by Dr Samuel Hahnemann (1755–1846). Symptoms are treated with microscopic doses of substances, selected on the basis that they produce similar symptoms when administered in normal doses to healthy people, in the belief that such treatment stimulates the natural inherent activity called healing. The claimed efficacy of the infinitesimally small doses that result from the extreme dilutions used in homeopathy defies scientific explanation. A meta-analysis of homeopathic treatments showed that the effects were not completely due to placebo, but there was no evidence that it was effective in any particular clinical condition.[30, 31] Many patients with advanced cancer take homeopathic medicine, probably without ill effect.

Bach flower remedies. The Bach flower remedies are a variant of homeopathy. Dr Edward Bach (1880–1936) developed a series of remedies made from extracts of flowers, diluted according to homeopathic principles, to be used to cure the ill-defined emotional origins of disease.

Traditional Chinese medicine

In traditional Chinese medicine, *Qi* is the life force and is affected by factors both hereditary and environmental. So long as *Qi* flows freely through the body, there will be balance between *yin* and *yang* and the person will be healthy. To maintain this state and to correct any imbalances, traditional Chinese medicine employs a combination of relaxation techniques, exercise (*T'ai chi*), acupuncture and a vast number of herbal preparations.

Mind–body interventions

The provision of good psychological care is of great importance in palliative care and a number of the techniques discussed below are very useful in the treatment of stress, anxiety and pain. However, the belief that cancer can be cured by psychic energy (spiritual healing) or by the patient's own mental effort (meditation and visualization), has not been scientifically documented. The available evidence regarding the effect of a patient's psychological attitude and the progression of cancer is that patients characterized as having a 'fighting spirit' *or* denial, fare best; patients with a resigned attitude or stoic acceptance fare worse.

Healing

Healing is the transmission of psychic energy for therapeutic purposes. It is practised throughout the world in countless ways ranging from conventional prayer to outrageous quackery. Faith healing, to activate the patient's own self-healing abilities, works by the power of suggestion or by hypnosis and requires the patient's belief in the healer. Spiritual or psychic healing involves the transmission of some form of energy from the healer to the patient and does not depend on the patient's belief. The healer may be a religious person, attributing his powers to God; others attribute the source of the energy to discarnate entities or departed spirits, or the fact that they themselves are able to focus natural forces. A systematic review of randomized and controlled trials of distant healing found that about half of the studies suggested it was effective, although methodological shortcomings prevent firm conclusions.[32]

Many patients with advanced cancer seek healing. Rare dramatic responses have been reported but are difficult to substantiate. The only adverse effect of healing is that there may be an escalation of depression when it becomes apparent that the treatment is not successful.

Psychological therapy

A wide range of techniques and methods are used including supportive counselling, relaxation therapy, meditation, visualization therapy, yoga, formal psychotherapy, and hypnosis. These treatments are all primarily aimed at promoting relaxation and controlling stress and anxiety, leading to improved coping and adjustment.[33] After initial training, patients themselves perform the treatment. These techniques will all lead to improved management of stress, anxiety and depression, and to improved insight and self-awareness. In some patients there may be improved pain control, whilst others may show better adjustment to their situation. There is no evidence that any of these treatments have anticancer activity.

Biologic-based therapies

Nutrition

A large number of different 'cancer diets' exist.[3, 34] The emphasis is on vegetarian food, although the benefits of this have been challenged.[35] The more conventional are designed to provide optimal nutrition to physically ill patients who may also be receiving anticancer therapy. The more extreme, with which malnutrition may be a concern, are described above.

Naturopathy

Traditional naturopathy uses natural remedies to help the body heal itself by strengthening the body's own vital curative energy and has been practised in one form or another since antiquity. It is based on three premises: that all disease is caused by an accumulation of waste material or toxins in the body; that there is a vital curative force within the human organism; and that the body has the power to heal itself, given the right circumstances. Naturopathic treatment depends on assessing the failure of the body's normal adaptive mechanisms and providing the optimal circumstances for the body to restore its own homeostasis. Assessment is necessarily holistic in approach, including not only the patient's physical symptoms but also psychosocial matters and lifestyle. It may also include analyses of the blood, urine and hair, looking for biochemical evidence of nutritional deficiency or the accumulation of toxic metals.

Naturopathy employs a range of nutritional, physical and psychological therapies. The nutritional therapy frequently starts with fasting or a restricted diet that is supposed to allow the body a physiological rest, during which time it has the opportunity to remove metabolic waste and restore homeostasis. Following this, an individually designed diet may be prescribed with an emphasis on the consumption of natural foods and with supplements of vitamins, trace elements, essential fatty acids and amino acids.

Many patients with advanced cancer receive naturopathic treatment. This may result in an improvement in their nutritional state, provided the initial restrictive phase is not too severe. Patients who have not received appropriate psychosocial treatment elsewhere may appreciate the support given by the holistic approach of naturopathy.

Herbal medicines

Herbal medications form an important part of naturopathy and traditional Chinese medicine. In addition, a number of herbs that are widely available as over-the-counter preparations are used for the treatment of particular symptoms.[36]

St John's wort. This is used for mild depression, although the evidence for it is inconclusive (see Chapter 26).

Kava. This extract of a Pacific islands plant is a popular over-the-counter anxiolytic and sedative. It has recently been withdrawn in a number of countries because of an association with hepatotoxicity, including a number of deaths.[37]

Ginseng. Prepared from the root of *Panax ginseng*, ginseng has been used in China for over 5,000 years as a panacea and revitalizing remedy. It has recently been shown to contain saponosides with hormone-like actions and may improve the ability of the adrenal cortex to respond to stress. It has no anticancer effect, but may lead to feelings of increased vitality in patients with debilitating disease. Used regularly over months or years, it can cause nervousness, insomnia, hypertension and depression. Amenorrhoea and mastalgia in women and gynaecomastia in men are also reported. Commercially available ginseng preparations are often adulterated with the roots of other plants and contain only trace amounts of ginseng.[38]

Hyperoxygenation therapies

Hyperoxygenation therapies are based on the concept that cancer is caused by oxygen deficiency and can be cured by exposing cancer cells to more oxygen than they can tolerate.

The use of germanium sesquioxide has been associated with renal failure in humans and there is no evidence that it is effective against cancer. Likewise, oral or intravenous hydrogen peroxide has never been shown to be effective against cancer and is not without side effects. Ozone therapy, using medically pure oxygen with 10% ozone given intravenously or per rectum, is similarly without foundation.[3]

Manual healing methods

Chiropractic

This involves the diagnosis and treatment of mechanical disorders of the joints, particularly the spine. Assessment usually involves both physical and radiological examination. Treatment is by manipulation, pressure techniques and massage. Patients with advanced cancer may benefit from chiropractic manipulation providing the possibility of local metastatic disease is first excluded.

Massage

Remedial massage may provide relaxation, a lessening of anxiety and an improvement in the feeling of well being. For patients who are confined to bed or have reduced mobility, massage may be important in maintaining muscle tone and movement. Patients with advanced cancer reported improvement in physical symptoms as well as reduced anxiety and tension, lasting for several days after each massage. Simple foot massage may improve patients' pain, nausea and anxiety.[39]

Reflexology. Reflexology is an ancient Chinese art of massaging pressure points on the soles of the feet to relieve symptoms elsewhere in the body and to relieve stress and tension.

Shiatsu. Shiatsu is a Japanese therapy that combines massage with finger pressure to acupuncture points and meridians (acupressure).

Aromatherapy. Aromatherapy is the therapeutic use of essential oils extracted from plants, applied externally by massage. Aromatherapy reduces anxiety and tension and produces a calming effect.[40]

Osteopathy

Osteopathy specializes in the treatment of abnormalities of the musculoskeletal system by soft tissue massage, joint therapy and manipulation. Patients with cancer and musculoskeletal pain may benefit from osteopathic therapy, provided there is no skeletal instability due to metastatic disease.

Energy therapies

Bioelectromagnetics involves treatment with electromagnetic fields that penetrate the body and can heal damaged tissues, including cancers. The insertion of electrodes and the passage of an electric current through tumours is under investigation and has been used to treat cancer in humans in China.

Radionics. Radionics measures abnormalities of the energy waves emitted from the patient for diagnosis and treatment. A special instrument with electrical dials is used (the Black Box), although it probably serves only to focus the therapist's mind. The patient's presence is not required and the technique is a form of psychic healing.

Reiki. This is a Japanese hands-on treatment used to manipulate energy fields within and around the body in order to liberate the body's natural healing powers.

Therapeutic touch. This involves an energy field interaction between two people, aimed at rebalancing or re-patterning the patient's energy fields to promote relaxation and pain relief, and activate self-healing. Despite its name, it involves no direct contact. It is performed by moving the hands a few inches away from the patient's body to detect and correct imbalances and blockages in the patient's energy fields.

References

1 Ernst, E. and Cassileth, B.R. (1998). The prevalence of complementary/ alternative medicine in cancer: a systematic review. *Cancer* 83, 777–82.

2 Cassileth, B.R. (1999). Complementary and alternative cancer medicine. *Journal of Clinical Oncology* 17, 44–52.

3 Ernst, E., et al. (2001). *The Desktop Guide to Complimentary and Alternative Medicine*. Edinburgh, Mosby.

4 Ernst, E. (2001). A primer of complementary and alternative medicine commonly used by cancer patients. *Medical Journal of Australia* 174, 88–92.

5 White, J.D. (2001). Complementary, alternative, and unproven methods of cancer treatment. In *Cancer. Principles and Practice of Oncology. 6th edition* (ed. V.T. De Vita, S. Hellman and S.A. Rosenberg). Philadelphia, Lippincott Williams Wilkins.

6   National Council for Complementary and Alternative Medicines (2003). <http://www.nccam.nih.gov/>

7   Owen, D.K., Lewith, G. and Stephens, C.R. (2001). Can doctors respond to patients' increasing interest in complementary and alternative medicine? *British Medical Journal* 322, 154–8.

8   Paltiel, O., et al. (2001). Determinants of the use of complementary therapies by patients with cancer. *Journal of Clinical Oncology* 19, 2439–48.

9   Burstein, H.J. (2000). Discussing complementary therapies with cancer patients: what should we be talking about? *Journal of Clinical Oncology* 18, 2501–4.

10 Jacobson, J.S., Workman, S.B. and Kronenberg, F. (2000). Research on complementary/alternative medicine for patients with breast cancer: a review of the biomedical literature. *Journal of Clinical Oncology* 18, 668–83.

11 Nahin, R.L. and Straus, S.E. (2001). Research into complementary and alternative medicine: problems and potential. *British Medical Journal* 322, 161–4.

12 Mason, S., Tovey, P. and Long, A.F. (2002). Evaluating complementary medicine: methodological challenges of randomised controlled trials. *British Medical Journal* 325, 832–4.

13 Cassileth, B.R., et al. (1991). Survival and quality of life among patients receiving unproven as compared with conventional cancer therapy. *New England Journal of Medicine* 324, 1180–5.

14 Ernst, E. (1997). Thymus therapy for cancer? A criteria-based, systematic review. *European Journal of Cancer* 33, 531–5.

15 Downer, S.M., et al. (1994). Pursuit and practice of complementary therapies by cancer patients receiving conventional treatment. *British Medical Journal* 309, 86–9.

16 Bagenal, F.S., et al. (1990). Survival of patients with breast cancer attending Bristol Cancer Help Centre. *Lancet* 336, 606–10.

17 Kaegi, E. (1998). Unconventional therapies for cancer: 3. Iscador. Task Force on Alternative Therapies of the Canadian Breast Cancer Research Initiative. *Canadian Medical Association Journal* 158, 1157–9.

18 Grossarth-Maticek, R., et al. (2001). Use of Iscador, an extract of European mistletoe (Viscum album), in cancer treatment: prospective nonrandomized and randomized matched-pair studies nested within a cohort study. *Alternative Therapies in Health and Medicine*. 7, 57–66, 68–72, 74–6.

19 Small, E.J., et al. (2000). Prospective trial of the herbal supplement PC-SPES in patients with progressive prostate cancer. *Journal of Clinical Oncology* 18, 3595–603.

20 Sovak, M., et al. (2002). Herbal composition PC-SPES for management of prostate cancer: identification of active principles. *Journal of the National Cancer Institute* 94, 1275–81.

21 Moertel, C.G., et al. (1982). A clinical trial of amygdalin (Laetrile) in the treatment of human cancer. *New England Journal of Medicine* 306, 201–6.

22 Creagan, E.T., et al. (1979). Failure of high-dose vitamin C (ascorbic acid) therapy to benefit patients with advanced cancer. A controlled trial. *New England Journal of Medicine* 301, 687–90.

23 Moertel, C.G., et al. (1985). High-dose vitamin C versus placebo in the treatment of patients with advanced cancer who have had no prior chemotherapy. A randomized double-blind comparison. *New England Journal of Medicine* 312, 137–41.

24 Italian Study Group for the Di Bella Multitherapy Trials (1999). Evaluation of an unconventional cancer treatment (the Di Bella multitherapy): results of phase II trials in Italy. *British Medical Journal* 318, 224–8.

25 Buiatti, E., et al. (1999). Results from a historical survey of the survival of cancer patients given Di Bella multitherapy. *Cancer* 86, 2143–9.

26 Miller, D.R., et al. (1998). Phase I/II trial of the safety and efficacy of shark cartilage in the treatment of advanced cancer. *Journal of Clinical Oncology* 16, 3649–55.

27 Lagman, R. and Walsh, D. (2003). Dangerous nutrition? Calcium, vitamin D, and shark cartilage nutritional supplements and cancer-related hypercalcemia. *Supportive Care in Cancer* 11, 232–5.

28 Lissoni, P. (2002). Is there a role for melatonin in supportive care? *Supportive Care in Cancer* 10, 110–16.

29 Gertz, M.A. and Bauer, B.A. (2001). Caring (really) for patients who use alternative therapies for cancer. *Journal of Clinical Oncology* 19, 4346–9.

30 Linde, K., et al. (1997). Are the clinical effects of homeopathy placebo effects? A meta-analysis of placebo-controlled trials. *Lancet* 350, 834–43.

31 Linde, K., et al. (1999). Impact of study quality on outcome in placebo-controlled trials of homeopathy. *Journal of Clinical Epidemiology* 52, 631–6.

32 Astin, J.A., Harkness, E. and Ernst, E. (2000). The efficacy of 'distant healing': a systematic review of randomized trials. *Annals of Internal Medicine* 132, 903–10.

33 Targ, E.F. and Levine, E.G. (2002). The efficacy of a mind-body-spirit group for women with breast cancer: a randomized controlled trial. *General and Hospital Psychiatry* 24, 238–48.

34 Ernst, E. and Cassileth, B.R. (1996). Cancer diets, fads and facts. *Cancer Prevention and Control* 2, 181–87.

35 Key, T.J., et al. (1999). Mortality in vegetarians and nonvegetarians: detailed findings from a collaborative analysis of 5 prospective studies. *American Journal of Clinical Nutrition* 70, 516S-24S.

36 Ernst, E. (2002). The risk-benefit profile of commonly used herbal therapies: Ginkgo, St. John's Wort, Ginseng, Echinacea, Saw Palmetto, and Kava. *Annals of Internal Medicine* 136, 42–53.

37 Gow, P.J., et al. (2003). Fatal fulminant hepatic failure induced by a natural therapy containing kava. *Medical Journal of Australia* 178, 442–3.

38 Vogler, B.K., Pittler, M.H. and Ernst, E. (1999). The efficacy of ginseng. A systematic review of randomised clinical trials. *European Journal of Clinical Pharmacology* 55, 567–75.

39 Grealish, L., Lomasney, A. and Whiteman, B. (2000). Foot massage. A nursing intervention to modify the distressing symptoms of pain and nausea in patients hospitalized with cancer. *Cancer Nursing* 23, 237–43.

40 Cooke, B. and Ernst, E. (2000). Aromatherapy: a systematic review. *British Journal of General Practice* 50, 493–6.

Index

Page numbers followed by f refer to figures, by t to tables.